Autoimmune Disorders

Autoimmune Disorders

Adjuvants and Other Risk Factors in Pathogenesis

EDITED BY

Abdulla Watad

Rheumatology Unit and Zabludowicz Center for Autoimmune Diseases
Sheba Medical Center
Tel Aviv University
Tel-Hashomer
Israel

Nicola Luigi Bragazzi

Laboratory for Industrial and Applied Mathematics (LIAM)
Department of Mathematics and Statistics
York University
Toronto
Canada

Postgraduate School of Public Health
Department of Health Sciences (DISSAL)
University of Genoa
Genoa
Italy

Yehuda Shoenfeld

Reichman University
Herzliya
Israel

Zabludowicz Center for Autoimmune Diseases (Founder)
Sheba Medical Center
Tel-Hashomer
Israel

WILEY

This edition first published 2024

Registered Offices
John Wiley & Sons, Inc., 111 River Street, Hoboken, NJ 07030, USA
John Wiley & Sons Ltd, The Atrium, Southern Gate, Chichester, West Sussex, PO19 8SQ, UK

For details of our global editorial offices, customer services, and more information about Wiley products visit us at www.wiley.com.

Wiley also publishes its books in a variety of electronic formats and by print-on-demand. Some content that appears in standard print versions of this book may not be available in other formats.

Library of Congress Cataloging-in-Publication Data
Names: Watad, Abdulla, editor. | Bragazzi, Nicola Luigi, editor. | Shoenfeld, Yehuda, 1948- editor.
Title: Autoimmune disorders : adjuvants and other risk factors in pathogenesis / edited by Abdulla Watad, Nicola Luigi Bragazzi, Yehuda Shoenfeld.
Other titles: Autoimmune disorders (Watad)
Description: Hoboken, NJ : Wiley, 2024. | Includes bibliographical references and index.
Identifiers: LCCN 2024007509 (print) | LCCN 2024007510 (ebook) | ISBN 9781119858416 (hardback) | ISBN 9781119858423 (adobe pdf) | ISBN 9781119858447 (epub)
Subjects: MESH: Autoimmune Diseases—etiology | Autoimmune Diseases—physiopathology | Adjuvants, Immunologic—adverse effects
Classification: LCC RC600 (print) | LCC RC600 (ebook) | NLM QW 545 | DDC 616.97/8—dc23/eng/20240325
LC record available at https://lccn.loc.gov/2024007509
LC ebook record available at https://lccn.loc.gov/2024007510

Cover Design: Wiley
Cover Image: © Ruslan Batiuk /Adobe Stock Photos

Set in 8.75/11pt MeridienLTStd by Straive, Chennai, India

Contents

List of Contributors, vii
Introduction, xiii
Abdulla Watad, Nicola Luigi Bragazzi, and Yehuda Sheonfeld

1 Hyperstimulation of the Immune System, 1
Hadas Hodadov and Abdulla Watad

2 Autoimmune/Inflammatory Syndrome Induced by Adjuvants (ASIA): Genetics, Immunization, and Autoimmunity, 7
Carlo Perricone, Elena Bartoloni Bocci, and Roberto Gerli

3 Vaccine Adjuvants: History, Role, Mechanisms of Action, and Side Effects, 15
Nicola Luigi Bragazzi, Abdulla Watad, and Yehuda Shoenfeld

4 Commonly Used Food Additives Are Nutritional Adjuvants in ASIA Syndrome, 29
Aaron Lerner and Carina Benzvi

5 Silicone Implant Incompatibility Syndrome, 51
Vânia Borba and Yehuda Shoenfeld

6 Silicone Breast Implants (SBIs) and Autoimmune Dysautonomya, 63
Gilad Halpert, Abdulla Watad, Howard Amital, and Yehuda Shoenfeld

7 Autoimmune/Inflammatory Syndrome Induced by Adjuvants (ASIA or Shoenfeld's Syndrome) Due to Polypropylene Mesh Implants, 67
Jan Willem Cohen Tervaert and Mohammed Osman

8 Vaccines, Vaccinosis, and Autoimmunity, 85
Nicola Luigi Bragazzi, Abdulla Watad, and Yehuda Shoenfeld

9 Sustained Immune Activation in ASIA Syndrome – A Bridge to Lymphomagenesis, 91
Dana Butnaru

10 Chronic Fatigue Syndrome, 107
Kassem Sharif

11 Autoantibodies and Autonomic Nervous System, 117
Iana Leineman, Varvara Ryabkova, and Natalia Gavrilova

12 Postural Orthostatic Tachycardia Syndrome (POTS) as a Part of ASIA Syndrome, 129
Paula David

13 Role of the Small-fiber Neuropathy in the Pathogenesis of ASIA Syndrome, 137
N. Gavrilova, E. Kamaeva, M. Lukashenko, and L. Soprun

14 Tattoo as a Possible Trigger for Autoimmune Syndrome Induced by Adjuvants, 147
Paula David

15 The Sick Building Syndrome as a Part of the Autoimmune (Autoinflammatory) Syndrome Induced by Adjuvant, 155
Asher Pardo and Eitan Israeli

16 Gulf War Syndrome (GWS) and ASIA Syndrome, 167
Efrosiniia Talalai

17 Vaccinations in Patients with Autoimmune Diseases, 181
Isa Seida and Naim Mahroum

18 Autoimmune Phenomena in Cancer Patients Treated with Immune Checkpoint Inhibitors, 191
Milena Tocut, Michael Ehrenfeld, and Gisele Zandman-Goddard

19 Heavy Metals in Autoimmune Diseases: Too Much Noise in Autoimmunity, 201
Kassem Sharif and Howard Amital

20 The Role of Bisphenol A in ASIA Syndrome, 225
Zora Lazurova

21 Sarcoidosis and Autoimmune Inflammatory Syndrome Induced by Adjuvants: Is There a Connection?, 247
Anna Malkova, Yulia Zinchenko, Anna Starshinova, Igor Kudryavtsev, Piotr Yablonskiy, and Yehuda Shoenfeld

22 Sjögren's Syndrome as a Proof of Concept of the Hyperstimulation Syndrome, 265
Vânia Borba and Yehuda Shoenfeld

23 Gluteal Biopolymer Injections as a Case of ASIA Syndrome, 283
Rojas-Villarraga Adriana, María Alejandra Martínez-Ceballos, Uribe Rosa, and Montealegre Giovanni

24 The Chemical and Social Landscape of the Modern World and Increased Risk of ASIA, 305
Albert Pinhasov, Elena Shmerkin, and Michael Kirby

25 Oil Injections and ASIA Syndrome, 323
Olga Vera-Lastra, Alberto Ordinola-Navarro, Abihai Lucas Hernández, Gabriela Medina, María P. Cruz-Domínguez, Gabriel M. Ramírez, and Luis J. Jara

26 Metals in Dental Implants as a Trigger of Autoimmunity, 337
Arad Dotan and Yehuda Shoenfeld

27 Conclusions: State of the Art and Prospects, 341
Abdulla Watad, Nicola Luigi Bragazzi, and Yehuda Shoenfeld

Index, 345

List of Contributors

Rojas-Villarraga Adriana
Research Institute
Fundación Universitaria de Ciencias de la Salud (FUCS)
Bogotá
Colombia

María Alejandra Martínez-Ceballos
Fundación Oftalmológica Nacional
Bogotá
Colombia

School of Medicine and Health Sciences
Universidad del Rosario
Bogotá
Colombia

Howard Amital
Zabludowicz Center for Autoimmune Diseases
Sheba Medical Center
Tel-Hashomer
Israel

Sackler Faculty of Medicine
Tel Aviv University
Tel Aviv
Israel

Department of Internal Medicine 'B'
Sheba Medical Center
Tel-Hashomer
Israel

Carina Benzvi
Zabludowicz Center for Autoimmune Diseases
Sheba Medical Center
Tel-Hashomer
Israel

Elena Bartoloni Bocci
Reumatologia
Dipartimento di Medicina e Chirurgia
Università di Perugia
Perugia
Italy

Vânia Borba
Internal Medicine Departmente
Rehaklik Dussnang AG
Dussnang
Thurgau
Switzerland

Nicola Luigi Bragazzi
Laboratory for Industrial and Applied Mathematics (LIAM)
Department of Mathematics and Statistics
York University
Toronto
Canada

Postgraduate School of Public Health
Department of Health Sciences (DISSAL)
University of Genoa
Genoa
Italy

Dana Butnaru
Department of Clinical Immunology
Hospital Clínico San Carlos
Complutense University of Madrid
Madrid
Spain

María P. Cruz-Domínguez
Internal Medicine Department
Unidad Médica de Alta Especiad
Hospital de Especialidades
"Dr. Antonio Fraga Mouret"
Centro Médico Nacional
"La Raza". Instituto Mexicano del Seguro Social
México City
México

Internal Medicine Department
División de Estudios de Posgrado
Facultad de Medicina
Universidad Nacional Autónoma de México
México City
México

Paula David
Department of Internal Medicine 'B'
Sheba Medical Center
Tel-Hashomer
Israel

Arad Dotan
Zabludowicz Center for Autoimmune Diseases
Sheba Medical Center
Tel-Hashomer
Israel

Sackler Faculty of Medicine
Tel Aviv University
Tel Aviv
Israel

Michael Ehrenfeld
Sackler Faculty of Medicine
Tel Aviv University
Tel Aviv
Israel

Zabludowicz Center for Autoimmune Diseases
Sheba Medical Center
Tel-Hashomer
Israel

Natalia Gavrilova
Federal State Budget Educational Institution of Higher Education "St. Petersburg State University"
University Emb.
7-9
Saint Petersburg
Russia

St Petersburg State University Hospital
Saint Petersburg
Russia

Roberto Gerli
Reumatologia
Dipartimento di Medicina e Chirurgia
Università di Perugia
Perugia
Italy

Montealegre Giovanni
Fundación Universitaria de Ciencias de la Salud (FUCS)
Hospital San José
Bogotá
Colombia

Gilad Halpert
Zabludowicz Center for Autoimmune Diseases
Sheba Medical Center
Tel-Hashomer
Israel

Department of Molecular Biology
Ariel University
Ariel
Israel

Abihai Lucas Hernández
Internal Medicine Department
Unidad Médica de Alta Especiad
Hospital de Especialidades
"Dr. Antonio Fraga Mouret"
Centro Médico Nacional
"La Raza". Instituto Mexicano del Seguro Social
México City
México

Hadas Hodadov
Sackler Faculty of Medicine
Tel Aviv University
Tel Aviv
Israel

Eitan Israeli
Zabludowicz Center for Autoimmune Diseases
Sheba Medical Center
Tel-Hashomer
Israel

Luis J. Jara
Research Division
Instituto Nacional de Rehabilitación
Mexico City
México

Yehuda Shoenfeld
Reichman University
Herzliya
Israel

Zabludowicz Center for Autoimmune Diseases
Sheba Medical Center
Tel-Hashomer
Israel

L. Soprun
Federal State Budget Educational Institution of Higher Education "St. Petersburg State University"
University Emb.
7-9
Saint Petersburg
Russia

St Petersburg State University Hospital
Saint Petersburg
Russia

Anna Starshinova
Almazov National Medical Research Centre
The Research Department
Saint Petersburg
Russia

Efrosiniia Talalai
Sackler Faculty of Medicine
Tel Aviv University
Tel Aviv
Israel

Zabludowicz Center for Autoimmune Diseases
Sheba Medical Center
Tel-Hashomer
Israel

Jan Willem Cohen Tervaert
Division of Rheumatology
Department of Medicine
University of Alberta
Edmonton
Alberta
Canada

Emeritus Professor of Medicine and Immunology
Maastricht University
Maastricht
The Netherlands

Milena Tocut
Department of Internal Medicine C
Wolfson Medical Center
Holon
Israel

Sackler Faculty of Medicine
Tel Aviv University
Tel Aviv
Israel

Olga Vera-Lastra
Internal Medicine Department
Unidad Médica de Alta Especiad
Hospital de Especialidades
"Dr. Antonio Fraga Mouret"
Centro Médico Nacional
"La Raza". Instituto Mexicano del Seguro Social
México City
México

Internal Medicine Department
División de Estudios de Posgrado
Facultad de Medicina
Universidad Nacional Autónoma de México
México City
México

Abdulla Watad
Rheumatology Unit and Zabludowicz Center for Autoimmune Diseases
Sheba Medical Center
Tel-Hashomer
Israel

Sackler Faculty of Medicine
Tel Aviv University
Tel Aviv
Israel

Section of Musculoskeletal Disease
Leeds Institute of Molecular Medicine
University of Leeds
Leeds
UK

Department of Internal Medicine 'B'
Sheba Medical Center
Tel-Hashomer
Israel

Institute of Oncology
Sheba Medical Center
Tel-Hashomer
Israel

Piotr Yablonskiy
Laboratory of the Mosaic of Autoimmunity
St. Petersburg State University
Saint Petersburg
Russia

St. Petersburg Research Institute of Phthisiopulmonology
Saint Petersburg
Russia

Gisele Zandman-Goddard
Department of Internal Medicine C
Wolfson Medical Center
Holon
Israel

Sackler Faculty of Medicine
Tel Aviv University
Tel Aviv
Israel

Yulia Zinchenko
St. Petersburg Research Institute of Phthisiopulmonology
Saint Petersburg
Russia

Introduction

"The Autoimmune/Inflammatory Syndrome Induced by Adjuvants (ASIA)" is a term introduced by one of the editors of this book, Prof. Yehuda Shoenfeld, to characterize a cluster of autoimmune and inflammatory disorders incited by exposure to various adjuvants [1]. These adjuvants can be encountered in diverse contexts, including vaccinations, silicone implants, and other materials, culminating in a spectrum of symptoms and medical conditions [2]. Given its relatively recent emergence in the medical landscape, with its introduction in 2011, ASIA remains a complex and evolving syndrome, with many facets yet to be fully elucidated. However, an accumulating body of evidence underscores the potential of specific adjuvants to incite autoimmune and inflammatory responses in susceptible individuals, often associated with HLA-DRB1 genetic factors [3]. Consequently, growing apprehension surrounds the safety of adjuvants integrated into certain vaccines and medical products. It is imperative to underscore that vaccines play a pivotal role in safeguarding public health. Over the years, they have played an instrumental role in eradicating lethal diseases such as smallpox, significantly reducing the prevalence of maladies such as measles and polio. Vaccines operate by invigorating the immune system to mount a defense against specific pathogens, all while sparing the individual from the disease itself. This herd immunity not only extends protection to vaccinated individuals but also shields the broader community, including those who cannot receive vaccines themselves. While vaccines can indeed elicit rare side effects, the immense benefits they confer decisively outweigh the associated risks, making them an indispensable tool in the preservation of public health. This book serves as a comprehensive exploration of ASIA and the diverse adjuvants capable of inciting autoimmune and inflammatory responses. We embark on a journey to decipher the substances implicated in ASIA syndrome, the array of symptoms and conditions it encompasses, and the current state of research in this realm. Our narrative commences by delving into the role of adjuvants in vaccines and the controversies regarding their safety. Though infrequent, some individuals exhibit heightened susceptibility to autoimmune and inflammatory reactions prompted by adjuvants in vaccines, culminating in an array of conditions including Guillain–Barré syndrome, multiple sclerosis, and lupus. We further scrutinize the involvement of silicone implants in the initiation of autoimmune and inflammatory responses. For years, silicone has been a cornerstone of breast implants [4], and though the safety of these implants has been subject to scrutiny [5], the connection between silicone and autoimmune maladies remains enigmatic. Nevertheless, a mounting body of evidence underscores that silicone exposure can incite autoimmune and inflammatory reactions, giving rise to conditions such as silicone implant syndrome, which can manifest with symptoms including fatigue, joint pain, and more. Beyond vaccines and silicone, we cast a spotlight on other adjuvants capable of inciting autoimmune and inflammatory reactions, encompassing commonly employed materials such as aluminum, prevalent in vaccines, and additional substances such as mesh and metals. We also conduct an exploration of autoimmune dysautonomia, a condition that has garnered substantial attention in recent years. Finally, we engage in a comprehensive discussion surrounding the diagnosis and treatment of ASIA as well as the prevailing controversies that encircle this syndrome. It is important to note that skepticism still pervades some medical circles regarding the existence of ASIA, with its symptoms and linkage to adjuvants often escaping recognition. Nonetheless, with an escalating awareness and an expanding body of research, the reality of ASIA as a genuine phenomenon affecting numerous individuals is becoming increasingly evident. In summation, this book aspires to provide an exhaustive overview of ASIA and the manifold adjuvants capable of triggering autoimmune and inflammatory responses. Our hope is that this volume will raise awareness about this intricate syndrome and empower individuals to make informed decisions regarding their health and the medical products they encounter.

References

1. Shoenfeld, Y. and Agmon-Levin, N. (2011). 'ASIA' – autoimmune/inflammatory syndrome induced by adjuvants. *J. Autoimmun.* 36 (1): 4–8.
2. Seida, I., Alrais, M., Seida, R. et al. (2023). Autoimmune/inflammatory syndrome induced by adjuvants (ASIA): past, present, and future implications. *Clin. Exp. Immunol.* uxad033.
3. Arango, M.-T., Perricone, C., Kivity, S. et al. (2017). HLA-DRB1 the notorious gene in the mosaic of autoimmunity. *Immunol. Res.* 65 (1): 82–98.
4. Watad, A., Rosenberg, V., Tiosano, S. et al. (2018). Silicone breast implants and the risk of autoimmune/rheumatic disorders: a real-world analysis. *Int. J. Epidemiol.* 47 (6): 1846–1854.
5. Watad, A., Bragazzi, N.L., Amital, H., and Shoenfeld, Y. (2019). Hyperstimulation of Adaptive Immunity as the Common Pathway for Silicone Breast Implants, Autoimmunity, and Lymphoma of the Breast. *Isr. Med. Assoc. J.* 21 (8): 517–519.

1 Hyperstimulation of the Immune System

Hadas Hodadov[1] and Abdulla Watad[1,2,3,4,5]

[1]Sackler Faculty of Medicine, Tel Aviv University, Tel Aviv, Israel
[2]Department of Medicine 'B', Sheba Medical Center, Tel-Hashomer, Israel
[3]Rheumatology Unit and Zabludowicz Center for Autoimmune Diseases, Sheba Medical Center, Tel-Hashomer, Israel
[4]Section of Musculoskeletal Disease, Leeds Institute of Molecular Medicine, University of Leeds, Leeds, UK
[5]Institute of Oncology, Sheba Medical Center, Tel-Hashomer, Israel

Background

The immune system safeguards living organisms against constant assaults from both external and internal environments, detecting a wide variety of pathogens, cancer cells, and drugs (i.e., "non-self") and distinguishing them from the organism's own healthy tissue ("self") [1]. Two main subsections constitute the immune system: innate immunity, which provides immediate though incomplete protection against intruders and, at best, has only short-term memory; and adaptive immunity, offering a tailored response to each stimulus by learning to recognise previously encountered molecules [2]. Dysfunction of the immune system can lead to autoimmune diseases, autoinflammatory disorders, and cancer. Autoimmunity results from a complex interplay between genetic predisposition and environmental factors [3]. Adjuvants are molecules capable of triggering an immune response against specific or nonspecific antigens [4]. Biomaterials are routinely employed to address various conditions in nearly every medical specialty. However, certain substances within this category have been reported to possess adjuvanticity, thereby potentially accelerating or initiating autoimmune phenomena [5].

Biomaterials that are lined to hyperstimulation of the immune system (silicone, mesh and heavy metals)

Biomaterials play a pivotal role in addressing various healthcare issues, including tissue engineering, drug delivery, and medical implants. Their significance lies in the broad potential of these materials to offer support (i.e., scaffolds), allow modifications of chemical properties, and protect biologically active products (i.e., cells, proteins, and chemicals). Biomaterials encompass a diverse range of compounds with varying functions and structural features, ranging from naturally occurring biological macromolecules to fully synthetic coatings [6]. However, a noteworthy aspect,

Autoimmune Disorders: Adjuvants and Other Risk Factors in Pathogenesis, First Edition.
Edited by Abdulla Watad, Nicola Luigi Bragazzi, and Yehuda Shoenfeld.

though rare, is that certain biomaterials can chronically stimulate the immune system, resulting in excessive inflammation, fibrotic encapsulation, impaired healing, tissue destruction, or even rejection of medical devices [5]. The implantation of biomaterial elicits a host reaction that determines the integration outcome and the biological response of the implant. Upon implantation, the material interacts with the blood, causing protein adsorption to the biomaterial surface and the development of a temporary matrix that forms on and around the biomaterial. This matrix serves as the initial thrombus at the tissue-material interface. Protein adsorption and fibrin-predominant temporary matrix formation are closely linked in their mechanistic responses [7]. Injury to vascularized connective tissue initiates inflammatory responses by the innate immune system, leading to thrombus formation. The temporary matrix contributes components to foreign body reactions and wound healing. Cytokines, growth factors, mitogens, and other bioactive materials within the matrix create a rich environment of activating and inhibiting substances capable of modulating macrophage activity, along with the proliferation of other cell populations involved in inflammatory and wound-healing responses. Following the initial blood-material interactions and temporary matrix formation, both acute and chronic inflammation responses ensue [8].

Hyperstimulation syndrome induced by silicone breast implants

One significant biomaterial is silicone, a polymeric compound forming rubber-like materials used in various applications, including dental procedures, medical implants, and insulation. Silicone breast implants (SBIs), introduced in 1962, have been widely implanted in millions of individuals [9]. While there was an earlier perception that silicone is a biologically inert material, this notion has been refuted, with reported immunological effects induced by silicone. Silicone gel particles can migrate outside the outer shell post-rupture, and even migration through an intact shell has been demonstrated, known as "gel bleed" [10]. Silicon-containing particles captured by macrophages induce the release of IL-1, activate the NALP3 inflammasome and B cells, leading to an imbalance of regulatory T cells, responder T cells, and Th17 cells [11]. Animal studies have demonstrated that SBIs induce an adjuvant effect, increasing susceptibility to autoimmune/rheumatic disorders. The mechanisms by which SBIs induce autoimmune phenomena are numerous, involving dysregulation of both innate and adaptive immunity in individuals genetically predisposed to autoimmunity [9]. In recent years, inconsistent findings on the safety of SBIs have emerged. A large population-based study involving over 24,000 women with SBIs and approximately 100,000 age-matched controls revealed a significantly increased risk of autoimmune disease in women with SBIs, with an adjusted odds-ratio (OR) of 1.22 ([95% CI 1.18–1.26], $p < 0.001$). The risk was even higher (OR>1.5, $p < 0.05$) in specific conditions such as sarcoidosis, systemic sclerosis, and Sjögren's syndrome [11]. Other studies have linked carrying SBIs with systemic clinical symptoms suggestive of rheumatic disorders, including fatigue, weakness, musculoskeletal pain, morning stiffness, and dry eyes and mouth [12]. Plausible mechanisms explaining the link between SBIs and autoimmune phenomena have been proposed, as supported by animal model studies. For example, injecting silicone gel in NZB mice induced proteinuria and autoimmune hemolytic anemia [13], while implanting silicone gel or silicone oil in MRL lpr/lpr mice increased anti-Ds-DNA antibodies [14]. In a rat model study, five genes (Fes, Aif1, Gata3, Tlr6, and Tlr2) were identified as hub genes likely linked to the immune responses induced by silicone. Four of these genes (Aif1, Gata3, Tlr6, and Tlr2) have been associated with autoimmunity as target genes or disease markers [15]. Thus, SBIs may trigger immune responses, with various immune reactions detected after silicone implantation.

Hyperstimulation syndrome induced by mesh

Mesh, a loosely woven sheet, constitutes another crucial biomaterial, with the commonly used polypropylene (PP) mesh being a strong yet flexible synthetic implant. PP, the second most widely manufactured type of plastic globally, finds application in various products such as furniture, electronic components, and medical devices [16]. Utilized since the 1960s for hernia repair surgeries and since the 1990s for urinary incontinence and pelvic organ prolapse, PP implants have enhanced surgical outcomes and reduced recurrence risks. Initially considered an inert plastic, chemically inactive to minimize patient complications, a contrasting notion has emerged, suggesting mesh-related complications, particularly the body's immunological reaction to the implanted material [17]. Some researchers propose that PP mesh may induce a systemic autoimmune inflammatory disorder, akin to women with SBIs induced by adjuvants. PP implants elicit a rapid and effective acute inflammatory response followed by a chronic body reaction. Local inflammatory reactions after mesh insertion may lead to systemic upregulation of inflammatory mediators, primarily regulated by monocytes and macrophages at the implant tissue interface. These cells, known to produce various cytokines, particularly IL-6, play a crucial role in the acute phase of the inflammatory process, regulating local and systemic responses [18]. One theory explaining the chronic foreign body response to mesh involves oxidative processes, with oxidation causing PP degradation, resulting in chronic inflammation and a subsequent systemic autoimmune inflammatory disorder. Supporting evidence for mesh acting as an adjuvant includes the appearance of systemic autoimmune symptoms shortly after mesh placement and the remission of symptoms after mesh removal [19]. A recent study evaluated patients with implanted PP for the development of systemic illness. Thirty-nine out of 40 patients presented with chronic fatigue, and 38 of 40 patients had myalgia, both occurring shortly after surgery. All patients fulfilled the diagnostic criteria for ASIA syndrome. In 45% of patients, there was a diagnosis of a well-established autoimmune disease, suggesting that PP mesh implants increase the risk of developing autoimmune diseases by acting as an adjuvant [20].

Hyperstimulation syndrome induced by metals

Metals and metal alloys, combinations of metal elements, have been widely utilized as medical implants for over a century across various medical specialties. They find application in a diverse range of medical devices, from solid metal implants in orthopedics to bioelectronics such as pacemakers or neurostimulators [21]. These metal implants are chosen as biomedical materials due to their numerous advantages over other materials, including high mechanical strength, good electrical conductivity, durability, and excellent biological compatibility. Ideally, metal implants should not cause any undesired reactions; however, interactions between the implant and the surrounding tissue can lead to complications, including infection, inflammation, and foreign body response. While heavy metals and their salts have previously been demonstrated to play a role in causing allergic diseases, recent evidence suggests their key involvement in the induction or exacerbation of autoimmune diseases [22]. The mechanism by which heavy metals trigger autoimmunity is not fully understood, but its comprehension is not necessary for establishing an association between them. Manifestations of autoimmunity may include the production of autoantibodies, an increase in serum IgG and IgE, polyclonal activation of B and T lymphocytes, infiltration of destructive inflammatory cells into different target organs, and the deposition of immune complexes in vascular sites [22]. Another suggested mechanism is that metal compounds may exert toxic effects on the immune system, leading to the malfunctioning of the system as a whole. Despite an incomplete understanding of the mechanism, there is a growing notion supported by extensive research that the interaction of metals with the immune system may lead to immunodysregulation, resulting in autoimmune diseases [23].

Link among foreign bodies, chronic stimulation, and lymphoproliferative disorders

Following acute inflammation, chronic inflammation at the implant site is characterized by the presence of mononuclear cells, including monocytes and lymphocytes. An implant may continue to elicit a chronic inflammatory response lasting for months or longer, marked by a broader immune cell infiltration, encompassing both myeloid and lymphoid cells. After the resolution of acute and chronic inflammatory responses, granulation tissue, identified by the presence of macrophages, infiltration of fibroblasts, and neovascularization, is observed in the new healing tissue [5]. It is hypothesized that any breast implant, whether saline or silicone, may release silicone corpuscles over time. Factors such as trauma causing microfractures, exposure to temperature or pressure, ultraviolet radiation, oxidation, and chemical reactions can accelerate this process. When the permeability of the elastomer is impaired, the physiological seroma in the space between the elastomer surface and the fibrous capsule reacts and transports the resulting polydimethylsiloxane compound from the implant surface, encountering the fibrous capsule [24]. The fibrous capsule acts as a physiological protective barrier against products from the intracapsular environment. If met with silicone particles, regardless of the mechanism, an immune response may be generated, potentially leading to a silicone-induced granuloma. If the fibrous capsule ruptures and exposes its contents to the extracapsular space, the immune reaction can trigger a systemic immune response [24]. Some patients may develop an autoimmune reaction to silicone components. A common finding related to silicone implant complications is a silicone-induced granuloma of the breast implant capsule (SIGBIC). Histologically, SIGBIC is formed by extracellular and/or intracellular silicone, numerous histiocytes, chronic granulomatous inflammatory infiltrate with multinucleated giant cells, and an infiltrate of mixed lymphocytes – T and B without atypia [25]. Another rare but serious complication is anaplastic large cell lymphoma (ALCL), a subtype of non-Hodgkin lymphoma of T cells [26]. An association between ALCL and saline and silicone implants exists. The first case of ALCL associated with breast implants was published in 1997 [27], and by 2011, the Food and Drug Administration published a statement confirming 60 cases of ALCL associated with prostheses. ALCL affects the fibrous capsule around the implant, rarely appears as a solid mass, and does not involve the breast parenchyma. As in SIGBIC, the mechanism of ALCL may involve an immune response induced by the silicone material in the implant, leading to an immune overreaction and monoclonal neoplasia with activated T lymphocytes. Additionally, in saline or silicone implants, the capsules may be responsible for chronic local inflammation with T-cell activation and clonal expansion [28]. Furthermore, in case of capsular disruption, silicone-containing particles are transported to the regional lymph nodes, causing a marked adjuvant effect. Silica particles induce a type-2 inflammatory response characterized by an increase in IgE and IgG1 and chronic activation of T cells [25]. The pathophysiology of ALCL and SIGBIC is very similar, with the only difference being the monoclonal neoplasia induced by the activation of T lymphocytes in ALCL, prompting consideration of whether ALCL is an evolution of SIGBIC. Clinically, ALCL may present as fluid filling within the intracapsular space (seroma), while SIGBIC is most often present as an intracapsular mass. Both conditions usually have an excellent prognosis once the fibrous capsule is excised and the implant is removed [28].

Studies on silicone, metals, and the risk of lymphoma

Due to evidence on breast implant-associated ALCL, some reports propose a possible development of ALCL in relation to other implants, such as metal. Examples include ALCL associated with a stainless-steel fixation plate for tibial fracture repair or after the placement of dental implants [29, 30]. Chronic inflammation and antigenic stimulation caused by the presence of implants (such as silicone, metal, or others) are suggested as possible neoplastic triggers. Resembling lymphomas associated with other inflammatory conditions, implant-associated lymphomas are believed to share similar features, including development after prolonged inflammation, localization to a confined body space, and a latency period until the development of lymphoid malignancy. This can be attributed to ongoing inflammation and chronic stimulation of adaptive immune cells with polyclonal activation, which may result in monoclonality and ultimately lead to the development of lymphoma in genetically susceptible hosts [21]. The relationship between SBIs and lymphoma can be demonstrated by the well-established link between Epstein–Barr virus (EBV) infection and the risk of lymphoma. The pathogenesis of EBV-associated lymphomas involves dysregulation between inflammatory and inflammation-neutralizing processes, leading to the production of radical oxygen species that can cause the impairment of critical oncogenic pathways, such as p53, promoting lymphomagenesis and eventually lymphomas [31]. As mentioned, silicone particles are capable of infiltrating lymph nodes, not only local but also distal ones, and enhancing antigen-specific immune reactions. Thus, the presence of SBIs is comparable to latent infection, with EBV leading to chronic nonspecific stimulation of adaptive immunity, polyclonal activation, monoclonal activation, and eventually, the development of lymphoma.

References

1. Nicholson, L.B. (2016). The immune system. *Essays Biochem.* 60 (3): 275–301.
2. Yatim, K.M. and Lakkis, F.G. (2015). A brief journey through the immune system. *Clin. J. Am. Soc. Nephrol.* 10 (7): 1274–1281.
3. Brodin, P. and Davis, M.M. (2017). Human immune system variation. *Nat. Rev. Immunol.* 17 (1): 21–29.
4. Watad, A., Sharif, K., and Shoenfeld, Y. (2017). The ASIA syndrome: basic concepts. *Mediterr. J. Rheumatol.* 28 (2): 64–69.
5. Anderson, J.M., Rodriguez, A., and Chang, D.T. (2008). Foreign body reaction to biomaterials. *Semin. Immunol.* 20 (2): 86–100.
6. Mariani, E., Lisignoli, G., Borzì, R.M., and Pulsatelli, L. (2019). Biomaterials: foreign bodies or tuners for the immune response? *Int. J. Mol. Sci.* 20 (3): 636.
7. Veiseh, O. and Vegas, A.J. (2019). Domesticating the foreign body response: recent advances and applications. *Adv. Drug Deliv. Rev.* 144: 148–161.
8. Higgins, D.M., Basaraba, R.J., Hohnbaum, A.C. et al. (2009). Localized immunosuppressive environment in the foreign body response to implanted biomaterials. *Am. J. Pathol.* 175 (1): 161–170.
9. Hajdu, S.D., Agmon-Levin, N., and Shoenfeld, Y. (2011). Silicone and autoimmunity: silicone and autoimmunity. *Eur. J. Clin. Investig.* 41 (2): 203–211.
10. Maijers, M.C., de Blok, C.J.M., Niessen, F.B. et al. (2013). Women with silicone breast implants and unexplained systemic symptoms: a descriptive cohort study. *Neth. J. Med.* 71 (10): 534–540.
11. Watad, A., Rosenberg, V., Tiosano, S. et al. (2018). Silicone breast implants and the risk of autoimmune/rheumatic disorders: a real-world analysis. *Int. J. Epidemiol.* 47 (6): 1846–1854.
12. Balk, E.M., Earley, A., Avendano, E.A., and Raman, G. (2016). Long-term health outcomes in women with silicone gel breast implants: a systematic review. *Ann. Intern. Med.* 164 (3): 164.
13. McDonald, A.H., Schneider, M., Gudenkauf, L. et al. (1998). Silicone gel enhances the development of autoimmune disease in New Zealand black mice but fails to induce it in BALB/cAnPt mice. *Clin. Immunol. Immunopathol.* 87 (3): 248–255.
14. Schaefer, C.J. and Wooley, P.H. (1999). The influence of silicone implantation on murine lupus in MRL lpr/lpr mice. *J. Rheumatol.* 26 (10): 2215–2221.
15. Huang, X., Zhou, Y., Liu, W. et al. (2017). Identification of hub genes related to silicone-induced immune response in rats. *Oncotarget* 8 (59): 99772–99783.
16. Kowalik, C.R., Zwolsman, S.E., Malekzadeh, A. et al. (2022). Are polypropylene mesh implants associated with systemic autoimmune inflammatory syndromes? A systematic review. *Hernia* 26 (2): 401–410. 12 [cited 2022 Mar 2]. https://link.springer.com/10.1007/s10029-021-02553-y.
17. Dias, E.R.M., Pivetta, L.G.A., de Carvalho, J.P.V. et al. (2021). Autoimmune [auto-inflammatory] syndrome induced by adjuvants (ASIA): case report after inguinal hernia repair with mesh. *Int. J. Surg. Case Rep.* 84: 106060.
18. Di Vita, G., Patti, R., Sparacello, M. et al. (2008). Impact of different texture of polypropylene mesh on the inflammatory response. *Int. J. Immunopathol. Pharmacol.* 21 (1): 207–214.
19. Chughtai, B., Sedrakyan, A., Mao, J. et al. (2017). Is vaginal mesh a stimulus of autoimmune disease? *Am. J. Obstet. Gynecol.* 216 (5): 495.e1–495.e7.

20. Tervaert, J.W.C. (2018). Autoinflammatory/autoimmunity syndrome induced by adjuvants (Shoenfeld's syndrome) in patients after a polypropylene mesh implantation. *Best Pract. Res. Clin. Rheumatol.* 32 (4): 511–520.
21. U.S Food & Drug Administration (FDA) (2019). Biological responses to metal implants.
22. Mishra, K.P. (2020). Heavy metals exposure and risk of autoimmune diseases: a review. *Arch. Immunol. Allergy* 3 (2): 22–26.
23. Pollard, K.M. (2015). Environment, Autoantibodies, and Autoimmunity. *Front. Immunol.* 6: 60. 11 [cited 2022 Mar 2];6. http://journal.frontiersin.org/Article/10.3389/fimmu.2015.00060/abstract.
24. de Faria Castro Fleury, E., D'Alessandro, G.S., and Lordelo Wludarski, S.C. (2018). Silicone-induced granuloma of breast implant capsule (SIGBIC): histopathology and radiological correlation. *J Immunol Res* 2018: 1, 9.
25. de Fleury, E.F.C. (2020). Synchronous breast implant associated anaplastic large cell lymphoma (BIA-ALCL) and silicone induced granuloma of breast implant capsule (SIGBIC): What to learn. *Radiol. Case Rep.* 15 (10): 1736–1742.
26. Kim, B., Predmore, Z.S., Mattke, S. et al. (2015). Breast implant–associated anaplastic large cell lymphoma: updated results from a structured expert consultation process. *Plast. Reconstr. Surg. Glob. Open* 3 (1): e296.
27. Keech, J.A. and Creech, B.J. (1997). Anaplastic T-cell lymphoma in proximity to a saline-filled breast implant. *Plast. Reconstr. Surg.* 100 (2): 554–555.
28. de Fleury, E.F.C., Rêgo, M.M., Ramalho, L.C. et al. (2017). Silicone-induced granuloma of breast implant capsule (SIGBIC): similarities and differences with anaplastic large cell lymphoma (ALCL) and their differential diagnosis. *Breast Cancer (Dove Med. Press)* 9: 133–140.
29. Palraj, B., Paturi, A., Stone, R.G. et al. (2010). Soft tissue anaplastic large T-cell lymphoma associated with a metallic orthopedic implant: case report and review of the current literature. *J. Foot and Ankle Surg.* 49 (6): 561–564.
30. Yoon, H.-J., Choe, J.-Y., and Jeon, Y.K. (2015). Mucosal CD30-positive T-cell lymphoproliferative disorder arising in the oral cavity following dental implants: report of the first case. *Int. J. Surg. Pathol.* 23 (8): 656–661.
31. Bizjak, M., Selmi, C., Praprotnik, S. et al. (2015). Silicone implants and lymphoma: the role of inflammation. *J. Autoimmun.* 65: 64–73.

2 Autoimmune/Inflammatory Syndrome Induced by Adjuvants (ASIA): Genetics, Immunization, and Autoimmunity

Carlo Perricone, Elena Bartoloni Bocci, and Roberto Gerli
Reumatologia, Dipartimento di Medicina e Chirurgia, Università di Perugia, Perugia, Italy

Introduction

Shoenfeld and Agmon-Levin in 2011 coined the term "ASIA – Autoimmune/inflammatory Syndrome Induced by Adjuvants" [1] to describe several clinical conditions, namely siliconosis, Gulf War Syndrome (GWSy), Macrophage Myofasciitis (MMF) syndrome, sick building syndrome (SBS), and postvaccination phenomena, which share similar signs or symptoms [2] and that have as a common denominator the presence of an adjuvant that triggers a disreactivity of the immune system.

Clustering of autoimmune diseases (AID) in families is well recognized, supporting a common genetic background [3]. Environmental factors (infectious agents, dust, vaccines, etc.) or other agents acting as adjuvants (dust, silicone, aluminum salts, etc.) cooperate on a genetically prone individual triggering autoimmune phenomena [4–9]. Enhanced immunogenicity might lead to reactogenicity in a process that does not always begin involving pathological stimulation [10]. Interestingly, several autoimmune conditions, such as Sjögren's syndrome [11], undifferentiated connective tissue disease [12], and silicone implant incompatibility syndrome [13], share pathogenetic aspects with ASIA syndrome. The mechanisms that have been proposed as instrumental in ASIA are different (Table 2.1).

Genetic background

The presence of a favoring genetic background as a prerequisite for the development of such conditions may explain their rarity [14]. Notably, loci in the human leukocyte antigen (HLA),

Autoimmune Disorders: Adjuvants and Other Risk Factors in Pathogenesis, First Edition.
Edited by Abdulla Watad, Nicola Luigi Bragazzi, and Yehuda Shoenfeld.

Table 2.1 Mechanism of adjuvant-induced autoimmunity.

Mechanisms of adjuvants-induced autoimmunity
• Alteration of the host's immune system
• Polyclonal activation of B cells
• Activation of autoreactive T cells
• Effects on immune regulatory cells
• Effects on virus-induced antibodies
• Molecular mimicry
• Bystander activation
• Epitope spreading
• Anti-idiotypic network
• Changing the host's antigens
• Expression of HLA family antigens
• Modification of surface antigens
• Induction of novel antigens
• Interaction with TLRs
• Antigens translocation
• Release of inflammatory cytokines

HLA, Human leukocyte antigen; TLRs, Toll-like receptors.

which have been shown to be associated with the development of AID, have been suggested to be associated with the classical ASIA syndrome conditions [3]. An in silico study has shown that six genes (TGFB1, interferon-γ, CD4, FCGR3A, FCGR2A, and HLA-DRB1) and 33 pathways seem to be common to Guillain–Barré Syndrome (GBS), Rheumatoid Arthritis (RA), Systemic Lupus Erythematosus (SLE), and Idiopathic (or immune) Thrombocytopenic Purpura (ITP) [15]. Not surprisingly, all these genes are well-known participants to the immune response: for instance, CD4 and interferon-γ implicate the response mediated by Th1 lymphocytes, TGFB1 suggests a role for T-regulatory cells, the two IgG FC receptors suggest an antibody-mediated immunopathology or immunomodulation, and finally, HLA-DRB1 suggests antigen processing for presentation to T cells [15].

GWSy has been associated with two genetic polymorphic sites of the enzyme paraxonase, involved in the hydrolysis of organophosphate pesticides and nerve gases, influencing their toxicity to mammals and man [16, 17], while MMS has been associated with the HLA class II allele DRB1*01 [18]. Indeed, HLA-DRB1*01 allele was highly represented in people with MMS who had received in the previous decade immunization against hepatitis B or A viruses or tetanus toxoid, all containing aluminum hydroxide as adjuvant. Kappel et al. evaluated three sisters carrying the BRCA-1 gene mutation who had a preventive mastectomy and were reconstructed with silicone breast implants. In all sisters within a period of four years, symptoms suggesting ASIA were observed, suggesting a possible common genetic background [19].

Young et al. reported that silicone breast-implanted women with autoimmune symptoms were more frequently displaying HLA-DR5 and HLA-DQ2 when compared to asymptomatic women with silicone implants [20]. This raises the possibility that HLA genotype might serve as a marker for women who are predisposed to develop autoimmune symptoms following exposure to silicone gel breast implants.

Postvaccination phenomena are more likely to occur in patients with genetic predisposition. A recent study suggested that giant cell arteritis/polymyalgia rheumatica can represent a very rare event developing postinfluenza vaccination, especially in persons at higher spontaneous risk such as those carrying DRB1*13:01 haplotype [21]. Narcolepsy is a chronic disabling neurologic disorder characterized by severe irresistible daytime sleepiness and abnormal sleep–wake patterns [22]. The disorder is uncommon in children younger than five years. However, in 2010, an increased incidence of narcolepsy was observed in Finland and Sweden in children and adolescents immunized with the H1N1 AS03-adjuvanted pandemic influenza vaccine. The European Medicines Agency confirmed the existence of this association, which has since been detected in England, Ireland, France, and Norway [23]. In these cases, narcolepsy appeared associated with HLA DQB1*0602, which is more common in Northern countries than elsewhere [24].

Post-SARS-CoV-2 vaccination autoimmune phenomena are extremely rare, strengthening the safety of the vaccines. Following vaccination, the most commonly reported diseases associated with new-onset events were immune thrombocytopenia, Guillain–Barré syndrome, and myocarditis. Immune thrombocytopenia, psoriasis, IgA nephropathy, and SLE, on the other hand, were the most reported illnesses associated with relapsing episodes. Both occurrences were widely linked to the mRNA-1273 SARS-CoV-2 vaccine, which was followed by Sinovac-CoronaVac and ChAdOx1 nCoV-19 vaccine (AZD1222). Germano et al. described cases of Guillain–Barrè syndrome following SARS-CoV-2 vaccination [25] usually presenting as an acute inflammatory demyelinating polyradiculoneuropathy and occurring after the first vaccine dose. Ramdas et al. reported seven cases of new-onset myasthenia gravis in timely association with SARS-CoV-2 vaccination, including a pediatric case [26]. Şendur et al. [27] suggested that the frequencies of HLA-B*35 and HLA-C*04 alleles could be higher in SARS-CoV-2 vaccine-induced subacute thyroiditis compared with controls [HLA-B*35: 13 (93%) versus 40 (40%), $p<0.001$; HLA-C*04: 13 (93%) versus 43 (43%), $p<0.001$, respectively]. Moreover, more severe thyrotoxicosis was seen in patients having HLA-B*35 and HLA-C*04 homozygous alleles [free thyroxine: 4.47 ng/dL (3.77–5.18) versus 1.41 ng/dL (1.22–2.63), $p = 0.048$]. Interestingly, already in 2011, an association among influenza vaccine, HLA-B*35, and subacute thyroiditis was suggested [28].

Thus, vaccination effects may clearly differ substantially due to the genetic background of the recipient individual, and the vaccination schedule would be better if personalized [29]. Thomas et al. have revised this issue gathering a number of examples of genotype/gene polymorphisms mainly in the HLA gene family, related to interindividual variation to vaccination [30]. The advances in the fields of immunology, genetics, molecular biology, bioinformatics, and the Human Genome Project have allowed for the emergence of the field of vaccinomics that encompasses the fields of immunogenetics and immunogenomics as applied to understanding the mechanisms of heterogeneity in immune responses to vaccines [31].

Hence, it is imperative to pursue the aim of implementing the tools of genomics and proteomics to allow the prediction of those population sets more likely to be nonresponsive or develop adverse reactions to vaccines.

Immunity

The trigger of a dysregulated immune response is different according to the agent serving as "adjuvant." Noteworthy, those vaccines that are associated with postvaccination phenomena are usually targeted toward an infectious agent that is per se capable of triggering that specific phenomenon. This suggests similar immunopathogenic mechanisms between vaccines and infectious agents as triggering factors of autoimmune diseases (ADs). Usually, the phenomena occur much more frequently following the infection than following vaccination [32]. For instance, this is the case of the recently described myocarditis following anti-SARS-CoV-2 vaccines that occurs at a much lower frequency than in patients affected by COVID-19 [33]. At the same extent, Guillain–Barré occurs at a greater frequency after influenza virus infection than it does after vaccination [34].

The anti-idiotype immune response can explain the common increased prevalence of certain reactions to vaccines and the infectious agent. Indeed, a specific antigen can trigger the production of second particular antibodies against the first ones [35]. Surprisingly, these second antibodies may be capable of binding to receptors that the initial antigen may attach to. This is significant since many autoimmune or -inflammatory reactions elicited by COVID-19 vaccinations have previously been reported with vaccines, whose principal immunopathogenic mechanism is the anti-idiotype immune response [36, 37].

Another possible mechanism by which an altered immune response may occur is due to molecular mimicry. This refers to the concept that an immune response, initially directed at bacterial or viral antigens, can target host molecules that share sequence homology or structural similarities with microbial epitopes [38]. Adjuvants accomplish this task by mimicking specific sets of evolutionarily conserved molecules (liposomes, lipopolysaccharides (LPSs), unmethylated CpG dinucleotide-containing DNA, etc.). On the other hand, the adjuvant may induce autoimmunity through the polyclonal activation of B cells [39], through an enhanced cytokine production and the expansion of autoreactive T cells [40].

For instance, SARS-CoV-2 might trigger AIDs [41] through molecular mimicry [42, 43]. Moreover, the history of past infections can alter the reactogenicity of mRNA vaccines through a cross-reactivity mechanism [44]. A greater reactogenicity may confer higher protection but could generate more adverse events. It is relevant to underline that patients with AIDs are not at increased risk of adverse events associated with vaccination [45], possibly due to the effect of immunomodulatory drugs on vaccine immunogenicity.

Concerning the case of narcolepsy, it is possible that molecular mimicry involving cross-reactivity of H1N1-specific T cells and hypocretin-producing neurons is the key pathogenic mechanism. Cross-reactive $CD4^+$ T cells that recognize both a foreign H1N1 epitope and an epitope present on hypocretin-producing cells and presented by HLA-DQB1*06:02 by antigen presenting cells could, however, be involved with a major overall alteration of T-cell subsets [46].

Other mechanisms that may be involved in postvaccination phenomena include neutrophil activation facilitated by NETosis and platelet activation especially in vaccine-induced immune thrombotic thrombocytopenia (VITT) [47]. VITT has also been related to the activation of the NF-kB pathway in which plasminogen activator inhibitor-1 (PAI-1) plays a relevant role in thrombotic events. The NF-kB may exert a direct effect on monocytes, leading to the production of cytokines, such as interleukin 1β, that in turn generate a procoagulant state [48, 49].

Autoimmunity

A full-blown autoimmune disease has been occasionally described following exposure to adjuvants, and several autoimmune conditions including Sjögren's syndrome and undifferentiated connective tissue disease seem to share pathogenetic aspects with ASIA syndrome. Despite debated [50], pollution dust seems to be capable of eliciting an autoimmune response in people experiencing the terroristic attack at the World Trade Center in New York on 11 September 2001 [51–53]. The debris and dust were composed of an amalgam of glass fibers, silica, asbestos, polycyclic aromatic hydrocarbons, dioxin, furans, and polychlorinated biphenyls, and the firefighters and the policemen who worked at the site of the attack later developed autoimmune diseases at an increased incidence than general population.

VITT is a thrombotic thrombocytopenia developing in a very small proportion of patients after exposure to ChAdOx1 and Ad26.COV.2 vaccines anti-SARS-CoV-2 [54]. In these patients, mostly females <50 years old, the presence of platelet-activating antibodies directed against platelet factor 4 (PF4) has been documented, suggesting a similarity to Heparin-associated thrombocytopenia, which is characterized by the presence of antibodies against the heparin/(PF4) complex, generating thrombocytopenia and thrombosis due to platelet activation. Indeed, the binding of PF4 with endothelial cells and platelets facilitates platelet aggregation and thrombus formation [55]. PF4 can interact with the double-stranded DNA of the vaccine vector, and the PF4/DNA vector complex recognized by the antigen-presenting cells allows in some patients the production of antibodies against PF4 [56].

SARS-CoV-2 infection and vaccines have represented an interesting model for the possible development of autoimmunity. In this context, García-Bravo et al. [57] have shown that myositis-related autoantibodies were more frequent during the pandemic, in particular anti-MDA5. In contrast, in 2021, after the vaccination campaigns, the most common antibodies were anti-PL7 and/or anti-PL12.

Other evidence of increased reactogenicity in patients with chronic inflammatory diseases vaccinated with anti-SARS-CoV-2 vaccines have been aroused. These patients may report more myalgia and fatigue after exposure to vaccines [58].

A recent study suggested that SARS-CoV-2 vaccines may trigger neurological autoimmunity including central nervous system demyelinating diseases, inflammatory peripheral neuropathies, myositis, myasthenia, limbic encephalitis, and giant cell arteritis, usually with a favorable outcome and good tolerance to revaccinations [59].

Conclusion

The panorama that we are now facing has dramatically changed. Vaccines save millions of lives each year, improving the quality of life, and this has proved even more true in these times of COVID-19 pandemic. If we consider the billions of doses of anti-SARS-CoV-2 vaccines administered, these can be considered extremely safe, as well as all the vaccines that are recommended in the general population. The novel vaccines technology, including the mRNA-based vaccinations, has significantly contributed to this generational leap in terms of vaccines safety, even in patients already suffering from an autoimmune disease [60].

Still, in the view of personalized medicine, a better knowledge of the relationships among a specific vaccine, the genetic background, and the immune milieu would even allow to avoid the occurrence of any autoimmune-rheumatic adverse events. At the same extent, although silicone implants are safe for the vast majority of subjects, screening for preexisting autoimmune phenomena and genetic testing appear useful tools for risk stratification before the implantation in predisposed subjects to dodge autoimmune phenomena and subsequent explanation surgeries [61].

References

1. Shoenfeld, Y. and Agmon-Levin, N. (2011). ASIA–autoimmune/inflammatory syndrome induced by adjuvants. *J. Autoimmun.* 36: 4–8.
2. Perricone, C., Colafrancesco, S., Mazor, R.D. et al. (2013). Autoimmune/inflammatory syndrome induced by adjuvants (ASIA) 2013: unveiling the pathogenic, clinical and diagnostic aspects. *J. Autoimmun.* 47: 1–16. https://doi.org/10.1016/j.jaut.2013.10.004.
3. Arango, M.T., Perricone, C., Kivity, S. et al. (2017). HLA-DRB1 the notorious gene in the mosaic of autoimmunity. *Immunol. Res.* 65 (1): 82–98. https://doi.org/10.1007/s12026-016-8817-7.
4. Carvalho, J.F., Barros, S.M., Branci, J.C., and Fonseca, J.E. (2011). ASIA or Shoenfeld's syndrome: highlighting different perspective for diffuse chronic pain. *Acta Rheumatol Port* 36: 10–12.
5. Meroni, P.L. (2011). Autoimmune or auto-inflammatory syndrome induced by adjuvants (ASIA): old truths and a new syndrome? *J. Autoimmun.* 36: 1–3.
6. Shoenfeld, Y., Huges, G.R.V., and Agmon-Levin, N. (2012). The spectrum of ASIA: 'autoimmune (auto-inflammatory) syndrome induced by adjuvants'. *Lupus* 21: 118–120.
7. Rosenblum, H., Shoenfeld, Y., and Amital, H. (2011). The common immunogenic etiology of chronic fatigue syndrome: from infections to vaccines via adjuvants to the ASIA syndrome. *Infect. Dis. Clin. N. Am.* 25: 851–863.
8. Israeli, E., Agmon-Levin, N., Blank, M., and Shoenfeld, Y. (2009). Adjuvants and autoimmunity. *Lupus* 18: 1217–1225.

9. Molina, V. and Shoenfeld, Y. (2005). Infection, vaccines and other environmental triggers of autoimmunity. *Autoimmunity* 38: 235–245. https://doi.org/10.1080/08916930500050277.
10. Watad, A., Quaresma, M., Brown, S. et al. (2017). Autoimmune/inflammatory syndrome induced by adjuvants (Shoenfeld's syndrome) – an update. *Lupus* 26: 675–681. https://doi.org/10.1177/0961203316686406.
11. Colafrancesco, S., Perricone, C., Priori, R. et al. (2014). Sjögren's syndrome: another facet of the autoimmune/inflammatory syndrome induced by adjuvants (ASIA). *J. Autoimmun.* 51: 10–16. https://doi.org/10.1016/j.jaut.2014.03.003.
12. Scanzi, F., Andreoli, L., Martinelli, M. et al. (2017). Are the autoimmune/inflammatory syndrome induced by adjuvants (ASIA) and the undifferentiated connective tissue disease (UCTD) related to each other? A case-control study of environmental exposures. *Immunol. Res.* 65 (1): 150–156. https://doi.org/10.1007/s12026-017-8912-4.
13. Cohen Tervaert, J.W. (2018). Autoinflammatory/autoimmunity syndrome induced by adjuvants (ASIA; Shoenfeld's syndrome): a new flame. *Autoimmun. Rev.* 17 (12): 1259–1264. https://doi.org/10.1016/j.autrev.2018.07.003.
14. Borba, V., Malkova, A., Basantsova, N. et al. (2020). Classical examples of the concept of the ASIA syndrome. *Biomolecules* 10 (10): 1436.
15. McGarvey, P.B., Suzek, B.E., Baraniuk, J.N. et al. (2014). In silico analysis of autoimmune diseases and genetic relationships to vaccination against infectious diseases. *BMC Immunol.* 15: 61. https://doi.org/10.1186/s12865-014-0061-0.
16. Haley, R.W., Billecke, S., and La Du, B.N. (1999). Association of low PON1 type Q (type A) arylesterase activity with neurologic symptom complexes in Gulf War veterans. *Toxicol. Appl. Pharmacol.* 157 (3): 227–233. https://doi.org/10.1006/taap.1999.8703.
17. Mackness, B., Durrington, P.N., and Mackness, M.I. (2000). Low paraoxonase in Persian Gulf War Veterans self-reporting Gulf war syndrome. *Biochem. Biophys. Res. Commun.* 276 (2): 729–733. https://doi.org/10.1006/bbrc.2000.3526.
18. Guis, S., Pellissier, J.F., Nicoli, F. et al. (2002). HLA-DRB1*01 and macrophagic myofasciitis. *Arthritis Rheum.* 46 (9): 2535–2537. https://doi.org/10.1002/art.10465.
19. Kappel, R.M., Cohen Tervaert, J.W., and Pruijn, G.J. (2014). Autoimmune/inflammatory syndrome induced by adjuvants (ASIA) due to silicone implant incompatibility syndrome in three sisters. *Clin. Exp. Rheumatol.* 32 (2): 256–258.
20. Young, V.L., Nemecek, J.R., Schwartz, B.D. et al. (1995). HLA typing in women with breast implants. *Plast. Reconstr. Surg.* 96 (7): 1497–1519.
21. Liozon, E., Parreau, S., Filloux, M. et al. (2021). Giant cell arteritis or polymyalgia rheumatica after influenza vaccination: a study of 12 patients and a literature review. *Autoimmun. Rev.* 20 (2): 102732. https://doi.org/10.1016/j.autrev.2020.102732.
22. Buonocore, S.M. and van der Most, R.G. (2022). Narcolepsy and H1N1 influenza immunology a decade later: what have we learned? *Front. Immunol.* 13: 902840. https://doi.org/10.3389/fimmu.2022.902840.
23. Juvodden, H.T., Viken, M.K., Nordstrand, S.E.H. et al. (2020). HLA and sleep parameter associations in post-H1N1 narcolepsy type 1 patients and first-degree relatives. *Sleep* 43 (3): zsz239. https://doi.org/10.1093/sleep/zsz239.
24. Viste, R., Lie, B.A., Viken, M.K. et al. (2021). Narcolepsy type 1 patients have lower levels of effector memory CD4+ T cells compared to their siblings when controlling for H1N1-(Pandemrix™)-vaccination and HLA DQB1*06:02 status. *Sleep Med.* 85: 271–279. https://doi.org/10.1016/j.sleep.2021.07.024.
25. Germano F, Bellucci M, Grisanti S, Beronio A, Grazzini M, Coco E, Tassinari T, Della Cava F, De Michelis C, Baldi O, Sivori G, Murialdo A, Cabona C, Durando P, Uccelli A, Schenone A, Franciotta D, Benedetti L. COVID-19 vaccine-related Guillain-Barré syndrome in the Liguria region of Italy: a multicenter case series. *J. Neurol. Sci.* 2022;440:120330. https://doi.org/10.1016/j.jns.2022.120330).
26. Ramdas, S., Hum, R.M., Price, A. et al. (2022). SARS-CoV-2 vaccination and new-onset myasthenia gravis: a report of 7 cases and review of the literature. *Neuromuscul. Disord.* 32 (10): 785–789.
27. Şendur, S.N., Özmen, F., Oğuz, S.H. et al. (2022). Association of human leukocyte antigen genotypes with severe acute respiratory syndrome coronavirus 2 vaccine-induced subacute thyroiditis. *Thyroid* 32 (6): 640–647. https://doi.org/10.1089/thy.2022.0010.

28. Hernán Martinez, J., Corder, E., Uzcategui, M. et al. (2011). Subacute thyroiditis and dyserythropoesis after influenza vaccination suggesting immune dysregulation. *Bol. Asoc. Med. P. R.* 103 (2): 48–52.
29. Nanishi, E., Dowling, D.J., and Levy, O. (2020). Toward precision adjuvants: optimizing science and safety. *Curr. Opin. Pediatr.* 32 (1): 125–138. https://doi.org/10.1097/MOP.0000000000000868.
30. Thomas, C. and Moridani, M. (2010). Interindividual variations in the efficacy and toxicity of vaccines. *Toxicology* 278 (2): 204–210. https://doi.org/10.1016/j.tox.2009.10.008.
31. Poland, G.A., Ovsyannikova, I.G., Jacobson, R.M., and Smith, D.I. (2007). Heterogeneity in vaccine immune response: the role of immunogenetics and the emerging field of vaccinomics. *Clin. Pharmacol. Ther.* 82 (6): 653–664. https://doi.org/10.1038/sj.clpt.6100415.
32. Nahra, V., Makandura, M., Anthony, D.D., and Mattar, M. (2022). A case series on the COVID-19 vaccines and possible immune-related adverse events: a new challenge for the rheumatologists. *Cureus* 14 (9): e29660. https://doi.org/10.7759/cureus.29660.
33. Heidecker, B., Dagan, N., Balicer, R. et al. (2022). Myocarditis following COVID-19 vaccine: incidence, presentation, diagnosis, pathophysiology, therapy, and outcomes put into perspective. A clinical consensus document supported by the Heart Failure Association of the European Society of Cardiology (ESC) and the ESC Working Group on Myocardial and Pericardial Diseases. *Eur. J. Heart Fail.* 24 (11): 2000–2018. https://doi.org/10.1002/ejhf.2669.
34. Salmon, D.A., Proschan, M., Forshee, R. et al. (2013). Association between Guillain-Barré syndrome and influenza A (H1N1) 2009 monovalent inactivated vaccines in the USA: a meta-analysis. *Lancet* 381 (9876): 1461–1468. https://doi.org/10.1016/S0140-6736(12)62189-8.
35. Murphy, W.J. and Longo, D.L. (2022). A possible role for anti-idiotype antibodies in SARS-CoV-2 infection and vaccination. *N. Engl. J. Med.* 386 (4): 394–396. https://doi.org/10.1056/NEJMcibr2113694.
36. Shukla, A.K. and Misra, S. (2022). Clinical implications of anti-idiotype antibodies in COVID-19. *J. Basic Clin. Physiol. Pharmacol.* https://doi.org/10.1515/jbcpp-2022-0123.
37. Bellucci, M., Germano, F., Grisanti, S. et al. (2022). Case report: post-COVID-19 vaccine recurrence of Guillain-Barré syndrome following an antecedent parainfectious COVID-19-related GBS. *Front. Immunol.* 13: 894872. https://doi.org/10.3389/fimmu.2022.894872.
38. Segal, Y. and Shoenfeld, Y. (2018). Vaccine-induced autoimmunity: the role of molecular mimicry and immune crossreaction. *Cell. Mol. Immunol.* 15 (6): 586–594. https://doi.org/10.1038/cmi.2017.151.
39. Tovey, M.G., Lallemand, C., Meritet, J.F., and Maury, C. (2006). Adjuvant activity of interferon alpha: mechanism(s) of action. *Vaccine* 24 (Suppl 2): S2-46-7. https://doi.org/10.1016/j.vaccine.2005.01.117.
40. van Aalst, S., Ludwig, I.S., van der Zee, R. et al. (2017). Bystander activation of irrelevant $CD4^+$ T cells following antigen-specific vaccination occurs in the presence and absence of adjuvant. *PLoS One* 12 (5): e0177365. https://doi.org/10.1371/journal.pone.0177365.
41. Rodríguez, Y., Rojas, M., Beltrán, S. et al. (2022). Autoimmune and autoinflammatory conditions after COVID-19 vaccination. New case reports and updated literature review. *J. Autoimmun.* 132: 102898. https://doi.org/10.1016/j.jaut.2022.102898.
42. Liu, Y., Sawalha, A.H., and Lu, Q. (2021). COVID-19 and autoimmune diseases. *Curr. Opin. Rheumatol.* 33: 155–162. https://doi.org/10.1097/BOR.0000000000000776.
43. Anaya, J.-M., Herrán, M., Beltrán, S., and Rojas, M. (2022). Is post-COVID syndrome an autoimmune disease? *Expet Rev. Clin. Immunol.* https://doi.org/10.1080/1744666X.2022.2085561. [
44. Vizcarra, P., Haemmerle, J., Velasco, H. et al. (2021). BNT162b2 mRNA COVID-19 vaccine Reactogenicity: the key role of immunity. *Vaccine* 39: 7367–7374. https://doi.org/10.1016/j.vaccine.2021.10.074.
45. Wieske, L., Kummer, L.Y.L., van Dam, K.P.J. et al. (2022). Risk factors associated with short-term adverse events after SARS-CoV-2 vaccination in patients with immune-mediated inflammatory diseases. *BMC Med.* 20: 100. https://doi.org/10.1186/s12916-022-02310-7.
46. Singh, A.K., Mahlios, J., and Mignot, E. (2013). Genetic association, seasonal infections and autoimmune basis of narcolepsy. *J. Autoimmun.* 43: 26–31. https://doi.org/10.1016/j.jaut.2013.02.003.
47. Holm, S., Kared, H., Michelsen, A.E. et al. (2021). Immune complexes, innate immunity, and NETosis in ChAdOx1 vaccine-induced thrombocytopenia. *Eur. Heart J.* 42: 4064–4072. https://doi.org/10.1093/eurheartj/ehab506.
48. Mattsson, E., Herwald, H., and Egesten, A. (2003). Superantigens from *Staphylococcus aureus* induce procoagulant activity and monocyte tissue factor expression in whole blood and mononuclear cells via IL-1 beta. *J. Thromb. Haemost.* 1: 2569–2576. https://doi.org/10.1111/j.1538-7836.2003.00498.x.

49. Iba, T., Umemura, Y., Wada, H., and Levy, J.H. (2021). Roles of coagulation abnormalities and microthrombosis in sepsis: pathophysiology, diagnosis, and treatment. *Arch. Med. Res.* 52: 788–797. https://doi.org/10.1016/j.arcmed.2021.07.003.
50. Sacks, H.S., Smirnoff, M., Carson, D. et al. (2022). Autoimmune conditions in the World Trade Center general responder cohort: a nested case-control and standardized incidence ratio analysis. *Am. J. Ind. Med.* 65 (2): 117–131. https://doi.org/10.1002/ajim.23313.
51. Webber, M.P., Moir, W., Zeig-Owens, R. et al. (2015). Nested case-control study of selected systemic autoimmune diseases in World Trade Center rescue/recovery workers. *Arthritis Rheumatol.* 67 (5): 1369–1376. https://doi.org/10.1002/art.39059.
52. Miller-Archie, S.A., Izmirly, P.M., Berman, J.R. et al. (2020). Systemic autoimmune disease among adults exposed to the September 11, 2001 terrorist attack. *Arthritis Rheumatol.* 72 (5): 849–859. https://doi.org/10.1002/art.41175.
53. Brite, J., Miller-Archie, S.A., and Cone, J. (2022). The relationship between 9/11 exposure, systemic autoimmune disease, and post-traumatic stress disorder: a mediational analysis. *Int. J. Environ. Res. Public Health* 19 (11): 6514. https://doi.org/10.3390/ijerph19116514.
54. Lavin, M., Elder, P.T., O'Keeffe, D. et al. (2021). Vaccine-induced immune thrombotic thrombocytopenia (VITT) – a novel clinico-pathological entity with heterogeneous clinical presentations. *Br. J. Haematol.* 195: 76–84. https://doi.org/10.1111/bjh.17613.
55. Cai, Z., Greene, M.I., Zhu, Z., and Zhang, H. (2020). Features structural, functions P.F.4. That occur in heparin-induced thrombocytopenia (HIT) complicated by COVID-19. *Antibodies* 9: 52. https://doi.org/10.3390/antib9040052.
56. McGonagle, D., De Marco, G., and Bridgewood, C. (2021). Mechanisms of immunothrombosis in vaccine-induced thrombotic thrombocytopenia (VITT) compared to natural SARS-CoV-2 infection. *J. Autoimmun.* 121: 102662. https://doi.org/10.1016/j.jaut.2021.102662.
57. García-Bravo, L., Calle-Rubio, M., Fernández-Arquero, M. et al. (2022). Association of anti-SARS-COV-2 vaccine with increased incidence of myositis-related anti-RNA-synthetases auto-antibodies. *J. Transl. Autoimmun.* 5: 100160. https://doi.org/10.1016/j.jtauto.2022.100160.
58. Yang, M.M., Taylor, K.E., Paez, D. et al. (2022). Reactogenicity of the messenger RNA SARS-CoV-2 vaccines associated with immunogenicity in patients with autoimmune and inflammatory disease. *Arthritis Care Res.* 74: 1953–1960. https://doi.org/10.1002/acr.24894.
59. Doubrovinskaia, S., Mooshage, C.M., Seliger, C. et al. (2022). Neurological autoimmune diseases following vaccinations against severe acute respiratory syndrome coronavirus 2 (SARS-CoV-2): a follow-up study. *Eur. J. Neurol.* https://doi.org/10.1111/ene.15602.
60. Assawasaksakul, T., Lertussavavivat, T., Sathitratanacheewin, S. et al. (2022). Comparison of immunogenicity and safety of inactivated, adenovirus-vectored, and heterologous adenovirus-vectored/mRNA vaccines in patients with systemic lupus erythematosus and rheumatoid arthritis: a prospective cohort study. *Vaccines (Basel).* 10 (6): 853. https://doi.org/10.3390/vaccines10060853.
61. Ribeiro, P.D.C. and Sato, E.I. (2022). Autoimmune/autoinflammatory syndrome induced by adjuvants: a focus on silicone. *Clin. Rheumatol.* 41 (11): 3275–3283. https://doi.org/10.1007/s10067-022-06274-0.

3 Vaccine Adjuvants: History, Role, Mechanisms of Action, and Side Effects

Nicola Luigi Bragazzi[1,2], Abdulla Watad[3,4,5,6,7], and Yehuda Shoenfeld[8,9]

[1]Laboratory for Industrial and Applied Mathematics (LIAM), Department of Mathematics and Statistics, York University, Toronto, Canada
[2]Postgraduate School of Public Health, Department of Health Sciences (DISSAL), University of Genoa, Genoa, Italy
[3]Rheumatology Unit and Zabludowicz Center for Autoimmune Diseases, Sheba Medical Center, Tel-Hashomer, Israel
[4]Section of Musculoskeletal Disease, Leeds Institute of Molecular Medicine, University of Leeds, Leeds, UK
[5]Sackler Faculty of Medicine, Tel Aviv University, Tel Aviv, Israel
[6]Department of Internal Medicine 'B', Sheba Medical Center, Tel-Hashomer, Israel
[7]Institute of Oncology, Sheba Medical Center, Tel-Hashomer, Israel
[8]Reichman University, Herzliya, Israel
[9]Zabludowicz Center for Autoimmune Diseases, Sheba Medical Center, Tel-Hashomer, Israel

Introduction

An "adjuvant" can be defined as a component incorporated into vaccines with the primary purpose of eliciting an immune response and magnifying its strength and duration [1].

In this chapter, we offer a comprehensive overview of vaccine adjuvants, delving into the "known knowns" and "known unknowns" of adjuvants and their historical and present-day developments. More specifically, we shed light on the emerging concepts in the field, provide fresh insights, and discuss how our expanding knowledge concerning human immunity (in particular, the innate immune system) and the burgeoning disciplines of immunoinformatics and systems vaccinology are reinvigorating the science behind adjuvant development.

This revitalization holds immense promise not only for old vaccines but especially for the novel ones, including those against the "Coronavirus Disease 2019" (COVID-19), potentially addressing the challenges posed by future infectious outbreaks and pandemics [2].

Autoimmune Disorders: Adjuvants and Other Risk Factors in Pathogenesis, First Edition.
Edited by Abdulla Watad, Nicola Luigi Bragazzi, and Yehuda Shoenfeld.

Materials and methods

To conduct the present review, we extensively searched MEDLINE via its freely available PubMed interface, using the following search string: "adjuvant* AND (vaccin* OR immuniz* OR immunis*) AND (safe* OR tolerab* OR 'adverse event*' OR 'side effect*' OR reactogenic*) NOT (cancer OR neoplasm OR tumor OR malignanc*) AND human*," specifically looking for systematic reviews and meta-analyses. We focused on preventative (or preventive or prophylactic) and not on therapeutic vaccines. We excluded vaccination products designed in the field of veterinary medicine.

The literature search was conducted at the beginning of January 2023 and updated on 9 September 2023.

Etymology of adjuvants

The term "adjuvant" is used in the context of vaccines to describe substances or components that assist and enhance the vaccine's effectiveness. Indeed, the word "adjuvant" was coined by Gaston Ramon, a prominent French veterinary scientist, during his staying at the Pasteur Institute, from 1920 to 1924/1925 [3], and has its origins in Latin, coming from the Latin word "*adjuvans,*" which is the present participle of the verb "*adjuvare.*" This is a compound word formed from "*ad,*" meaning "to" or "toward," and "*juvare,*" meaning "to help," "to aid," or "to assist." From an etymological standpoint, "adjuvant" essentially means "helping," "aiding," or "assisting," which well reflects its role in vaccines, where adjuvants help boost the immune response to the vaccine's active components.

Classification of adjuvants

Adjuvants can be classified into several ways based on (i) their physicochemical properties, (ii) molecular and cellular mechanisms of action, or (iii) chemical composition [4] (Table 3.1).

Table 3.1 An overview of major vaccine adjuvants.

Adjuvant family	Examples of adjuvants
Mineral salts	Aluminum salts (alum)
	Calcium phosphate
Lipid particles/ liposomes	Incomplete Freund's adjuvant
	Oil-based emulsions (MF59, AS03, AS04, AS01E, squalene-in-water emulsions or SWEs, stable emulsions or SEs, such as GLA-SE and SLA-SE, Montanide ISA™51, Montanide ISA™720, and CoVaccine)
	Cochleates/nano(structured) cochleates
Microparticles	Virus-like particles (VLPs)
	Virosomes, including immunopotentiating reconstituted influenza virosomes (IRIVs)
	PLA (polylactic acid), PLG (poly[lactide-coglycolide])
Immune potentiators	dsRNA: Poly(I:C), Poly-IC:LC
	Monophosphoryl lipid A (MPL-A), LPS
	Flagellin
	Imidazoquinolines, including imiquimod (R837), resiquimod (848)
	CpG oligodeoxynucleotides (ODN)
	Muramyl dipeptide (MDP)
	Saponins (QS-21)
Mucosal adjuvants	Cholera toxin subunit B (CT-B)
	Heat-labile enterotoxin (LTK3 and LTR72)
	Bordetella pertussis toxin
	Chitosan

A general classification of adjuvants subdivides them into the broad categories of traditional and novel adjuvants. The former includes mineral salts.

Mineral salts

There exist two broad classes of mineral salts that act as vaccine adjuvants, namely (i) aluminum and (ii) calcium salts. Aluminum salts include aluminum oxyhydroxide or AlO(OH), aluminum hydroxyphosphate or $HAlO_5P$, aluminum phosphate or $Al(PO_4)_3$, and aluminum potassium sulfate or $AlK(SO_4)_2$. These compounds are derivatives of the historical solution of alum, potassium aluminum sulfate [$KAl(SO_4)_2 \cdot 12H_2O$], which was deployed to purify tetanus and diphtheria toxoids by precipitation of the proteins. Since the 1920s—1930s, they have been used in vaccines for many decades and are known for their ability to enhance the antibody response [5]. Despite being old, aluminum is currently being utilized to create the next generation of enhanced adjuvants through the adsorption and delivery of various immunopotentiators [5].

Calcium salts include calcium phosphate [4], a naturally occurring compound in the human body, which served as an adjuvant in diphtheria, tetanus, pertussis, and poliomyelitis vaccines. Even though, in the late 1980s, it was entirely replaced by alum salts, it is currently being considered as a potential substitute for alum salts in vaccines, as it shows an excellent safety profile.

Emulsions

More recent adjuvants consist of oil-in-water emulsions; these adjuvants, such as MF59 and AS03, are composed of oil droplets suspended in water. They are able to enhance both antibody and cellular immune responses [6].

Bacterial- or microbial-derived adjuvants

Other compounds are bacterial-derived adjuvants: examples include *Bordetella pertussis* toxin, heat-labile enterotoxin (LTK3 and LTR72), and *Cholera* toxin subunit B (CT-B). These are derived from bacteria and can stimulate strong immune responses [7].

TLR agonists

Novel adjuvants [7, 8] include the Toll-like receptor (TLR) agonists. These adjuvants activate specific receptors (TLRs) located on immune cells, triggering an immune response. Examples include monophosphoryl lipid A (MPL-A) and CpG oligodeoxynucleotides (CpG ODNs). Another example of novel adjuvants is saponins, natural compounds found in plants such as *Quillaja saponaria* (soapbark, a tree commonly found in Chile) and *Gypsophila paniculata* (baby's breath, common gypsophila or panicled baby's breath, a plant particularly abundant in central and eastern Europe). They can enhance immune responses and are used in some experimental vaccines, still under investigation. Another example is given by flagellins, which represent the major structural protein of Gram-negative flagella and were first identified by Ciacci-Woolwine et al. [9] in 1998. They are able to broadly mobilize T and B lymphocytes to secondary lymphoid organs, along with the activation of $TLR5^+CD11c^+$ cells and T lymphocytes, which occurs in a manner distinct from the recognition of specific antigens. The adaptability of flagellin has enabled the creation of various fusion proteins combining flagellin with antigens, which have demonstrated effectiveness as vaccines in animal studies.

Lipid particles/liposomes

Liposomes are lipid-based vesicles that can carry antigens and improve their delivery to immune cells. Liposome-based adjuvants are under investigation for various vaccines, while virosomes are lipid vesicles incorporating viral proteins that can mimic viral infections and stimulate strong immune responses [10].

Microparticles/nanoparticles

Microparticles/nanoparticles or particulate structures, such as virus-like particles (VLPs) and other microparticles/nanoparticles, can serve as adjuvants by presenting antigens in a way that enhances immune recognition [11].

Cytokine- and interleukin-based adjuvants

In some cases, the antigen itself can serve as an adjuvant, especially if it has inherent immunostimulatory properties. Some recent vaccines include specific cytokine-based adjuvants, such as interleukins, to boost the immune response [12].

Adjuvant delivery systems

Adjuvants can also be classified based on their delivery systems, including nanoparticles [13], liposomes, or other carriers designed to improve antigen delivery and presentation. Finally, as previously mentioned, an emerging category is represented by pathogen-derived adjuvants; certain components derived from pathogens, such as viral vectors or bacterial proteins, can function as adjuvants in vaccines. It is important to note that adjuvant research is ongoing, and new adjuvants are continually being developed and tested to improve the effectiveness and safety of vaccines. As such, the classification of adjuvants is constantly under flux.

The choice of adjuvant depends on the specific vaccine, target pathogen, and desired immune response. Additionally, regulatory agencies such as the US Food and Drug Administration (FDA) and the World Health Organization (WHO) evaluate and approve adjuvants for use in vaccines to ensure their safety and efficacy, which will be overviewed in the following sections.

History of adjuvants

The exploration of adjuvants' origins traces back to the pioneering work of Ramon, who made the pivotal observation that horses developing abscesses at the injection site exhibited significantly higher levels of specific antibodies. To test this hypothesis in a methodologically robust fashion, Ramon conducted a series of experiments wherein he intentionally induced sterile abscesses at the injection site by combining starch, tapioca, or breadcrumbs with inactivated toxins. His findings rigorously proved the link between substances capable of instigating localized inflammation and the enhanced production of antisera [14]. This groundbreaking work laid the foundation for our understanding of adjuvants' capacity to boost immune responses [15, 16].

Subsequent to Ramon's pioneering work, Glenny and his colleagues [17] embarked on further investigations in 1926, marking a further significant milestone. Their experiments revealed that precipitating diphtheria toxoid with aluminum salts led to a substantial augmentation of the immune response to the toxoid. Subsequent experiments conducted in 1932 by Park and Schroder [18] and in 1934 by Harrison [19] showed that alum can enhance diphtheria toxoid immunization in humans, and immunization of guinea pigs with alum plus pollen extracts increases allergic sensitization, respectively [20]. As a result, aluminum salts were introduced in the late 1930s as adjuvants in human vaccines against diphtheria, pertussis, tetanus, and poliovirus, with Alhydrogel becoming commercially available in 1939, and marking a historic breakthrough [21]. Today, they are integral components of vaccines against various diseases, including hepatitis A and B, *Haemophilus influenzae* type b, meningococcus, pneumococcus, and human papillomavirus.

It is important to underscore that the inclusion of an adjuvant in these vaccines is indispensable for their efficacy. Salts of aluminum, a compound usually and commonly found in air, soil, and water, have firmly established their role in facilitating stronger and longer-lasting immunity, increasing local inflammation, improving antigen uptake by antigen-presenting cells (APCs), and enhancing antibody production [20]. Remarkably, for approximately six decades, aluminum salts remained the sole adjuvants employed in licensed vaccines. Aluminum is also utilized in the development of medicines and cosmetics as well as in the food industry. It can be inhaled or ingested, and, then, undergoes a three-stage process, resulting into its (partial) elimination and urinary excretion, in that approximately less than 3% and 1% of inhaled and consumed aluminum can diffuse throughout the organism, respectively.

After the introduction of aluminum salts, the landscape of vaccine adjuvants underwent a transformative shift starting in the early 1990s. This period witnessed the licensing of several vaccines featuring novel adjuvants. These innovations have expanded the arsenal of adjuvanted vaccines and contributed to enhanced immune responses. Notable examples include the Fluad® and Fluad® Pediatric vaccines [21], incorporating the squalene emulsion-based adjuvant MF59, as well as the Epaxal® [22] and Inflexal® vaccines [21], which utilize immunopotentiating reconstituted influenza virosomes (IRIVs) [23]. Additionally, the human papillomavirus (HPV) vaccine Cervarix® integrates AS04, an aluminum hydroxide adjuvant combined with immunostimulatory MPL-A [24, 25]. The Pandemrix® vaccine includes AS03, a squalene emulsion enriched with the immunopotentiating α-tocopherol (a form of vitamin E) [26]. Malaria vaccine RTS,S/AS01 (Mosquirix®), on the other hand, features AS01E, a liposomal adjuvant comprising MPL-A and immunostimulatory saponin QS-21 [27].

These advances signify a dynamic era in adjuvant research and underscore the critical role adjuvants play in bolstering vaccine efficacy, offering promising avenues for further vaccine development and the potential to address pressing global health challenges [28].

The demand for innovative adjuvants tailored to elicit robust T-cell immunity and localized immunity within mucosal tissues remains substantial [29]. Mucosal tissues serve as the primary entry points for numerous pathogens, making it imperative to develop adjuvants capable of enhancing immune responses at these sites. Robust T-cell responses play a pivotal role in combating a wide range of infections, including but not limited to tuberculosis, dengue, human immunodeficiency virus (HIV), *Chlamydia, Streptococcus,* hepatitis C virus, and respiratory syncytial virus (RSV). It is noteworthy, however, that the clinical development of adjuvant candidates designed to specifically induce potent T-cell responses in humans remains relatively limited.

A select few adjuvants have emerged as promising candidates with documented efficacy in this regard. One such candidate is the IC31® adjuvant, a unique formulation composed of an 11-mer cationic antibacterial peptide intricately linked to synthetic immunostimulatory oligodeoxynucleotides (ODN). This adjuvant holds the potential to stimulate robust T-cell responses, offering promise in the fight against infections necessitating strong cellular immunity, including pneumococcal disease and tuberculosis, among others.

Another notable contender is the "cationic adjuvant formulation" (CAF01) adjuvant, which is composed of cationic liposomes formed by *N,N'*-dimethyl-*N,N'*-dioctadecylammonium (DDA) incorporating the synthetic mycobacterial immunostimulatory α,α'-trehalose 6,6'-dibeheneate (TDB). This formulation demonstrates the ability to bolster T-cell responses, showing promising results in three animal disease models of *Mycobacterium tuberculosis, Chlamydia trachomatis,* and blood-stage malaria, presenting a valuable tool in the quest to combat infectious diseases with T cell, humoral, or mixed/combined immunity components [30].

Furthermore, as previously mentioned, the AS01E adjuvant has been recognized for its effectiveness. This liposomal adjuvant, featuring MPL-A and immunostimulatory saponin QS-21, stands out as a robust inducer of T-cell immunity. In conclusion, there is a growing imperative to develop novel adjuvants that can specifically elicit potent T-cell responses, especially at mucosal sites crucial for pathogen entry. While the number of adjuvant candidates with demonstrated efficacy in inducing strong T-cell immunity in humans remains limited, promising formulations such as IC31®, CAF01, and AS01E are advancing the field and hold significant potential in the fight against a range of infectious diseases, which represent significant public and global health concerns.

Role and mechanisms of actions of adjuvants

Adjuvants constitute vital components of vaccines, amplifying the strength, scope, and endurance of the immune response they elicit. The historical context reveals that for over seven decades since its debut in the 1920s–1930s, alum stood as the sole adjuvant authorized for human vaccination.

However, the past three decades have witnessed the inclusion of additional adjuvants in licensed vaccines, even though the precise molecular and cellular mechanisms underlying their actions remain only partly elucidated.

Nonetheless, recent advancements in our comprehension of how the innate immune system is triggered through pattern recognition receptors (PRRs) and other molecules are progressively improving our grasp of adjuvants' actions and effects [31]. Notably, recent conceptual breakthroughs have drawn attention to the idea that factors such as tissue damage, diverse types of cell death, and the activation of metabolic and nutrient sensors can collectively influence the innate immune system, thereby stimulating the adaptive immune response. Furthermore, in the realm of vaccine research, the application of systems biology to probe the intricate molecular networks governing immune reactions to vaccines – often referred to as "systems vaccinology" [32, 33] – is now yielding valuable mechanistic insights.

This approach is anticipated to herald a new era in vaccine discovery and development, reshaping traditional paradigms.

Safety and side effects

Adjuvants are included in vaccines to enhance the body's immune response to the antigens (harmless pieces of the pathogen) in the vaccine. While adjuvants are generally safe and well tolerated, they can sometimes cause mild side effects, similar to the side effects of vaccines themselves. It is important to note that the benefits of vaccination in preventing serious diseases typically far outweigh the potential side effects.

Commonly reported side effects of adjuvanted vaccines may include local reactions, which are the most common side effects and usually occur at the injection site. Injection site pain or soreness is common and usually mild. Some people may experience redness or mild swelling at the injection site. Hardness or a small, firm lump at the injection site can occur and is generally harmless. Another category of potential side effects is represented by systemic reactions: these side effects can affect the whole body and are usually mild and temporary. These include fever (usually a low-grade fever, particularly in children), fatigue (feeling tired or fatigued is common after vaccination), headache (some individuals may experience a mild headache), muscle aches or joint pain (this side effect can occur but is usually short-lived), and nausea (some people may feel slightly nauseated). Serious side effects from adjuvants are rare. The rigorous testing and regulatory oversight of vaccines help ensure their safety. Health care providers and regulatory agencies closely monitor vaccine safety and investigate any reports of adverse events.

Finally, it is essential to remember that the risk of severe disease or complications from the actual infectious diseases that vaccines prevent is much higher than the risk of side effects from the vaccines themselves. Vaccination is a critical public health measure for preventing the spread of infectious diseases and protecting individuals and communities. If you or your child experience any concern or unusual symptoms after receiving a vaccine, it is important to contact your health care provider or report it to the U.S. Vaccine Adverse Event Reporting System (VAERS) or the equivalent system in other countries. Health care professionals are trained to recognize and manage potential vaccine-related adverse events.

Safety and side effects of aluminum-adjuvanted vaccines

In terms of evidence-based vaccinology [34], aluminum-adjuvanted diphtheria, tetanus, and pertussis vaccines show a good safety profile. Jefferson et al. [35] have conducted a comprehensive analysis of adverse events following diphtheria, tetanus, and pertussis immunization, whether provided individually or in combination with each other. An extensive, methodologically robust literature search was carried out across various databases, including the Cochrane Vaccines Field

Register, the Cochrane Library, MEDLINE, Embase, Biological Abstracts, Science Citation Index, and the VAERS website. The authors looked for randomized and semirandomized trials as well as for comparative cohort studies that provided sufficient data to extract critical information such as the concentration of aluminum, vaccine composition, and safety outcomes. The assessment encompassed 35 reports/studies, three of which were randomized trials, four semirandomized trials, and one cohort study. The meta-analysis concerned two primary comparisons: vaccines containing aluminum hydroxide versus those without any adjuvant in children aged up to 18 months and vaccines containing various types of aluminum versus those without adjuvants in children aged 10–16 years. In the case of young children, vaccines with aluminum hydroxide elicited significantly more cases of erythema and induration compared to nonadjuvanted vaccines, with an odds ratio (OR) of 1.87 [95% confidence interval (CI) 1.57–2.24]). However, they resulted in significantly fewer adverse reactions of all types, with an odds ratio of 0.21 [95% CI 0.15–0.28]. Notably, the frequencies of local reactions of all types, including collapse or convulsions, and persistent crying or screaming did not exhibit significant differences between the two cohorts of trials. Conversely, among older children, no notable association was found between exposure to aluminum-containing vaccines and the onset of local induration, swelling, or a raised temperature. However, there was an association observed with local pain lasting up to 14 days, with an OR of 2.05 [95% CI 1.25–3.38]. In conclusion, the analysis did not uncover any substantial evidence indicating that aluminum salts used in vaccines give rise to serious or long-lasting adverse events. Despite the paucity of high-quality evidence, the authors did not recommend further research on this topic be undertaken.

Concerning aluminum-adjuvanted vaccines against poliovirus, evidence was reviewed and appraised by Hawken and Troy [36], who performed an extensive scan of the literature. In 1960, an Italian study conducted an investigation involving guinea pigs, where they administered aluminum phosphate-adjuvanted inactivated polio vaccine (IPV) and compared it to IPV alone. The animals received two subcutaneous doses, spaced 14 days apart. The study observed higher antibody titers in the group receiving aluminum phosphate-adjuvanted IPV compared to the group receiving IPV alone. In the same year, a German study focused on infants and their immune response to a combination vaccine containing diphtheria, pertussis, tetanus, and polio, adjuvanted with aluminum hydroxide. This vaccine was administered subcutaneously in three doses, with four-week intervals between each dose. Although the study did not include a control group, it noted a substantial 4–16-fold increase in median antibody titers against each serotype of the poliovirus three months after vaccination. Moving to 1962, researchers explored the use of aluminum oxide as an adjuvant for monovalent IPV using a rhesus monkey model. They conducted a comparison between adjuvanted and nonadjuvanted vaccines, administering them subcutaneously or intramuscularly with various dosing schedules. The results showed that the aluminum-adjuvanted vaccine achieved significantly higher geometric mean titers overall. After vaccination, the monkeys were challenged with live poliovirus and immunosuppressive corticosteroids. Interestingly, in the adjuvanted vaccine group, only 2 out of 16 monkeys (12%) developed paralytic poliomyelitis, whereas 15 out of 19 monkeys (79%) in the nonadjuvanted group developed paralytic polio postchallenge. A similar study in 1967 assessed the adjuvant effect of aluminum oxide with trivalent IPV in rhesus monkeys, yielding consistent results – adjuvanted vaccines exhibited higher geometric mean titers and provided superior protection after intramuscular challenge with live virus of each of the three serotypes. In 1985, a study compared the adjuvant capabilities of aluminum hydroxide with Freund's complete adjuvant for polio-derived peptides in rabbits, rats, and guinea pigs. Although the study did not incorporate a nonadjuvanted control group, it found that Freund's adjuvant induced higher levels of peptide-specific antibody titers than aluminum. However, both adjuvants were similarly ineffective in inducing polio neutralizing antibodies. Currently, aluminum-based adjuvants are widely employed in combination vaccines containing IPV and have undergone extensive evaluation for safety and efficacy in humans. Recent studies have compared standalone IPV with combination vaccines containing IPV adjuvanted with aluminum. In a 2001 pediatric study, a combination vaccine comprising diphtheria–tetanus–acellular pertussis, hepatitis B, and IPV (Pediarix®), adjuvanted with aluminum hydroxide and aluminum phosphate, was compared to standalone IPV. The results showed no significant difference in local reactions between the combination and control groups. Both the combination and standalone IPV, administered in three doses at two, four, and six months of age, achieved protective levels of antibody titers in over 98% of participants. Antibody titers were higher in the combination vaccine group for all three serotypes after three injections, although the difference was statistically significant for serotypes 1 and 3. Another study from China compared the immunogenicity and safety of Pentaxim®, a combination vaccine containing diphtheria–tetanus–acellular pertussis, *Haemophilus influenzae*, and IPV, adjuvanted with aluminum hydroxide, to standalone vaccines. Both groups, when given at three, four, and five months of age, achieved seroconversion rates of over 99%. However, antibody titers were significantly higher in the combination vaccine group for all three serotypes. This study also reported more frequent erythema and swelling in the combination vaccine group compared to the control group. Similarly, another study found seroprotective titers in 99.4–100% of toddlers immunized with either standalone IPV or Pentacel®, a combination vaccine containing aluminum phosphate-adjuvanted diphtheria–tetanus–acellular pertussis, *H. influenzae*, and IPV (DTaP-IPV-Hib). Local reactions to combination vaccines were not significantly higher than those observed in the control group. Geometric mean antibody titers were roughly equivalent between the combination and traditional vaccine groups for all three serotypes. However, it is worth noting that this trial did not specify whether the separate injections were administered in separate limbs, which could potentially influence the immune response against IPV due to the aluminum present in the DTaP component. Despite its efficacy as an adjuvant, aluminum does have limitations. It is less immunogenic than some other adjuvants, has limited capacity to induce CD8 T-cell responses, and can occasionally lead to localized adverse reactions.

Overall, these results were corroborated by an analysis recently conducted by Krauss et al. [37], who evaluated the advantages and disadvantages of aluminum adjuvants compared to a placebo or no intervention in randomized clinical trials concerning human vaccine development. The comprehensive approach involved carrying out a systematic review, meta-analysis, and trial sequential analysis, along with the assessment of evidence certainty using the Grading of Recommendations Assessment, Development, and Evaluation (GRADE) framework. Data sources for this investigation included searches of CENTRAL, MEDLINE, Embase, LILACS, BIOSIS, Science Citation Index Expanded, and Conference Proceedings Citation Index-Science as well as Chinese databases. The analysis incorporated 102 randomized clinical trials, totaling 26,457 participants. The comparison of aluminum adjuvants versus placebo or no intervention yielded the following findings: aluminum adjuvants may not have a discernible effect on serious adverse events (with a risk ratio (RR) of 1.18 [95% CI 0.97–1.43]; very low certainty) or all-cause mortality (RR 1.02 [95% CI 0.74–1.41]; very low certainty). Quality-of-life outcomes were not reported in any of the trials. Aluminum adjuvants may potentially increase the occurrence of adverse events (RR 1.13 [95% CI 1.07–1.20]; very low certainty). There was limited or no evidence indicating a significant difference between aluminum adjuvants and placebo or no intervention in assessments of serology based on geometric mean titers or concentrations as well as participants' seroprotection status. In conclusion, based on very low-certainty evidence, the analysis was not able to identify any clear benefits associated with the use of aluminum adjuvants. Additionally, their use may be linked to nonserious adverse events.

Nevertheless, despite these drawbacks, aluminum remains the most widely used adjuvant in the United States, Europe, and globally.

Safety and side effects of emulsion-adjuvanted vaccines

Camilloni et al. [38] assessed the immunogenicity and safety profiles of intramuscular (IM) MF59-adjuvanted (Fluad) and intradermal (ID) administered influenza enhanced (Intanza) vaccines in subjects aged over 60. When examining injection-site reactions during the first 6–7 days postvaccination, findings corroborated prior research, suggesting that these reactions were more prevalent in the ID group compared to the IM-MF59 group. Specifically, erythema (local redness) and local inflammation emerged as the most frequently reported symptoms among ID recipients, with Van Damme et al. [39] reporting rates of 63.1%, and Scheifele et al. [40] documenting rates of 76.2%, as compared to 13.4% and 13.0% among IM-MF59 recipients, respectively. Additionally, the incidence of swelling and induration (localized hardening) was notably higher in the ID group compared to IM-MF59. For instance, the prevalence of swelling was recorded at 34.2% versus 8.6% and 49.2% versus 12.0% in the ID group compared to IM-MF59, respectively. Similarly, induration was reported in 32.9% versus 10.6% and 46.5% versus 8.0% among ID versus IM-MF59 recipients, respectively. Regarding injection site pain, the data from Van Damme et al. [39] indicated comparable rates between the IM-MF59 and ID groups (20.9% versus 19.8%). However, Scheifele et al. [40] reported slightly higher rates of injection site pain in the IM-MF59 group (37.9% versus 29.7%). Importantly, systemic adverse events were generally mild, transient, and exhibited a similar occurrence in both the IM-MF59 and ID groups.

van Doorn et al. [41] also reviewed the safety profile of Montanide ISA™51 (ISA 51), a vaccine adjuvant that has undergone testing in both therapeutic and prophylactic vaccine trials. A systematic search of the literature was conducted using PubMed, EMBASE, and clinicaltrials.gov. The analysis consisted of 91 studies, which were uncontrolled studies involving individuals with underlying health conditions, controlled studies involving individuals with underlying health conditions, or controlled studies involving healthy individuals. Commonly observed adverse events encompassed reactions at the injection site, injection site pain, myalgia (muscle pain), headache, gastrointestinal issues, fatigue, and fever. These side effects were reported irrespective of the administration route and the characteristics of the subjects. Importantly, specific adverse events, such as injection site reactions and rashes, were more frequently noted in subjects receiving vaccines adjuvanted with ISA 51 compared to those who received the antigen alone or ISA 51 without the antigen. Furthermore, the reported side effects were generally of mild to moderate intensity. Serious adverse events were reported in 27% of the uncontrolled trials and in two trials involving healthy subjects. Notably, two other trials conducted with healthy subjects had to be prematurely halted due to unacceptable adverse events. It is worth noting that certain studies suggest that the process of mixing the antigen and adjuvant might influence the occurrence of side effects. Reports of serious adverse events and the termination of two trials underscore the need for caution when considering the use of ISA 51. However, it is important to acknowledge that side effects might be preventable through proper mixing of the vaccine and adjuvant to create a stable emulsion. The authors concluded that, in order to provide a fair assessment of adjuvant safety, further trials that include an active control group are warranted.

Safety and side effects of novel adjuvants

Kompier et al. [42] conducted a systematic review of clinical trials involving a low-dose inactivated influenza vaccine enhanced with azoximer bromide (AZB, also known as polyoxidonium). The objective of the authors was to compare the vaccine's reactogenicity to nonadjuvanted vaccines and to evaluate whether the reduced antigen content per viral strain in AZB-adjuvanted vaccines influenced antibody responses. Through a rigorous search strategy, the research team identified scientific publications reporting data from 30 clinical trials, encompassing a total of 11,736 participants and comprising 86 trial arms for inclusion in the analysis. The rates of local reactions following vaccination appeared to be lower in the treatment arms using AZB-adjuvanted vaccines compared to those using comparator vaccines. Furthermore, the analysis revealed that postvaccination geometric mean titers in individuals exposed to AZB-adjuvanted vaccines were comparable to those in comparator vaccine treatment arms. This similarity was observed in both children and adults aged 18–60 years. This suggests that AZB may have an antigen-sparing effect. To strengthen the findings, the authors conducted a meta-regression analysis using a literature search that encompassed records and reports of clinical trials involving AZB and the inactivated subunit of influenza, conducted between 1998 and 2018. This analysis, conducted online in January 2019 and subsequently updated in August 2019, covered trials conducted from 1993 to 2016. The results of this extended search indicated that AZB did not contribute to vaccine reactogenicity.

Evidence concerning other novel adjuvants is still lacking, and systematic reviews and meta-analyses, if feasible, should be conducted, even though from available data novel adjuvants appear to have a good safety profile.

Overall synthesis of safety and side effects of adjuvanted vaccines

Gidengil et al. [43] conducted a literature search to update a review previously conducted by the Agency for Healthcare Research and Quality in 2014. This update involved integrating newly available data from studies that compared vaccines and reported the presence or absence of specific adverse events. The authors followed the methodology established by the Evidence-based Practice Center and assessed the strength of evidence for all statements based on the collected evidence. Among the 56,603 citations reviewed, 338 studies that met the inclusion criteria were identified, and these were reported in 518 publications. In the case of children, the authors found high strength of evidence indicating no increased risk of autism following the measles, mumps, and rubella vaccines. On the contrary, high strength of evidence was observed for an increased risk of febrile seizures with the measles, mumps, and rubella vaccines. Regarding the rotavirus vaccine, there was moderate strength of evidence showing no increased risk of intussusception at the latest follow-up and high strength of evidence suggesting no increased risk of diabetes. For newer vaccines such as the 9-valent human papillomavirus and meningococcal B vaccines, there was either no evidence of increased risk or insufficient evidence for key adverse events. Turning to adults, the analysis revealed no evidence of increased risk for key adverse events, with varying levels of strength of evidence, or insufficient evidence for the new adjuvanted inactivated influenza vaccine and recombinant adjuvanted zoster vaccine.

The authors also found no evidence of increased risk, with varying levels of strength of evidence for key adverse events among pregnant women following the tetanus, diphtheria, and acellular pertussis vaccines, including stillbirth, with a moderate strength of evidence. In conclusion, the authors' comprehensive review of a substantial body of research identified only few associations between vaccines and serious key adverse events. It is important to note that rare events are challenging to study. In assessing any adverse events, it is crucial to weigh them against the protective benefits that vaccines offer.

Conclusions and future directions

Adjuvants are integral to vaccination; indeed, they play a crucial role in enhancing the effectiveness of vaccines by bolstering immune responses. While alum has historically been the primary adjuvant, recent decades have witnessed the introduction of diverse adjuvants, broadening our options for vaccine formulation. Recent breakthroughs in understanding the mechanisms behind adjuvants, particularly their interactions at the molecular level, have provided valuable insights. This knowledge is essential for optimizing adjuvant design and vaccine efficacy. The emergence of systems vaccinology, which investigates complex molecular networks governing immune responses to vaccines, represents a paradigm shift in vaccine research. This holistic approach promises to refine our understanding of adjuvants and vaccine development. The revitalization of adjuvant science holds immense promise not only for addressing current challenges, such as vaccines against COVID-19, but also for future pandemics. Adjuvants can potentially expedite vaccine development and enhance the effectiveness of pandemic vaccines.

Future directions include the development of tailored or precision vaccine adjuvants [44]; customized adjuvant selection based on the specific vaccine and target pathogen is a promising area of ongoing research. Developing adjuvants tailored to specific vaccines can optimize immune responses and improve vaccine safety profiles. Continued research into the precise mechanisms of adjuvant action, particularly in the context of innate immunity and molecular interactions, is essential. This will enable the rational design of adjuvants for novel vaccines. "Integrative systems vaccinology" is anticipated to further revolutionize the way adjuvants are conceived, designed, and produced. Expanding the application of systems vaccinology to investigate adjuvant–vaccine interactions will provide a deeper understanding of immune responses, guiding the development of more effective vaccines and adjuvants. As adjuvants evolve, rigorous safety assessments and regulatory evaluations must remain at the forefront. Ensuring the safety of adjuvanted vaccines is paramount for public confidence in vaccination programs. Adjuvants are poised to play a pivotal role in accelerating vaccine development during pandemics. Research efforts should focus on adjuvants that can enhance the rapid production of effective vaccines in response to emerging infectious threats.

New approaches, such as adversomics [45], vaccine informatics and vaccine adjuvant informatics, and Artificial Intelligence and big data analytics (BDA) applied to vaccinovigilance, appear to be promising. Adversomics is a term introduced for the first time in 2009, which encompasses the examination of vaccine-related adverse reactions through the lenses of immunogenomics and systems biology methodologies. The landscape of adversomics research is continuously burgeoning and evolving. We propose "adjuvantomics," as a specialized branch stemming from adversomics, which would combine cutting-edge, sophisticated epidemiological and molecular biology techniques.

In conclusion, adjuvants are essential components of modern vaccines, and ongoing research is expanding our knowledge of their mechanisms and applications. The integration of systems vaccinology and the development of tailored adjuvants represent promising avenues for advancing vaccine science and addressing future public health challenges.

However, safety and regulatory considerations must remain central as we harness the potential of adjuvants for pandemic preparedness and vaccine optimization.

References

1. Christensen, D. (2016). Vaccine adjuvants: why and how. *Hum. Vaccin. Immunother.* 12 (10): 2709–2711. https://doi.org/10.1080/21645515.2016.1219003.
2. Pulendran, B., Arunachalam, P.S., and O'Hagan, D.T. (2021). Emerging concepts in the science of vaccine adjuvants. *Nat. Rev. Drug Discov.* 20 (6): 454–475. https://doi.org/10.1038/s41573-021-00163-y.
3. Apostólico Jde, S., Lunardelli, V.A., Coirada, F.C. et al. (2016). Adjuvants: classification, modus operandi, and licensing. *J. Immunol. Res.* 2016: 1459394. https://doi.org/10.1155/2016/1459394.
4. Masson, J.D., Thibaudon, M., Bélec, L., and Crépeaux, G. (2017). Calcium phosphate: a substitute for aluminum adjuvants? *Expert Rev. Vaccines* 16 (3): 289–299. https://doi.org/10.1080/14760584.2017.1244484.
5. Laera, D., HogenEsch, H., and O'Hagan, D.T. (2023). Aluminum adjuvants-'back to the future'. *Pharmaceutics* 15 (7): 1884. https://doi.org/10.3390/pharmaceutics15071884.
6. Shah, R.R., Taccone, M., Monaci, E. et al. (2019). The droplet size of emulsion adjuvants has significant impact on their potency, due to differences in immune cell-recruitment and -activation. *Sci. Rep.* 9 (1): 11520. https://doi.org/10.1038/s41598-019-47885-z.
7. Fan, J., Jin, S., Gilmartin, L. et al. (2022). Advances in infectious disease vaccine adjuvants. *Vaccines (Basel)* 10 (7): 1120. https://doi.org/10.3390/vaccines10071120.
8. Facciolà, A., Visalli, G., Laganà, A., and Di Pietro, A. (2022). An overview of vaccine adjuvants: current evidence and future perspectives. *Vaccines (Basel)* 10 (5): 819. https://doi.org/10.3390/vaccines10050819.
9. Ciacci-Woolwine, F., Blomfield, I.C., Richardson, S.H., and Mizel, S.B. (1998). Salmonella flagellin induces tumor necrosis factor alpha in a human promonocytic cell line. *Infect. Immun.* 66 (3): 1127–1134. https://doi.org/10.1128/IAI.66.3.1127-1134.1998.

10. Verma, S.K., Mahajan, P., Singh, N.K. et al. (2023). New-age vaccine adjuvants, their development, and future perspective. *Front. Immunol.* 14: 1043109. https://doi.org/10.3389/fimmu.2023.1043109.
11. Tretiakova, D.S. and Vodovozova, E.L. (2022). Liposomes as adjuvants and vaccine delivery systems. *Biochem. (Mosc.) Suppl. Ser. A Membr. Cell Biol.* 16 (1): 1–20. https://doi.org/10.1134/S1990747822020076.
12. Nooraei, S., Bahrulolum, H., Hoseini, Z.S. et al. (2021). Virus-like particles: preparation, immunogenicity and their roles as nanovaccines and drug nanocarriers. *J. Nanobiotechnol.* 19 (1): 59. https://doi.org/10.1186/s12951-021-00806-7.
13. Rahman, T., Das, A., Abir, M.H. et al. (2023). Cytokines and their role as immunotherapeutics and vaccine adjuvants: the emerging concepts. *Cytokine* 169: 156268. https://doi.org/10.1016/j.cyto.2023.156268.
14. Garg, A. and Dewangan, H.K. (2020). Nanoparticles as adjuvants in vaccine delivery. *Crit. Rev. Ther. Drug Carrier Syst.* 37 (2): 183–204. https://doi.org/10.1615/CritRevTherDrugCarrierSyst.2020033273.
15. Vogel, F. and Hem, S.L. (2004). Immunologic adjuvants. In: *Vaccines*, 69–79. Philadelphia, PA: Saunders Elsevier.
16. Di Pasquale, A., Preiss, S., Tavares Da Silva, F., and Garçon, N. (2015). Vaccine adjuvants: from 1920 to 2015 and beyond. *Vaccines (Basel)* 3 (2): 320–343. https://doi.org/10.3390/vaccines3020320.
17. Glenny, A.T., Pope, C.G., Waddington, H., and Wallace, U. (1926). Immunological notes. XVII.-XXIV. *J. Pathol. Bacteriol.* 29: 31–40. https://doi.org/10.1002/path.1700290106.
18. Park, W.H. and Schroder, M.C. (1932). Diphtheria toxin-antitoxin and toxoid: a comparison. *Am. J. Public Health Nations Health* 22: 7–16.
19. Harrison, W.T. (1934). Effect of alum-precipitated ragweed pollen extract on guinea pigs. *Public Health Rep.* 49: 462–464.
20. Marrack, P., McKee, A.S., and Munks, M.W. (2009). Towards an understanding of the adjuvant action of aluminium. *Nat. Rev. Immunol.* 9 (4): 287–293. https://doi.org/10.1038/nri2510.
21. Gasparini, R., Amicizia, D., Lai, P.L. et al. (2013). Effectiveness of adjuvanted seasonal influenza vaccines (Inflexal V® and Fluad®) in preventing hospitalization for influenza and pneumonia in the elderly: a matched case-control study. *Hum. Vaccin. Immunother.* 9 (1): 144–152. https://doi.org/10.4161/hv.22231.
22. Bovier, P.A. (2008). Epaxal: a virosomal vaccine to prevent hepatitis A infection. *Expert Rev. Vaccines* 7 (8): 1141–1150. https://doi.org/10.1586/14760584.7.8.1141.
23. Glück, R. (1992). Immunopotentiating reconstituted influenza virosomes (IRIVs) and other adjuvants for improved presentation of small antigens. *Vaccine* 10 (13): 915–919. https://doi.org/10.1016/0264-410x(92)90325-e.
24. McKeage, K. and Romanowski, B. (2011). AS04-adjuvanted human papillomavirus (HPV) types 16 and 18 vaccine (Cervarix®): a review of its use in the prevention of premalignant cervical lesions and cervical cancer causally related to certain oncogenic HPV types. *Drugs* 71 (4): 465–488. https://doi.org/10.2165/11206820-000000000-00000.
25. Panatto, D., Amicizia, D., Bragazzi, N.L. et al. (2015). Human papillomavirus vaccine: state of the art and future perspectives. *Adv. Protein Chem. Struct. Biol.* 101: 231–322. https://doi.org/10.1016/bs.apcsb.2015.08.004.
26. O'Hagan, D.T., van der Most, R., Lodaya, R.N. et al. (2021). "World in motion" – emulsion adjuvants rising to meet the pandemic challenges. *NPJ Vaccines* 6 (1): 158. https://doi.org/10.1038/s41541-021-00418-0. Erratum in: (2008). *NPJ Vaccines*. 8(1): 7.
27. Laurens, M.B. (2020). RTS,S/AS01 vaccine (Mosquirix™): an overview. *Hum. Vaccin. Immunother.* 16 (3): 480–489. https://doi.org/10.1080/21645515.2019.1669415.
28. Castrodeza-Sanz, J., Sanz-Muñoz, I., and Eiros, J.M. (2023). Adjuvants for COVID-19 vaccines. *Vaccines (Basel)* 11 (5): 902. https://doi.org/10.3390/vaccines11050902.
29. Lavelle, E.C. and Ward, R.W. (2022). Mucosal vaccines – fortifying the frontiers. *Nat. Rev. Immunol.* 22 (4): 236–250. https://doi.org/10.1038/s41577-021-00583-2. Erratum in: (2021). *Nat. Rev. Immunol.*
30. Agger, E.M., Rosenkrands, I., Hansen, J. et al. (2008). Cationic liposomes formulated with synthetic mycobacterial cordfactor (CAF01): a versatile adjuvant for vaccines with different immunological requirements. *PLoS One* 3 (9): e3116. https://doi.org/10.1371/journal.pone.0003116.
31. Suresh, R. and Mosser, D.M. (2013). Pattern recognition receptors in innate immunity, host defense, and immunopathology. *Adv. Physiol. Educ.* 37 (4): 284–291. https://doi.org/10.1152/advan.00058.2013.
32. Pulendran, B., Li, S., and Nakaya, H.I. (2010). Systems vaccinology. *Immunity* 33 (4): 516–529. https://doi.org/10.1016/j.immuni.2010.10.006.

33. Raeven, R.H.M., van Riet, E., Meiring, H.D. et al. (2019). Systems vaccinology and big data in the vaccine development chain. *Immunology* 156 (1): 33–46. https://doi.org/10.1111/imm.13012.
34. Nalin, D.R. (2002). Evidence based vaccinology. *Vaccine* 20 (11–12): 1624–1630. https://doi.org/10.1016/s0264-410x(01)00481-9.
35. Jefferson, T., Rudin, M., and Di Pietrantonj, C. (2004). Adverse events after immunisation with aluminium-containing DTP vaccines: systematic review of the evidence. *Lancet Infect. Dis.* 4 (2): 84–90. https://doi.org/10.1016/S1473-3099(04)00927-2.
36. Hawken, J. and Troy, S.B. (2012). Adjuvants and inactivated polio vaccine: a systematic review. *Vaccine* 30 (49): 6971–6979. https://doi.org/10.1016/j.vaccine.2012.09.059.
37. Krauss, S.R., Barbateskovic, M., Klingenberg, S.L. et al. (2022). Aluminium adjuvants versus placebo or no intervention in vaccine randomised clinical trials: a systematic review with meta-analysis and trial sequential analysis. *BMJ Open* 12 (6): e058795. https://doi.org/10.1136/bmjopen-2021-058795.
38. Camilloni, B., Basileo, M., Valente, S. et al. (2015). Immunogenicity of intramuscular MF59-adjuvanted and intradermal administered influenza enhanced vaccines in subjects aged over 60: a literature review. *Hum. Vaccin. Immunother.* 11 (3): 553–563. https://doi.org/10.1080/21645515.2015.1011562.
39. Van Damme, P., Arnou, R., Kafeja, F. et al. (2010). Evaluation of non-inferiority of intradermal versus adjuvanted seasonal influenza vaccine using two serological techniques: a randomised comparative study. *BMC Infect. Dis.* 10: 134. https://doi.org/10.1186/1471-2334-10-134.
40. Scheifele, D.W., McNeil, S.A., Ward, B.J. et al. (2013 Nov). PHAC /CIHR influenza research network. Safety, immunogenicity, and tolerability of three influenza vaccines in older adults: results of a randomized, controlled comparison. *Hum. Vaccin. Immunother.* 9 (11): 2460–2473. https://doi.org/10.4161/hv.25580.
41. van Doorn, E., Liu, H., Huckriede, A., and Hak, E. (2016). Safety and tolerability evaluation of the use of Montanide ISA™51 as vaccine adjuvant: a systematic review. *Hum. Vaccin. Immunother.* 12 (1): 159–169. https://doi.org/10.1080/21645515.2015.1071455.
42. Kompier, R., Neels, P., Beyer, W. et al. (2022). Analysis of the safety and immunogenicity profile of an azoximer bromide polymer-adjuvanted subunit influenza vaccine. *F1000Res* 11: 259. https://doi.org/10.12688/f1000research.75869.2.
43. Gidengil C, Goetz MB, Newberry S, Maglione M, Hall O, Larkin J, Motala A, Hempel S. Safety of vaccines used for routine immunization in the United States: an updated systematic review and meta-analysis. *Vaccine* 2021 Jun 23;39(28):3696-3716. doi: https://doi.org/10.1016/j.vaccine.2021.03.079.
44. Nanishi E, Angelidou A, Rotman C, Dowling DJ, Levy O, Ozonoff A. Precision vaccine adjuvants for older adults: a scoping review. *Clin. Infect. Dis.* 2022 Aug 15;75(Suppl 1):S72-S80. doi: https://doi.org/10.1093/cid/ciac302.
45. Whitaker JA, Ovsyannikova IG, Poland GA. Adversomics: a new paradigm for vaccine safety and design. *Expert. Rev. Vaccines* 2015 Jul;14(7):935-47. doi: https://doi.org/10.1586/14760584.2015.1038249.

4 Commonly Used Food Additives Are Nutritional Adjuvants in ASIA Syndrome

Aaron Lerner[1,2] and Carina Benzvi[1]

[1]Zabludowicz Center for Autoimmune Diseases,
Sheba Medical Center, Tel-Hashomer, Israel
[2]Campus Ariel, Ariel University, Ariel, Israel

Introduction

Epidemiological surveys on the prevalence of autoimmune diseases (ADs) provide convincing evidences for a steady rise in those diseases throughout Westernized societies over the past three decades [1–3]. Rheumatoid arthritis, celiac disease, multiple sclerosis, systemic lupus erythematosus, type 1 diabetes, inflammatory bowel diseases, autoimmune thyroiditis, autoimmune hepatitis, primary biliary cirrhosis, bullous pemphigoid, myasthenia gravis, and antiphospholipid diseases are such several examples [1, 3, 4]. Genetics plays a well-established contributing factor; hence, environment is a major factor in their evolvement. The relationship to socioeconomic status, the geoepidemiological distribution, the worldwide West–East and North–South gradients, and their rapid increase in migrant populations and developed countries testify for environmental impact, rather than genetic factors, impacting those rapid and recent evolutionary processes [1, 3]. Infections and the dysbiome, toxins, chemicals, pollution, psychological stress, global warming, and processed food are gaining attention in recent years for their role in ADs' induction [1, 3, 5]. However, it appears that nutrients might be an additional environmental factor that enhance ADs [6–8]. During the past decade, a new entity, namely the autoimmune/inflammatory syndrome induced by adjuvants (ASIA), is being forwarded [9–12]. The present review introduces a novel aspect to the syndrome, highlighting the place of nutritional adjuvants in autoimmunogenesis.

ASIA syndrome

Based on four entities linked to previous exposure to adjuvants (the Gulf War syndrome, silicosis, the macrophagic myofasciitis syndrome, and postvaccination phenomena) sharing comparable signs and symptoms, Shoenfeld et al. [9] coined a new syndrome named ASIA or Shoenfeld's syndrome [9–12]. It highlights the common dominator and the role of various adjuvants in the pathogenesis of immune-mediated diseases [11]. As for 2020, more than 4400 cases were reported, illustrating the heterogeneous symptomatology, signs, and outcome of the affected patients. Since its presentation in 2011 [11], many adjuvants-related medical conditions were added to the list,

Autoimmune Disorders: Adjuvants and Other Risk Factors in Pathogenesis, First Edition.
Edited by Abdulla Watad, Nicola Luigi Bragazzi, and Yehuda Shoenfeld.

the most recent ones being Sjögren's syndrome, sarcoidosis, undifferentiated connective tissue disease, silicone implant incompatibility syndrome, immune-related adverse events, biomaterial injections, and prostheses, mainly silicone, hyaluronic acid, acrylamides and methacrylate compounds, and gluteal biopolymer remodeling injections, and the list is constantly expanding [11, 13–17]. In parallel to the expanding list of conditions, the list of the offending adjuvants is growing up. Vaccines' adjuvants include alum, silicone implants, squalene, drugs, infections, metals and foreign bodies, ink components used for making tattoos, and biopolymers [8–20]. Several mechanisms were suggested to explain those multifactorial conditions included in the ASIA syndrome, namely genetics, innate immune dysregulation, immune hyperstimulation, release of inflammatory cytokines, T-cell failure, unbalanced Th1/Th2 immune response ratio with excessive Th1 response, antigen-driven local immune response through Th17 cells activation, B-cell activation, and epigenetic modifications [11–16, 21]. Given the dynamic expansion of the syndrome, the increased number of publications and patient's registries, the definition criteria of ASIA syndrome were recently redefined [11]. They include major and minor criteria, spanning clinical manifestations, removal of inciting agents inducing improvement, typical biopsy of involved organs, specific human leukocyte antigen (HLA), evolvement of an autoimmune disease, other clinical manifestations, and appearance of autoantibodies or antibodies directed at the suspected adjuvants [11]. With respect to the last point of circulating autoantibodies, some new autonomic autoantibodies (autoantibodies against adrenergic receptors, acetylcholine receptors, muscarinic receptors, G-protein-coupled receptors, and angiotensin II receptor type 1) and anatomopathological aspects of small-fiber neuropathy (SFN) in skin biopsies of patients with silicone breast implants were recently described, thus opening a new objective marker of those entities [22, 23]. The present review discusses a novel aspect of ASIA syndrome, extending the list of adjuvants by adding five groups of food additives to the list.

Increased usage of food additives in the processed food industries

The transition from agricultural societies toward industrial ones, in the past two centuries, changes completely the food productivity, diversity, composition, and decreased seasonal dependency [24]. This process is accompanied by a substantial surge in industrially processed food production and consumption [1]. The "Western diet" and the increased consumption of fast foods, characterized by high fat, trans fatty acids, cholesterol, proteins, sugars, salt intake, and food additives, are boosting even in the developing countries [25, 26]. The increased consumption of Western diet and fast and processed foods is associated with a plethora of chronic and morbid human conditions, including inflammatory, metabolic, overweight, hepatic steatosis, neurodegenerative, cancerous, and all-cause mortality at least in the United States, and even autoimmune diseases [1, 27, 28]. It appears that it is not only the caloric access, but not less, it is also the food processing [28]. Before plunging into the food additive adjuvanticity, the following sections deal with five nutritional constituents that are increasingly applied by the industrial food processing companies.

Gluten

Gluten is a major food ingredient heavily consumed by the processed food manufacturers. Being a cheap stabilizer and a thickener, having emulsifying capacity and increasing shelf life, it is used, not only in the bakeries but literally, in hundreds of processed foods and nondietary products. It is the dough-forming protein of wheat flour and the major wheat protein comprising 80% of its proteins. Its consumption surpasses all other crops combined, representing the world's most favored staple food. In the previous century, global wheat output expanded by about fivefold. Since then, there has been a dramatic 10-fold increase in the rate of wheat yield improvement per year. In parallel to its increased agricultural production, the processed food industry took its share. It was estimated that the net fold % increases/year of gluten usage as an industrial food additive, over the past fout to six decades, reach 1.8 ± 0.4 [1]. The Global Vital Wheat Gluten Market accounted for \$2 billion in 2019 and is expected to reach \$2.74 billion by 2027, growing at a compound annual growth rate of 4% during the forecast period [29].

Microbial transglutaminase

Officially and practically, transglutaminase (EC 2.3.2.13), i.e. protein-glutamine γ-glutamyltransferase, catalyzes the formation of an isopeptide bond between the group of γ-carboxamides of glutamine residues (the donor) and the first-order ε-amine groups of different compounds, such as proteins or peptides (the acceptors of an acyl residue). It is considered as a natural glue, and its most popular name is meat glue, due to its incredible ability to "glue" meat proteins together [30]. Interestingly, its applications spread to other food and textile industries, biomedical engineering, diagnostic applications, and even to biotherapy [31]. Not only in the bakery, with time, the application extended to many food products. This biological glue improves meat texture, appearance, hardness, and preservability; improves quality and texture of milk and dairy products; increases fish product hardness; decreases calories intake; and improves protein film stability and appearance, elasticity and texture of sweet foods, and extension of shelf time in the supermarkets. This is probably one of the fastest-growing areas, as reflected by the increasing number of patent applications filed on mTG. The demand for baked goods and food and beverage enzymes is forecasted to grow by 0.22–0.32-fold per year, between 2000 and 2020. Altogether, a maximum daily intake of mTG could range up to 15 mg. Dosing for restructuring is about 50–100 mg of mTG for each kilogram of treated food [1, 32–34].

Nanoparticles

The accepted definition of nanoparticles is any particles of matter that are between 1 and 100 nm in diameter. They are distinguished from microparticles that have the diameter of 1–1000 μm and are much smaller than the wavelengths of visible light (400–700 nm). Nowadays, they are used in multiple domains including foods processing, production and packaging, functional food development, detection of foodborne microbes, shelf-life extension of food products, and food safety [35]. One of those are the nanoemulsions, increasingly consumed in the processed food industries to protect, encapsulate, and deliver lipophilic functionally active. The average net increase in nanoparticle usage, as an industrial food additive, is estimated to be 25.8% per year [1]. According to a new market research study by Technavio, the global food nanotechnology market projects the market to grow at a compound annual growth rate of more than 24% during the period 2019–2023 [36]. It is estimated that, at least in the developed countries, more than 10^{12} inorganic nanoparticles are taken into the human body per day [37].

Emulsifiers

Emulsifiers are food additives that encourage the suspension of one liquid in another, as in the mixture of oil and water. Concentrating at the interface between water and oil, the emulsifiers reduce the surface or interfacial tension, thereby making the emulsions more stable. They stabilize multiple processed foods products such as margarine, shortening, ice cream, and salad dressing [38], playing a role in improving food appearance, delivery, texture, and mouthfeel; disguising flavors; and achieving palatable low-fat foods [39]. Often, they are referred as surfactants, an abbreviation of surface-active agents. The alimentary emulsifiers market is a fast-growing one due to the growing trend toward reducing fat content in food products. It is largely driven by diglycerides and derivatives, lecithin, polysorbates, stearoyl lactylates, polyglycerol esters (PGE), polyglycerol polyricinoleate (PGPR), and various sucrose esters. Notably, many other synthetics as well as natural emulsifiers are gaining momentum constantly [38, 39]. According to news reports, the global food emulsifiers market reached a value of USD 3 billion in 2020. It is expected to grow at a CAGR over 5% in the forecast period of 2021–2026 to reach USD 4 billion by 2026 [40, 41].

Food colorants

Food colors, dyes, or pigments are added to numerous types of food products to increase their visual attractiveness, compensate for natural color variations, and preserve the appearance for a longer period. Food colorants constitute an important part of food additives. For the past

10–15 years, natural colorants are expended as an alternative to the synthetic ones due to an existing health concern of the latter [42]. The main users are the food producers of beverages, bakery, dairy and frozen products, sauces and condiments, meat, poultry and seafood, and confectionery industries. The main approved food colorants are for red/pink: Ponceau 4R, Carmoisine, Allura red, and Erythrosine; for yellow: Tartrazine and sunset yellow; for blue: Indigo Carmine and Brilliant Blue; and for green: Fast Green [43]. The global food colors market size was USD 2.55 billion in 2018 and is projected to reach USD 4.77 billion by 2026, exhibiting a CAGR of 8.19% during the forecast period [44]. Human nature prefer products that are more attractive, delightful, nutritive, nice looking, and healthy, were "fun-foods" is spreading worldwide. Hence, food colorants deliver those goods.

Gluten is a nutritional adjuvant

Before describing the adjuvant effects of gluten, its detrimental and side effects should be detailed.

Gluten side effects

Numerous in vitro studies have confirmed the cytotoxicity of various gliadins' peptides originating from the mother molecule gluten. The in vitro and ex/in vivo side effects were recently reviewed [45–47]. In short, gluten is pro-inflammatory, pro-oxidative, apoptotic, immunogenic, and cytotoxic; decreases cell viability; and alters differentiation. It affects epigenetics, influences the microbiome, and increases intestinal permeability [45]. Most recently, antibody's cross-reactivity and sequence homology were demonstrated between gluten/wheat and human body antigens, thus reinforcing gluten as a food additive with potential multiple molecular mimicries repertoire [46–48]. Those findings further extend the list of food components that express autoimmunogenic capacities. Since the leaky gut is frequently associated with a large range of ADs [49], the place of gluten in compromising the tight junction functional integrity should be detailed. By binding to its epithelial CXCR3 receptor, gliadin induces zonulin release, via a MyD88-dependent pathway, resulting in transactivation of epidermal growth factor receptor (EGFR) by PAR2, leading to small intestine tight junction disassembly [1, 50]. Gluten impacts several pathways and branches of the immune system [45, 46]. It increases Th-17 activity, TLR4 signaling, NKG2P expression, and neutrophil migration. Intriguingly, it affects the innate and reactive immune functions and impacts Treg performances [45]. In fact, and as a proof of concept, in certain nonceliac ADs, withdrawing gluten may help curtail the adverse effects of gluten [45, 51–53]. Finally, gluten was shown to increase intestinal permeability not only in nonceliac gluten sensitivity but also in normal controls [54].

Gluten-depended autoimmunity

The classical list of gluten-depended disease is growing. The hallmark conditions are celiac disease and gluten allergy, but dermatitis herpetiformis, gluten ataxia, and nonceliac gluten sensitivity are on the list [55, 56]. Since the undiagnosed/diagnosed celiac disease (CD) patient's ratio is 7:1, many are a/hyposymptomatic, and extraintestinal manifestations are more prevalent [57], many patients do not know that gluten might induce their symptoms. Irritable bowel disease is such an example [58].

Gluten fulfills the diagnostic criteria of ASIA syndrome

Taken together and based on the above, the food components, and food additives, gluten fulfills all the major and minor diagnostic criteria [11]. In the major ones, gluten is a classical external stimulus; induces typical clinical manifestations, be it allergic, intestinal, or extraintestinal, targeting various remote organs and tissues [57, 59]; and its removal in gluten-depended autoimmune conditions leads definitely to improvement. Screening the minor criteria, antigluten/antigliadin antibodies are prevalent in gluten-related and non-celiac-related ADs and chronic conditions [60, 61]. Despite controversies about their specificity and sensitivity [62], when gluten/gliadins are posttranslationally modified by tissue or microbial transglutaminases, their cross-linked complexes induce very specific antibodies, namely anti-neo-epitope tissue transglutaminase and anti-neo-epitope microbial transglutaminase antibodies [63–65]. Celiac disease is a typical HLA-DQ-2/8-dependent condition, and gluten is a well-documented offending environmental factor. As mentioned above, gluten is related to several ADs. In summary, gluten fulfills all the ASIA diagnostic criteria and is a nutritional-based adjuvant.

Microbial transglutaminase is a potential new adjuvant

Microbial transglutaminase is a potential inducer of autoimmune disease

Secreted by bacteria, mTG is considered as a protective factor for prokaryotes, executed by its ability to deamidate or transamidate its substrates by posttranslational modification of proteins (PTMP) [66, 67]. Interestingly, it functionally imitates tissue transglutaminase, the autoantigen of CD [32–34, 63–71], and is currently suspected as a new environmental inducer of CD, based on the following observations. (i) Epidemiologically, its annual increased usage in the processed food industries coincides with the annual increased incidences of CD and ADs in general, in the past decades [3, 4, 32–34]. (ii) Rich in glutamine and proline, gluten is a prime substrate for mTG cross-linking, turning a naïve molecule to an immunogenic one [32–34]. (iii) Serologically, only naïve CD patients mount the specific antibodies: anti-neo-epitope mTG against the gluten-mTG cross-linked complex [63–65, 69]. (iv) Gluten and mTG were demonstrated recently to comigrate trans-epithelialy, to be deposited below the epithelial monolayer, facing the local immune cells [72]. (v) *Streptococcus suis*-originated mTG was shown to suppress phagocytosis, thus protecting the microbe from the human phagocytes and compromising the immune protection, including the antigen-presenting macrophages [73–75]. (vi) It appears that frequently used processed food products contain mTG, thus increasing the enzyme luminal load for nutrients cross-linking [76]. (vii) mTG-deamidated gluten peptides were recognized by gluten-specific T cells, thus potentiating gluten immunogenic capacity [77]. More so, mTG-treated gluten peptides applied to ex vivo cultures of celiac patients' intestinal biopsies induced a 15-fold increase in INFγ secretion and 2.5- and 2.1-fold increases in tissue transglutaminase antibody levels and antiendomysial antibody positivity, respectively, as measured in the culture medium [78]. It can be concluded that both mTG-gliadin cross-linked complexes and mTG-treated gluten peptides are immunogenic to the celiac population. (viii) The immunological reactivity gap between process and raw food nutrients was highlighted by Vojdani [79]. Human sera antibodies' titers are significantly higher against the industrial processed food than to its raw components. When raw wheat was compared to its processed combinations, the immune reactivity was very high. (ix) Gliadin uptake is facilitated by mTG when checked on intestinal-originated human cell line [66]. Several mechanisms can be forwarded for the mTG-induced enhanced gut permeability. Gluten/gliadins peptides are major compromisers of tight-junction integrity. Their mTG cross-linking might potentiate this phenomenon. mTG possesses emulsifier activity, resulting in the functional failure of the lining mucus by breaking its stability. mTG is a survival factor for the luminal pathobionts. Finally, several tight junction's key proteins are ideal substrates for the mTG. Their cross-linking might compromise their activities. All of those mTG-related detrimental pathways can join forces to increase intestinal permeability [1, 32–34, 63, 64, 68–71, 80]. (x) Notably, mTG creates covalent isopeptide bonds that are highly resistant to the luminal proteases, reducing substances, bile acids, and detergents, resulting in their half-life extension, to exert their harmful activities [32–34, 68, 69, 80]. Finally, the frequently used mTG cross-linked complexes, in multiple processed food industries (and not exclusively in the bakery in the treated prolamins or crude gluten), are immunogenic, provoking specific antibodies, inducing pro-inflammatory cytokines, and generating clones of committed and active T cells that drive the intestinal injury in CD [32–34, 70, 71, 77, 80–82].

Microbial transglutaminase fulfills the diagnostic criteria of ASIA syndrome

Based on the above, the frequently consumed food additives, namely mTG, fulfill all the major and minor diagnostic criteria [11]. Facing the major diagnostic criteria, no doubt that the mTG is an external stimulus [1, 32], induces typical clinical manifestations by its post-translation-modified substrates, turning naïve gluten to an immunogenic one and actively participating in CD induction [32–34, 46, 61, 63, 64, 66–71]. Furthermore, the enzyme transmigration through the enterocyte and its subepithelial contact with the mucosal immune cells originate secretion of systemic antibodies, namely anti-neo-epitope mTG against the gluten-mTG cross-linked complex [72]. Those antibodies are accepted as new serological markers for CD diagnosis and follow-up [61]. Only few naïve CD patients mount specific antibodies against the enzyme itself; hence, when CD patients consume gluten, their immune cells overreact and secrete high levels of those anti-neo-epitope mTG against the gluten-mTG cross-linked complex [63, 64, 69]. The mTG is targeting the small bowel, and the removal of gluten leads to clinical and pathological intestinal improvements [34, 45, 69, 72]. It is suggested that the unresponsive CD patients, despite adhering to gluten withdrawal, might improve on mTG-free nutrients. As regard the minor criteria, anti-neo-epitope mTG against the gluten-mTG cross-linked complex are frequently detected in naïve CD patients [61, 63, 64]. In fact, they reach a specificity of 78–98% and sensitivity of 64–95% for CD diagnosis, pending on the immunoglobulin isotype checked [61, 63, 64, 69]. Celiac disease is a classical HLA-DQ-2/8-dependent condition, and gluten is a well-documented offending external factor. It can be concluded that the food additive, mTG, fulfills all the ASIA diagnostic criteria and is a nutritional-based adjuvant.

Nanoparticle complexes are potential new adjuvants

Nanotheranostics is one of the exponentially emerging research areas in the field of nanobiotechnology offering exciting promises for diagnosis, therapy, and many other uses. Several nanoparticles (NPs) are used in food preservation since they form an impassable barrier against humidity, gases, and other factors that could affect food stability. More so, their antibacterial capacity and antioxidant activities are additional reasons for their food usage [83, 84], but the present review concentrates on the nanoparticles that are applied in the food industries. Extensive applications of nanostructured materials, with bioactive agents, are today an integral part of the food industries. The nanoparticles found in foods can be divided into two categories: inorganic (e.g. titanium oxide, silver, iron oxide, zinc oxide, and silicon dioxide) and organic components (e.g. lipids, proteins, and carbohydrates). Their enteric fate is determined by their composition, charges, and other chemical–physical properties [85–87]. Despite the well-described advantages that the nanotechnology offers, emerging concerns regarding nanoparticles usage are accumulating [88, 89]. Nanoparticles are foreign bodies and can be regarded as xenobiotics. The nanostructured materials can accumulate in the environment and penetrate into the human bodies, resulting in several health and safety hazards [37, 85–90]. Increased intestinal permeability is a common feature of ADs. In this regard, nanoparticles join multiple food additives that brake mucus, disrupt brush border, and compromise tight junction functional integrity [1, 91–93]. Finally, food-processed nanoparticles increase oxidative stress, resulting in gastropathy, hepatotoxicity, and alteration in animal behavior [85, 89].

Nanoparticles fulfill the criteria of ASIA syndrome

There are three major diagnostic criteria in ASIA syndrome. The NPs fulfill all the three. Nanoparticles are external factors. In fact, the NPs can be divided into three environmental categories: artificially produced, accidentally formed, or naturally produced [84]. NPs expose typical clinical manifestations. Depending on the carrier NPs and the carried molecules, compound NPs are associated with many human diseases and pathologies. The metal\molecule involved, the exposure dose, particle size, aggregation state, and coating of the nanoparticles, as well as the carrier cell type or organism on which it is tested, are all important factors impacting the effect, side effects, and potential toxicity of NPs. The following paragraphs summarize some of the organs, tissues, and cells that could be damaged by them. They can penetrate and aggregate many organs' functions, including brain. They can damage neurons, in particular dopaminergic neurons, and recently suspected to drive Parkinson's disease [94, 95]. Silica nanoparticles are heavily used in dietary supplements. It appears that they might have immunotoxicity. They have toxic effects on phagocytes, particularly macrophages, T-lymphocytes, and dendritic cells [96]. More so, ingested silica NPs were shown to exacerbate intestinal inflammation [97] and induce cell death of hepatocytic cells by apoptosis [98] or by disrupting mitochondrial functions [99]. Intriguingly, NPs induce ferroptosis, which is an iron-dependent cell death mechanism [100]. Growing body of evidences is accumulating, substantiating their cytotoxic and unfortunately the genotoxic cellular effects. NPs affects epigenetics. They can induce histone modifications and alter DNA methylation patterns and miRNA expressions [101–103]. Other NPs extensively used in food products are titanium dioxide particles. Their toxic effects are carried by increased reactive oxygen species production, resulting in oxidative stress, genotoxicity, inflammation, metabolic change, and even potentially carcinogenesis [103, 104]. They might affect fertility and even damage microglial cells [104, 105]. Importantly, titanium dioxide can exacerbate dextran sulfate sodium (DSS)-induced colitis, by involving the NLRP3 inflammasome [106]. It was suggested that this NP may represent an additional environmental food additive that drive human inflammatory bowel disease (IBD). There are much more publications on the toxic and the side effects of NPs usage, performed on ex or in vivo animal and human models [107]. The third major criteria are the removal of the triggers that leads to improvement. Screening the available scientific literature, there are no studies on NP-free diets and health improvement. However, since vegan, natural, and organic diets are low or devoid of processed foods, they consume much less artificial or engineered nanoparticles. Despite the fact that they face environmental nanoparticles, they consume less food NPs, and many are organic, less-harmful NPs [108]. It is well accepted that vegan, natural, and organic foods prevent morbidity, are healthier, and avoid chronic human diseases, including neurologic, neurodegenerative, and autoimmune ones [109–111]. Interestingly, several strategies were offered to reduce NP toxicities. Designing NPs that discourage binding with a cell surface, reducing the toxic levels by replacing with less-toxic elements that have similar effects, and minimizing the surface area, thus minimizing dissolution, chelating agents can be introduced onto the nanomaterial's surface or measures to reduce the oxidative stress [112]. All those findings, epidemiological data, nutritional manipulations, and redesigning healthier NPs suggest that removal of harmful NPs might lead to less toxicity and health improvement. As for the minor criteria for ASIA, as for autoantibody or antibody to the adjuvant, there are observation describing various antibodies against cross-linked NPs. Polyethylenimine-coated poly lactic-co-glycolic acid (PLGA) nanoparticles-encapsulated *Angelica sinensis* polysaccharide is suggested as an adjuvant to enhance immune responses, and specific antibodies were produced after immunization [113]. Similarly, antibodies against cross-linked gelatin nanoparticles [114], trimethyl chitosan nanoparticles [115], low NPs-coated molecular weight molecules [116], and many more. Despite the fact that the antigenicity to NPs is not well understood, when fullerene derivatives are conjugated to a protein carrier such as Bovine serum albumin (BSA), particle-specific antibodies were generated [117]. Furthermore, polyamidoamine dendrimers conjugated to BSA showed increased antigenic properties, and as a result, dendrimer-specific antibodies were generated in vivo [118]. It was hypothesized that water-soluble nanoparticles may behave as haptens. They become antigenic only after they bind to protein carriers [119]. Interestingly, specific HLAs can be related to NP adjuvants. Nano-APC with engineered HLA alleles and IL-2 deliver peptide–MHC complexes and can activate T-cell receptor (TCR) signaling pathways [120]. The interplay between specific HLAs and NPs allows controlling the dose and the location of immunomodulating molecules, thus specifically addressing unique receptors through targeted compound binding [121]. Many studies were performed on NPs as inducers of tolerance and activating the Tregs to treat ADs. However, NPs are also involved in ADs' initiation and progression. Nanoparticles can be recognized as foreign by the immune cells, may result in adverse immune response against them and lead to toxicity in the host, and/or suppress therapeutic efficacy. It was reported that granulomas can be formed in various organs in animals exposed to carbon nanotubes [122]. Finally, in addition to immune stimulation, NPs can drive several classical autoimmune pathways. They impact the microbiome [123], compromise tight junction functions [1], can be posttranslationally modified by luminal enzymes [67, 124], and generate cytokine secretion and inflammation [125, 126]. It can be concluded that the immunogenic properties of various PNs and their capacity to conjugate weak antigens make them ideal adjuvants [113, 127]. On the other hand, it should be stressed that NPs are being developed to treat ADs, using their tolerogenic immune-modifying capacities [128, 129].

Food colorants are potential new adjuvants

Additives are commonly added to industrially processed and much more to ultraprocessed food products, heavily consumed in Westernized countries [130]. Among these, colorants are extensively used and are responsible for 62–90% of the consumer's assessment, before buying the product [131]. This fact makes food colorant professionals a very profitable job. The major food categories containing colors were liquor and beverages for adults and beverages, ice cream, and chocolate for children. However, there are some dark sides to those colorants. Their consumption can drive the inflammatory cascade, enhance intestinal permeability to larger antigenic molecules, and induce human self-cross-reactive antibodies with the colorants, thus pushing toward autoimmunogenesis [48, 132]. Even neurobehavioral disorders such as attention-deficit disorder and attention-deficit/hyperactivity disorder are attributed to colorant's intake [132, 133]. Food colorants were shown to alter the microbiome toward a dysbiotic profile [134]. Basic colorants such as pararosaniline, auramine O, and rhodamine B are unauthorized food additives because of their toxicity; despite this, they find their way to the markets. All three, and some other colorants such as caramel coloring used in soft drinks, are carcinogenic and toxic to humans and animals [135]. Azo food dyes were shown to elicit pro-inflammatory responses when applied to neutrophils [136]. In addition, the azo dye, Metanil Yellow, is a synthetic food color used extensively in India and developing countries as food additive. It is shown to be toxic to hepatic and kidney tissues, is carcinogenic, and impairs the estrous cycle physiology and ovarian folliculogenesis, and its metabolite, p-Anilinoaniline, classified as a moderate acute toxic agent is shown to induce DNA damage and cell cycle arrest [137–139]. More so, artificial food coloring binds to food proteins. The luminal digestive enzymes cannot break down many of these proteins once they are bound to food dyes, thus creating gut inflammation and damage, leading to leaky gut. Posttranslational modification of proteins is a well-known mechanism to turn naïve peptides to immunogenic one, by losing their tolerance [66, 67]. Food colorants are associated with allergic reactions [140]. Xanthene food dyes are toxic by inhibition of human drug-metabolizing enzymes, thus affecting pharmacological activities [141]. Caramel color class IV modified the methylation status of HL-60 cell line, suggesting an epigenetic modulation by food, thus food colorant [142]. Daily food brilliant blue dyes antagonize purinergic receptors, and this receptor family is critical not only for cellular homeostasis but also for inflammation and even cell death [143]. Tartazine is a common colorant in processed food and causes major side effects such as urticaria, angioedema, and asthma and is possibly embroiled in conduct behaviors [144]. The immunotoxic potential of the food dye Orange II was shown on splenocytes [145]. Intriguingly, laboratory mice also consume food dyes, and some of them suffered from neurotoxicity [146]. Most recently, it was reported that the heavily used food colorants, such as Red 40 and Yellow 6, induce colitis in mice overexpressing IL-23. Interestingly, the elevated IL-23 stimulated pathogenic $CD4^+$ T cells to secret IFN-γ, and the colitis depended on the commensal bacteria: *Bacteroides ovatus* and *Enterococcus faecalis*. It appears that those microbes metabolize the food dyes to create ANSA-Na, which induces a relapse of the colitis [147]. In conclusion, food colorants/dyes can be regarded as adjuvants since they can be immunostimulant for human lymphocytes, activate cell-mediated immune responses and increase immunoglobulin's secretion, and induce cross-reactive antibodies [132, 148–150]. Finally, some experts suggested that "the evidence for carcinogenicity, genotoxicity, and hypersensitivity, coupled with the fact that dyes do not improve the safety or nutritional quality of foods, indicates that all of the currently used dyes should be removed from the food supply and replaced, if at all, by safer colorings" [151]. Or, "we strongly believe that the use of these potentially toxic colors in food needs to be reconsidered" [152].

Food colorants fulfill the criteria of ASIA syndrome

Taking into considerations the major criteria of the syndrome, food colorants fulfill all the three. No doubt they are classical environmental external factors. They can induce typical clinical manifestations ranging from urticaria, angioedema, asthma, and conducting abnormal behaviors to IBD-type colitis [132, 133, 140, 144]. Removing some nutritional dyes has ameliorated some attention-deficit or hyperactivity disorder symptoms [143, 153–155]. Restricted diet of food additives is a frequent clinical practice. Eliminating food dyes can ameliorate urticaria [156], asthma [157, 158], and even prevent anaphylactic reactions [159]. Finally, based on in vivo and in vitro studies, it was suggested that "high chronic intake of food colorings throughout the entire life is not advisable" [160]. As for the minor criteria, antibodies are produced in food colorant-treated animals. IgG, IgM, and overall antibody were significantly increased in tartrazine-treated rats, compared to controls [150]. Food dye effects are not related to specific HLAs; however, allergy, various cancers, and IBD-type, dextran sodium sulfate-induced colitis are HLA dependent [161, 162]. Finally, no specific ADs were directly connected to processed food dyes, except for the titanium dioxide color used in a plethora of different foods to make them brighter and whiter [104]. As mentioned above, this dye exacerbates DSS-induced colitis by activating the NLRP3 inflammasome intracellular pathway [106]. In conclusion, food colorants act as adjuvants, are immune stimulators, and fulfill the major and partially the minor criteria of the ASIA syndrome.

Emulsifiers are potential new adjuvants

Surfactants is the abbreviation for "surface-active agents," heavily used in pharmacy and in the processed food industries as food emulsifiers. The most used ones are polysorbate 80, mono/di glycerides, and lecithin. The most frequently processed food applications are in spreads, creams, dressings, sauces, dips, and beverages. Surfactant-coated nanoparticles are a developing aspect in food nanotechnology, mainly in food processing, functional foods, drinking water purification, food preservation, texture improvement, and extending shelf life [163]. Food emulsifiers maintain the texture, consistency, hydration, viscosity, structural integrity, heat resistance and mold resistance, color, and taste of multiphase processed food and beverages. All those beneficial properties are counteracted by their drawbacks and questionable safety. Emulsifier toxicity was summarized by multiple reviews [39, 164–166]. They are involved in IBD evolution, mainly Crohn's disease [167–169]; their usage is linked to obesity [170]; they exacerbate the development of spontaneous enteric adenoma [171]; act as pro-inflammatory and might promote colon carcinogenesis [172]; increase intestinal permeability [173], impact microbiome/dysbiome ratio [174]; alter intestinal mucus and increase pathobionts translocation [169, 175], and promote metabolic syndrome [176] and IBS [177]. Various emulsifiers are immune stimulants. They can activate immune myeloid cells [173], and emulsifier-based vaccines stimulate several branches of the animal and human immune systems. Not surprising, high toxicity is associated with many experimental adjuvants, thus hindering their usage. Self-adjuvanting and nanoemulsifiers are increasingly used as vaccine adjuvants. Trying to replace the aluminum salts, squalene nanoemulsions represent the frequently employed class of adjuvants in approved vaccines. It appears that they stimulate human cells cytokine production from human cells in vitro and enhance antigen-specific immune responses in several animal models [178]. Vaccines emulsified in vegetable oil adjuvants are increasingly developed and are efficient in stimulating various immune responses [179, 180]. Self-adjuvanting lipopeptide vaccines incorporate immunostimulatory lipids into peptide antigens and were reported to elicit adequate immune response in human clinical trials. They have the advantage over alum salts since they can be administered via mucosal routs, they provoke antigen-specific cytotoxic T lymphocytes and activate mucosal immunity, and induce little-to-no toxicity and side effects [181–183]. More so, hydrocarbon oil structures are adjuvants and induce autoimmunity [184]. Arthritis can be induced in animals by several oil adjuvants (hexadecane, heptadecane, squalene, and Arlacel) [184]. Being adjuvants, mineral oils were shown to be involved in ADs' initiation. Hence, increased risk of developing rheumatoid arthritis and possibly lupus was reported [185, 186]. In summary, food emulsifiers are immune stimulants and have adjuvant properties, and surface-active agents are increasingly used in the current vaccines.

Emulsifiers fulfill the criteria of ASIA syndrome

Considering the major criteria of the syndrome, food emulsifiers fulfill all the three of them. Emulsifiers are natural or artificially designed molecules and as such are classical environmental external factors. They can induce typical clinical manifestations ranging from IBD-type manifestation, obesity, colonic polyps and cancer, leaky gut, mucus lysis, metabolic syndrome, IBS, and occupational or allergic asthma to even acute urticaria [39, 167–177, 187–190]. Food emulsifiers were shown to disrupt tight junctions' function and aggravate testicular toxicity [191]. Removing some environmental or food emulsifiers will prevent the hypersensitivity reaction. Emulsifier-free diets ameliorated ulcerative colitis and decreased clinical disease index and IL-6 and fecal calprotectin levels inflammatory parameters [192]. When unexposed to two emulsifiers, carboxymethylcellulose and polysorbate-80, the control mice had normal microbiome, unaffected intestinal permeability, decreased inflammatory markers, normal flagellin levels, no carcinogenesis, and even no anxiety, compared to the treated groups [193]. Titanium dioxide is an NP; however, it possesses emulsifying activity. Titanium oxide-free diets showed improvement in animal-induced colitis, normal immune cells behavior, no fibrosis, and no oxidative stress accumulation [193]. Paleolithic diet excludes ultraprocessed foods but allows wild meats, and a noncereal, plant-based diet was reported to ameliorate unresponsive Crohn's disease patients [193, 194]. It seems that eliminating dietary emulsifiers is beneficial in many aspects. Screening the minor criteria, antibodies are produced, very efficiently, to proteins or tissue homogenates emulsified in complete Freund's adjuvant vaccinated animals or humans [178–183]. Being an adjuvant, the emulsified inoculum fulfills its immune-stimulating function and produces antigen-specific antibodies. Isolated emulsifiers' effects are not related to specific HLAs; however, many emulsifier-based vaccines injected to animals or humans are HLA depended [195–199]. Interestingly, using several frequently used oil adjuvant emulsifiers, the induced arthritis was linked to 33-kb Ltab-Ncr3 haplotype in MHC-III [200]. Finally, several specific ADs were directly connected to processed food emulsifiers. Titanium dioxide has dual application as an emulsifier and a dye, used in a plethora of different foods [107, 193]. This emulsifier exacerbates DSS-induced colitis by activating the NLRP3 inflammasome intracellular pathway [109]. In addition, titanium dioxide induced colitis, activated immune cells, increased oxidative stress, and was associated with animal tissue fibrosis [193]. Emulsifiers are associated with multiple animal or human diseases; some of them are ADs such as Crohn's disease and ulcerative colitis and arthritis [189, 191, 193]. More so, they induce several dysfunctions that are typically autoimmunogenic such as increased intestinal permeability and leaky gut, altered microbiome, increased bacterial translocation tissue inflammation, and obesity [39, 169, 170, 173–175, 201]. Emulsified complete Freund's adjuvants are routinely used to induce ADs in laboratory animals. In this regard, they were shown to be effective in collagen-induced arthritis, rheumatoid arthritis, and Sjögren's syndrome [202–204]. In conclusion, processed food emulsifiers act as adjuvants, they are immune stimulators, and fulfill the major and the minor criteria of the ASIA syndrome. It can be summarized that all the above-described five food additives can act as adjuvants, thus fulfilling the ASIA syndrome inclusion criteria. The present review reenforces Mancuso and Barisani, conclusions that "Food additives could play an important role in the pathogenesis of CD" [205]. They are autoimmunogenic and add to the growing list of adjuvants of ASIA syndrome.

Conclusions

Based on the above, the five frequently consumed, industrial food additives, namely gluten, mTG, NPs, colorants, and emulsifiers, have immune-stimulation activities, are often used as adjuvants, and fulfill the major as well as the minor criteria of ASIA syndrome. Figure 4.1 schematically describes those nutritional adjuvant, and Table 4.1 lists their fulfillment of the syndrome's criteria.

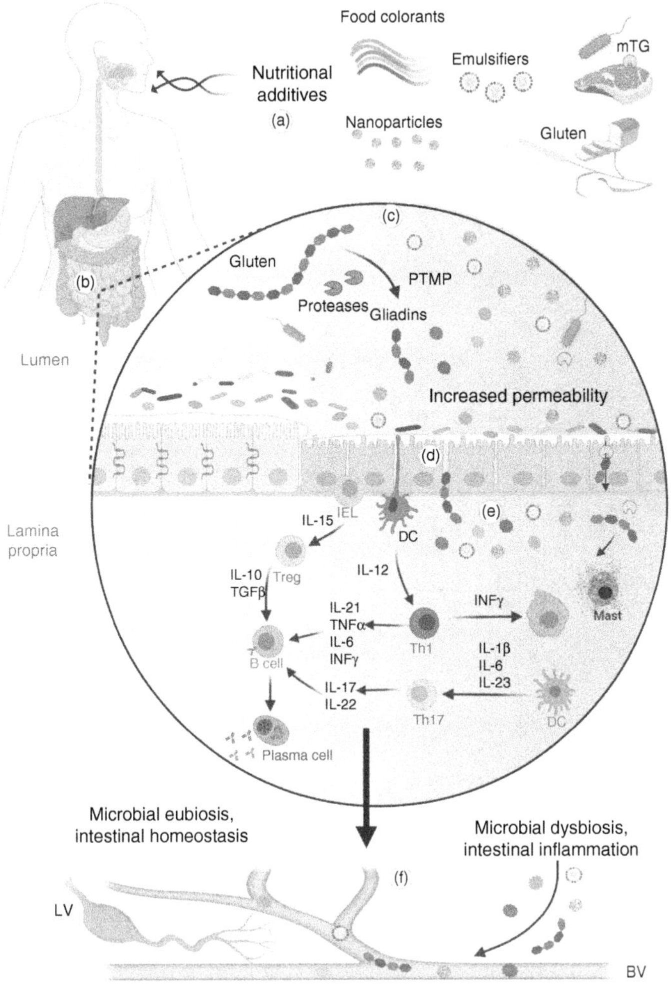

Figure 4.1 A schematic presentation of five frequently used food additives as part of the nutritional adjuvants in ASIA syndrome. (a) Oral consumption of the five food additives, namely gluten, NPs, colorants, emulsifiers, and food products that were processed by mTG, such as meat, dairy, and bread. (b) NPs, colorants and emulsifiers, Gliadins' peptides, and mTG peptides' complexes reach the gut lumen. (c) Gliadins are rich in glutamine and proline and thus are prime substrates for mTG cross-linking, turning a naïve molecule to an immunogenic one. More so, other mTG-processed food products increase the enzyme luminal load for nutrients cross-linking. The result is an increase in PTMP by the ability of mTG to deamidate or transamidate its substrates. Furthermore, luminal digestive peptidases cannot break down the resistant bonds between artificial food additives and food proteins, thus inducing gut inflammation and damage to the intestinal epithelium. (d) NPs, mTG, emulsifier, and colorants can potentially damage the lining mucus by breaking its stability and compromise tight junction functional integrity. Gluten increases intestinal permeability by binding to its epithelial CXCR3 receptor inducing zonulin release. Gliadin-mTG and other small peptide complexes might penetrate into the lamina propria through the open junctions or trans-enterocytically. (e) In the lamina propria, all these food additives were found to have toxic and pro-inflammatory effects. For instance, gluten increases Th-17 activity, TLR4 signaling, NKG2P expression, and neutrophil migration. mTG cross-linked complexes induce pro-inflammatory cytokines that drive T cells activation. Th1 secretes IFNγ that activates macrophages. Th17 secretes IL-17 and IL-22, which activate B cells. Two types of DCs are present, the subepithelial one senses the lumen and regulates gut microbiota, and another mucosal one supports Th1 immunity. (f) Small particles that escaped the immune system can enter blood vessels (BV) and lymphatic vessels (LV). They can eventually reach distant organs and have a toxic effect or trigger an autoimmune response.

Table 4.1 Nutritional adjuvants fulfill the diagnostic criteria of the ASIA syndrome's criteria.

Criteria	Gluten	Microbial transglutaminase	Nanoparticles	Food colorants	Emulsifiers
		Major criteria for ASIA			
Exposure to external stimuli	√	√	√	√	√
	[57, 59]	[1, 32]	[84]	[131]	[38, 39]
Typical clinical manifestations	√	√	√	√	√
	[55, 56, 57]	[32–34, 46, 61, 63, 64, 66–71]	[94, 95, 97, 106]	[132, 133, 140, 144]	[170–177, 187–191]
Removal of triggers leads to improvement	√	√	√	√	√
	[45, 51, 52, 53, 55, 56]	[56]	[108, 109–111]	[143, 153–155, 158]	[192–194]
		Minor criteria for ASIA			
Autoantibody or antibody to the adjuvant	√	√	√	√	√
	[60, 61, 63–65]	[61, 63, 64]	[113, 118]	[149]	[178–183]
Specific HLA	√	√	√	√	√
	[4, 57, 61, 80]	[32, 34]	[120, 121]	[161, 162]	[195–200]
Autoimmune disease	√	√	√	√	√
	[55–57]	[32–34, 46, 61, 63, 64, 66–71]	[122–126]	[106, 132, 140, 144, 147]	[106, 184, 201, 202–204]

The numbers above are specific references.

They can be added to the increasing list of environmental factors that induce inflammation and ADs' postadjuvant exposure. It is not only infectious agents, breast implants, and many other foreign bodies, drugs, metals, or vaccines' adjuvants. The presently added nutritional adjuvants should be included in the ASIA syndrome.

Abbreviations

CD	celiac disease
ASIA	the autoimmune/inflammatory syndrome induced by adjuvants

ADs	autoimmune diseases
mTG	microbial transglutaminase
NPs	nanoparticles
PTMP	posttranslational modification of proteins

Author contributions

AL screened the literature and designed and wrote the chapter; CB screened the literature, edited and revised the chapter, and designed the figure. The two authors agreed to the published version of the chapter.

References

1. Lerner, A. and Matthias, T. (2015). Changes in intestinal tight junction permeability associated with industrial food additives explain the rising incidence of autoimmune disease. *Autoimmun. Rev.* 14: 479–489. https://doi.org/10.1016/j.autrev.2015.01.009.
2. Selmi, C. (2010). The worldwide gradient of autoimmune conditions. *Autoimmun. Rev.* 9: A247–A250.
3. Lerner, A., Jeremias, P., and Matthias, T. (2015). The world incidence and prevalence of autoimmune diseases is increasing. *Int. J. Celiac Dis.* 3: 151–155.
4. Lerner, A., Jermias, P., and Matthias, T. (2015). The world incidence of celiac disease is increasing: a review. *Int. J. Recent Sci. Res.* 7: 5491–5496.
5. Khan, M.F. and Wang, H. (2020). Environmental exposures and autoimmune diseases: contribution of gut microbiome. *Front. Immunol.* 10: 3094. https://doi.org/10.3389/fimmu.2019.03094.
6. Manzel, A., Muller, D.N., Hafler, D.A. et al. (2014). Role of "Western diet" in inflammatory autoimmune diseases. *Curr. Allergy Asthma Rep.* 14: 404. https://doi.org/10.1007/s11882-013-0404-6.
7. Alpízar-Rodríguez, D., Finckh, A., and Gilbert, B. (2020). The role of nutritional factors and intestinal microbiota in rheumatoid arthritis development. *Nutrients* 13: 96. https://doi.org/10.3390/nu13010096.
8. Kivity, S., Agmon-Levin, N., Blank, M., and Shoenfeld, Y. (2009). Infections and autoimmunity——friends or foes? *Trends Immunol.* 30: 409–414.
9. Shoenfeld, Y. and Agmon-Levin, N. (2011). 'ASIA' – autoimmune/inflammatory syndrome induced by adjuvants. *J. Autoimmun.* 36: 4–8. https://doi.org/10.1016/j.jaut.2010.07.003.
10. Watad, A., Quaresma, M., Brown, S. et al. (2017). Autoimmune/inflammatory syndrome induced by adjuvants (Shoenfeld's syndrome) – an update. *Lupus* 26: 675–681. https://doi.org/10.1177/0961203316686406.
11. Borba, V., Malkova, A., Basantsova, N. et al. (2020). Classical examples of the concept of the ASIA syndrome. *Biomol. Ther.* 10: 1436. https://doi.org/10.3390/biom10101436.
12. Cohen Tervaert, J.W. (2018). Autoinflammatory/autoimmunity syndrome induced by adjuvants (ASIA; Shoenfeld's syndrome): a new flame. *Autoimmun. Rev.* 17: 1259–1264. https://doi.org/10.1016/j.autrev.2018.07.003.
13. Alijotas-Reig, J., Esteve-Valverde, E., Gil-Aliberas, N., and Garcia-Gimenez, V. (2018). Autoimmune/inflammatory syndrome induced by adjuvants-ASIA-related to biomaterials: analysis of 45 cases and comprehensive review of the literature. *Immunol. Res.* 66: 120–140. https://doi.org/10.1007/s12026-017-8980-5.
14. Montealegre, G., Uribe, R., Martínez-Ceballos, M.A., and Rojas-Villarraga, A. (2021). ASIA syndrome symptoms induced by gluteal biopolymer injections: case-series and narrative review. *Toxicol. Rep.* 8: 303–314. https://doi.org/10.1016/j.toxrep.2021.01.011.
15. Cohen Tervaert, J.W. and Kappel, R.M. (2013). Silicone implant incompatibility syndrome (SIIS): a frequent cause of ASIA (Shoenfeld's syndrome). *Immunol. Res.* 56: 293–298. https://doi.org/10.1007/s12026-013-8401-3.
16. Watad, A., Rosenberg, V., Tiosano, S. et al. (2018). Silicone breast implants and the risk of autoimmune/rheumatic disorders: a real-world analysis. *Int. J. Epidemiol.* 47: 1846–1854. https://doi.org/10.1093/ije/dyy217.

17. Hajdu, S.D., Agmon-Levin, N., and Shoenfeld, Y. (2011). Silicone and autoimmunity. *Eur. J. Clin. Investig.* 41: 203–211. https://doi.org/10.1111/j.1365-2362.2010.02389.x.
18. Stolarczyk, J., Kubiś, M., and Brzosko, M. (2016). Autoimmune/inflammatory syndrome induced by adjuvants, ASIA. *Pomeranian J. Life Sci.* 62: 35–39.
19. Lerner, A. (2007). Aluminum is a potential environmental factor for Crohn's disease induction: extended hypothesis. *Ann. N. Y. Acad. Sci.* 1107: 329–345. https://doi.org/10.1196/annals.1381.035.
20. Lerner, A. (2012). Aluminum as an adjuvant in Crohn's disease induction. *Lupus* 21: 231–238. https://doi.org/10.1177/0961203311430090.
21. Alijotas-Reig, J. (2015). Human adjuvant-related syndrome or autoimmune/inflammatory syndrome induced by adjuvants. Where have we come from? Where are we going? A proposal for new diagnostic criteria. *Lupus* 24: 1012–1018. https://doi.org/10.1177/0961203315579092.
22. Watad, A., Bragazzi, N.L., McGonagle, D. et al. (2019). Autoimmune/inflammatory syndrome induced by adjuvants (ASIA) demonstrates distinct autoimmune and autoinflammatory disease associations according to the adjuvant subtype: insights from an analysis of 500 cases. *Clin. Immunol.* 203: 1–8. https://doi.org/10.1016/j.clim.2019.03.007.
23. Shoenfeld, Y., Ryabkova, V.A., Scheibenbogen, C. et al. (2020). Complex syndromes of chronic pain, fatigue and cognitive impairment linked to autoimmune dysautonomia and small fiber neuropathy. *Clin. Immunol.* 214: 108384. https://doi.org/10.1016/j.clim.2020.108384.
24. Kearney, J. (2010). Food consumption trends and drivers. *Philos. Trans. R. Soc. Lond. Ser. B Biol. Sci.* 365: 2793–2807.
25. Azzam, A. (2021). Is the world converging to a 'Western die'? *Public Health Nutr.* 24: 309–317. https://doi.org/10.1017/S136898002000350X.
26. Baker, P. and Friel, S. (2014). Processed foods and the nutrition transition: evidence from Asia. *Obes. Rev.* 15: 564–577. https://doi.org/10.1111/obr.12174.
27. Laster, J., Bonnes, S.L., and Rocha, J. (2019). Increased use of emulsifiers in processed foods and the links to obesity. *Curr. Gastroenterol. Rep.* 21: 61. https://doi.org/10.1007/s11894-019-0723-4.
28. Laster, J. and Frame, L.A. (2019). Beyond the calories-is the problem in the processing? *Curr. Treatm. Opt. Gastroenterol.* 17: 577–586. https://doi.org/10.1007/s11938-019-00246-1.
29. Wood, L. (2020). Global Vital Wheat Gluten Industry Assessment 2018–2020, Dublin. Accessed Jan 2023. https://www.globenewswire.com/news-release/2020/06/30/2055191/0/en/Global-Vital-Wheat-Gluten-Industry-Assessment-2018-2020-2024-2027.html.
30. Chan, S.K. and Lim, T.S. (2019). Bioengineering of microbial transglutaminase for biomedical applications. *Appl. Microbiol. Biotechnol.* 103: 2973–2984. https://doi.org/10.1007/s00253-019-09669-3.
31. Doti, N., Caporale, A., Monti, A. et al. (2020). A recent update on the use of microbial transglutaminase for the generation of biotherapeutics. *World J. Microbiol. Biotechnol.* 36: 53. https://doi.org/10.1007/s11274-020-02829-y.
32. Lerner, A. and Matthias, T. (2015). Possible association between celiac disease and bacterial transglutaminase in food processing: a hypothesis. *Nutr. Rev.* 73: 544–552.
33. Lerner, A. and Matthias, T. (2019). Microbial transglutaminase is beneficial to food industries but a caveat to public health. *Med. One* 4 (1): e190001.
34. Lerner, A. and Matthias, T. (2020). Processed food additive microbial transglutaminase and its cross-linked gliadin complexes are potential public health concerns in celiac disease. *Int. J. Mol. Sci.* 21: 1127. https://doi.org/10.3390/ijms21031127.
35. Singh, T., Shukla, S., Kumar, P. et al. (2017). Application of nanotechnology in food science: perception and overview. *Front. Microbiol.* 8: 1501. https://doi.org/10.3389/fmicb.2017.01501.
36. Maida, J. (2019). Global Food Nanotechnology Market 2019-2023 | Growing Applications in Nutraceuticals to Boost the Market | Technavio | Business Wire [Internet]. London. https://www.businesswire.com/news/home/20190610005263/en/Global-Food-Nanotechnology-Market-2019-2023-Growing-Applications-in-Nutraceuticals-to-Boost-the-Market-Technavio.
37. Buzea, C., Pacheco, I.I., and Robbie, K. (2007). Nanomaterials and nanoparticles: sources and toxicity. *Biointerphases* 2: MR17–MR71. https://doi.org/10.1116/1.2815690.
38. Cox S, Sandall A, Smith L, Rossi M, Whelan K. Food additive emulsifiers: a review of their role in foods, legislation and classifications, presence in food supply, dietary exposure, and safety assessment. *Nutr. Rev.* 2021;79:726-741. Doi https://doi.org/10.1093/nutrit/nuaa038.

39. Halmos, E.P., Mack, A., and Gibson, P.R. (2019). Review article: emulsifiers in the food supply and implications for gastrointestinal disease. *Aliment. Pharmacol. Ther.* 49: 41–50. https://doi.org/10.1111/apt.15045.
40. (2021). Food Emulsifiers Market Report, Size, Share, Trends 2021–2026 [Internet]. Accessed Jan 2023. https://www.expertmarketresearch.com/reports/food-emulsifiers-market.
41. (2021). Global Food Emulsifiers Market valuation to surge at 4.7% CAGR through 2027 - Market Study Report [Internet]. Accessed Jan 2023. https://www.marketstudyreport.com/news/food-emulsifiers-market-size.
42. Luzardo-Ocampo, I., Ramírez-Jiménez, A.K., Yañez, J. et al. (2021). Technological applications of natural colorants in food systems: a review. *Foods* 10: 634. https://doi.org/10.3390/foods10030634.
43. Shanmugasundaram, P. and Bavenro, T.R. (2019). A review on food coloring agents – safe or unsafe? *Res. J. Pharm. Tech.* 12 (5): 2503–2505. https://doi.org/10.5958/0974-360X.2019.00421.9.
44. (2021). The global food colors market size was USD 2.55 billion in 2018 and is projected to reach USD 4.77 billion by 2026, exhibiting a CAGR of 8.19% during the forecast period. Read More at: https://www.fortunebusinessinsights.com/food-colors-market-102644.
45. Lerner, A., Shoenfeld, Y., and Matthias, T. (2017). Adverse effects of gluten ingestion and advantages of gluten withdrawal in nonceliac autoimmune disease. *Nutr. Rev.* 75: 1046–1058. https://doi.org/10.1093/nutrit/nux054.
46. Lerner, A. and Benzvi, C. (2021). "Let food be thy medicine": gluten and potential role in neurodegeneration. *Cell* 10: 756. https://doi.org/10.3390/cells10040756.
47. Vojdani, A., Lerner, A., and Vojdani, E. (2021). Cross-reactivity and sequence homology between alpha-synuclein and food products: a step further for Parkinson's disease synucleinopathy. *Cell* 10: 1111. https://doi.org/10.3390/cells10051111.
48. Vojdani, A., Gushgari, L.R., and Vojdani, E. (2020). Interaction between food antigens and the immune system: association with autoimmune disorders. *Autoimmun. Rev.* 19: 102459. https://doi.org/10.1016/j.autrev.2020.102459.
49. Kinashi, Y. and Hase, K. (2021). Partners in leaky gut syndrome: intestinal dysbiosis and autoimmunity. *Front. Immunol.* 12: 673708. https://doi.org/10.3389/fimmu.2021.673708.
50. Fasano, A. (2020). All disease begins in the (leaky) gut: role of zonulin-mediated gut permeability in the pathogenesis of some chronic inflammatory diseases. *F1000Res* 9: F1000. Faculty Rev-69. https://doi.org/10.12688/f1000research.20510.1.
51. Lerner, A., Ramesh, A., and Matthias, T. (2018). Going gluten free in non-celiac autoimmune diseases: the missing ingredient. *Expert. Rev. Clin. Immunol.* 14: 873–875. https://doi.org/10.1080/1744666X.2018.1524757.
52. Lerner, A., Ramesh, A., and Matthias, T. (2017). Are non-celiac autoimmune diseases responsive to gluten-free diet? *Int. J. Celiac Dis.* 5: 164–167.
53. Lerner, A., Freire de Carvalho, J., Kotrova, A., and Shoenfeld, Y. (2021). Gluten free diet can improve non-celiac autoimmune diseases. *Nutr. Rev.* 80: 525–543.
54. Hollon, J., Puppa, E.L., Greenwald, B. et al. (2015). Effect of gliadin on permeability of intestinal biopsy explants from celiac disease patients and patients with non-celiac gluten sensitivity. *Nutrients* 7: 1565–1576. https://doi.org/10.3390/nu7031565.
55. Taraghikhah, N., Ashtari, S., Asri, N. et al. (2020). An updated overview of spectrum of gluten-related disorders: clinical and diagnostic aspects. *BMC Gastroenterol.* 20: 258. https://doi.org/10.1186/s12876-020-01390-0.
56. O'Bryan, T. and Lerner, A. (2021). Nonresponsive celiac disease treated with a unique functional medical approach. *Int. J. Celiac Dis.* 9: 41–64. https://doi.org/10.12691/ijcd-9-2-7.
57. Lerner, A., Matthias, T., and Wusterhausen, P. (2019). Autoimmunity in celiac disease: extra-intestinal manifestations. *Autoimmun. Rev.* 18: 241–246. https://doi.org/10.1016/j.autrev.2018.09.010.
58. Irvine, A.J., Chey, W.D., and Ford, A.C. (2017). Screening for celiac disease in irritable bowel syndrome: an updated systematic review and meta-analysis. *Am. J. Gastroenterol.* 112: 65–76. https://doi.org/10.1038/ajg.2016.466.
59. Lerner, A. and Matthias, T. (2016). GUT-the trojan horse in remote organs autoimmunity. *J. Clin. Cell Immunol.* 7: 401.
60. Shaoul, R. and Lerner, A. (2007). Associated autoantibodies in celiac disease. *Autoimmun. Rev.* 6: 559–565. https://doi.org/10.1016/j.autrev.2007.02.006.

61. Lerner, A., Ramesh, A., and Matthias, T. (2019). Serologic diagnosis of celiac disease: new biomarkers. *Gastroenterol. Clin. N. Am.* 48: 307–317. https://doi.org/10.1016/j.gtc.2019.02.009.
62. Lerner, A. and Lebenthal, E. (1991). The controversy of the use of anti-gluten antibody (AGA) as a diagnostic tool in celiac disease. *J. Pediatr. Gastroenterol. Nutr.* 12: 407–409.
63. Lerner, A., Jeremias, P., Neidhöfer, S., and Matthias, T. (2017). Comparison of the reliability of 17 celiac disease associated bio-markers to reflect intestinal damage. *J. Clin. Cell Immunol.* 8: 486.
64. Agardh, D., Matthias, T., Wusterhausen, P. et al. (2020). Antibodies against neo-epitope of microbial and human transglutaminases' complexes as biomarkers of childhood celiac disease. *Clin. Exp. Immunol.* 199: 294–302.
65. Lerner, A., Jeremias, P., Neidhöfer, S., and Matthias, T. (2016). Antibodies against neo-epitope tTg complexed to gliadin are different and more reliable then anti-tTg for the diagnosis of pediatric celiac disease. *J. Immunol. Methods* 429: 15–20. https://doi.org/10.1016/j.jim.2015.12.006.
66. Lerner, A., Aminov, R., and Matthias, T. (2017). Intestinal dysbiotic transglutaminases are potential environmental drivers of systemic autoimmunogenesis. *Front. Microbiol.* 8: 3389.
67. Lerner, A., Aminov, R., and Matthias, T. (2016). Dysbiosis may trigger autoimmune diseases via inappropriate posttranslational modification of host proteins. *Front. Microbiol.* 7: 84.
68. Lerner, A. and Matthias, T. (2019). Microbial transglutaminase: a new potential player in celiac disease. *Clin. Immunol.* 199: 37–43.pii: S1521-6616(18)30717-4. https://doi.org/10.1016/j.clim.2018.12.008.
69. Matthias, T. and Lerner, A. (2018). Microbial transglutaminase is immunogenic and potentially pathogenic in pediatric celiac disease. *Front. Pediatr.* 6: 389. https://doi.org/10.3389/fped.2018.00389.
70. Lerner, A. and Matthias, T. (2019). Microbial transglutaminase should be considered as an environmental inducer of celiac disease. *World J. Clin. Cases* 7: 3912–3914.
71. Lerner, A. and Matthias, T. (2016). Don't forget the exogenous microbial transglutaminases: it is immunogenic and potentially pathogenic. *AIMS Biophys.* 3: 546–552.
72. Stricker, S., de Laffolie, J., Rudloff, S. et al. (2019). Intracellular localization of microbial transglutaminase and its influence on the transport of gliadin in enterocytes. *J. Pediatr. Gastroenterol. Nutr.* 68: e43–e50. https://doi.org/10.1097/MPG.0000000000002171.
73. Fittipaldi, N., Segura, M., Grenier, D., and Gottschalk, M. (2012). Virulence factors involved in the pathogenesis of the infection caused by the swine pathogen and zoonotic agent *Streptococcus suis*. *Future Microbiol.* 7: 259–279. https://doi.org/10.2217/fmb.11.149.
74. Xu, B., Zhang, P., Li, W. et al. (2017). *hsdS*, Belonging to the type I restriction-modification system, contributes to the *Streptococcus suis* serotype 2 survival ability in phagocytes. *Front. Microbiol.* 8: 1524. https://doi.org/10.3389/fmicb.2017.01524.
75. Pian, Y., Wang, P., Liu, P. et al. (2015). Proteomics identification of novel fibrinogen-binding proteins of *Streptococcus suis* contributing to antiphagocytosis. *Front. Cell. Infect. Microbiol.* 5: 19. https://doi.org/10.3389/fcimb.2015.00019. eCollection 2015.
76. Kaufmann, A., Koppel, R., and Widmer, M. (2012). Determination of microbial transglutaminase in meat and meat products. *Food Addit. Contam. Part A Chem. Anal. Control Expo. Risk Assess.* 29: 1364–1373.
77. Dekking, E.H.A., Van Veelen, P.A., de Ru, A. et al. (2008). Microbial transglutaminase generate T cell stimulatory epitopes involved in celiac disease. *J. Cereal Sci.* 47: 339–346.
78. Elli, L., Roncoroni, L., Hils, M. et al. (2012). Immunological effects of transglutaminase-treated gluten in coeliac disease. *Hum. Immunol.* 73: 992–997.
79. Vojdani, A. (2009). Detection of IgE, IgG, IgA and IgM antibodies against raw and processed food antigens. *Nutr. Metab. (Lond.)* 6: 22.
80. Lerner, A. and Matthias, T. (2019). Gluten and autoimmunogenesis. In: *Musaic of Autoimmunity, The Novel Factors of Autoimmune Diseases Revisited*, 2e (ed. Y. Shoenfield and C. Perricone), 315–321. Elsevier.
81. Lerner, A. and Matthias, T. (2015). Food industrial microbial transglutaminase in celiac disease: treat or trick. *Int. J. Celiac Dis.* 3: 1–6.
82. Gerrard, J.A. and Sutton, K.H. (2008). Addition of transglutaminase to cereal products may generate the epitope responsible for coeliac disease. *Trends Food Sci. Technol.* 16: 510–512.
83. Rhim, J.W., Park, H.M., and Ha, C.S. (2013). Bio-nanocomposites for food packaging applications. *Prog. Polym. Sci.* 38: 1629–1652. https://doi.org/10.1016/j.progpolymsci.2013.05.008.
84. Martínez, G., Merinero, M., Pérez-Aranda, M. et al. (2021). Environmental impact of nanoparticles' application as an emerging technology: a review. *Materials (Basel)* 14 (1): 166. https://doi.org/10.3390/ma14010166.

85. McClements, D.J. and Xiao, H. (2017). Is nano safe in foods? Establishing the factors impacting the gastrointestinal fate and toxicity of organic and inorganic food-grade nanoparticles. *NPJ Sci. Food* 1: 6. https://doi.org/10.1038/s41538-017-0005-1.
86. McClements, D.J., Xiao, H., and Demokritou, P. (2017). Physicochemical and colloidal aspects of food matrix effects on gastrointestinal fate of ingested inorganic nanoparticles. *Adv. Colloid Interf. Sci.* 246: 165–180. https://doi.org/10.1016/j.cis.2017.05.010.
87. Huang, Y.-W., Cambre, M., and Lee, H.-J. (2017). The toxicity of nanoparticles depends on multiple molecular and physicochemical mechanisms. *Int. J. Mol. Sci.* 18: 2702. https://doi.org/10.3390/ijms18122702.
88. Bajpai, V.K., Kamle, M., Shukla, S. et al. (2018). Prospects of using nanotechnology for food preservation, safety, and security. *J. Food Drug Anal.* 26: 1201–1214. https://doi.org/10.1016/j.jfda.2018.06.011.
89. Medina-Reyes, E.I., Rodríguez-Ibarra, C., Déciga-Alcaraz, A. et al. (2020). Food additives containing nanoparticles induce gastrotoxicity, hepatotoxicity and alterations in animal behavior: the unknown role of oxidative stress. *Food Chem. Toxicol.* 146: 111814. https://doi.org/10.1016/j.fct.2020.111814.
90. Lin, M.-H., Lin, C.-f., Yang, S.-C. et al. (2018). The interplay between nanoparticles and neutrophils. *J. Biomed. Nanotechnol.* 14: 66–85. https://doi.org/10.1166/jbn.2018.2459.
91. Faust, J.J., Masserano, B.M., Mielke, A.H. et al. (2014). Engineered nanoparticles induced brush border disruption in a human model of the intestinal epithelium. *Adv. Exp. Med. Biol.* 811: 55–72. https://doi.org/10.1007/978-94-017-8739-0_4.
92. Gamazo, C., Martín-Arbella, N., Brotons, A. et al. (2015). Mimicking microbial strategies for the design of mucus-permeating nanoparticles for oral immunization. *Eur. J. Pharm. Biopharm.* 96: 454–463. https://doi.org/10.1016/j.ejpb.2015.01.010.
93. Lama, S., Merlin-Zhang, O., and Yang, C. (2020). In vitro and in vivo models for evaluating the oral toxicity of nanomedicines. *Nanomaterials (Basel)* 10 (11): 2177. https://doi.org/10.3390/nano10112177.
94. Mohammadipour, A., Haghir, H., and Bideskan, A.E. (2020). A link between nanoparticles and Parkinson's disease. Which nanoparticles are most harmful? *Rev. Environ. Health* 35: 545–556. https://doi.org/10.1515/reveh-2020-0043.
95. Boyes, W.K. and van Thriel, C. (2020). Neurotoxicology of nanomaterials. *Chem. Res. Toxicol.* 33 (5): 1121–1144. https://doi.org/10.1021/acs.chemrestox.0c00050.
96. Liangjiao, C., Yiyuan, K., Hongbing, G. et al. (2019). The current understanding of immunotoxicity induced by silica nanoparticles. *Nanomedicine* 14: 1227–1229. https://doi.org/10.2217/nnm-2019-0107.
97. Ogawa, T., Okumura, R., Nagano, K. et al. (2021). Oral intake of silica nanoparticles exacerbates intestinal inflammation. *Biochem. Biophys. Res. Commun.* 534: 540–546. https://doi.org/10.1016/j.bbrc.2020.11.047.
98. Yang, Y., Du, X., Wang, Q. et al. (2019). Mechanism of cell death induced by silica nanoparticles in hepatocyte cells is by apoptosis. *Int. J. Mol. Med.* 44 (3): 903–912. https://doi.org/10.3892/ijmm.2019.4265.
99. Qi, Y., Ma, R., Li, X. et al. (2020). Disturbed mitochondrial quality control involved in hepatocytotoxicity induced by silica nanoparticles. *Nanoscale* 12: 13034–13045. https://doi.org/10.1039/d0nr01893g.
100. Zheng, H., Jiang, J., Xu, S. et al. (2021). Nanoparticle-induced ferroptosis: detection methods, mechanisms and applications. *Nanoscale* 13: 2266–2285. https://doi.org/10.1039/d0nr08478f.
101. Smolkova, B., El Yamani, N., Collins, A.R. et al. (2015). Nanoparticles in food. Epigenetic changes induced by nanomaterials and possible impact on health. *Food Chem. Toxicol.* 77: 64–73. https://doi.org/10.1016/j.fct.2014.12.015.
102. Wong, B.S.E., Hu, Q., and Baeg, G.H. (2017). Epigenetic modulations in nanoparticle-mediated toxicity. *Food Chem. Toxicol.* 109 (Pt 1): 746–752. https://doi.org/10.1016/j.fct.2017.07.006.
103. Grande, F. and Tucci, P. (2016). Titanium dioxide nanoparticles: a risk for human health? *Mini Rev. Med. Chem.* 16: 762–769. https://doi.org/10.2174/1389557516666160321114341.
104. Winkler, H.C., Notter, T., Meyer, U., and Naegeli, H. (2018). Critical review of the safety assessment of titanium dioxide additives in food. *J. Nanobiotechnol.* 16: 51. https://doi.org/10.1186/s12951-018-0376-8.
105. Rihane, N., Nury, T., M'rad, I. et al. (2016). Microglial cells (BV-2) internalize titanium dioxide (TiO_2) nanoparticles: toxicity and cellular responses. *Environ. Sci. Pollut. Res. Int.* 23 (10): 9690–9699. https://doi.org/10.1007/s11356-016-6190-7.
106. Ruiz, P.A., Morón, B., Becker, H.M. et al. (2017). Titanium dioxide nanoparticles exacerbate DSS-induced colitis: role of the NLRP3 inflammasome. *Gut* 66: 1216–1224. https://doi.org/10.1136/gutjnl-2015-310297.

107. Yang, W., Wang, L., Mettenbrink, E.M. et al. (2021). Nanoparticle toxicology. *Ann. Rev. Pharmacol. Toxicol.* 61: 269–289. https://doi.org/10.1146/annurev-pharmtox-032320-110338.
108. Peters, R., Dam, G., Bouwmeester, H. et al. (2011). Identification and characterization of organic nanoparticles in food. *Trends Anal. Chem.* 30: 100–112.
109. Sharma, D., Chaubey, P., and Suvarna, V. (2021). Role of natural products in alleviation of rheumatoid arthritis-a review. *J. Food Biochem.* 45: e13673. https://doi.org/10.1111/jfbc.13673.
110. McCarty, M.F. and Lerner, A. (2021). Perspective: low risk of Parkinson's disease in quasi-vegan cultures may reflect GCN2-mediated upregulation of parkin. *Adv. Nutr.* 12: 355–362. https://doi.org/10.1093/advances/nmaa112.
111. Null, G., Pennesi, L., and Feldman, M. (2017). Nutrition and lifestyle intervention on mood and neurological disorders. *J. Evid. Based Complementary Altern. Med.* 22: 68–74. https://doi.org/10.1177/2156587216637539.
112. Buchman, J.T., Hudson-Smith, N.V., Landy, K.M., and Haynes, C.L. (2019). Understanding nanoparticle toxicity mechanisms to inform redesign strategies to reduce environmental impact. *Acc. Chem. Res.* 52 (6): 1632–1642. https://doi.org/10.1021/acs.accounts.9b00053.
113. Gu, P., Wusiman, A., Wang, S. et al. (2019). Polyethylenimine-coated PLGA nanoparticles-encapsulated *Angelica sinensis* polysaccharide as an adjuvant to enhance immune responses. *Carbohydr. Polym.* 223: 115128. https://doi.org/10.1016/j.carbpol.2019.115128.
114. Dehalu, V., Weigel, S., Rebe, S. et al. (2012). Production and characterization of antibodies against crosslinked gelatin nanoparticles and first steps toward developing an ELISA screening kit. *Anal. Bioanal. Chem.* 403: 2851–2857. https://doi.org/10.1007/s00216-012-5793-1.
115. Joshi, H., Malik, A., Aggarwal, S. et al. (2019). In-vitro detection of phytopathogenic fungal cell wall by polyclonal sera raised against trimethyl chitosan nanoparticles. *Int. J. Nanomed.* 14: 10023–10033. https://doi.org/10.2147/IJN.S220488.
116. George, S.E., Elliott, C.T., McLaughlin, D.P. et al. (2012). An investigation into the potential use of nanoparticles as adjuvants for the production of polyclonal antibodies to low molecular weight compounds. *Vet. Immunol. Immunopathol.* 149: 46–53. https://doi.org/10.1016/j.vetimm.2012.06.002.
117. Braden, B.C., Goldbaum, F.A., Chen, B.X. et al. (2000). Erlanger BF X-ray crystal structure of an anti-Buckminsterfullerene antibody fab fragment: biomolecular recognition of C(60). *Proc. Natl. Acad. Sci. U. S. A.* 97: 12193–12197.
118. Lee, S.C., Parthasarathy, R., Botwin, K. et al. (2004). Biochemical and immunological properties of cytokines conjugated to dendritic polymers. *Biomed. Microdevices* 6: 191–202.
119. Zolnik, B.S., González-Fernández, A., Sadrieh, N., and Dobrovolskaia, M.A. (2010). Nanoparticles and the immune system. *Endocrinology* 151: 458–465. https://doi.org/10.1210/en.2009-1082.
120. Liu, M., Miao, T., Zhu, H. et al. (2012). IL-2-engineered nano-APC effectively activates viral antigen-mediated T cell responses from chronic hepatitis B virus-infected patients. *J. Immunol.* 188: 1534–1543. https://doi.org/10.4049/jimmunol.1102709.
121. Raker, V.K., Becker, C., Landfester, K., and Steinbrink, K. (2020). Targeted activation of T cells with IL-2-coupled nanoparticles. *Cells* 9: 2063. https://doi.org/10.3390/cells9092063.
122. Poland, C.A., Duffin, R., Kinloch, I. et al. (2008). Carbon nanotubes introduced into the abdominal cavity of mice show asbestos-like pathogenicity in a pilot study. *Nat. Nanotechnol.* 3: 423–428.
123. Ghebretatios, M., Schaly, S., and Prakash, S. (2021). Nanoparticles in the food industry and their impact on human gut microbiome and diseases. *Int. J. Mol. Sci.* 22: 1942. https://doi.org/10.3390/ijms22041942.
124. Mohamed, B.M., Verma, N.K., Davies, A.M. et al. (2012). Citrullination of proteins: a common post-translational modification pathway induced by different nanoparticles in vitro and in vivo. *Nanomedicine (Lond.)* 7: 1181–1195. https://doi.org/10.2217/nnm.11.177.
125. Shvedova, A.A., Kisin, E.R., Mercer, R. et al. (2005). Unusual inflammatory and fibrogenic pulmonary responses to single-walled carbon nanotubes in mice. *Am. J. Physiol. Lung Cell. Mol. Physiol.* 289: L698–L708.
126. Vallhov, H., Qin, J., Johansson, S.M. et al. (2006). The importance of an endotoxin-free environment during the production of nanoparticles used in medical applications. *Nano Lett.* 6: 1682–1686.
127. Gheibi Hayat, S.M. and Darroudi, M. (2019). Nanovaccine: a novel approach in immunization. *J. Cell. Physiol.* 234: 12530–12536. https://doi.org/10.1002/jcp.28120.

128. Pearson, R.M., Podojil, J.R., Shea, L.D. et al. (2019). Overcoming challenges in treating autoimmuntity: development of tolerogenic immune-modifying nanoparticles. *Nanomedicine* 18: 282–291. https://doi.org/10.1016/j.nano.2018.10.001.
129. Freitag, T.L., Podojil, J.R., Pearson, R.M. et al. (2020). Gliadin nanoparticles induce immune tolerance to gliadin in mouse models of celiac disease. *Gastroenterology* 158: 1667–1681.e12. https://doi.org/10.1053/j.gastro.2020.01.045.
130. Aguayo-Patrón, S.V. and Calderón de la Barca, A.M. (2017). Old fashioned vs. ultra-processed-based current diets: possible implication in the increased susceptibility to type 1 diabetes and celiac disease in childhood. *Foods* 6 (11): 100. https://doi.org/10.3390/foods6110100.
131. Singh, S. (2006). Impact of color on marketing. *Manag. Decis.* 44: 783–789. https://doi.org/10.1108/00251740610673332.
132. Vojdani, A. and Vojdani, C. (2015). Immune reactivity to food coloring. *Altern. Ther. Health Med.* 21 (Suppl 1): 52–62.
133. Stevens, L.J., Kuczek, T., Burgess, J.R. et al. (2013). Mechanisms of behavioral, atopic, and other reactions to artificial food colors in children. *Nutr. Rev.* 71: 268–281. https://doi.org/10.1111/nure.12023.
134. Gultekin, F., Oner, M.E., Savas, H.B., and Dogan, B. (2020). Food additives and microbiota. *North Clin. Istanb.* 7 (2): 192–200. https://doi.org/10.14744/nci.2019.92499.
135. Sato, K. and Akiyama, H. (2014). A simple and rapid chromatographic method to determine unauthorized basic colorants (rhodamine B, auramine O, and pararosaniline) in processed foods. *Food Sci. Nutr.* 2: 547–556. https://doi.org/10.1002/fsn3.127.
136. Leo, L., Loong, C., Ho, X.L. et al. (2018). Occurrence of azo food dyes and their effects on cellular inflammatory responses. *Nutrition* 46: 36–40. https://doi.org/10.1016/j.nut.2017.08.010.
137. Sharma, U.K., Kumar, R., Gupta, A. et al. (2019). Ameliorating efficacy of eugenol against metanil yellow induced toxicity in albino Wistar rats. *Food Chem. Toxicol.* 126: 34–40. https://doi.org/10.1016/j.fct.2019.01.032.
138. Nath, P.P., Sarkar, K., Mondal, M., and Paul, G. (2016). Metanil yellow impairs the estrous cycle physiology and ovarian folliculogenesis in female rats. *Environ. Toxicol.* 31: 2057–2067. https://doi.org/10.1002/tox.22205.
139. Elliott, A. and Reiners, J.J. Jr. (2008). Suppression of autophagy enhances the cytotoxicity of the DNA-damaging aromatic amine p-anilinoaniline. *Toxicol. Appl. Pharmacol.* 232: 169–179. https://doi.org/10.1016/j.taap.2008.06.017.
140. Feketea, G. and Tsabouri, S. (2017). Common food colorants and allergic reactions in children: myth or reality? *Food Chem.* 230: 578–588. https://doi.org/10.1016/j.foodchem.2017.03.043.
141. Mizutani, T. (2009). Toxicity of xanthene food dyes by inhibition of human drug-metabolizing enzymes in a noncompetitive manner. *J. Environ. Public Health* 2009: 953952. https://doi.org/10.1155/2009/953952.
142. Mateo-Fernández, M., Alves-Martínez, P., Del Río-Celestino, M. et al. (2019). Food safety and nutraceutical potential of caramel colour Class IV using in vivo and in vitro assays. *Foods* 8: 392. https://doi.org/10.3390/foods8090392.
143. Ferreira, L.G.B., Faria, R.X., da Silva Ferreira, N.C., and Soares-Bezerra, R.J. (2016). Brilliant blue dyes in daily food: how could purinergic system be affected? *Int. J. Food Sci.* 2016: 7548498. https://doi.org/10.1155/2016/7548498.
144. Manjunatha, J.G. (2018). A novel voltammetric method for the enhanced detection of the food additive tartrazine using an electrochemical sensor. *Heliyon* 4: e00986. https://doi.org/10.1016/j.heliyon.2018.e00986.
145. Yadav, A., Kumar, A., Dwivedi, P.D. et al. (2012). In vitro studies on immunotoxic potential of Orange II in splenocytes. *Toxicol. Lett.* 208 (3): 239–245. https://doi.org/10.1016/j.toxlet.2011.11.014.
146. Weiskirchen, S., Weiper, K., Tolba, R.H., and Weiskirchen, R. (2020). All you can feed: some comments on production of mouse diets used in biomedical research with special emphasis on non-alcoholic fatty liver disease research. *Nutrients* 12: 163. https://doi.org/10.3390/nu12010163.
147. He, Z., Chen, L., Catalan-Dibene, J. et al. (2021). Food colorants metabolized by commensal bacteria promote colitis in mice with dysregulated expression of interleukin-23. *Cell Metab.* 33: 1358–1371.e5. https://doi.org/10.1016/j.cmet.2021.04.015.

148. Valverde, E., Vich, J.M., García-Calderón, J.V., and García-Calderón, P.A. (1980). In vitro stimulation of lymphocytes in patients with chronic urticaria induced by additives and food. *Clin. Allergy* 10: 691–698. https://doi.org/10.1111/j.1365-2222.1980.tb02153.x.

149. Warrington, R.J., Sauder, P.J., and McPhillips, S. (1986). Cell-mediated immune responses to artificial food additives in chronic urticaria. *Clin. Allergy* 16: 527–533. https://doi.org/10.1111/j.1365-2222.1986.tb01991.x.

150. Shakoor, S., Ismail, A., Sabran, M. et al. (2022). In-vivo study of synthetic and natural food colors effect on biochemical and immunity parameters. *Food Sci. Technol. Int.* 42: 41420. https://doi.org/10.1590/fst.41420.

151. Kobylewski, S. and Jacobson, M.F. (2012). Toxicology of food dyes. *Int. J. Occup. Environ. Health* 18: 220–246. https://doi.org/10.1179/1077352512Z.00000000034.

152. Demirkol, O., Zhang, X., and Ercal, N. (2012). Oxidative effects of Tartrazine (CAS No. 1934-21-0) and New Coccin (CAS No. 2611-82-7) azo dyes on CHO cells. *J. Verbr. Lebensm.* 7: 229–236. https://doi.org/10.1007/s00003-012-0782-z.

153. Nigg, J.T., Lewis, K., Edinger, T., and Falk, M. (2012). Meta-analysis of attention-deficit/hyperactivity disorder or attention-deficit/hyperactivity disorder symptoms, restriction diet, and synthetic food color additives. *J. Am. Acad. Child Adolesc. Psychiatry* 51 (1): 86.e8–97.e8. https://doi.org/10.1016/j.jaac.2011.10.015.

154. Schab, D.W. and Trinh, N.-H.T. (2004). Do artificial food colors promote hyperactivity in children with hyperactive syndromes? A meta-analysis of double-blind placebo-controlled trials. *J. Dev. Behav. Pediatr.* 25 (6): 423–434. https://doi.org/10.1097/00004703-200412000-00007.

155. Millichap, J.G. and Yee, M.M. (2012). The diet factor in attention-deficit/hyperactivity disorder. *Pediatrics* 129 (2): 330–337. https://doi.org/10.1542/peds.2011-2199.

156. Kotobuki, Y., Azukizawa, H., Nishida, Y. et al. (2007). Case of urticaria due to cochineal dye in red-colored diet. *Arerugi* 56: 1510–1514.

157. Gultekin, F. and Doguc, D.K. (2013). Allergic and immunologic reactions to food additives. *Clin. Rev. Allergy Immunol.* 45: 6–29. https://doi.org/10.1007/s12016-012-8300-8.

158. Takeo, N., Nakamura, M., Nakayama, S. et al. (2018). Cochineal dye-induced immediate allergy: review of Japanese cases and proposed new diagnostic chart. *Allergol. Int.* 67: 496–505. https://doi.org/10.1016/j.alit.2018.02.012.

159. DiCello, M.C., Myc, A., Baker, J.R. Jr., and Baldwin, J.L. (1999). Anaphylaxis after ingestion of carmine colored foods: two case reports and a review of the literature. *Allergy Asthma Proc.* 20: 377–382. https://doi.org/10.2500/108854199778251816.

160. Merinas-Amo, R., Martínez-Jurado, M., SJurado-Güeto, S. et al. (2019). Biological effects of food coloring in in vivo and in vitro model systems. *Foods* 8: 176. https://doi.org/10.3390/foods8050176.

161. Gonzalez, A. and Sarna, S.K. (2001). Different types of contractions in rat colon and their modulation by oxidative stress. *Am. J. Physiol. Gastrointest. Liver Physiol.* 280: G546–G554. https://doi.org/10.1152/ajpgi.2001.280.4.G546.

162. Turton, C.W., Morris, L., Buckingham, J.A. et al. (1979). Histocompatibility antigens in asthma: population and family studies. *Thorax* 34: 670–676. https://doi.org/10.1136/thx.34.5.670.

163. Miyazawa, T., Itaya, M., Burdeos, G.C. et al. (2021). A critical review of the use of surfactant-coated nanoparticles in nanomedicine and food nanotechnology. *Int. J. Nanomed.* 16: 3937–3999. https://doi.org/10.2147/IJN.S298606.

164. Pitkänen, L., Heinonen, M., and Mikkonen, K.S. (2018). Safety considerations of plant polysaccharides for food use: a case study on phenolic-rich softwood galactoglucomannan extract. *Food Funct.* 9: 1931–1943. https://doi.org/10.1039/c7fo01425b.

165. Nerin, C., Canellas, E., Vera, P. et al. (2018). A common surfactant used in food packaging found to be toxic for reproduction in mammals. *Food Chem. Toxicol.* 113: 115–124. https://doi.org/10.1016/j.fct.2018.01.044.

166. McClements, D.J. and Rao, J. (2011). Food-grade nanoemulsions: formulation, fabrication, properties, performance, biological fate, and potential toxicity. *Crit. Rev. Food Sci. Nutr.* 51: 285–330. https://doi.org/10.1080/10408398.2011.559558.

167. Roberts, C.L., Rushworth, S.L., Richman, E., and Rhodes, J.M. (2013). Hypothesis: increased consumption of emulsifiers as an explanation for the rising incidence of Crohn's disease. *J. Crohns Colitis* 7: 338–341. https://doi.org/10.1016/j.crohns.2013.01.004.

168. Sandall, A.M., Cox, S.R., Lindsay, J.O. et al. (2020). Emulsifiers impact colonic length in mice and emulsifier restriction is feasible in people with Crohn's disease. *Nutrients* 12: 2827. https://doi.org/10.3390/nu12092827.
169. Roberts, C.L., Keita, A.V., Duncan, S.H. et al. (2010). Translocation of Crohn's disease *Escherichia coli* across M-cells: contrasting effects of soluble plant fibres and emulsifiers. *Gut* 59: 1331–1339. https://doi.org/10.1136/gut.2009.195370.
170. Laster, J., Bonnes, S.L., and Rocha, J. (2019). Increased use of emulsifiers in processed foods and the links to obesity. *Curr. Gastroenterol. Rep.* 21: 61. https://doi.org/10.1007/s11894-019-0723-4.
171. Viennois, E. and Chassaing, B. (2021). Consumption of select dietary emulsifiers exacerbates the development of spontaneous intestinal adenoma. *Int. J. Mol. Sci.* 22: 2602. https://doi.org/10.3390/ijms22052602.
172. Viennois, E., Merlin, D., Gewirtz, A.T., and Chassaing, B. (2017). Dietary emulsifier-induced low-grade inflammation promotes colon carcinogenesis. *Cancer Res.* 77: 27–40. https://doi.org/10.1158/0008-5472.CAN-16-1359.
173. Oscarsson, E., Lindberg, T., ZellerK, S. et al. (2020). Changes in intestinal permeability ex vivo and immune cell activation by three commonly used emulsifiers. *Molecules* 25: 5943. https://doi.org/10.3390/molecules25245943.
174. Naimi, S., Viennois, E., Gewirtz, A.T., and Chassaing, B. (2021). Direct impact of commonly used dietary emulsifiers on human gut microbiota. *Microbiome* 9: 66. https://doi.org/10.1186/s40168-020-00996-6.
175. Lock, J.Y., Carlson, T.L., Wang, C.-M. et al. (2018). Acute exposure to commonly ingested emulsifiers alters intestinal mucus structure and transport properties. *Sci. Rep.* 8: 10008. https://doi.org/10.1038/s41598-018-27957-2.
176. Chassaing, B., Koren, O., Goodrich, J. et al. (2015). Dietary emulsifiers impact the mouse gut microbiota promoting colitis and metabolic syndrome. *Nature* 519 (7541): 92–96. https://doi.org/10.1038/nature14232.
177. Rinninella, E., Cintoni, M., Raoul, P. et al. (2020). Food additives, gut microbiota, and irritable bowel syndrome: a hidden track. *Int. J. Environ. Res. Public Health* 17: 8816. https://doi.org/10.3390/ijerph17238816.
178. Fox, C.B., Hoeven, N.V., Granger, B. et al. (2019). Vaccine adjuvant activity of emulsified oils from species of the Pinaceae family. *Phytomedicine* 64: 152927. https://doi.org/10.1016/j.phymed.2019.152927.
179. Cui, X., Wang, Y., Guan, R. et al. (2020). Enhanced immune responses with serum proteomic analysis of hu sheep to foot-and-mouth disease vaccine emulsified in a vegetable oil adjuvant. *Vaccines (Basel)* 8: 180. https://doi.org/10.3390/vaccines8020180.
180. Yuan, L., Wang, Y., Li, Z. et al. (2020). Sunflower seed oil containing ginseng stem-leaf saponins (E515-D) is a safe adjuvant for Newcastle disease vaccine. *Poult. Sci.* 99: 4795–4803. https://doi.org/10.1016/j.psj.2020.06.063.
181. Moyle, P.M. and Toth, I. (2008). Self-adjuvanting lipopeptide vaccines. *Curr. Med. Chem.* 15: 506–516. https://doi.org/10.2174/092986708783503249.
182. Lodaya, R.N., Kanitkar, A.P., Friedrich, K. et al. (2019). Formulation design, optimization and in vivo evaluations of an alpha-tocopherol-containing self-emulsified adjuvant system using inactivated influenza vaccine. *J. Control. Release* 316: 12–21. https://doi.org/10.1016/j.jconrel.2019.10.042.
183. Bastola, R., Seo, J.E., Noh, G. et al. (2019). Determination of *Mycoplasma hyopneumoniae*-specific IgG, IgG1, and IgG2a titers in BALB/c mice induced by mineral oil-based oil-in-water emulsion adjuvants prepared using a self-emulsifying drug delivery system. *AAPS PharmSciTech* 20: 31. https://doi.org/10.1208/s12249-018-1245-3.
184. Yau, A.C.Y., Lönnblom, E., Zhong, J., and Holmdahl, R. (2017). Influence of hydrocarbon oil structure on adjuvanticity and autoimmunity. *Sci. Rep.* 7: 14998. https://doi.org/10.1038/s41598-017-15096-z.
185. Sverdrup, B., Källberg, H., Bengtsson, C. et al. (2005). Association between occupational exposure to mineral oil and rheumatoid arthritis: results from the Swedish EIRA case-control study. *Arthritis Res. Ther.* 7: R1296–R1303. https://doi.org/10.1186/ar1824.
186. Dahlgren, J., Takhar, H., Anderson-Mahoney, P. et al. (2007). Cluster of systemic lupus erythematosus (SLE) associated with an oil field waste site: a cross sectional study. *Environ. Health* 6: 8. https://doi.org/10.1186/1476-069X-6-8.

187. Massin, N., Bohadana, A.B., Wild, P. et al. (1996). Airway responsiveness, respiratory symptoms, and exposures to soluble oil mist in mechanical workers. *Occup. Environ. Med.* 53: 748–752. https://doi.org/10.1136/oem.53.11.748.
188. Yokoyama, A., Hamazaki, T., Ohshita, A. et al. (2000). Effect of aerosolized docosahexaenoic acid in a mouse model of atopic asthma. *Int. Arch. Allergy Immunol.* 123: 327–332. https://doi.org/10.1159/000053645.
189. Béliveau, S., Gaudreault, P., Goulet, L. et al. (2008). Type I hypersensitivity in an asthmatic child allergic to peanuts: was soy lecithin to blame? *J. Cutan. Med. Surg.* 12: 27–30. https://doi.org/10.2310/7750.2007.00031.
190. Hend, M.S., Beattie, B.E., and Burge, P.S. (1985). Occupational asthma due to an emulsified oil mist. *Br. J. Ind.* 42: 51–54. https://doi.org/10.1136/oem.42.1.51.
191. Xia, L., Yang, M., and Jiang, M. (2021). Food emulsifier glycerin monostearate aggravates phthalates' testicular toxicity by disrupting tight junctions' barrier function in rates. *Food Qual. Saf.* 5: fyab002. https://doi.org/10.1093/fqsafe/fyab002.
192. Bhattacharyya, S., Shumard, T., Xie, H. et al. (2017). A randomized trial of the effects of the no-carrageenan diet on ulcerative colitis disease activity. *J. Nutr. Healthy Aging* 4: 181–192. https://doi.org/10.3233/NHA-170023.
193. Marion-Letellier, R., Amamou, A., Savoye, G., and Ghosh, S. (2019). Inflammatory bowel diseases and food additives: to add fuel on the flames! *Nutrients* 11: 1111. https://doi.org/10.3390/nu11051111.
194. Tóth, C., Dabóczi, A., Howard, M. et al. (2016). Crohn's disease successfully treated with the paleolithic ketogenic diet. *Int. J. Case Rep. Images* 7: 570–578. https://doi.org/10.5348/ijcri-2016102-CR-10690.
195. Cong, H., Mui, E.J., Witola, W.H. et al. (2010). Human immunome, bioinformatic analyses using HLA supermotifs and the parasite genome, binding assays, studies of human T cell responses, and immunization of HLA-A*1101 transgenic mice including novel adjuvants provide a foundation for HLA-A03 restricted CD8+T cell epitope based, adjuvanted vaccine protective against Toxoplasma gondii. *Immunome Res.* 6: 12. https://doi.org/10.1186/1745-7580-6-12.
196. Alexander, J., Oseroff, C., Sidney, J., and Sette, A. (2003 Feb). Derivation of HLA-B*0702 transgenic mice: functional CTL repertoire and recognition of human B*0702-restricted CTL epitopes. *Hum. Immunol.* 64 (2): 211–223. https://doi.org/10.1016/s0198-8859(02)00786-3.
197. Arellano, B., Hussain, R., Zacharias, T. et al. (2012). Human aquaporin 4281-300 is the immunodominant linear determinant in the context of HLA-DRB1*03:01: relevance for diagnosing and monitoring patients with neuromyelitis optica. *Arch. Neurol.* 69 (9): 1125–1131. https://doi.org/10.1001/archneurol.2012.1300.
198. Schuhmacher, J., Heidu, S., Balchen, T. et al. (2020). Vaccination against RhoC induces long-lasting immune responses in patients with prostate cancer: results from a phase I/II clinical trial. *J. Immunother. Cancer* 8 (2): e001157. https://doi.org/10.1136/jitc-2020-001157.
199. Daiko, H., Marafioti, T., Fujiwara, T. et al. (2020). Exploratory open-label clinical study to determine the S-588410 cancer peptide vaccine-induced tumor-infiltrating lymphocytes and changes in the tumor microenvironment in esophageal cancer patients. *Cancer Immunol. Immunother.* 69: 2247–2257. https://doi.org/10.1007/s00262-020-02619-3.
200. Yau, A.C.Y., Tuncel, J., and Holmdahl, R. (2017). The major histocompatibility complex class III haplotype Ltab-Ncr3 regulates adjuvant-induced but not antigen-induced autoimmunity. *Am. J. Pathol.* 187: 987–998. https://doi.org/10.1016/j.ajpath.2016.12.022.
201. Akdis, C.A. (2021). Does the epithelial barrier hypothesis explain the increase in allergy, autoimmunity and other chronic conditions? *Nat. Rev. Immunol.* 21: 739–751. https://doi.org/10.1038/s41577-021-00538-7.
202. Song, H.P., Li, X., Yu, R. et al. (2015). Phenotypic characterization of type II collagen-induced arthritis in Wistar rats. *Exp. Ther. Med.* 10: 1483–1488. https://doi.org/10.3892/etm.2015.2667.
203. de Molon, R.S., Hsu, C., Bezouglaia, O. et al. (2016 Aug). Rheumatoid arthritis exacerbates the severity of osteonecrosis of the jaws (ONJ) in mice. A randomized, prospective, controlled animal study. *J. Bone Miner. Res.* 31 (8): 1596–1607. https://doi.org/10.1002/jbmr.2827.
204. Yin, J., Zheng, J., Deng, F. et al. (2018). Gene expression profiling of lacrimal glands identifies the ectopic expression of MHC II on glandular cells as a presymptomatic feature in a mouse model of primary Sjögren's syndrome. *Front. Immunol.* 9: 2362. https://doi.org/10.3389/fimmu.2018.02362.
205. Mancuso, C. and Barisani, D. (2019). Food additives can act as triggering factors in celiac disease: current knowledge based on a critical review of the literature. *World J. Clin. Cases* 7: 917–927. https://doi.org/10.12998/wjcc.v7.i8.917.

5 Silicone Implant Incompatibility Syndrome

Vânia Borba[1] and Yehuda Shoenfeld[2,3]

[1]Internal Medicine Departmente, Rehaklik Dussnang AG, Dussnang, Thurgau, Switzerland
[2]Zabludowicz Center for Autoimmune Diseases, Sheba Medical Center, Tel-Hashomer, Israel
[3]Reichman University, Herzliya, Israel

Highlights

- Silicone can act as an immunologic adjuvant, enhancing, accelerating, and/or prolonging an antigen-specific immune response.
- SBI cause characteristic systemic reactions in certain women with variable morbidity, frequently leading to symptoms of sufficient severity to warrant the silicone explantation.
- Clinical manifestations have been frequently misdiagnosed by the medical community, basing their conclusions in normal diagnostic tests.
- Symptoms such as chronic fatigue, depression, cognitive impairment, and sleep disturbances were recently found to be associated with SFN and dysregulated levels of circulating autoantibodies.
- The hyperactivation of the immune system can culminate in immune deficiencies, autoimmune reactions, and a chronic inflammatory state, leading in some cases to malignant transformation.
- To date, more than 500 women worldwide have developed anaplastic large cell lymphoma around breast implants, strongly suggesting a cause-and-effect relationship.
- The decision surrounding silicone implantation should be made based on an individualized analysis of each patient and its clinical history.

Introduction

Since 1960s, silicone breast implants (SBI) have been widely used in the medical field for both cosmetic and reconstruction purposes. To date, more than one million breast augmentation procedures using SBI have been performed worldwide [1]. Despite years of technological advancement in the composition and manufacturing, the basic design largely remains the same [2]. Silicone is a branched polymer that has been obtained from silica atoms, which means it cannot be found in

Autoimmune Disorders: Adjuvants and Other Risk Factors in Pathogenesis, First Edition.
Edited by Abdulla Watad, Nicola Luigi Bragazzi, and Yehuda Shoenfeld.

nature. Interestingly, long exposure of humans to silica has already shown to trigger the development of autoimmune diseases (AID) [3, 4].

At the beginning, medical societies have mistakenly considered silicone to be an inert material in relation to the human body and the immune system. Nevertheless, following numerous new reports claiming association of SBI with various health conditions, the safety of silicone has resurged as a major public health crisis [5]. In 2020, the *Food and Drug Administration* (FDA) declared to have received 2497 medical device reports of SBI causing symptoms consistent with Breast Implant Illness (BII) between November 2018 and October 2019, illustrating the growing scope of this problem [6]. Since 2017, SBI removal has increased overall by 34.4%, while breast augmentation procedures have decreased by 14.9% [7].

The autoimmune syndrome induced by adjuvants (ASIA) illustrates the role of environmental immune stimulating agents, or adjuvants, in the instigation of complex autoimmune reactions among individuals bearing a genetic preponderance [8]. Hence, the emergence of ASIA syndrome is associated with individual genetic predisposition, for instance those carrying HLA-DRB1*01 or HLA-DRB4, and results from exposure to external and/or endogenous adjuvants [5, 9]. All five clinical entities of the ASIA syndrome share similar clinical manifestations, as mentioned before [10]. In addition, they might be associated with the appearance of autoantibodies and tend to improve once the inciting agent is removed [11]. Consequently, the hyperactivation of the immune system can culminate in immune deficiencies, autoimmune reactions, or a chronic inflammatory state, leading in some cases to malignancy, such as non-Hodgkin lymphoma [9, 12–15]. Adjuvants have demonstrated to be able to induce autoimmune phenomena in both animal models and humans via diverse mechanisms including effects on cellular immunity, polyclonal activation of B cells, and alteration of the host's immune system [16, 17]. Their influence, both on the innate and adaptive arms of the immune system, encourages the initiation and perpetuation of aberrant immune response by the activation of pattern recognition receptors [18].

Silicone as an immunologic adjuvant

Silicone implantations have led to a significant increase in heterogeneous and enigmatic symptoms such as severe fatigue, widespread pain, impaired cognition, sleep disturbances, depression, headache, dry eyes and/or mouth, hair loss, morning stiffness, paresthesia, lymphadenopathy, and fever, resembling chronic fatigue syndrome (CFS) and fibromyalgia (Figure 5.1) [5]. In the past years, those complaints in patients with SBI have been named differently: adjuvant breast disease, silicone-related symptom complex, siliconosis, and, more recently, ASIA syndrome due to SIIB [19]. There is not of a doubt that silicone can act as an immunologic adjuvant, enhancing, accelerating, and/or prolonging an antigen-specific immune response. As part of an inflammatory response to a foreign body, a capsule around the implant is formed following SBI insertion, which is an expectable reaction to a nondegradable material too large to be engulfed by macrophages. Even in the absence of implant rupture signs, "bleeding" of silicone into the surrounding tissues comprises another possible, and not rare, complication [20]. Yu et al. calculated that the silicone diffusion of several implant models was approximately 300 mg/year [21]. Since then, several reports have described how silicone originating from ruptured SBI can cause subcutaneous nodules and lead to the development of siliconomas [22–24]. Furthermore, the continued stimulus of silicone particles leads to chronic immune activation, BII/ASIA, AID, allergies, immune deficiencies, and even malignancy (Figure 5.2) [25]. To date, more than 500 women worldwide have developed a $CD30^+$ T-cell lymphoma around SBI, designated as breast implant-associated anaplastic large cell lymphoma (BIA-ALCL), strongly suggesting a cause-and-effect relationship. In this manner, the World Health Organization (WHO) has recognized it in 2016 as a rare type of non-Hodgkin's lymphoma that can occur after SBI placement, regardless of the cosmetic or reconstructive purpose of the surgery [26].

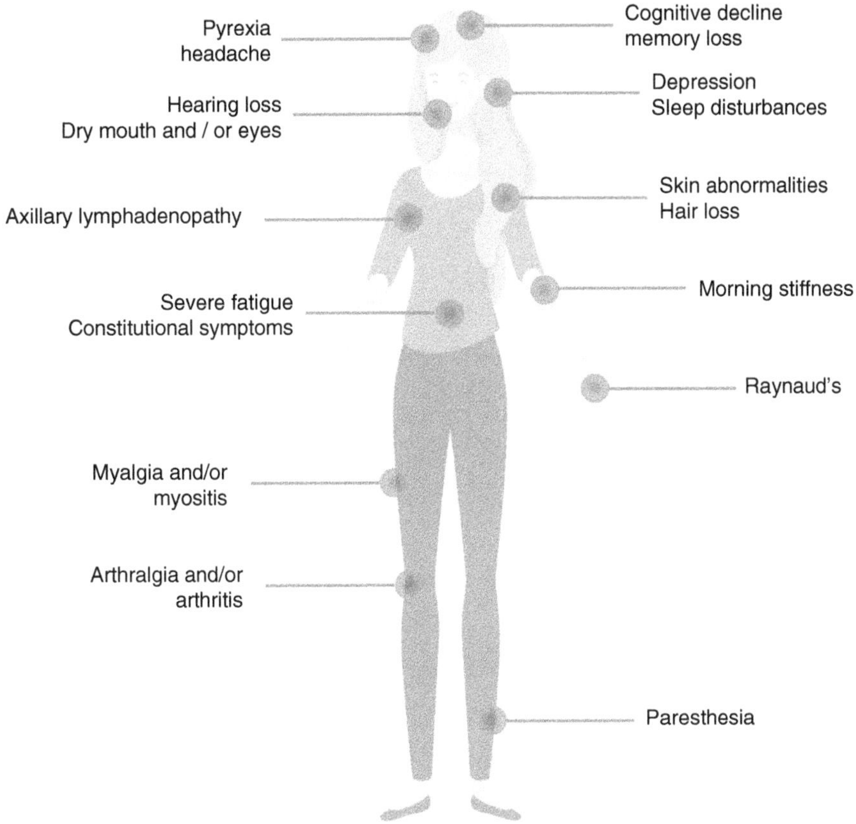

Figure 5.1 Commonly associated clinical manifestations in patients with SIIS.

Pathophysiological mechanisms of inflammatory/immunological disturbances related to SBI

SBI are associated with acute and further chronic, and granulomatous, inflammation processes, leading to capsule formation and fibrosis [27]. Indeed, capsular fibrosis has been seen to result from fibroblast proliferation. Moreover, silicone may also induce an immunogenic response via cross-reactions with glucosaminoglycans, natural, and silicone-containing molecules found in connective tissues [28]. There is still some debate as whether silicon-based reaction is an acquired or cross-reactive entity or even a direct immune reaction stimulated after nonspecific polyclonal activation. Hence, silicone has proven to be immunogenic for delayed-type hypersensitivity reactions [28–30].

The rupture of an SBI or the migration of silicone compounds through the implant's envelope leads to the mount of an inflammatory reaction with recruitment of antigen presenting cells (APCs). These, in turn, proliferate and can develop oncogenic mutations. In addition, silicone can also provoke B-cell stimulation through dysregulated expression of B-cell activating factor (BAFF) by dendritic cells, exhilarating autoantibody formation, polyclonal hypergammaglobulinemia which can progress to monoclonality, and subsequently development of lymphoma [14, 27, 31].

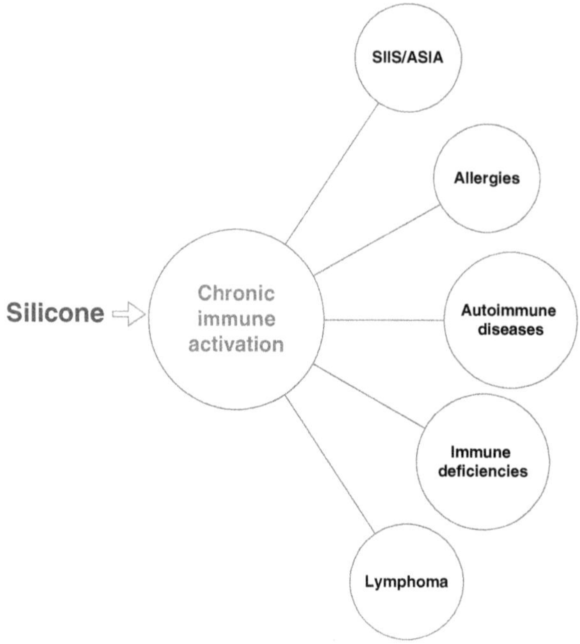

Figure 5.2 Clinical entities related with chronic immune activation due to silicone stimulus as an adjuvant.

Some authors report that the inflammatory triggering process can also be secondary to the formation of a biofilm in the SBI surface. Both the silicone and the biofilm can enhance the inflammasome, prompting the release of pro-inflammatory cytokines such as interleukin (IL)-1 and IL-18, which trigger the inflammatory reactions. In a long-term stimulation, it would lead to a more significant response of activated TH1/TH17 cells, promoting the production of profibrotic cytokines as a result of a failure in the capacity of regulatory T cells [31]. Th1/Th17-derived cytokines (i.e. IL-17, IL-6, IL-8, transforming growth factor-β1, and interferon-γ) perpetuate the immune reaction, eventually leading to polyclonal/monoclonal lymphocytic activation [27]. Additionally, the presence of eosinophils and mast cells covered with Immunoglobulin (Ig) E in tumor tissue of patients with BIA-ALCL (characteristic of the allergic inflammation associated with IL-13) supports the pathogenesis being based on an amplified immune response with characteristics of a chronic allergic reaction (features typically absent in systemic ALCL, without association with SBI) [32].

Silicone implant incompatibility syndrome

In September 2020, the FDA published recommendations to incorporate the BII as part of the informed consent form and as a boxed warning for all types of SBI [6]. The silicones present in the breast implants represent an external nonself, chronic stimulus that may lead to hyperstimulation of the immune system, and appearance of nonspecific subjective clinical manifestations, and autoantibody production [33]. Both autoinflammatory and -immune disorders are characterized by aberrant changes in innate and adaptive immunity that may result in organ-specific damage. Nevertheless, a genetic predisposition has been found to be condition *sine qua non* in the development of autoimmunity. Almost 30 years ago, Young et al. reported that silicone breast-implanted women with autoimmune symptoms were positive for HLA-DR5 and HLA-DQ2 when compared to asymptomatic women with SBI, raising the possibility that HLA genotype might serve as a marker for women who are predisposed to develop autoimmune symptoms following exposure to SBI [34].

Parallel to the myriad of symptoms associated with SBI, increased risk of developing AID has also been observed. Suh et al. performed an extensive review of epidemiological studies in the past 10 years and exhibited evidence affirming an association between SBI and AID [35]. The most recognized diseases were Sjögren's syndrome, rheumatoid arthritis, systemic sclerosis, CFS, and Raynaud's phenomena [9, 36–40].

Subjective/autonomic-related manifestations complained by symptomatic women with SBI are known to be reported also in patients with other suspected autoimmune dysautonomic-related disorders such as CFS, postural orthostatic tachycardia syndrome, and fibromyalgia syndrome [5]. Zandman-Goddard et al. investigated the frequency of autoantibody production in asymptomatic compared to symptomatic women with SBI. The authors found that the incidence of increased titers of autoantibodies ranged from 2% to 13% for 13 different autoantibodies among asymptomatic women. Polyclonality was more prominent in the group of symptomatic women with SBI but also evident in asymptomatic women. Interestingly, the development of autoantibodies may be related to implant duration, since the mean duration of implant in the asymptomatic group was significantly less compared with the symptomatic group ($p < 0.01$) [41]. More recently, Shoenfeld et al. [42] proposed a novel common explanation to the nonspecific clinical manifestations reported by women with SBI and other ASIA-related entities, small-fiber neuropathy (SFN), and the appearance of circulating autonomic autoantibodies in patients with SBI [43, 44]. Circulating autoantibodies against G protein-coupled receptors (anti-GPCR) of the autonomic nervous systems, such as adrenergic and muscarinic acetylcholine receptors, have been found in the sera of women with SBI, which might be the common denominator to the enigmatic, subjective, and undefined symptomatology [42, 45]. Several functional IgG autoantibodies targeting GPCRs are associated with AID, including antiadrenergic receptors (α1AR, α2AR, β1AR, and β2AR), antimuscarinic acetylcholine receptors (M1R–M5R), anti-endothelin receptor type A (ETAR), and antitype 1 angiotensin II receptor (AT1R) [46]. Tocut et al. explored the potential association between circulating autoantibodies against the autonomic nervous system and cognitive impairment, memory deficit, and depressive symptoms. Significant changes in the titters of anti-β1AR, anti-AT1R, and anti-ETAR autoantibodies in women with SBI, as compared with age-matched healthy women, were detected. Notably, anti-β1AR autoantibody was found to be significantly associated with autonomic-related manifestations such as depression and sleep disorders [47]. Importantly, anti-GPCR autoantibody and SFN could serve as probable new biomarkers for these subgroups.

Assorted patients with silicone implant incompatibility syndrome (SIIS) also fulfill the criteria for CFS, fibromyalgia, sarcoidosis, and/or undifferentiated connective tissue disease (UCTD) [48]. In 2013, Tervaert et al. reported 32 cases of patients with ASIA due to SIIS. The median time between the start of complaints and the time of SBI was 10 years (2–24 years); 53% of the ASIA patients had an established systemic AID, 22% of patients had an organ-specific AID, and 47% of patients had a humoral immunodeficiency (either hypogammaglobulinemia or a IgG subclass deficiency) [49].

Autoimmune diseases in patients with SIIS

Since the recognition of ASIA, more than 4400 documented cases have been reported so far, showing heterogeneous clinical manifestations and diverse severity of the complains [50]. Nevertheless, the exact prevalence of symptomatology in patients with SBI is unknown [40]. In order to better understand the link between different adjuvants and the spectrum of inflammation against self, an international registry of ASIA syndrome was created in 2011. By 2016, more than 200 cases of ASIA syndrome were identified following exposure to SBI. Despite modifications in the SBI components during the past half century, silicone still produces a chronic stimulus of the immune system, yielding similar clinical manifestations as observed in many large cohorts of patients [51]. A meta-analysis presented by Balk et al., which pooled outcomes from 32 observational studies, found statistically significant increased incidence of autoimmune/rheumatic disorders, such as Sjögren's syndrome, systemic sclerosis, and sarcoidosis in women with SBI [40]. More recently, Watad et al. has performed a large cross-sectional study, using the computerized database system of the *Maccabi Healthcare Services* (Israel), which provides data of 2 million clients with a mean follow-up of 20 years. The study enrolled 24,651 women with SBI matched with 98,604 women without SBI. The adjusted OR between being recipient of the implant and being diagnosed with any autoimmune/rheumatic diseases was 1.22 [95% CI 1.18–1.26], with the strongest associations with SBI being found for Sjögren' syndrome (OR 1.58), systemic sclerosis (OR 1.63), and sarcoidosis (OR 1.98) [9], supporting previous findings of published studies. Furthermore, the presence of positive antibodies was evident in up to 54.4% of the cases of women with SIIS [52]. In 2019, Khoos et al. aimed to relate clinical manifestations of fibromyalgia, depression, and CFS in patients with SBI, when compared with a control group of systemic lupus erythematosus and scleroderma patients. Significantly more patients with fibromyalgia and/or CFS in the SBI case group were found, when matched to the controls (20.0% of cases versus 2.2% of scleroderma controls, $p = 0.01$) [38]. In addition, a great coin supporting the concept of the ASIA syndrome has been recently presented by Burja et al. on a case report of a patient with granulomatosis with polyangiitis and $PR3^+$ ANCA antibodies, with three years history of SBI and five weeks after COVID-19 vaccination. Interestingly, the symptoms were initially mainly localized to implanted breast tissue along with constitutional symptoms, primarily suggesting silicone-induced autoimmune reaction. Indeed, silicone implants could presumably induce chronic adverse reaction of immune system that was acutely exacerbated by vaccine-trigged immune activation, culminating in a severe granulomatosis with polyangiitis [53].

Nevertheless, such a wide array of clinical manifestations is still today frequently misdiagnosed by the medical community who examined those patients, basing their conclusions in normal diagnostic tests (routine serologies, electromyography, etc.).

Effectivity of SBI explantation in improving symptoms and laboratory findings

A pivotal study reflecting the results of SBI removal in patients with silicone-related complaints and/or AID was recently performed by Boer et al., who performed a critical review of the existing literature. The authors analyzed previously published studies and concluded that explantation was able to improve silicone-related complaints in approximately 75% of the patients [19]. Likewise, 56% of women with established AID ameliorated the disease course. However, subjects who have already developed AID needed additional treatment with immunosuppressive drugs to induce remission of the disease [54].

Hence, some reports also related the implant-removal effect with the laboratory findings. Interestingly, antinuclear antibodies (ANA) remained positive in all presented case reports after the SBI explantation [54–57]. This raises the question of whether those autoantibodies can predict and precede the development of AID in women with SBI. Unfortunately, few data are available with respect to the effect of reconstruction after implant removal. For example, the explantation of the SBI in three symptomatic sisters, and subsequently replacement of hydrocellulose-filled implants, was followed by full recovery evaluated 2.5 years later. Indeed, the generation of ASIA in three sisters supports that the susceptibility to the development of SIIS may be genetically determined [57]. Another study enrolling 35 patients who underwent explantation of the SBI (with or without capsulectomy), followed by immediate reconstruction with a hydrocellulose-filled implants, revealed significant improvement in symptoms [58]. In contrast, a case of a 53-year-old woman with morphea who underwent replacement of a silicone implant by a saline-filled implant with a polyurethane capsule did not result in disease improvement [59]. Further, in another cohort, only 32, 4% of the 37 patients who underwent replacement of SBI and subsequently reconstruction with autologous tissue (*transverse rectus abdominis* flap or *latissimus dorsi* flap), presented ameliorated symptoms six months postoperative [60].

Assorted possibilities could explain why women improve their clinical condition after SBI removal [19]:

1. Explantation of the SBI results in reduction in the autoimmune/inflammatory response.
2. SBI removal decreases nociceptive signals, in which a disturbed pain signaling pathway due to the silicone nociceptive stimulus, cause excessive stimulation of neurotransmitters in the central nervous system and therefore provoke the systemic complaints.

In the same manner, the unsuccessful removal of SBI in improving symptoms and laboratory findings could be explained by the silicone particles migration into the periprosthetic tissue, lymph nodes, and other tissues [24, 61]. This implies that silicone particles remain present in the body after explantation, perpetuating the detrimental stimulus. Migration of silicone from implant "bleeds" typically follows the lymphatic pathway; however, it can spread widely. Additionally, there is also a possibility that surgical removal of the SBI may lead to dissemination of silicone or other substances in the whole body, thereby worsening the patient symptoms and/or disease course [24].

SIIS, who might be at risk?

Development of autoimmunity is believed to result from complex multifactorial interactions, involving both a genetic predisposition and an additional trigger. Since ASIA is considered to be a group of exacerbated immune responses resulting from chronic immune stimulation by adjuvants, the following patients are considered to be at risk of developing SIIS when exposed to silicones [20, 62]:

1. Patients with prior documented autoimmune reaction to an adjuvant (coadjuvant effect) [63–65].
   a. Vaccines, implants, etc.
2. Patients with established autoimmune conditions [66–68].
   a. Higher risk of developing another AID.
   b. Prone to develop autoantibodies upon presentation of exogenous adjuvants.
3. Individuals who are susceptible to develop autoimmunity: genetic predisposition and/or exposure to relevant environmental triggers [56, 69–71].
   a. HLA-DR4, DRB1, DR53, DQA1*0102, and HLA-C.
   b. Clustering of AID in the family.
   c. Active smoking, obesity, infections, toxics, etc.
4. Patients with history of allergic conditions/atopic disorders [72].
   a. Up to 75% of women who developed silicone-induced ASIA reported preexisting allergic conditions prior to silicone implantation.
   b. Eczema, hay fever, pollen and dust mite's allergy, drug allergy, rubber or latex allergy, etc.

In this manner, the decision surrounding silicone implantation should be made based on an individualized analysis of each patient and its clinical history.

Conclusion

The safety of SBI has stirred an intense debate, concerning their potential for induction of autoimmunity and lymphoma. With currently significant increase in public awareness, SIIS is perhaps becoming the most controversial subject in aesthetic and reconstructive breast surgery. SBI cause characteristic systemic reactions in certain women with variable morbidity, frequently leading to symptoms of sufficient severity to warrant the silicone explantation. Nevertheless, such a wide array of manifestations has been frequently misdiagnosed by the medical community who examined those patients, basing their conclusions in normal diagnostic tests (routine serologies, electromyography, etc.). The importance of recognizing this panoply of symptoms resulting from adjuvant exposure is twofold: (i) for the patients who without a clear medical definition may wander endlessly though health care systems with no validation for their diseases and, more importantly, without proper treatment and (ii) perhaps most significantly, the urgent need to start adequately adjusted epidemiological studies to obtain not only better evidence but also possible preventive and curative measures.

Abbreviations

ANA	Antinuclear antibodies
AID	Autoimmune diseases
Anti-GPCR	Autoantibodies against G protein-coupled receptor
APC	Antigen presenting cells
ASIA	Autoimmune/Inflammatory Syndrome Induced by Adjuvants
BIA-ALCL	Breast implant-associated anaplastic large cell lymphoma
BII	Breast implant illness
CFS	Chronic fatigue syndrome
COVID-19	Coronavirus disease 2019
FDA	Food and Drug Administration
Ig	Immunoglobulin
IL	Interleukin
SBI	Silicone breast implants
SIIS	Silicone implant incompatibility syndrome
SNF	Small-fiber neuropathy
UCTD	Undifferentiated connective tissue disease
WHO	World Health Organization

References

1. Maldonado, G., Guerrero, R., Intriago, M., and Rios, C. (2021). Autoinflammatory/autoimmunity syndrome induced by adjuvants (ASIA) due to silicone incompatibility syndrome. *Case Rep. Rheumatol.* 2021: 5595739.
2. Maxwell, G.P. and Gabriel, A. (2017). Breast implant design. *Gland Surg.* 6 (2): 148–153.
3. Boudigaard, S.H., Schlünssen, V., Vestergaard, J.M. et al. (2021). Occupational exposure to respirable crystalline silica and risk of autoimmune rheumatic diseases: a nationwide cohort study. *Int. J. Epidemiol.* 50 (4): 1213–1226.
4. Pollard, K.M. (2016). Silica, silicosis, and autoimmunity. *Front. Immunol.* 7: 97.
5. Halpert, G., Amital, H., and Shoenfeld, Y. (2022). Silicone breast illness as a classical example of autoimmune/inflammatory syndrome induced by adjuvant (ASIA). *Isr. Med. Assoc. J.* 24 (6): 357–359.
6. U.S. FDA. (2020). Breast Implants - Certain labeling recommendations to improve patient communication - Guidance for Industry and Food and Drug Administration Staff.

7. Ranieri, J., Fiasca, F., Guerra, F. et al. (2021). Examining the post-operative well-being of women who underwent mammoplasty: a cross-sectional study. *Front. Psychiatry* 12: 645102.
8. Shoenfeld, Y. and Agmon-Levin, N. (2011). "ASIA" - autoimmune/inflammatory syndrome induced by adjuvants. *J. Autoimmun.* 36 (1): 4–8.
9. Watad, A., Rosenberg, V., Tiosano, S. et al. (2018). Silicone breast implants and the risk of autoimmune/rheumatic disorders: a real-world analysis. *Int. J. Epidemiol.* 47 (6): 1846–1854.
10. Segal, Y., Dahan, S., Sharif, K. et al. (2018). The value of autoimmune syndrome induced by adjuvant (ASIA) - shedding light on orphan diseases in autoimmunity. *Autoimmun. Rev.* 17 (5): 440–448.
11. Watad, A., Sharif, K., and Shoenfeld, Y. (2017). The ASIA syndrome: basic concepts. *Mediterr. J. Rheumatol.* 28 (2): 64–69.
12. Moling, O., Piccin, A., Tauber, M. et al. (2016). Intravascular large B-cell lymphoma associated with silicone breast implant, HLA-DRB1*11:01, and HLA-DQB1*03:01 manifesting as macrophage activation syndrome and with severe neurological symptoms: a case report. *J. Med. Case Rep.* 10 (1): 254.
13. Groth, K. and A, Graf R. (2020). Breast implant-associated anaplastic large cell lymphoma (BIA-ALCL) and the textured breast implant crisis. *Aesthet. Plast. Surg.* 44 (1): 1–12.
14. Fleming, D., Stone, J., and Tansley, P. (2018). Spontaneous regression and resolution of breast implant-associated anaplastic large cell lymphoma: implications for research, diagnosis and clinical management. *Aesthet. Plast. Surg.* 42 (3): 672–678.
15. Patzelt, M., Zarubova, L., Klener, P. et al. (2018). Anaplastic large-cell lymphoma associated with breast implants: a case report of a transgender female. *Aesthet. Plast. Surg.* 42 (2): 451–455.
16. Schaefer, C.J. and Wooley, P.H. (1999). The influence of silicone implantation on murine lupus in MRL lpr/lpr mice. *J. Rheumatol.* 26 (10): 2215–2221.
17. McDonald, A.H., Weir, K., Schneider, M. et al. (1998). Silicone gel enhances the development of autoimmune disease in New Zealand black mice but fails to induce it in BALB/cAnPt mice. *Clin. Immunol. Immunopathol.* 87 (3): 248–255.
18. Naim, J.O., Satoh, M., Buehner, N.A. et al. (2000). Induction of hypergammaglobulinemia and macrophage activation by silicone gels and oils in female A.SW mice. *Clin. Diagn. Lab. Immunol.* 7 (3): 366–370.
19. de Boer, M., Colaris, M., van der Hulst, R.R.W.J., and Cohen Tervaert, J.W. (2017). Is explantation of silicone breast implants useful in patients with complaints? *Immunol. Res.* 65 (1): 25–36.
20. Perricone, C., Colafrancesco, S., Mazor, R.D. et al. (2013). Autoimmune/inflammatory syndrome induced by adjuvants (ASIA) 2013: unveiling the pathogenic, clinical and diagnostic aspects. *J. Autoimmun.* 47: 1–16.
21. Yu, L.T., Latorre, G., Marotta, J. et al. (1996). In vitro measurement of silicone bleed from breast implants. *Plast. Reconstr. Surg.* 97 (4): 756–764.
22. Sagi, L., Baum, S., Lyakhovitsky, A. et al. (2009). Silicone breast implant rupture presenting as bilateral leg nodules. *Clin. Exp. Dermatol.* 34 (5): e99–e101.
23. Dragu, A., Theegarten, D., Bach, A.D. et al. (2009). Intrapulmonary and cutaneous siliconomas after silent silicone breast implant failure. *Breast J.* 15 (5): 496–499.
24. Todorov, T.I., de Bakker, E., Smith, D. et al. (2021). A case of silicone and sarcoid granulomas in a patient with "highly cohesive" silicone breast implants: a histopathologic and laser Raman microprobe analysis. *Int. J. Environ. Res. Public Health* 18 (9): 4526.
25. Cohen Tervaert, J.W., Mohazab, N., Redmond, D. et al. (2022). Breast implant illness: scientific evidence of its existence. *Expert. Rev. Clin. Immunol.* 18 (1): 15–29.
26. Swerdlow, S.H., Campo, E., Pileri, S.A. et al. (2016). The 2016 revision of the World Health Organization classification of lymphoid neoplasms. *Blood* 127 (20): 2375–2390.
27. Bizjak, M., Selmi, C., Praprotnik, S. et al. (2015). Silicone implants and lymphoma: the role of inflammation. *J. Autoimmun.* 65: 64–73.
28. Watad, A., Quaresma, M., Brown, S. et al. (2017). Autoimmune/inflammatory syndrome induced by adjuvants (Shoenfeld's syndrome) - an update. *Lupus* 26 (7): 675–681.
29. Cimolai, N. (2020). Mast cell biology and linkages for non-clonal mast cell activation and autoimmune/inflammatory syndrome induced by adjuvants. *SN Compr. Clin. Med.* 2 (11): 2310–2323.
30. André, D., Gouveia, F., Nascimento, R. et al. (2022). ASIA syndrome: adverse reaction or autoimmunity? *J. R. Soc. Med. Open* 13 (4): 20542704221086170.

31. Turner, S.D., Inghirami, G., Miranda, R.N., and Kadin, M.E. (2020). Cell of origin and immunologic events in the pathogenesis of breast implant-associated anaplastic large-cell lymphoma. *Am. J. Pathol.* 190 (1): 2–10.
32. Kadin, M.E., Morgan, J., Xu, H. et al. (2018). IL-13 is produced by tumor cells in breast implant-associated anaplastic large cell lymphoma: implications for pathogenesis. *Hum. Pathol.* 78: 54–62.
33. Borba, V., Malkova, A., Basantsova, N. et al. (2020). Classical examples of the concept of the ASIA syndrome. *Biomol. Ther.* 10 (10): E1436.
34. Young, V.L., Nemecek, J.R., Schwartz, B.D. et al. (1995). HLA typing in women with breast implants. *Plast. Reconstr. Surg.* 96 (7): 1497–1519. discussion 1520.
35. Suh, L.J., Khan, I., Kelley-Patteson, C. et al. (2022). Breast implant-associated immunological disorders. *J. Immunol. Res.* 2022: 8536149.
36. Singh, N., Picha, G.J., Hardas, B. et al. (2017). Five-year safety data for more than 55,000 subjects following breast implantation: comparison of rare adverse event rates with silicone implants versus national norms and saline implants. *Plast. Reconstr. Surg.* 140 (4): 666–679.
37. Lee, I.M., Cook, N.R., Shadick, N.A. et al. (2011). Prospective cohort study of breast implants and the risk of connective-tissue diseases. *Int. J. Epidemiol.* 40 (1): 230–238.
38. Khoo, T., Proudman, S., and Limaye, V. (2019). Silicone breast implants and depression, fibromyalgia and chronic fatigue syndrome in a rheumatology clinic population. *Clin. Rheumatol.* 38 (5): 1271–1276.
39. Coroneos, C.J., Selber, J.C., Offodile, A.C. et al. (2019). US FDA breast implant postapproval studies: long-term outcomes in 99,993 patients. *Ann. Surg.* 269 (1): 30–36.
40. Balk, E.M., Earley, A., Avendano, E.A., and Raman, G. (2016). Long-term health outcomes in women with silicone gel breast implants: a systematic review. *Ann. Intern. Med.* 164 (3): 164–175.
41. Zandman-Goddard, G., Blank, M., Ehrenfeld, M. et al. (1999). A comparison of autoantibody production in asymptomatic and symptomatic women with silicone breast implants. *J. Rheumatol.* 26 (1): 73–77.
42. Shoenfeld, Y., Ryabkova, V.A., Scheibenbogen, C. et al. (2020). Complex syndromes of chronic pain, fatigue and cognitive impairment linked to autoimmune dysautonomia and small fiber neuropathy. *Clin. Immunol.* 214: 108384.
43. Halpert, G., Watad, A., Tsur, A.M. et al. (2021). Autoimmune dysautonomia in women with silicone breast implants. *J. Autoimmun.* 120: 102631.
44. Gavrilova, N.Y., Lukashenko, M., Churilov, L., and Shoenfeld, Y. (2022). Autoimmune small fiber neuropathy: is there a place for the confocal microscopy? *Isr. Med. Assoc. J.* 24 (4): [cited 2022 Jul 11]. https://www.ima.org.il/MedicineIMAJ/viewarticle.aspx?year=2022&month=04&page=271.
45. Halpert, G., Amital, H., and Shoenfeld, Y. (2020). Dysregulation of G protein-coupled receptors of the autonomic nervous system, adrenergic and muscarinic acetylcholine receptors, in patients with autoimmune dysautonomic-related disorders. *Brain. Behav. Immun. Health* 4: 100056.
46. Cabral-Marques, O. and Riemekasten, G. (2017). Functional autoantibodies targeting G protein-coupled receptors in rheumatic diseases. *Nat. Rev. Rheumatol.* 13 (11): 648–656.
47. Tocut, M., Halpert, G., Tsur, A.M. et al. (2022). Cognitive impairment, sleep disturbance, and depression in women with silicone breast implants: association with autoantibodies against autonomic nervous system receptors. *Biomol. Ther.* 12 (6): 776.
48. Tervaert, J.W.C., Colaris, M.J., and van der Hulst, R.R. (2017). Silicone breast implants and autoimmune rheumatic diseases: myth or reality. *Curr. Opin. Rheumatol.* 29 (4): 348–354.
49. Cohen Tervaert, J.W. and Kappel, R.M. (2013). Silicone implant incompatibility syndrome (SIIS): a frequent cause of ASIA (Shoenfeld's syndrome). *Immunol. Res.* 56 (2–3): 293–298.
50. Jara, L.J., García-Collinot, G., Medina, G. et al. (2017). Severe manifestations of autoimmune syndrome induced by adjuvants (Shoenfeld's syndrome). *Immunol. Res.* 65 (1): 8–16.
51. Colaris, M.J.L., de Boer, M., van der Hulst, R.R., and Cohen Tervaert, J.W. (2017). Two hundreds cases of ASIA syndrome following silicone implants: a comparative study of 30 years and a review of current literature. *Immunol. Res.* 65 (1): 120–128.
52. Watad, A., Bragazzi, N.L., McGonagle, D. et al. (2019). Autoimmune/inflammatory syndrome induced by adjuvants (ASIA) demonstrates distinct autoimmune and autoinflammatory disease associations according to the adjuvant subtype: insights from an analysis of 500 cases. *Clin. Immunol.* 203: 1–8.
53. Burja, B., Hočevar, A., Šekoranja, D. et al. (2022). PR3-ANCA vasculitis as manifestation of ASIA syndrome following aesthetic breast augmentation: a new kid on the block? *Clin. Exp. Rheumatol.* 40 (4): 865–866.

54. Kivity, S., Katz, M., Langevitz, P. et al. (2012). Autoimmune syndrome induced by adjuvants (ASIA) in the Middle East: morphea following silicone implantation. *Lupus* 21 (2): 136–139.
55. Jara, L.J., Medina, G., Gómez-Bañuelos, E. et al. (2012). Still's disease, lupus-like syndrome, and silicone breast implants. A case of "ASIA" (Shoenfeld's syndrome). *Lupus* 21 (2): 140–145.
56. Levy, Y., Rotman-Pikielny, P., Ehrenfeld, M., and Shoenfeld, Y. (2009). Silicone breast implantation-induced scleroderma: description of four patients and a critical review of the literature. *Lupus* 18 (13): 1226–1232.
57. Kappel, R.M., Cohen Tervaert, J.W., and Pruijn, G.J.M. (2014). Autoimmune/inflammatory syndrome induced by adjuvants (ASIA) due to silicone implant incompatibility syndrome in three sisters. *Clin. Exp. Rheumatol.* 32 (2): 256–258.
58. Kappel, R.M. and Pruijn, G.J.M. (2012). The monobloc hydrogel breast implant, experiences and ideas. *Eur. J. Plast. Surg.* 35 (3): 229–233.
59. Granel, B., Serratrice, J., Gaudy, C. et al. (2001). Localized morphea after silicone-gel-filled breast implant. *Dermatology* 202 (2): 143–144. [cited 2022 Jul 9]; https://www.scienceopen.com/document?vid=3518a90e-079d-477e-bb28-978770049ca4.
60. Godfrey, P.M. and Godfrey, N.V. (1996). Response of locoregional and systemic symptoms to breast implant replacement with autologous tissues: experience in 37 consecutive patients. *Plast. Reconstr. Surg.* 97 (1): 110–116.
61. Hajdu, S.D., Agmon-Levin, N., and Shoenfeld, Y. (2011). Silicone and autoimmunity. *Eur. J. Clin. Investig.* 41 (2): 203–211.
62. Goren, I., Segal, G., and Shoenfeld, Y. (2015). Autoimmune/inflammatory syndrome induced by adjuvant (ASIA) evolution after silicone implants. Who is at risk? *Clin. Rheumatol.* 34 (10): 1661–1666.
63. Vera-Lastra, O., Medina, G., Cruz-Dominguez, M.D.P. et al. (2013). Autoimmune/inflammatory syndrome induced by adjuvants (Shoenfeld's syndrome): clinical and immunological spectrum. *Expert. Rev. Clin. Immunol.* 9 (4): 361–373.
64. Konstantinou, D., Paschalis, C., Maraziotis, T. et al. (2001). Two episodes of leukoencephalitis associated with recombinant hepatitis B vaccination in a single patient. *Clin. Infect. Dis.* 33 (10): 1772–1773.
65. Nancy, A.L. and Shoenfeld, Y. (2008). Chronic fatigue syndrome with autoantibodies--the result of an augmented adjuvant effect of hepatitis-B vaccine and silicone implant. *Autoimmun. Rev.* 8 (1): 52–55.
66. Wallace, D.J., Basbug, E., Schwartz, E. et al. (1996). A comparison of systemic lupus erythematosus and scleroderma patients with and without silicone breast implants. *J. Clin. Rheumatol.* 2 (5): 257–261.
67. Al Aranji, G., White, D., and Solanki, K. (2014). Scleroderma renal crisis following silicone breast implant rupture: a case report and review of the literature. *Clin. Exp. Rheumatol.* 32 (2): 262–266.
68. Lazzaroni, M.G., Campochiaro, C., Bertoldo, E. et al. (2021). Association of anti-RNA polymerase III antibody with silicone breast implants rupture in a multicentre series of Italian patients with systemic sclerosis. *Clin. Exp. Rheumatol.* 39 (4): 25–28.
69. Somers, E.C., Thomas, S.L., Smeeth, L., and Hall, A.J. (2006). Autoimmune diseases co-occurring within individuals and within families: a systematic review. *Epidemiology* 17 (2): 202–217.
70. Kawai, V.K., Shi, M., Feng, Q. et al. (2020). Pleiotropy in the genetic predisposition to rheumatoid arthritis: a phenome-wide association study and inverse variance-weighted meta-analysis. *Arthritis Rheumatol.* 72 (9): 1483–1492.
71. Versini, M., Jeandel, P.Y., Rosenthal, E., and Shoenfeld, Y. (2014). Obesity in autoimmune diseases: not a passive bystander. *Autoimmun. Rev.* 13 (9): 981–1000.
72. Maijers, M.C., de Blok, C.J.M., Niessen, F.B. et al. (2013). Women with silicone breast implants and unexplained systemic symptoms: a descriptive cohort study. *Neth. J. Med.* 71 (10): 534–540.

6 Silicone Breast Implants (SBIs) and Autoimmune Dysautonomya

Gilad Halpert[1,2], Abdulla Watad[3,4,5,6,7], Howard Amital[1,5,6], and Yehuda Shoenfeld[1,8]

[1]Zabludowicz Center for Autoimmune Diseases, Sheba Medical Center, Tel-Hashomer, Israel
[2]Department of Molecular Biology, Ariel University, Ariel, Israel
[3]Rheumatology Unit and Zabludowicz Center for Autoimmune Diseases, Sheba Medical Center, Tel-Hashomer, Israel
[4]Section of Musculoskeletal Disease, Leeds Institute of Molecular Medicine, University of Leeds, Leeds, UK
[5]Sackler Faculty of Medicine, Tel Aviv University, Tel Aviv, Israel
[6]Department of Internal Medicine 'B', Sheba Medical Center, Tel-Hashomer, Israel
[7]Institute of Oncology, Sheba Medical Center, Tel-Hashomer, Israel
[8]Reichman University, Herzliya, Israel

Silicone is a foreign material to our body and cannot be found in nature. Silicone is a polymer, created from some chemical modifications of silica. Silica, or crystalline silica, does exist in nature and has been found to be associated with autoimmune diseases in subjects who experience long-term exposure to this material [1, 2].

Silicone breast implants have been in use, for breast augmentation and reconstruction purposes, since 1960. On those days, silicone has been considered as an inert material to the human body [3–5]. Not surprisingly, following the first augmentation mammoplasty procedure, Kumagai et al. were among the first to describe the occurrence of connective tissue disease after cosmetic surgery [6, 7]. Increasing evidence for the appearance of inflammatory, autoimmune, and connective tissue diseases in women with silicone breast implants have been reported in the following decades, until today [4–6, 8–14].

As the silicone implants being located in the body for many years, the silicone material can act as an adjuvant and cause chronic hyperstimulation of the immune system in genetically predisposed subjects [13, 15]. Our group, among others, showed that silicone microparticles can "bleed" and migrate out of the implants toward many tissues in the body such as lymph nodes [16], thyroid, spinal cord, and even the brain [17], emphasizing the potential harmful capabilities of silicone material, outside the implants. Indeed, silicone implants have been found to affect both innate and adaptive immunity, both in vitro and in vivo, in animals and human subjects [18–21]. In line with these findings, our group reported dysregulation in the production of classical autoantibodies

Autoimmune Disorders: Adjuvants and Other Risk Factors in Pathogenesis, First Edition.
Edited by Abdulla Watad, Nicola Luigi Bragazzi, and Yehuda Shoenfeld.

in asymptomatic and symptomatic women with silicone breast implants [22]. Importantly, in a large-population-based study, we found a significant increased risk for women with silicone breast implants to develop autoimmune diseases such as Sjögren's syndrome, systemic sclerosis, sarcoidosis, and rheumatoid arthritis [14].

Recently, we thoroughly interviewed symptomatic women with silicone breast implant who suffered from various enigmatic, subjective, and autonomic-related manifestations such as severe fatigue, widespread pain, depression, cognitive impairment, sleep disorders, palpitations, hearing loss, and dry mouth and eyes. These symptomatic women with silicone breast implants (SBIs) have been interviewed before by many physicians who could not find solution to their devastating situation [23]. Notably, clinical routine blood tests were found to be normal in these symptomatic women, and in fact, many physicians prescribed antidepressants and/or antipsychotic drugs for these women. Unfortunately, these drugs caused side effects and sometimes even aggravated the clinical manifestations of these patients.

Unique autoantibodies directed against G-protein-coupled receptors (GPCRs) of the autonomic nervous system have been already described to play a significant role in the development of autoimmune disease (such as Sjögren's syndrome, multiple sclerosis, and rheumatoid arthritis) [24, 25] and in other suspected autoimmune dysautonomia-related disorders such as chronic fatigue syndrome, postural orthostatic tachycardia syndrome, and complex regional pain syndrome [26]. As of such, we hypothesized that dysregulation in the level and function of these anti-GPCR autoantibodies might explain, at least in part, some of the clinical manifestations reported by silicone breast illness patients. Indeed, we recently reported a significant reduction in the circulating titter of anti-GPCRs IgG autoantibodies directed against autonomic nervous system autoantigens such as anti-β1 adrenergic receptor, anti-angiotensin II type 1 receptor, and anti-endothelin receptor type A in symptomatic women with SBIs as compared with age-matched healthy women. Furthermore, anti-β1 adrenergic receptor autoantibody was found to significantly correlate with autonomic-related manifestations such as depression and sleep disorders in women with SBIs [23]. Importantly, we showed that passive transfer of IgG antibodies, isolated from symptomatic women with SBIs who suffered from autonomic-related manifestations (such as severe fatigue, widespread pain, depression, cognitive impairment, and sleep disorders), into mice brain affects anxiety and reduced locomotor activity of the mice, indicating apathic/depression-like behavior of the animals [27]. Moreover, we also found that IgG derived from symptomatic women with SBI cannot reduce the production of pro-inflammatory mediators from lipopolysaccharides (LPS)-induced activated human peripheral blood mononuclear cells, as compared to healthy IgGs, which significantly reduces such mediators [27] (as already described previously with regard to the anti-inflammatory activity of intravenous immunoglobulins [28]). It is worth mentioning that we found that symptomatic women with SBIs who decided to remove their implants reported a significant improvement in their subjective and autonomic-related manifestations, as already been suggested by others [11, 29, 30].

Overall, we would like to present silicone breast illness syndrome as a classic example of autoimmune/inflammatory syndrome induced by adjuvants (ASIA) syndrome [31]. Specifically, as suggested in the major criteria for ASIA syndrome [32], external stimuli to our body, such as the silicone material, act as an adjuvant and cause clinical manifestations such as fatigue, sleep disturbance, cognitive impairment, and memory loss. The removal of the adjuvants from the body, in this case, the removal of the silicone implants, significantly improves the clinical status of silicone breast illness patients [17, 29, 30]. Moreover, as suggested in the minor criteria for ASIA syndrome [32], silicone material acts as an adjuvant [13] in genetically predisposed women (e.g. human leukocyte antigen [HLA]) [15] to overactivate the immune system to produce antibodies toward the silicone itself but also classical [22] and nonclassical autoantibodies toward peripheral and central autoantigens [23]. This hyperstimulation of immune system might lead to the development of autoimmune diseases as has already been reported by us [14].

References

1. Sanchez-Roman, J., Wichmann, I., Salaberri, J. et al. (1993). Multiple clinical and biological autoimmune manifestations in 50 workers after occupational exposure to silica. *Ann. Rheum. Dis.* 52 (7): 534–538.
2. Ueki, A., Isozaki, Y., Tomokuni, A. et al. (2001). Different distribution of HLA class II alleles in anti-topoisomerase I autoantibody responders between silicosis and systemic sclerosis patients, with a common distinct amino acid sequence in the HLA-DQB1 domain. *Immunobiology* 204 (4): 458–465.
3. Bridges, A.J. and Vasey, F.B. (1993). Silicone breast implants. History, safety, and potential complications. *Arch. Intern. Med.* 153 (23): 2638–2644.
4. Shons, A.R. and Schubert, W. (1992). Silicone breast implants and immune disease. *Ann. Plast. Surg.* 28 (5): 491–499; discussion 499–501.
5. Zandman-Goddard, G., Ehrenfeld, M., and Shoenfeld, Y. (1993). Silicone implants for breast augmentation and autoimmune disease. *Harefuah* 125 (10): 360–364.
6. Kumagai, Y., Abe, C., and Shiokawa, Y. (1979). Scleroderma after cosmetic surgery: four cases of human adjuvant disease. *Arthritis Rheum.* 22 (5): 532–537.
7. Kumagai, Y., Shiokawa, Y., Medsger, T.A. Jr., and Rodnan, G.P. (1984). Clinical spectrum of connective tissue disease after cosmetic surgery. Observations on eighteen patients and a review of the Japanese literature. *Arthritis Rheum.* 27 (1): 1–12.
8. Aharon-Maor, A., Levy, Y., and Schoenfeld, Y. (1998). Fibrosarcoma after silicone breast augmentation: is there a connection? *Harefuah* 134 (5): 339–341, 424.
9. Ehrenfeld, M. and Shoenfeld, Y. (1998). Breast silicone implant and autoimmunity--coincidence or cause and effect relationship? *Harefuah* 134 (5): 361–364.
10. Gabriel, S.E., O'Fallon, W.M., Kurland, L.T. et al. (1994). Risk of connective-tissue diseases and other disorders after breast implantation. *N. Engl. J. Med.* 330 (24): 1697–1702.
11. Meier, L.G., Barthel, H.R., and Seidl, C. (1997). Development of polyarthritis after insertion of silicone breast implants followed by remission after implant removal in 2 HLA-identical sisters bearing rheumatoid arthritis susceptibility genes. *J. Rheumatol.* 24 (9): 1838–1841.
12. Sanchez-Guerrero, J., Colditz, G.A., Karlson, E.W. et al. (1995). Silicone breast implants and the risk of connective-tissue diseases and symptoms. *N. Engl. J. Med.* 332 (25): 1666–1670.
13. Watad, A., Bragazzi, N.L., Amital, H., and Shoenfeld, Y. (2019). Hyperstimulation of adaptive immunity as the common pathway for silicone breast implants, autoimmunity, and lymphoma of the breast. *Isr. Med. Assoc. J.* 21 (8): 517–519.
14. Watad, A., Rosenberg, V., Tiosano, S. et al. (2018). Silicone breast implants and the risk of autoimmune/rheumatic disorders: a real-world analysis. *Int. J. Epidemiol.* 47 (6): 1846–1854.
15. Young, V.L., Nemecek, J.R., Schwartz, B.D. et al. (1995). HLA typing in women with breast implants. *Plast. Reconstr. Surg.* 96 (7): 1497–1519; discussion 1520.
16. Nesher, G., Soriano, A., Shlomai, G. et al. (2015). Severe ASIA syndrome associated with lymph node, thoracic, and pulmonary silicone infiltration following breast implant rupture: experience with four cases. *Lupus* 24 (4-5): 463–468.
17. Dijkman, H., Slaats, I., and Bult, P. (2021). Assessment of silicone particle migration among women undergoing removal or revision of silicone breast implants in the Netherlands. *JAMA Netw. Open* 4 (9): e2125381.
18. Bizjak, M., Selmi, C., Praprotnik, S. et al. (2015). Silicone implants and lymphoma: the role of inflammation. *J. Autoimmun.* 65: 64–73.
19. Caravantes-Cortes, M.I., Roldan-Valadez, E., Zwojewski-Martinez, R.D. et al. (2020). Breast prosthesis syndrome: pathophysiology and management algorithm. *Aesthet. Plast. Surg.* 44: 1423–1437.
20. Ojo-Amaize, E.A., Lawless, O.J., and Peter, J.B. (1996). Elevated concentrations of interleukin-1 beta and interleukin-1 receptor antagonist in plasma of women with silicone breast implants. *Clin. Diagn. Lab. Immunol.* 3 (3): 257–259.
21. Schaefer, C.J. and Wooley, P.H. (1999). The influence of silicone implantation on murine lupus in MRL lpr/lpr mice. *J. Rheumatol.* 26 (10): 2215–2221.
22. Zandman-Goddard, G., Blank, M., Ehrenfeld, M. et al. (1999). A comparison of autoantibody production in asymptomatic and symptomatic women with silicone breast implants. *J. Rheumatol.* 26 (1): 73–77.

23. Halpert, G., Watad, A., Tsur, A.M. et al. (2021). Autoimmune dysautonomia in women with silicone breast implants. *J. Autoimmun.* 120: 102631.
24. Cabral-Marques, O., Marques, A., Giil, L.M. et al. (2018). GPCR-specific autoantibody signatures are associated with physiological and pathological immune homeostasis. *Nat. Commun.* 9 (1): 5224.
25. Cabral-Marques, O. and Riemekasten, G. (2017). Functional autoantibodies targeting G protein-coupled receptors in rheumatic diseases. *Nat. Rev. Rheumatol.* 13 (11): 648–656.
26. Shoenfeld, Y., Ryabkova, V.A., Scheibenbogen, C. et al. (2020). Complex syndromes of chronic pain, fatigue and cognitive impairment linked to autoimmune dysautonomia and small fiber neuropathy. *Clin. Immunol.* 214: 108384.
27. Talalai, E., Gorobets, D., Halpert, G. et al. (2023). Functional IgG autoantibodies against autonomic nervous system receptors in symptomatic women with silicone breast implants. *Cells* 12 (11): 1510.
28. Siedlar, M., Strach, M., Bukowska-Strakova, K. et al. (2011). Preparations of intravenous immunoglobulins diminish the number and proinflammatory response of $CD14^{+}CD16^{++}$ monocytes in common variable immunodeficiency (CVID) patients. *Clin. Immunol.* 139 (2): 122–132.
29. de Boer, M., Colaris, M., van der Hulst, R., and Cohen Tervaert, J.W. (2017). Is explantation of silicone breast implants useful in patients with complaints? *Immunol. Res.* 65 (1): 25–36.
30. Peters, W., Smith, D., Fornasier, V. et al. (1997). An outcome analysis of 100 women after explantation of silicone gel breast implants. *Ann. Plast. Surg.* 39 (1): 9–19.
31. Borba, V., Malkova, A., Basantsova, N. et al. (2020). Classical examples of the concept of the ASIA syndrome. *Biomol. Ther.* 10 (10).
32. Shoenfeld, Y. and Agmon-Levin, N. (2011). 'ASIA' - autoimmune/inflammatory syndrome induced by adjuvants. *J. Autoimmun.* 36 (1): 4–8.

7 Autoimmune/Inflammatory Syndrome Induced by Adjuvants (ASIA or Shoenfeld's Syndrome) Due to Polypropylene Mesh Implants

Jan Willem Cohen Tervaert[1,2] and Mohammed Osman[1]

[1]Division of Rheumatology, Department of Medicine, University of Alberta, Edmonton, Alberta, Canada
[2]Emeritus Professor of Medicine and Immunology, Maastricht University, Maastricht, The Netherlands

Introduction

The implantation of synthetic mesh to repair weak tissue started in the 1940s. In 1963, polypropylene (PP) mesh was initially used to perform a tensionless hernia repair of abdominal wall defects [1]. The tension-free prosthetic repairs of groin and/or abdominal hernia were further popularized in the 1980s and constitute a major and indispensable share of such defects since then. At present, it is estimated that there are over 20 million hernia repair procedures performed every year worldwide with PP mesh repair utilized for most of them.

From the early 1990s, transvaginal implantation of PP mesh was also used to reinforce a weak pelvic muscle floor stemming from stress urinary incontinence (SUI) and pelvic organ prolapse (POP). In addition, midurethral mesh slings using a PP tension-free vaginal tape (TVT) have been utilized globally for managing female SUI [2]. Hence, PP mesh use in hernia repair and in pelvic organ prolapse surgery clearly offers clinical benefits, but the efficacy of these implants is hindered by the body's immunologic reaction to the implanted material. Undesirable local effects have been extensively described. Systemic effects are also reported and will be discussed in this chapter.

Maladaptive immunological reactions to various external stimuli (e.g. foreign bodies, infections, or genotoxic environmental stressors) are associated with genetic risk factors, which result in hyperinflammatory reactions to these compounds. Well-studied examples of environmental factors in humans are infections, vaccines, and silica. Mercury has been extensively studied in experimental animals [3]. These factors promote an "adjuvant" effect to the immune system. In the past decade, it has become evident that implanted foreign body materials may also trigger an adjuvant

Autoimmune Disorders: Adjuvants and Other Risk Factors in Pathogenesis, First Edition.
Edited by Abdulla Watad, Nicola Luigi Bragazzi, and Yehuda Shoenfeld.

effect on the immune system, resulting in a systemic immune response [4]. These reactions may stem from genetic factors inherent to an individual patient (such as HLA-DRB1 or HLA-DQB1) and the nature of the foreign materials utilized for implantation.

The best studied foreign body materials that have been implicated in promoting maladaptive inflammatory reactions are silicones. Silicones are used in a variety of medical applications such as breast implants, hydrocephalus shunts, catheter lines, intraocular implants, rhinoplasty, hearing aids, laryngotracheal stenosis and various other stents, joint implants, and testicular prosthesis. Silicones were introduced in the 1960s and were initially thought to be biologically inert. However, in the past 50 years, it became clear that silicones can induce various immunological effects. These effects are best studied in patients with silicone breast implants (SBI) [5] where various inflammatory reactions have been described.

After SBI, local and distant complications of SBI have been reported. Local ones include pain, swelling, redness, infections, capsular contracture, implant rupture, and gel bleeding through the intact capsule. More systemic general complications may also occur and include joint pain and/or swelling, generalized muscle pain, fatigue, nonrefreshing sleep, postexertional malaise, and cognitive dysfunction; but more importantly, they also develop humoral immune dysfunction, systemic autoinflammatory symptoms (such as fever), and autoimmune diseases [5]. In addition, autoantibodies are produced and stroke-like and/or multiple sclerosis-like symptoms may be present [5, 6] (Figure 7.1).

The systemic symptoms that have been described in the past 50 years have been given different names such as human adjuvant disease, siliconosis, silicone incompatibility syndrome, silicone-induced toxicity, and, more recently, autoimmune/inflammatory syndrome induced by adjuvants (ASIA) [5–8]. Both patients and treaters suspect that these complaints are caused by the implants.

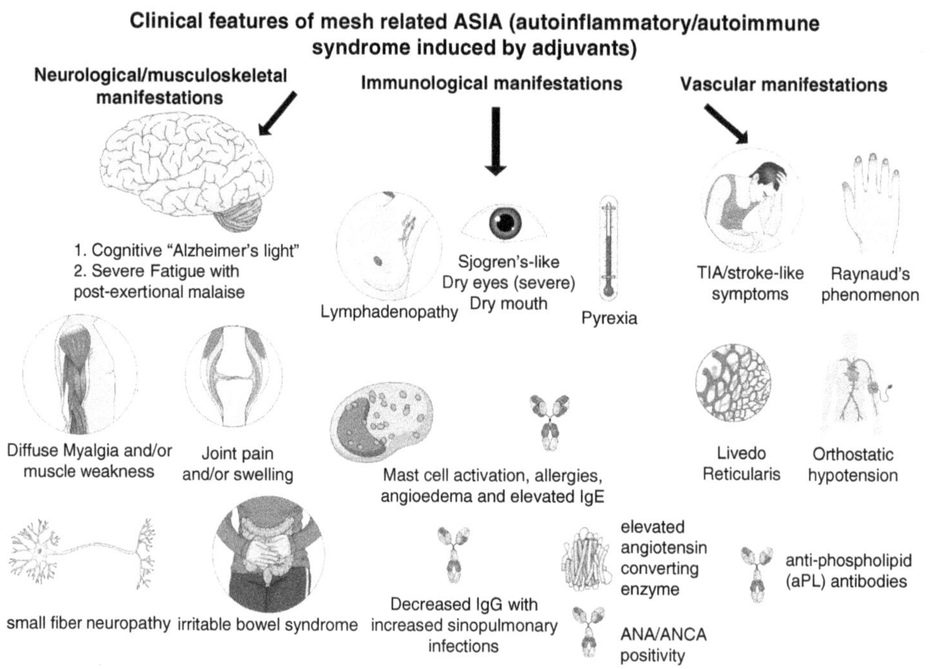

Figure 7.1 Mesh-induced ASIA (autoinflammatory/autoimmunity syndrome induced by adjuvants) presents with neurological/musculoskeletal, immunological, and/or vascular manifestations. ANA, antinuclear antibodies; ANCA, antineutrophil cytoplasmic antibodies.

Recently, we reviewed the evidence that there was indeed a causal relationship between the silicone implants and the ensuing symptoms that patients developed [9]. One of the most convincing properties supporting causality is the substantial improvement of patient-reported symptoms after implant removal in 60–80% of the patients studied [10, 11]. However, in patients with longer periods of silicone implantation, systemic symptoms persisted in spite of implant removal. Together, this may suggest that similar to other chronic inflammatory diseases, silicone implants may initially trigger the systemic disease, but over time, other mechanisms may promote subsequent inflammatory responses (e.g. altered protein posttranslational modification, epitope spreading, or epigenetic changes in somatic cells).

It is currently postulated that SBI cause an inflammatory reaction, and that silicone-containing particles are transported to regional lymph nodes, resulting in a pronounced adjuvant effect [5]. Also, other implanted biomaterials may act as adjuvants, resulting in enhanced adaptive immune responses to an autoantigen. During the past decade, it became clear that debris from medical implants, including joint implants, injectables such as silicones, and medical devices used for sterilization may act as adjuvants [5, 12–17] – although more studies are required to identify potential antigens promoting inflammatory responses.

Further to this, we and others have previously reported that polypropylene mesh could also act as a trigger for ASIA, immune deficiency, and autoimmunity [18, 19]. Intriguingly, most patients with systemic symptoms also describe more severe localized inflammatory reactions prior to the onset of their systemic ones – suggesting that the systemic symptoms may reflect persistent inflammatory reactions to mesh implantation.

Adverse events associated with mesh implants

A large number of ongoing adverse events have been reported to the FDA regarding mesh implants. Many of these adverse effects were severe and resulted in a large frequency of women requesting surgical removal of their mesh implants [20]. These include pain, mesh erosions through the vagina, infections, urinary problems, pain during sexual intercourse (dyspareunia), bleeding, and even visceral organ perforation. As a result, the FDA ordered postmarket surveillance investigations with nearly 522 ensuing studies by manufacturers of urogynecologic surgical mesh devices to address specific safety and effectiveness concerns related to minisling devices for SUI and surgical mesh used for transvaginal repair of POP. In 2018 (July 13), the FDA ordered the manufacturers of mesh surgical products on the market for the transvaginal repair of pelvic organ prolapse in the posterior compartment (rectocele) to stop selling and distributing their products based on safety issues.

In August 2021, 522 studies were completed, and the final reports (36-month follow-up data) were reviewed by the FDA. The study results showed that Boston Scientific transvaginal POP mesh had similar effectiveness and safety outcomes to native tissue repair at 36 months. However, patients with transvaginal POP mesh repair were exposed to additional risks, such as mesh exposure and erosion, compared to patients receiving a native tissue repair. Thus, the FDA continues to believe that these devices do not have a favorable benefit–risk profile.

Adverse events related to mesh implants can be categorized into four [4] subgroups:

(I) Local complications such as pain
(II) Surgical complications such as mesh exposure and erosion
(III) Allergy to components of the mesh
(IV) Systemic symptoms such as autoimmune-like symptoms.

Until recently, only 40 patients who developed symptoms of a systemic illness after mesh implantation have been described [18]. All 40 patients had complaints of fatigue, myalgias, and/or other symptoms suggestive of ASIA. In about half of the patients, an autoimmune disease developed, and in about a quarter of the patients, serological parameters consistent with a humoral immune deficiency [18]. Together, it was concluded that mesh may trigger downstream maladaptive inflammatory mechanisms that are associated with autoimmune/inflammatory syndrome induced by adjuvants. Since this study was published, we have subsequently described an additional 32 patients with similar signs and symptoms that were often (partially) reversible if the mesh could be totally removed (Cohen Tervaert, personal observation).

Systemic symptoms and signs of mesh-mediated systemic disease

Chronic fatigue is the most common symptom experienced by most patients suffering from mesh-mediated disease. Patients describe severe fatigue that does not resolve with sleep or rest. This severe fatigue is associated with a substantial reduction in the ability to engage premorbid levels of occupational, educational, social and/or personal activities. Importantly, most patients report postexertional malaise, also referred to as a symptom flare or "crash," which occurs following physical or cognitive exertion and can last for long periods (days to weeks) after engaging in exercise. Sleep disturbances, such as problems falling asleep and/or staying asleep, are also common. These symptoms may also potentiate the severity of fatigue and may be associated with cognitive impairment, resulting in memory deficits ("Alzheimer-light"), absentmindedness, word-finding difficulties, and difficulty paying attention.

Pain is also a common symptom most patients describe early in the course of their disease. These may include diffuse muscle pain compatible with fibromyalgia (FM). Indeed, most patients fulfill the 2016 criteria for FM (see Table 7.1) [21] and/or muscle weakness. Some weakness can be profoundly severe and may restrict patients from leaving their homes rendering them bedridden or wheelchair bound. Many patients also complain of joint pain and/or swelling. In fact, occasionally, some patients may present with a (symmetric) joint swelling (polyarthritis) that is compatible with a diagnosis of rheumatoid arthritis.

Other common systemic symptoms that affect patients with mesh-related illness include subjective night sweats or pyrexia. This is associated with significant persistently present lymphadenopathy, both near the site of implantation (i.e. inguinal) and also in other remote areas (axillary or cervical), lymph nodes are enlarged and tender in most (70–80%) patients. Many patients also suffer from dry mouth and dry eyes that are associated with "sand-like" sensations and even blurry vision. As these patients also have fatigue, sometimes they are mistaken for Sjögren's syndrome (SS) – although in contrast to patients with SS, patients with mesh-associated xerostomia rarely have a positive anti-Sjogren's syndrome related antigen A and anti-Sjogren's syndrome related antigen B antibodies (anti-SSA/SSB).

Vascular complications in mesh-related illness are common. Most commonly they include signs of orthostatic intolerance such as dizziness, disturbed balance, irregular heartbeat, and sometimes chest pain. In addition, many patients may develop new onset or worsening Raynaud's phenomenon. Although digital ulcers are rare, some of these patients may develop "systemic sclerosis spectrum disorder" changes that are detected using nailfold video capillaroscopy.

Many of these vascular manifestations are accompanied by cutaneous changes. A prominent livedo reticularis can be found in some patients, whereas mild livedo reticularis is present in most patients. Finally, patients may have ill-defined skin rashes, unexplained (sometimes severe) pruritus, and/or alopecia.

A spectrum of neurological manifestations that are distinct from cognitive impairment are also common in patients with mesh-induced ASIA. They may be mild in nature, such as sensory peripheral neuropathies characterized by "pins and needles" and (atypical) small-fiber neuropathy. Other patients may develop more severe symptoms such as ischemic cerebral disease, a multiple sclerosis-like syndrome, or even amyotrophic lateral sclerosis-like disease. Intriguingly, in patients with ischemic cerebral disease, anticardiolipin antibodies and/or lupus anticoagulant are detected in only a minority of the patients. Similarly, traditional risk factors, such as atrial fibrillation, diabetes, hypertension, or dyslipidemia, are often also absent.

Table 7.1 Fibromyalgia 2016 criteria.

Criteria

A patient satisfies modified 2016 fibromyalgia criteria if the following three conditions are met:

1. Widespread pain index (WPI) ≥ 7 and symptom severity scale (SSS) score ≥ 5 OR WPI of 4–6 and SSS score ≥ 9
2. Generalized pain, defined as pain in at least four of five regions, must be present. Jaw, chest, and abdominal pain are not included in generalized pain definition
3. Symptoms must have been present for at least 3 months
4. A diagnosis of fibromyalgia is valid irrespective of other diagnoses. A diagnosis of fibromyalgia does not exclude the presence of other clinically important illnesses

Notes

1. Widespread pain index (WPI): note the number of areas in which the patient has had pain over the last week. In how many areas has the patient had pain? Score will be between 0 and 19
2. Symptom severity scale (SSS) score

Fatigue, Waking unrefreshed. Cognitive symptoms.

For each of the three symptoms above, indicate the level of severity over the past week using the following scale:

0 = No problem.
1 = Slight or mild problems, generally mild or intermittent.
2 = Moderate, considerable problems, often present and/or at a moderate level.
3 = Severe: pervasive, continuous, life-disturbing problems.

The symptom severity scale (SSS) score is the sum of the severity scores of the three symptoms (fatigue, waking unrefreshed, and cognitive symptoms) (0–9) plus the sum (0–3) of the number of the following symptoms the patient has been bothered by that occurred during the previous 6 months:

(1) Headaches (0–1) (2) Pain or cramps in lower abdomen (0–1) (3) Depression (0–1)
The final symptom severity score (SSS) is between 0 and 12

A majority of patients with mesh-related illness suffer from atopic diseases. In many cases, however, patients report an exacerbation of allergic complaints after mesh surgery. Allergic complaints include sneezing, itching of the nose and eyes, red eyes, rhinorrhea, nasal congestion, and postnasal drip. Food allergies also occur, and patients may develop new-onset urticaria and/or angioneurotic (or Quincke's) edema. Alternatively, they develop oral hypersensitivity reactions. Asthmatic patients may also suffer from cough, wheeze, and shortness of breath; and sometimes even fibrotic changes are detected radiographically. Intriguingly, a remarkable and frequent (up to 50%) finding is metal allergy with nickel inducing a contact dermatitis. This dermatitis may be severe and cause pain at the site of exposure and severe rashes. Finally, a large frequency of patients may develop recurrent sinopulmonary infections. These symptoms may be mild but may also be severe and require the use of antibiotics or even hospitalization for pulmonary infections.

Gastrointestinal disease is very common. Most patients suffer from gastrointestinal symptoms such as abdominal pain associated with changes in bowel movement patterns as described in irritable bowel syndrome (IBS). Although IBS may be preexistent in many patients, an exacerbation of complaints is often reported in these patients after mesh implantation. Similarly, many patients may also develop difficulties with swallowing stemming from decreased salivary production, which may also become more apparent after mesh insertion.

Laboratory and radiological findings and other diagnostic procedures in mesh-induced disease

Based on our clinical experience, diagnostic delays associated with a multitude of clinical investigations are undertaken in most patients prior to obtaining a diagnosis. This is because the testing required to confirm mesh-related disease is not commonly understood by front-line medical practitioners. Although serological assessments of markers suggestive of inflammation (e.g. C-reactive protein) are within the normal range in most patients, they may be slightly more elevated [4, 18]. In contrast, angiotensin-converting enzyme and soluble interleukin-2 receptor levels are often elevated. Autoantibodies may be present in up to 40% of patients. Such antibodies may include anti-SSA/SSB, anti-dsDNA, anti-Scl-70, antipolymerase III, anti-Ku, anticardiolipin, anti-CCP antibodies, IgM-rheumatoid factor, antineutrophil cytoplasmic antibodies (ANCA), and/or cryoglobulins. Vitamin D insufficiency and/or deficiency is a frequent finding, and about 25% of patients have decreased levels of total IgG and/or IgG subclasses (particularly IgG1 and 2) [4, 18] (Figure 7.1).

Along with serological assessments, there are several other diagnostic procedures that are useful to further assess patients with suspected mesh-related illness. These include cardiopulmonary exercise testing by cycling until maximal exertion is achieved and then repeating the test 24 hours later to objectively measure postexertional malaise [22]. Similarly, overnight polysomnography may objectively capture poor sleep quality, while nailfold video capillaroscopy may help detect capillary abnormalities [23]. Skin biopsies may show reduced intraepidermal nerve fiber density whereas abnormal temperature threshold testing may also confirm small-fiber neuropathy [24]. Simple and high yield tests may also include measuring tear production, tear quality, and/or corneal surface evaluations via Schirmer testing, tear breakup time, and staining of the cornea and conjunctiva to confirm the impaired tear production, respectively. In contrast to patients with SS, labial salivary gland biopsies demonstrate only mild lymphocytic infiltration differentiating mesh-induced sicca symptoms from Sjögren's syndrome [4]. Finally, histological examinations of explanted mesh and lymph nodes may confirm granulomatous inflammation.

ASIA, autoimmune diseases, and lymphoma development

With the constellation of the aforementioned symptoms, mesh-induced illness has been coined a form of human adjuvant disease or ASIA [4]. This stems from the presence of chronic forms of immune activation, allergies, autoantibodies, IgG and/or IgG subclass deficiencies, and/or immune dysregulation, which may eventually lead to lymphoproliferative diseases in these patients. Unfortunately, there are no comprehensive population epidemiologic studies performed to calculate the risk of ASIA in mesh patients – underscoring the need for such studies to capture the potential impact of mesh-related ASIA.

Importantly, many patients with mesh-related disease fulfill the classification criteria for myalgic encephalomyelitis [myalgic encephalomyelitis/chronic fatigue syndrome (ME/CFS)] [25], FM [21], or unclassifiable connective tissue diseases. Furthermore, a substantial number of patients may develop well-defined systemic autoimmune diseases such as Sjögren's syndrome, rheumatoid arthritis, antiphospholipid syndrome, and/or eosinophilic granulomatosis with polyangiitis. Although the incidence of systemic autoimmune diseases in mesh patients has not been well studied in mesh-related illness, patients with silicone breast implant-related ASIA clearly have an increased frequency of autoimmune diseases [26, 27]. These ASIA patients with SBI may also develop lymphoma as a complication [28] – suggesting that chronic immune stimulation, such as described in other rheumatic diseases, may promote lymphoproliferations. Although the development of a lymphoma may occur as is suggested from reported cases [29, 30], large epidemiological studies in patients with mesh implants are still lacking.

ASIA: autoimmune/inflammatory syndrome induced by adjuvants (Shoenfeld's syndrome)

In 2011, a syndrome entitled ASIA was first described. The idea that adjuvants promote immune hyperactivation as a driver of this disease was not new but was derived from several lines of evidence. Silicones were well known to promote immune stimulatory factors in susceptible individuals [4, 31] since their introduction in the 1960s. Silicone, similar to other adjuvants, enhances specific immune reactions, resulting in higher titers of antibodies (like those targeting pathogens) [32]. Other examples of well-known adjuvants include aluminum hydroxide, squalene, and silica [33]. During the past decade, it became clear that implanted medical implants, including injectables such as silicones and polypropylene meshes, may act as adjuvants [4, 18].

As the lead author of the 2011 paper describing ASIA, Professor Shoenfeld stated: "The role of various environmental factors in the pathogenesis of immune mediated diseases is well established." [7] Dr. Shoenfeld did not describe a new phenomenon with his descriptions of ASIA. Rather, he aimed to restructure this clinical spectrum into a unifying umbrella where external environmental factors promote immune hyperactivation. This restructuring in turn facilitated the development of a better understanding for the mechanisms underpinning the inflammatory pathways. The inciting agents described by Shoenfeld include injectable silicones, aluminum salts, various implants, and various infectious agents. Further to this notion, there is support for this in the literature as patients developed ASIA following breast or testicular silicone implantation, rhinoplasty (with silicone implants), and with polypropylene mesh implantation for hernia repair, for the reinforcement of a weak pelvic floor, in patients with tension-free vaginal tape implantation for stress incontinence, and in patients with prosthetic materials for arthroplasty [4, 18].

Individually, as each one of the aforementioned adjuvants has already been linked to the development of autoimmunity, ASIA suggests a common and potentially shared mechanism of adjuvant-induced autoimmunity (Figure 7.2). This would suggest that similar to other autoimmune diseases, there is a shared genetic component in susceptible individuals. Although the factors promoting ASIA following medical device implantation to various materials are unclear, several clinical risk factors have been postulated. These include risk factors known to promote immune dysregulation such as obesity, smoking, or the inheritance of specific HLA alleles (particularly in the HLA DR and DQ beta loci). Similarly, patients with chronic atopic diseases, autoimmunity, or a family history of autoimmunity may be at increased risk of developing ASIA after implantation [4].

Pathophysiology of ASIA after foreign body implantation

In general, commonly used biomaterials for implantation are nonimmunogenic and nontoxic. Intriguingly, implanted biomaterials trigger a foreign body reaction resulting in granulomatous inflammation in some individuals [34, 35]. This may be explained in part by the presence of microbial biofilms on implants [36, 37], which promote the development of chronic inflammatory response. In this setting, these implanted biomaterials promote immune recognition, with subsequent enhancement and responsiveness to specific antigens within the implanted medical device [38] (see Figure 7.3).

Immediately after implantation of a biomaterial, a layer of host proteins is deposited onto the biomaterial surface, resulting in the attraction of phagocytes [predominantly macrophages polarized to produce pro-inflammatory cytokines such as interleukin 1 beta (IL-1β) and tumor necrosis factor alpha (TNFα)]. Importantly, this process is critically dependent on the presence of activated mast cells and histamine. Furthermore, biomaterials may act as an adjuvant, resulting in

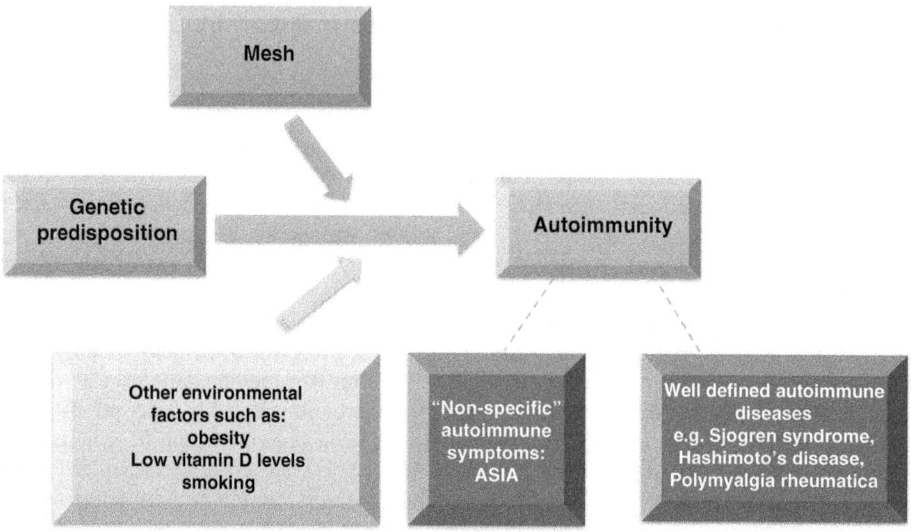

Figure 7.2 Schematic illustration of the process of autoimmunity development. ASIA may serve to describe the principle pathogenesis of all autoimmune conditions. This process entails an exposure of a genetically prone individual to an external immune stimulatory trigger such as mesh, resulting in overt autoimmunity, which may manifest as a well-recognized autoimmune disease such as Sjögren's syndrome, Hashimoto's disease, or polymyalgia rheumatica or in a collection of autoimmune symptoms, which may be referred to as ASIA. *Abbreviations*: ASIA, autoinflammatory/autoimmune syndrome induced by adjuvants.

the enhancement of the adaptive immune response to an autoantigen. The immune reactions are directed against the adjuvant (which comprises the implanted medical device) and adsorbed host proteins. Also, after implantation, a biofilm is formed, and the microorganisms in this biofilm may also act as adjuvants (see Figure 7.3) [39]. Mast cell-derived mediators such as histamine and prostaglandins are critical chemoattractants for other immune cells [40]. Histamine may also promote the development of pain at the site of implantation, as it may sensitize the transient reporter potential channel V1 (TRPV1), one of the nociceptors [41]. Furthermore, the biomaterials may directly serve as an adjuvant which further augments inflammatory cell functions and the development of downstream adaptive (T-cell) responses targeting specific autoantigen(s) [38].

Foreign materials such as silicone breast implants, silicones in other materials, polypropylene mesh, Essure devices (used for sterilization), and prosthetic materials used for arthroplasty are known to cause clinical features present in ASIA. Importantly, virtually all these materials promote the formation of foreign body giant cell reactions and granulomas [42]. Hence, the biomaterial, in a susceptible patient or in the presence of a biofilm, may deliver a "danger signal" to the immune system, subsequently resulting in maladaptive inflammation [38, 43, 44].

Several mechanisms have been proposed to explain how adjuvants potentiate inflammatory responses. These include:

- Induction of a progressive release of the antigen (Ag) to enhance antibody production via blocking its clearance and prolonging exposure by antigen-presenting cells (APCs) such as macrophages, dendritic cells (DCs), and B cells;
- Promotion of Ag translocation to lymph nodes where subsequent T-cell recognition ensues;
- Conversion of Ag into particulate forms that are more readily phagocytosed by APCs and eventually presented to Ag-specific T cells;

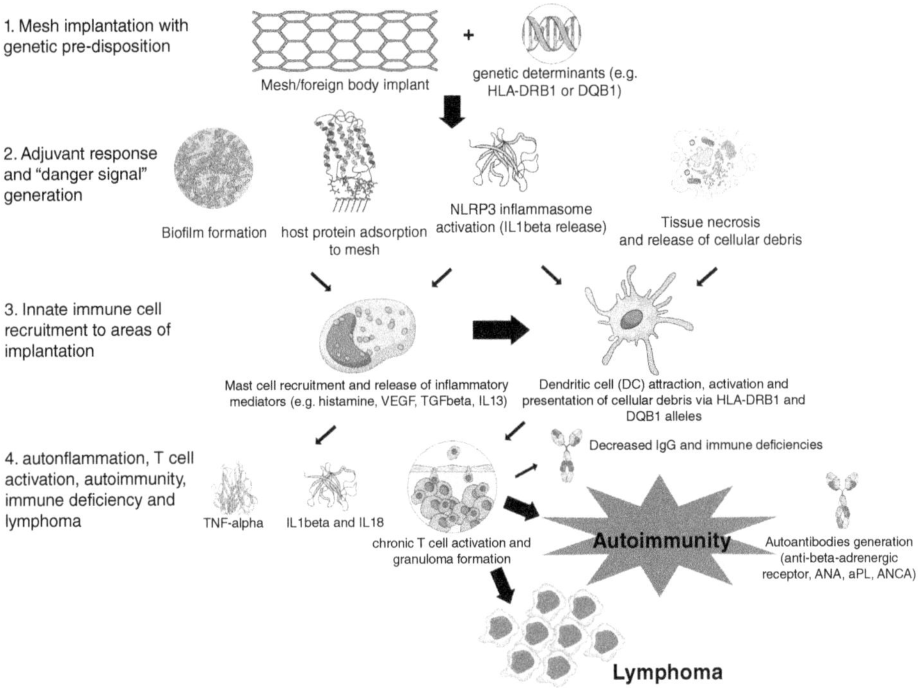

Figure 7.3 Pathogenesis of mesh-related ASIA. In genetically predisposed individuals (e.g. personal or family history of autoimmunity or severe allergic diseases), implantation (1) results in the initiation of a danger signal (2), which in turn results in mast cell activation and the activation of the NLRP3 inflammasome and the release of mediators such as Interleukin-1 beta and Interleukin 18 to attract antigen-presenting cells such as dendritic cells (DCs, 3). DCs potentiate a specific antigen response, which results in chronic T-cell activation (4), autoimmunity, immune deficiency, and lymphoma. *Abbreviations*: ASIA, autoinflammatory/autoimmune syndrome induced by adjuvants; ANA, antinuclear antibodies; aPL, antiphospholipid antibodies; ANCA, antineutrophil cytoplasmic antibodies.

- Increase in APC activation through danger signals such as inflammatory cytokines (e.g. TNFα, IL1β, and IL6), activations of the NLRP3 (NOD-, LRR-, and pyrin domain-containing protein 3) inflammasome, or interaction with Toll-like receptors (TLRs).

It is clear that most adjuvants stimulate the NLRP3 inflammasome. It is composed of a multi-protein complex containing NLRP3 and ASC [apoptosis-associated speck-like protein containing a C-terminal caspase-recruitment domain (CARD)] proteins which are responsible for a caspase1-dependent cleavage of IL1β and IL18 into their mature forms. The NLRP3 inflammasome is a primary sensing mechanism present in both somatic and myeloid cells that responds to metal debris, aluminum salts, silicones, and other adjuvants to induce the secretion of pro-inflammatory cytokines and recruit other myeloid-lineage cells [45].

Together, these lines of evidence indicate that these adjuvants are capable of evoking an adaptive immune response characterized by lymphocyte activation and immunological "memory." Lymphocyte lineages, particularly T cells and B cells, contain the amnestic, "memory" features of lasting acquired immunity through selective programming and dating of specific lymphocyte clones.

These lymphocyte memory responses are central in orchestrating the recruitment, activation, and effector functions of other cells of the immune system in an ongoing process of dynamic response through cellular and molecular cross talk. Lymphocytes often dominate implant-associated ectopic lymphoid structures. In joint implants, this is called *aseptic lymphocytic (lymphocyte-dominated) vasculitis-associated lesions* (ALVAL) [46].

Pattern recognition receptors, exemplified by Toll-like receptor 4 (TLR4), also serve as critical triggers of inflammation following recognition of endogenous "alarmin" molecules released in injured tissues. These include heat-shock proteins, biglycan fragments, and heparan sulfates, among others [47]. Adjuvants have been shown to directly activate TLR4, promoting local inflammation and tissue remodeling via the activation of the canonical NFκB pathway, leading to inflammatory cytokine production [48]. Release of alarm signals from injured tissues couples initial implantation to immediate inflammatory and innate immune responses. However, tissue injury particularly from failed or compromised implants may perpetuate these maladaptive pathways [49].

The association between implants and ASIA likely results in the following scenario: macrophages and, subsequently, inflammasomes are activated, resulting in the production of cytokines such as interleukin-1β. Reactive oxygen species (ROS) and reactive nitrogen species are also produced. Subsequently, apoptosis of macrophages occurs, and neutrophils are attracted. These neutrophils are activated, producing higher levels of ROS, and release enzymes such as myeloperoxidase. Additionally, materials from implants are transported to the regional lymph nodes, resulting in pronounced adjuvant effects and subsequent lymphocyte responses (Figure 7.3). In animal models that are genetically susceptible, it has been shown that implants such as silicone breast implants and polypropylene meshes are able to induce an adjuvant effect and in turn increase the susceptibility to and/or exacerbate autoimmune diseases. In nonsusceptible animals, however, autoimmunity could not be induced [50].

Table 7.2 Criteria for the diagnosis of autoimmune/inflammatory syndrome induced by adjuvants (ASIA) [4, 7]

Major criteria:

- Exposure to an external stimulus (implants such as silicone and mesh are classic adjuvants) prior to clinical manifestations
- The appearance of "typical" clinical manifestations such as:
  - Chronic fatigue, unrefreshing sleep, or sleep disturbances
  - Myalgia, myositis, or muscle weakness
  - Arthralgia and/or arthritis
  - Cognitive impairment and memory loss
  - Pyrexia
  - Sicca (dry mouth and dry eyes)
  - Neurological manifestations (especially associated with demyelination)
- Removal of the inciting agent induces improvement
- Typical biopsy of involved organs

Minor criteria:

- The appearance of autoantibodies or antibodies directed at the suspected adjuvant.
- Other clinical manifestations (i.e. irritable bowel syndrome and Raynaud's phenomenon)
- Specific HLA associations (i.e. HLA DRB1 and HLA DQB1)
- Evolvement of an autoimmune disease (i.e. multiple sclerosis, rheumatoid arthritis, Sjögren's syndrome, and systemic sclerosis)

Evidence that mesh can cause ASIA

Patients are considered to have ASIA when either two major or one major and two minor criteria are present [7]. Mesh implant patients with autoimmune symptoms generally satisfy at least two of the major criteria (Table 7.2).

The exposure to mesh implants precedes onset or worsening of symptoms; typical clinical manifestations appear; and removal of mesh implants induces improvement. The latter criteria is somewhat unique to ASIA, and is key to the discussion on causation, as these clinical manifestations generally do not spontaneously resolve, and these autoimmune symptoms would not be expected to resolve after surgery, absent the removal of some triggering stimulus. Each of these criteria will be discussed in detail.

Exposure to mesh implants precedes the onset or worsening of symptoms

Apart from the clinical trials, which did not systematically assess adverse events, research on adverse events associated with mesh implants relies upon self-report as to when the symptoms began. Although this introduces an element of *uncertainty* stemming from biases or poor memory, the consistency in the types of complaints reported after mesh implants provides some reassurance as to the validity of the reports.

The appearance of "typical" clinical manifestations

As discussed above, patients suffering from ASIA tend to present with a cluster of similar clinical characteristics including chronic fatigue, myalgia, arthralgia, neurological and skin manifestations, sicca (dry eyes and mouth), cognitive impairment ("brain fog"), and fever. This same diverse but predictable cluster of symptoms is seen in mesh-implant patients [18, 19]. ASIA symptoms can progress to full-blown autoimmune disease, and even to lymphoma, if the stimulus is not removed.

Angiotensin-converting enzyme and soluble interleukin-2 receptor levels are often elevated. These are well-established markers of granulomatous inflammation. Further to this, biopsies of lymph nodes and/or explanted implants show granulomatous inflammation. Chronic activation of the immune system in genetically prone patients may progress from experiencing ASIA to developing full-blown autoimmune diseases, humoral immune deficiencies, allergic diseases, and/or lymphomas. While mesh removal (at least where complete removal is possible) often resolves all ASIA symptoms (as will be discussed in the following section), once the person's autoimmune condition progresses to autoimmune disease (e.g. rheumatic arthritis and scleroderma), a full recovery after removal of the mesh is rare, and in these cases, additional treatment (e.g. with immune-suppressing drugs) is needed.

Removal of inciting agent induces improvement

Another major criteria of ASIA is that the symptoms and signs that began after implantation (such as chronic fatigue or widespread pain) improve after explantation of the inciting medical device. The cessation or reduction of symptoms after removal (also called "dechallenge") is an extremely important observation in diagnosing ASIA and in determining causation. Such improvement has been well documented in patients with surgical mesh implants [18, 19].

Hence, in patients with improved symptoms following mesh removal, it can be concluded that mesh implants may also promote ASIA – an observation that is corroborated by numerous studies. Improvement in the ASIA symptoms (fatigue, arthralgia, muscle pain and weakness, cognitive impairment, alopecia, widespread pain, and allergies) after removal of mesh implants also provides confirming evidence of causation. This constellation of symptoms did not resolve by chance – rather they improved after removal of mesh implants, suggesting that they were caused by the device. This observation is in contrast to patients with idiopathic chronic fatigue syndrome and fibromyalgia where spontaneous improvements are extremely rare.

Biological plausibility of mesh implants as a cause of ASIA

Apart from the general mechanisms by which implants induce a foreign body reaction (described above), specific components of mesh implants may exacerbate the above-described processes. Mesh implants cause a foreign body reaction ("FBR") creating a chronic inflammatory response that results in scarring around the device. These FBR are observed histologically in many explanted mesh devices. FBR occur quickly after implantation and can promote granulomatous inflammation around the device within a few days after implantation [51]. The chronic inflammation is characterized by persistent lymphocyte infiltration at the sites of medical device insertion even years after implantation.

Approaches to causation

While arguably the strongest evidence [52], randomized controlled trials are not always feasible or ethical when attempting to assess whether certain exposures "causally alter disease risk." For studies of etiology, a systematic review of prospective cohort studies is considered the highest level of evidence, but again, such studies may not be feasible for rare diseases. Instead, the assessment of causation may need to be inferred from the "harmony of evidence" – the accumulation of evidence from different, including multidisciplinary, approaches that consistently suggest the same story [53]. In determining causation in clinical medicine, Koch's postulates and the Bradford–Hill criteria have been historically implemented for extrapolating causation. The discussion of these approaches as they relate to mesh-associated ASIA is summarized below.

Koch's postulates

Koch's postulates are rigorous criteria that were proposed to assess the causal relationship between a microbe and a disease in 1884. In 2002, Koch's postulates were adapted in an attempt to assess which diseases with a suspected autoimmune etiology are in fact caused by an autoimmune reaction [54]. The adapted postulates are as follows:

- the specific adaptive immune response is directed to the affected organ or tissue;
- autoreactive T cells and/or autoantibodies are present in the affected organ or tissue;
- autoreactive T cells and/or autoantibodies can transfer the disease to healthy individuals or animals;
- immunization with the autoantigen induces the disease in animal models;
- elimination or suppression of the autoimmune response prevents disease progression or even ameliorates the clinical manifestation.

With this approach, accepted autoimmune diseases such as multiple sclerosis, celiac disease, myasthenia gravis, and granulomatosis with polyangiitis were evaluated using these postulates, and none were found to fully fulfill the demands of these postulates. One reason is that these conditions involve cofactors, such as infectious or triggering agents (such as Ebstein–Barr virus in multiple sclerosis, *Staphylococcus aureus* in granulomatosis with polyangiitis, gluten in celiac disease, or a foreign body in ASIA). Thus, it can be concluded that Koch's postulates are far too stringent and thus cannot reasonably be employed to determine causation for the wide array of diseases with a suspected autoimmune etiology.

Bradford–Hill criteria

As an alternative to Koch's postulates, scientists often consider the Bradford–Hill criteria to determine whether an association between a triggering event and an outcome is indeed causal [9, 55].

The Bradford–Hill criteria are consistent in many ways with the ASIA criteria (*described above*). For determination of whether there is a reasonable possibility that the product is etiologically related to the adverse event, different causality assessments are included, such as assessment of temporal relationships, dechallenge/rechallenge information, association with (or lack of association with) underlying disease, presence (or absence) of a more likely cause, and plausibility [56]. Not all of the causation criteria need to be met to draw reliable causal conclusions.

The Bradford–Hill criteria and relevant evidence regarding mesh implants and autoimmune symptoms are as follows:

Strength of association

Where available, randomized controlled studies that are properly powered to study an outcome of interest are a strong method for demonstrating an association between an exposure and an outcome. However, if not conducted during the preapproval stage for a drug or medical device, it is unusual for such studies to be conducted, for ethical and practical reasons [57]. Mesh implants were not evaluated in a randomized, double-blind, controlled studies prior to (FDA or EMEA) approval, and none have been conducted since approval.

In some circumstances, cross-sectional epidemiological studies of large populations can be used to show an association between an exposure and an outcome by quantifying the relative risk of exposure and nonexposure. But epidemiological calculation of relative risk is not always necessary to demonstrate an association. Some rarer and longer term effects of a drug, such as diabetes or birth defects, may require signal detection methods operating on large databases. But, for most adverse effects, seasoned clinicians allied with health literate patients are better placed than randomized controlled trials (RCTs) to determine causality [52]. To this end, peer-reviewed published cohort studies have been utilized to demonstrate an association between mesh implantation and ASIA. There are also several challenge–dechallenge studies that have suggested that the removal of mesh implants may result in relief of ASIA symptoms.

Causation has been shown by epidemiological studies linking environmental exposures with poor outcomes. This is best illustrated in lung cancer population studies. Unfortunately, no well-designed large-population epidemiological study of mesh implants has looked at the frequency of autoimmune conditions as a major endpoint.

Challenge–dechallenge–rechallenge evidence

If a woman with a mesh implant is experiencing pain in the area where the mesh is paced, and that pain disappears upon removal of the device, there is challenge–dechallenge evidence of a causal association between the mesh pain and the implants. If the woman wished to try a second mesh implant, and the pain reappeared, that "rechallenge" would provide additional evidence of causation. If large numbers of women show this same pattern, broader conclusions can be drawn about whether the mesh implant is causally associated with the symptoms described.

Bradford Hill himself acknowledged the role of challenge–dechallenge–rechallenge evidence in determining causality [52], and the FDA mentions it in its definition of causal assessment [56]. As can be seen in the example above, rechallenge evidence is often lacking. Particularly, it would be unethical to require an individual to undergo reexposure to a drug resulting in potential harm simply to confirm causation. Specifically, once an association is suspected based on challenge and dechallenge, a rechallenge should be undertaken to collect further evidence of causation *only with great caution and a compelling need,* because it may cause severe (or even fatal) reactions. Contraindications and ethical considerations must be taken into account, and an individual risk–benefit calculation must be performed in every case. With this limitation under consideration, it becomes more persuasive when the outcomes from challenge–dechallenge responses in many patients as observed by many treaters are the same.

Challenge–dechallenge can provide evidence of general causality, even in a case study of one patient. While case studies have historically been viewed as a lower level of causality evidence, that view is beginning to change. "[W]hen a form of medical therapy is being applied, a crucial question is whether it improves or heals the disease or symptom, ie, whether it yields *therapeutic causality*." Although case reports "have an ambivalent reputation," they are able to capture and describe instances of therapeutic causality in ways that are useful beyond the individual case. "In 2008, for instance, the publication of a few case reports revolutionized treatment for severe hemangioma in infants." [58]. We have systematically accumulated challenge–dechallenge evidence in the case of mesh implants, as described above. In many patients, autoimmune-like symptoms begin or worsen after mesh implants are placed; then they decreased or resolved when mesh implants were removed – strongly suggesting a causal association.

Upon review of the relevant literature, we find that the association between mesh implants and autoimmune symptoms is sufficiently robust to warrant consideration of the remaining Bradford–Hill criteria.

Consistency

Consistency refers to a result that can be replicated. A consistent cluster of autoimmune-like symptoms as well as a consistent pattern of challenge–dechallenge evidence has been reported by patients.

Specificity of association

Specificity is the idea that an exposure causes one disease or syndrome, not a group of diverse diseases or syndromes. In mesh implant patients, it is common to see a cluster of symptoms consistent with the diagnostic criteria for ASIA. It is not the case that mesh implants are associated with hair loss in some patients, fatigue in others, and joint pain in still others, but rather that patients tend to have a predictable cluster of symptoms consistent with an ASIA diagnosis [4]. This is what we call "specificity of association."

The concept of specificity also involves ruling out alternative explanations (the medical concept of differential diagnosis). As discussed above, alternative causes of autoimmune disease can easily be ruled out when a patient's symptoms begin after mesh implants are implanted, and cease when the implants are removed. To this end, when mesh implants are removed, symptoms such as fatigue and arthralgias/myalgias disappear, but concomitant autoimmune diseases that may have developed, such as Sjögren's syndrome and/or systemic sclerosis, still need to be treated according to our international guidelines.

Temporal relationship

Temporality is the idea that for an exposure to be considered causal, it must precede the onset of the disease. The published literature supports the conclusion that new autoimmune symptoms often appear for the first time after mesh implants are implanted. This is also an ASIA criteria, as was discussed above.

Dose–response

This criteria is applicable to drugs and not to devices.

Biological plausibility

The plausible biological mechanism by which mesh implants may cause ASIA has been discussed at length above.

Coherence

Coherence is related to biological plausibility and often involves a coherent set of findings from animal and human research. There is in vitro and in vivo experimental evidence in animal models that strongly suggest that mesh results in the activation of the immune system, as described above.

Experimental evidence (where available)

Evidence from controlled experimental studies, which attempt to isolate and manipulate single variables, can be strong causation evidence, although this can be concluded only if the study is designed and powered to study the primary outcome [52]. In the case of mesh implants and autoimmune disease development, no such studies have been conducted in animals or in humans. This is not unusual, which is why experimental evidence is just one factor among many as Bradford Hill outlined. That being said, mesh implant removal ("dechallenge") creates a "natural experiment" in that a single, possibly contributing variable is manipulated, while other factors remain the same for the individual who suffers from autoimmune symptoms.

Consistency with other scientific knowledge (analogy)

> "Hill implied that when there is strong evidence of a causal relationship between a particular agent and a specific disease, researchers should be more accepting of weaker evidence that a similar agent may cause a similar disease. Analogy has been interpreted to mean that when one causal agent is known, the standards of evidence are lowered for a second causal agent that is similar in some way." [49].

With mesh implants, peer-reviewed research demonstrates that patients may develop systemic autoimmune-like symptoms [18, 19]. Silicone breast implants are the prototype of implant-related autoimmune complaints, with a huge body of published literature and medical experience, spanning over 50 years, supporting a causal link between the implants and autoimmune-like symptoms in susceptible individuals. Well-designed animal studies provide additional support for these conclusions. In the study by McDonald et al., researchers used an animal model, and put breast implants into mice that were genetically predisposed to autoimmune disease, and compared them to other mice that were not predisposed [50, 59, 60]. In the predisposed mice, the breast implants accelerated the development of autoimmune disease and made it more severe than would otherwise be. No autoimmune disease developed in mice that were not predisposed.

In autoimmune diseases, the immune system attacks normal cells and tissues in the body that are generally recognized as "self" and do not normally trigger immune responses. In allergic diseases, the immune system overreacts to a harmless substance such as dust, mold, or pollen. The inappropriate immune response in both conditions results from a deficient regulation of the immune response. This defect is partially genetically and partially environmentally determined. An increased occurrence of both disorders has been observed in families with these disorders. As such, in humans with a history of extensive allergies, a personal or family history of an autoimmune condition, the use of silicone breast implants should be considered a contraindication [4]. Clinicians should discuss these potential complications with these patients prior to the procedures. In the Netherlands, there is a strong warning, but not a contraindication, against the use of silicone breast implants in women with a personal history of allergy. This warning was first provided on 23 December 2013 [61]. This was subsequently extended to patients with mesh implants with a personal history of allergic diseases [18]. In our opinion, the causal link between polypropylene mesh implants and autoimmune symptoms is likely. More studies are needed to support the causal relation between mesh implants and systemic autoimmune diseases.

Conclusion

A causal association between mesh implants and systemic reactions such as those observed in ASIA (autoimmune/inflammatory syndrome induced by adjuvants) is likely. Pathophysiology of the foreign body-induced immune reaction is established, and data from other medical implants support a causal relationship. Importantly, the associated morbidity suffered is variable and can be debilitating for some patients. Mesh implants may cause characteristic systemic reactions in certain patients, leading to symptoms of sufficient severity to warrant device removal. Removal resolves the symptoms in most patients and is the most effective treatment.

References

1. Usher, F.C. (1963). Hernia repair with knitted polypropylene mesh. *Surg. Gynecol. Obstet.* 117: 239–240.
2. Atherton, M.J. and Stanton, S.L. (2005). The tension-free vaginal tape reviewed: an evidence-based review from inception to current status. *BJOG* 112 (5): 534–546.
3. Crowe, W., Allsopp, P.J., Watson, G.E. et al. (2017). Mercury as an environmental stimulus in the development of autoimmunity – a systematic review. *Autoimmun. Rev.* 16 (1): 72–80.
4. Cohen Tervaert, J.W. (2018). Autoinflammatory/autoimmunity syndrome induced by adjuvants (ASIA; Shoenfeld's syndrome): a new flame. *Autoimmun. Rev.* 17 (12): 1259–1264.
5. Cohen Tervaert, J.W., Colaris, M.J., and van der Hulst, R.R. (2017). Silicone breast implants and autoimmune rheumatic diseases: myth or reality. *Curr. Opin. Rheumatol.* 29: 348–354.
6. Colaris, M.J., de Boer, M., van der Hulst, R.R., and Cohen Tervaert, J.W. (2017). Two hundreds cases of ASIA syndrome following silicone implants: a comparative study of 30 years and a review of current literature. *Immunol. Res.* 65 (1): 120–128.
7. Shoenfeld, Y. and Agmon-Levin, N. (2011). 'ASIA'-autoimmune/inflammatory syndrome induced by adjuvants. *J. Autoimmun.* 36: 4–8.
8. Cohen Tervaert, J.W. and Kappel, R.M. (2013). Silicone implant incompatibility syndrome (SIIS): a frequent cause of ASIA (Shoenfeld's syndrome). *Immunol. Res.* 56: 293–298.
9. Cohen Tervaert, J.W., Mohazab, N., Redmond, D. et al. (2022). Breast implant illness: scientific evidence of its existence. *Expert. Rev. Clin. Immunol.* 18 (1): 15–29.
10. de Boer, M., Colaris, M., van der Hulst, R.R., and Cohen Tervaert, J.W. (2017). Is explantation of silicone breast implants useful in patients with complaints? *Immunol. Res.* 65 (1): 25–36.
11. Wee, C.E., Younis, J., Isbester, K. et al. (2020). Understanding breast implant illness, before and after explantation: a patient-reported outcomes study. *Ann. Plast. Surg.* 85 (S1 Suppl 1): S82–S86.
12. Stejskal, V. (2014). Metals as a common trigger of inflammation resulting in non-specific symptoms: diagnosis and treatment. *Isr. Med. Assoc. J.* 16: 753–758.
13. Towers, W.S. and Kurtom, K. (2020). Rare systemic response to titanium spinal fusion implant: case report. *Cureus* 12 (2): e7109. https://doi.org/10.7759/cureus.7109.
14. Schiff, A. et al. (2021). A possible association of orthopedic metal implants and ASIA syndrome. *Rheumatology (Oxford)* 60 (3): e95–e96.
15. Loyo, E., Jara, L.J., López, P.D., and Puig, A.C. (2012). Autoimmunity in connection with a metal implant: a case of autoimmune/autoinflammatory syndrome induced by adjuvants. *Auto Immun. Highlights* 4 (1): 33–38.
16. Chauhan, U., Cassidy, B., and Cohen Tervaert, J.W. (2021). ASIA (Shoenfeld's Syndrome) due to hysteroscopic essure sterilization. *Autoimmun. Rev.* 20 (12): 102979.
17. Nunes, D.B.C., Nunes de Brito, J.B., Machado, A.K.L. et al. (2020). Autoimmune/autoinflammatory syndrome induced by adjuvants (Asia): morphea case report after metallic bone prosthesis. *Int. J. Dev. Res.* 10: 18326.
18. Cohen Tervaert, J.W. (2018). Autoinflammatory/autoimmunity syndrome induced by adjuvants (Shoenfeld's syndrome) in patients after a polypropylene mesh implantation. *Best Pract. Res. Clin. Rheumatol.* 32 (4): 511–520.

19. Dias, E.R.M., Pivetta, L.G.A., de Carvalho, J.P.V. et al. (2021). Autoimmune [auto-inflammatory] syndrome induced by adjuvants (ASIA): case report after inguinal hernia repair with mesh. *Int. J. Surg. Case Rep.* 84: 106060.
20. https://www.fda.gov/medical-devices/urogynecologic-surgical-mesh-implants/fdas-activities-urogynecologic-surgical-mesh. Accessed 10 May 2022.
21. Wolfe, F., Clauw, D.J., Fitzcharles, M.A. et al. (2016). 2016 Revisions to the 2010/2011 fibromyalgia diagnostic criteria. *Semin. Arthritis Rheum.* 46: 319–329.
22. Vermeulen, R.C., Kurk, R.M., Visser, F.C. et al. (2010). Patients with chronic fatigue syndrome performed worse than controls in a controlled repeated exercise study despite a normal oxidative phosphorylation capacity. *J. Transl. Med.* 8: 93.
23. Tariq, S., Cohen Tervaert, J.W., and Osman, M. (2019). Nailfold capillaroscopy in systemic lupus erythematosus (SLE): a point-of-care tool that parallels disease activity and predicts future complications. *Curr. Treat. Options Rheumatol.* 5 (4): 1–10.
24. Clauw, D.J. (2015). What is the meaning of 'small fiber neuropathy' in fibromyalgia? *Pain* 156: 2115–2116.
25. Sunnquist, M. et al. (2017). A comparison of case definitions for myalgic encephalomyelitis and chronic fatigue syndrome. *J. Chronic Dis. Manag.* 2 (2): 1013.
26. Watad, A., Rosenberg, V., Tiosano, S. et al. (2018). Silicone breast implants and the risk of autoimmune/rheumatic disorders: a real-world analysis. *Int. J. Epidemiol.* 47 (6): 1846–1854.
27. Coroneos, C.J., Selber, J.C., Offodile, A.C. 2nd et al. (2019). US FDA breast implant postapproval studies: long-term outcomes in 99,993 patients. *Ann. Surg.* 269 (1): 30–33.
28. de Boer, M., van Leeuwen, F.E., Hauptmann, M. et al. (2018). Breast implants and the risk of anaplastic large-cell lymphoma in the breast. *JAMA Oncol.* 4 (3): 335–341.
29. Pocard, M., Vaillant, J.C., Fritsch, S. et al. (1999). Possible first report of distant peritoneal metastases from a nodal mesenteric lymphoma after laparoscopic inguinal hernia repair. *Eur. J. Surg. Oncol.* 25 (6): 635–636.
30. Fujimoto, M., Haga, H., Okamoto, M. et al. (2008). EBV-associated diffuse large B-cell lymphoma arising in the chest wall with surgical mesh implant. *Pathol. Int.* 58 (10): 668–671.
31. Segal, Y. et al. (2018). The value of autoimmune syndrome induced by adjuvant (ASIA) – shedding light on orphan diseases in autoimmunity. *Autoimmun. Rev.* 17 (5): 440–448.
32. Coffman, R., Sher, A., and Seder, R. (2010). Vaccine adjuvants: putting innate immunity to work. *Immunity* 33 (4): 492–503.
33. Ruiz, J.T., Lujan, L., Blank, M., and Shoenfeld, Y. (2017). Adjuvants-and vaccines-induced autoimmunity: animal models. *Immunol. Res.* 65 (1): 55–65.
34. Major, M.R., Wong, V.W., Nelson, E.R. et al. (2015). The foreign body response: at the interface of surgery and bioengineering. *Plast. Reconstr. Surg.* 135 (5): 1489–1498.
35. Anderson, M., Rodriguez, A., and Chang, D.T. (2008). Foreign body reaction to biomaterials. *Semin. Immunol.* 20 (2): 86–100.
36. Ajdic, D., Zoghbi, Y., Gerth, D. et al. (2016). The relationship of bacterial biofilms and capsular contracture in breast implants. *Aesthet. Surg. J.* 36 (3): 297–309.
37. Langbach, O., Kristoffersen, A.K., Abesha-Belay, E. et al. (2016). Oral, intestinal, and skin bacteria in ventral hernia mesh implants. *J. Oral Microbiol.* 8: 31854.
38. Babensee, J.E. (2008). Interaction of dendritic cells with biomaterials. *Semin. Immunol.* 20: 101–108.
39. Nolfi, A.L., Brown, B.N., Liang, R. et al. (2016). Host response to synthetic mesh in women with mesh complications. *Am. J. Obstet. Gynecol.* 215 (2): 206.e1–206.e8.
40. Zdolsek, J.W. and Eaton, L.T. (2007). Histamine release and fibrinogen adsorption mediate acute inflammatory responses to biomaterial implants in humans. *J. Transl. Med.* 5: 31.
41. Wouters, M.M., Balemans, D., Van Wanrooy, S. et al. (2016). Histamine receptor H1-mediated sensitization of TRPV1 mediates visceral hypersensitivity and symptoms in patients with irritable bowel syndrome. *Gastroenterology* 150 (4): 875–887.
42. Junge, K., Binnebösel, M., von Trotha, K.T. et al. (2012). Mesh biocompatibility: effects of cellular inflammation and tissue remodelling. *Langenbeck's Arch. Surg.* 397 (2): 255–270.
43. Matzelle, M.M. and Babensee, J.E. (2004). Humoral immune responses to model antigen co-delivered with biomaterials used in tissue engineering. *Biomaterials* 25 (2): 295–304.

44. Bennewitz, N.L. and Babensee, J.E. (2005). The effect of the physical form of poly(lactic-co-glycolic acid) carriers on the humoral immune response to co-delivered antigen. *Biomaterials* 26 (16): 2991–2999.
45. Kool, M. (2008). Cutting edge: alum adjuvant stimulates inflammatory dendritic cells through activation of the NALP3 inflammasome. *J. Immunol.* 181 (6): 3755–3759.
46. See https://radiopaedia.org/articles/metal-on-metal-pseudotumour?lang=us. Accessed 10 May 2022.
47. Cobelli, N., Scharf, B., Crisi, G.M. et al. (2011). Mediators of the inflammatory response to joint replacement devices. *Nat. Rev. Rheumatol.* 7 (10): 600–608. https://doi.org/10.1038/nrrheum.2011.128.
48. Dowling, J. (2016). Toll-like receptors: the Swiss army knife of immunity and vaccine development. *Clin. Transl. Immunol.* 5: e85.
49. Grammatopoulos, G. et al. (2016). The diagnosis of infection in metal-on-metal hip arthroplasties. *J. Arthroplast.* 31 (11): 2569–2573. https://doi.org/10.1016/j.arth.2016.03.064.
50. McDonald, A.H., Weir, K., Schneider, M. et al. (1998). Silicone gel enhances the development of autoimmune disease in New Zealand black mice but fails to induce it in BALB/cAnPt mice. *Clin. Immunol. Immunopathol.* 87: 248–255.
51. See FDA Report: Biological Responses to Metal Implants (September 2019) at: https://www.fda.gov/media/131150/download. Accessed 10 May 2022.
52. Healy, D. and Mangin, D. (2019). Clinical Judgments, not algorithms, are key to patient safety. *BMJ* 367: I5777.
53. Lucas, R. and Rodney Harris, R. (2018). On the nature of evidence and 'Proving' causality: smoking and lung cancer vs. sun exposure, vitamin D and multiple sclerosis. *Int. J. Environ. Res. Public Health* 15 (8): E1726. https://doi.org/10.3390/ijerph15081726.
54. Damoiseaux, J.G.M.C. and Cohen Tervaert, J.W. (2002). The definition of autoimmune disease: are Koch's postulates applicable? *Neth. J. Med.* 60 (7): 266–268.
55. Fedak, K.M., Bernal, A., Capshaw, Z.A., and Gross, S. (2015). Applying the Bradford Hill criteria in the 21st century: how data integration has changed causal inference in molecular epidemiology. *Emerg. Themes Epidemiol.* 12: 14. https://doi.org/10.1186/s12982-015-0037-4.
56. "Guideline for Adverse Experience Reporting for Licensed Biological Products: Definitions" https://www.fda.gov/medwatch/report/cberguid/define.htm. Accessed 10 May 2022.
57. Song, J.W. and Chung, K.C. (2010). Observational studies: cohort and case-control studies. *Plast. Reconstr. Surg.* 126 (6): 2234–2242.
58. Kiene, H. et al. (2013). In support of clinical case reports: a system of causality assessment. *Glob. Adv. Health Med.* 2 (2): 64–75.
59. Schaefer, C.J., Lawrence, W.D., and Wooley, P.H. (1999). Influence of long term silicone implantation on type II collagen induced arthritis in mice. *Ann. Rheum. Dis.* 58: 503–509.
60. Schaefer, C.J. and Wooley, P.H. (1999). The influence of silicone implantation on murine lupus in MRL lpr/lpr mice. *J. Rheumatol.* 26 (10): 2215–2221.
61. https://www.medischcontact.nl/nieuws/laatste-nieuws/artikel/igz-check-voor-allergie-opborstprothese.htm. Accessed 10 May 2022

8 Vaccines, Vaccinosis, and Autoimmunity

Nicola Luigi Bragazzi[1,2], Abdulla Watad[3,4,5,6,7], and Yehuda Shoenfeld[8,9]

[1]Laboratory for Industrial and Applied Mathematics (LIAM), Department of Mathematics and Statistics, York University, Toronto, Canada
[2]Postgraduate School of Public Health, Department of Health Sciences (DISSAL), University of Genoa, Genoa, Italy
[3]Rheumatology Unit and Zabludowicz Center for Autoimmune Diseases, Sheba Medical Center, Tel-Hashomer, Israel
[4]Section of Musculoskeletal Disease, Leeds Institute of Molecular Medicine, University of Leeds, Leeds, UK
[5]Sackler Faculty of Medicine, Tel Aviv University, Tel Aviv, Israel
[6]Department of Internal Medicine 'B', Sheba Medical Center, Tel-Hashomer, Israel
[7]Institute of Oncology, Sheba Medical Center, Tel-Hashomer, Israel
[8]Reichman University, Herzliya, Israel
[9]Zabludowicz Center for Autoimmune Diseases, Sheba Medical Center, Tel-Hashomer, Israel

Vaccines and their epidemiological, clinical, societal, and economic impact

Vaccination stands as one of the most significant and transformative medical achievements in the annals of human history, as only a few public and global health intervention measures are comparable with the impact of vaccines, in terms of reduced burden of disease, comorbidities, and mortality [1].

Vaccines have played and still play a pivotal role in reducing the incidence and prevalence rates as well as the severity of numerous infectious diseases that were once widespread and devastating, such as smallpox and polio. Their virtual eradication has been made possible, thanks to mass vaccination campaigns [2, 3], while infectious diseases such as measles, mumps, rubella, and hepatitis have seen a significant decline, resulting in healthier populations and reduced suffering [4, 5].

Vaccines not only prevent specific diseases but also help prevent associated complications, sequelae, and comorbidities. For example, the influenza vaccine helps protect against seasonal flu, reducing the likelihood of developing pneumonia, being hospitalized, and dying, especially in vulnerable populations such as the frail elderly and individuals with underlying health conditions, meaning fewer people suffering from debilitating complications and a lower strain on healthcare systems [6].

Autoimmune Disorders: Adjuvants and Other Risk Factors in Pathogenesis, First Edition.
Edited by Abdulla Watad, Nicola Luigi Bragazzi, and Yehuda Shoenfeld.

Vaccines have been instrumental in saving countless lives: by preventing deadly diseases, they have directly contributed to a substantial decrease in mortality rates, especially among infants and children, who are particularly vulnerable to infectious diseases and have benefited tremendously from vaccines, as they are now shielded from the devastating consequences of diseases such as diphtheria, whooping cough, and tetanus [7, 8].

Beyond individual protection, vaccines also foster herd immunity. When a sufficient portion of a population is vaccinated, the spread of a disease is greatly curtailed. This not only protects those who cannot be vaccinated due to medical reasons but also contributes to the overall reduction in disease transmission. Herd immunity has been a key factor in the control of diseases such as measles and the "Coronavirus Disease 2019" (COVID-19) [9].

By preventing illness and reducing healthcare costs associated with treating infectious diseases, vaccines save governments and individuals billions of dollars annually. Additionally, they enable a more productive workforce by reducing absenteeism due to illness. Vaccination is not limited by borders: it is a public and global public health intervention that has improved the well-being of people worldwide. International vaccination efforts, such as those led by organizations such as the World Health Organization (WHO) and Gavi, the Vaccine Alliance, have reached underserved populations, helping to bridge healthcare disparities and improve health equity [10].

Vaccination represents a monumental milestone in the realm of medicine and human history; with such a profound impact, only a handful of other public health measures and global interventions can rival its significance [1].

In summary, vaccination is an unparalleled medical achievement that has significantly contributed to reshaping the course of human history by (i) reducing the burden of disease, (ii) preventing comorbidities, (iii) saving lives, (iv) fostering herd immunity, (v) spurring economic growth, and (vi) promoting public and global health. As such, vaccination is a cornerstone of modern medicine and a testament to human progress, innovation, and collaboration, standing as a shining example of how science and medicine can triumph over some of the most formidable challenges humanity faces. To quote Orenstein and Ahmed, "simply put: vaccination saves lives" [1].

Vaccines, vaccinosis, and autoimmunity

As previously said, the history of vaccination is replete with stories of triumph over affliction, from the eradication of smallpox to the curbing of polio's devastating reach. Vaccines, through the priming of the immune system with innocuous components of pathogens or weakened pathogens themselves, have enabled the building-up of immunological memory, which empowers the immune system to mount swift and robust defenses upon subsequent encounters with the actual pathogenic agents.

Yet, in some rare cases, rather than safeguarding the body, vaccination turns insidiously against its own tissues. The exploration into the potential correlations between vaccines and autoimmune disorders has resulted in two distinct but interwoven lines of scholarly inquiry. The first centers on the concept of molecular mimicry, wherein certain components of pathogens present in vaccines might resemble self-structures, inadvertently fostering a misguided immune attack on the body's own tissues. The second revolves around the notion that vaccine-triggered immune responses could potentially escalate preexisting autoimmune predispositions or unleash latent autoimmune reactions, thereby contributing to the onset or exacerbation of autoimmune conditions. Crucially, within these debates, vaccine adjuvants have emerged as a subject of meticulous scrutiny. They serve to amplify the immune system's recognition and response to the targeted pathogenic elements. For instance, aluminum salts have become a quintessential adjuvant, stimulating heightened immune reactions through the formation of a depot at the injection site and fostering a prolonged interaction between the immune cells and the antigen. However, as the discourse regarding vaccines and autoimmune diseases has gained traction, certain adjuvants, particularly those categorized as immune response modulators, have spurred discussion about their safety due to their potential to perturb the immune equilibrium. These adjuvants, including oil-in-water emulsions and toll-like receptor agonists, possess the capacity to elicit robust immune responses. While this attribute is the bedrock of their effectiveness, it also sparks concerns that they might inadvertently incite imbalances that could potentially contribute to autoimmune propensities or exacerbate existing autoimmune conditions in susceptible individuals. This symphony of factors – the awe-inspiring efficacy of vaccines, the intricacies of autoimmune disorders, and the nuanced properties of vaccine adjuvants – harmonizes in the realm of immune responses. The capacity of vaccine adjuvants to amplify and direct immune reactions is both a boon and a challenge, as their deliberate modulation may tip the balance in unpredictable ways, holding both the potential for enhanced protection and unforeseen consequences. The ongoing quest to comprehend the intricate interplay among vaccines, autoimmune diseases, and the pivotal role of vaccine adjuvants embodies a testament to the ceaseless pursuit of scientific understanding and the imperative to safeguard public and global health in a world replete with both promise and complexity.

Vaccines and immune system activation

Vaccines function by stimulating the immune system to recognize and mount defenses against specific pathogens. This involves introducing harmless components of the pathogen, such as proteins or genetic material, to trigger an immune response. The immune system then develops memory cells that provide rapid and targeted responses if reexposure to the pathogen occurs. While vaccines have been crucial in preventing infectious diseases, concerns have been raised about the potential for vaccines to trigger or exacerbate autoimmune diseases.

Autoimmune diseases: background and mechanisms

Autoimmune diseases result from a malfunctioning immune system that targets and damages the body's own tissues, mistaking them for foreign invaders. Examples include rheumatoid arthritis, multiple sclerosis, and lupus. Complex interactions involving genetic predispositions, environmental factors, and immune dysregulation contribute to the development of these conditions. The role of vaccines in precipitating autoimmune diseases has led to investigations into specific vaccine components, particularly adjuvants [11, 12].

Vaccine adjuvants: purpose and impact

Vaccine adjuvants are substances added to vaccines to enhance the immune response. They help activate immune cells, increase the persistence of antigens in the body, and promote the production of antibodies. Common adjuvants include aluminum salts and oil-in-water emulsions (Chapter 3). These adjuvants provoke stronger and longer-lasting immune reactions, ultimately improving vaccine efficacy. However, concerns have arisen regarding their potential to trigger autoimmune responses in susceptible individuals.

Adjuvants and autoimmunity: the body of currently available evidence

Scientific investigations into the relationship between adjuvants and autoimmune diseases have yielded mixed results. The majority of studies suggest that vaccine adjuvants are generally safe and do not significantly contribute to the development of autoimmune diseases in the general population. However, a small subset of individuals with specific genetic predispositions might exhibit adverse reactions to adjuvanted vaccines.

Autoimmune/Inflammatory Syndrome Induced by Adjuvants (ASIA) is a medical condition initially introduced by Shoenfeld et al. in 2011. The authors proposed a set of major and minor criteria, to assist in diagnosing ASIA syndrome. This syndrome encompasses a group of closely related immune-mediated diseases that share common clinical features and a history of previous exposure to adjuvant agents. These common factors are particularly evident in individuals who have experienced conditions such as Macrophagic Myofasciitis Syndrome (MMF), postvaccination phenomena, Gulf War Syndrome (GWS), and siliconosis. Postvaccination phenomena and MMF are primarily associated with the use of aluminum-based adjuvants. In contrast, squalene adjuvant exposure has been linked to the incidence of GWS. Clinically, these four diseases exhibit typical constitutional symptoms, including myalgia, arthralgia, chronic fatigue, and dry mouth, as well as neurological manifestations such as cognitive disturbances, memory loss, and neurological disabilities. Similar to other autoimmune disease entities, the etiology of these conditions involves a complex interplay between environmental factors and genetic predisposition, as evidenced by their association with specific Human Leukocyte Antigen (HLA) haplotypes. Since its identification as a distinct medical condition, more than 4000 documented cases of ASIA syndrome have been reported, showing varying clinical severity and diverse histories of adjuvant exposure. In this review, we aim to provide a comprehensive overview of the current literature concerning ASIA syndrome and its relationship with vaccines and compounds, such as adjuvants. Our goal is to elucidate fundamental concepts to increase physician awareness, thereby facilitating early diagnosis and preventing adjuvant exposure in individuals at high risk for autoimmunity.

As previously overviewed, the development of vaccines has been a significant milestone in public health, ranking among the most substantial advancements of the past century. Vaccinations offer protection against infectious diseases that were once associated with severe consequences, including high rates of illness and mortality. While vaccines are generally well tolerated, there have been instances where vaccine administration has been linked to the induction of autoimmune manifestations and the production of autoantibodies. Additionally, individuals with preexisting rheumatologic conditions have reported worsening of their diseases following vaccination. The phenomenon of postvaccination effects is believed to be primarily related to the immunological properties of adjuvants administered alongside vaccines. Adjuvants are extensively studied to ensure that they possess qualities such as stability, strong immunogenicity, and adequate bioavailability, all while being well tolerated. Aluminum salts, specifically aluminum phosphate or hydroxide, are among the most commonly used adjuvants. They have been shown to enhance antigen presentation, activate the innate immune system, and promote the activation of T-helper cells (TH)1 and TH2. Vaccines containing aluminum-based adjuvants have been associated with postvaccination phenomena and symptoms related to ASIA. Animal models have demonstrated an increase in seroconversion and antibody levels for systemic lupus erythematosus (SLE) following hepatitis B virus (HBV) vaccination in genetically susceptible mice. Furthermore, the administration of alum-based adjuvants in mice led to the development of Sjögren-like disease, characterized by higher antibody levels, reduced saliva production, and documented inflammatory responses in the salivary glands. Similar findings from animal studies have prompted numerous investigations into autoimmune adverse effects associated with vaccination administration. Many of these investigations have relied on safety surveillance data from the United States Vaccine Adverse Event Reporting System (VAERS). For instance, a case–control study revealed an increased risk of arthritis, vasculitis, SLE, and neurological conditions following the quadrivalent HPV vaccine administered over a six-year period. These effects typically occurred approximately 1–7 weeks after vaccination. The quadrivalent HPV vaccine contains virus-like particles of four HPV serotypes (6, 11, 16, and 18) in an aluminum-based adjuvanted formulation. Several other associations between vaccination and autoimmune phenomena have been documented, including Guillain–Barre syndrome outbreaks following H1N1 and HBV vaccinations, idiopathic thrombocytopenic purpura (ITP) following Measles–Mumps–Rubella (MMR) and varicella zoster vaccinations, arthritis following diphtheria–tetanus–pertussis (DTP) and MMR vaccinations, and influenza vaccine preceding Hashimoto's thyroiditis. Additionally, multiple cases of giant cell arthritis (GCA) were reported in otherwise healthy individuals who received adjuvanted influenza vaccination within the previous three months. Besides the proposed role of adjuvants in triggering autoimmune responses, other vaccine components such as neomycin and polymyxin have been implicated in influencing specific immunological responses. Several mechanisms have been suggested for how infections can induce autoimmune diseases, including molecular mimicry, which involves structural similarities between viral antigens (or vaccine components) and self-antigens, and the formation of immune complexes, which can lead to vasculitis and the exacerbation of existing autoimmune symptoms.

Regulatory measures and ongoing research

While most epidemiological studies do not indicate apparent safety concerns regarding vaccines, awareness of the development of ASIA syndrome and the identification of high-risk factors could help prevent adverse reactions in susceptible individuals.

Regulatory agencies, such as the WHO and the U.S. Food and Drug Administration (FDA), rigorously assess the safety of vaccine adjuvants before their approval for use in vaccines. Ongoing research seeks to better understand the mechanisms of adjuvant-induced immune responses and their potential implications for autoimmune diseases. Advances in personalized medicine are expected to shed light on the genetic factors that may render certain individuals more susceptible to adverse reactions.

Conclusion

The relationship among vaccines, autoimmune diseases, and vaccine adjuvants remains a complex and evolving field of study. While the majority of evidence indicates that adjuvanted vaccines are safe and effective, ongoing research strives to uncover potential links between specific adjuvants and autoimmune disorders. Understanding the underlying mechanisms and genetic factors that contribute to such relationships will guide the development of safer and more tailored vaccination strategies, ultimately benefiting public health. In the pursuit of these objectives, the imperative to prevent infectious diseases must be harmonized with the goal of safeguarding vulnerable individuals from potential adverse reactions.

References

1. Orenstein, W.A. and Ahmed, R. (2017). Simply put: vaccination saves lives. *Proc. Natl. Acad. Sci. U. S. A.* 114 (16): 4031–4033. https://doi.org/10.1073/pnas.1704507114.
2. Aylward, B. and Tangermann, R. (2011). The global polio eradication initiative: lessons learned and prospects for success. *Vaccine* 29 (Suppl 4): D80–D85. https://doi.org/10.1016/j.vaccine.2011.10.005.
3. Javed, H., Rizvi, M.A., Fahim, Z. et al. (2023). Global polio eradication; can we replicate the smallpox success story? *Rev. Med. Virol.* 33 (3): e2409. https://doi.org/10.1002/rmv.2409.
4. Elliman, D., Sengupta, N., El Bashir, H., and Bedford, H. (2009). Measles, mumps, and rubella: prevention. *BMJ Clin. Evid.* 2009: 0316.
5. Mohanty, P., Jena, P., and Patnaik, L. (2020). Vaccination against hepatitis B: a scoping review. *Asian Pac. J. Cancer Prev.* 21 (12): 3453–3459. https://doi.org/10.31557/APJCP.2020.21.12.3453.
6. Rémy, V., Zöllner, Y., and Heckmann, U. (2015). Vaccination: the cornerstone of an efficient healthcare system. *J. Mark. Access Health Policy.* 3 (1): 27041. https://doi.org/10.3402/jmahp.v3.27041.
7. Clem, A.S. (2011). Fundamentals of vaccine immunology. *J. Global Infect. Dis.* 3 (1): 73–78. https://doi.org/10.4103/0974-777X.77299.
8. Delany, I., Rappuoli, R., and De Gregorio, E. (2014). Vaccines for the 21st century. *EMBO Mol. Med.* 6 (6): 708–720. https://doi.org/10.1002/emmm.201403876.
9. McDermott, A. (2021). Core Concept: Herd immunity is an important-and often misunderstood-public health phenomenon. *Proc. Natl. Acad. Sci. U. S. A.* 118 (21): e2107692118. https://doi.org/10.1073/pnas.2107692118.
10. Ekezie, W., Awwad, S., Krauchenberg, A. et al. (2022). Access to vaccination among disadvantaged, isolated and difficult-to-reach communities in the WHO European Region: a systematic review. *Vaccines (Basel)* 10 (7): 1038. https://doi.org/10.3390/vaccines10071038.
11. Institute of Medicine (US) Board on Health Promotion and Disease Prevention (1997). *Vaccine Safety Forum: Summaries of Two Workshops.* Washington, DC: National Academies Press (US) https://www.ncbi.nlm.nih.gov/books/NBK233000/.
12. Watad, A., Sharif, K., and Shoenfeld, Y. (2017). The ASIA syndrome: basic concepts. *Mediterr. J. Rheumatol.* 28 (2): 64–69. https://doi.org/10.31138/mjr.28.2.64.

9 Sustained Immune Activation in ASIA Syndrome – A Bridge to Lymphomagenesis

Dana Butnaru

Department of Clinical Immunology, Hospital Clínico San Carlos, Complutense University of Madrid, Madrid, Spain

Background

If in the past the immune system has *mainly* been fighting foreign invaders (e.g. bacteria, viruses, and parasites), nowadays, the increasing incidence and prevalence of autoimmune and autoinflammatory diseases in our world show that we are facing a different battle –a battle in which the immune system unexpectedly turns against body's own organs and systems, opposing a different type of enemy – *the enemy within.*

Immune-mediated pathological conditions such as those arising within the autoimmune spectrum are a significant cause of morbidity and mortality worldwide and especially among young individuals [1]. Their increase is having a destabilizing impact upon society, shaking its two fundamental pillars: the workforce and the procreative potential. First, it does so by mainly targeting young and middle-aged adults and, secondly, by disproportionately affecting women.

It has long been acknowledged that infectious agents such as *Helicobacter pylori*, Epstein–Barr virus, and hepatitis C virus play an important role in the ethology of malignancies [2–4]. Lymphoma arising in the context of chronic/sustained activation of the immune system depends mainly on two factors: (i) the disease intensity and (ii) the accumulated inflammatory activity [5, 6]. It is associated not only with pathogens but also with sterile (pathogen-free) inflammation, as in the case of the classical autoimmune disorders as well as related to (perhaps) a less-known condition referred to as the autoimmune syndrome induced by adjuvants (ASIA *syndrome*) [7].

Introduction

Over a decade ago, in 2010, Shoenfeld and Agmon-Levin [7] observed that four "enigmatic" medical conditions including the Gulf War syndrome, macrophagic myofasciitis, siliconosis, and postvaccination phenomena share clinical manifestations and common mechanisms, being triggered by adjuvant exposure. The link between these four conditions and adjuvants was later validated in animal models [8–11], pointing, thus, to an underlying autoinflammatory/autoimmune

Autoimmune Disorders: Adjuvants and Other Risk Factors in Pathogenesis, First Edition.
Edited by Abdulla Watad, Nicola Luigi Bragazzi, and Yehuda Shoenfeld.

Table 9.1 Major and minor criteria for the diagnosis of the ASIA syndrome.

Major criteria
1 Exposure to an external stimuli (infection, vaccine, silicone, and adjuvant) prior to clinical manifestations
2 The appearance of "typical" clinical manifestations: – *Myalgia, Myositis, or muscle weakness* – *Arthralgia and/or arthritis* – *Chronic fatigue, unrefreshing sleep, or sleep disturbances* – *Neurological manifestations (especially associated with demyelination)* – *Cognitive impairment and memory loss* – *Pyrexia and dry mouth*
3 Removal of inciting agent induces improvement
4 Typical biopsy of involved organs
Minor criteria
a) Presence of antibodies or autoantibodies directed against the suspected adjuvant b) Other clinical manifestations (i.e. irritable bowel syndrome – IBS) c) Specific HLAs (i.e. HLA DRB1 and HLA DQB1) d) Initiation or evolvement toward an autoimmune disease (i.e. MS and SSc)

Source: Adapted from Shoenfeld and Agmon-Levin [7].

process as a common etiological denominator. The ASIA syndrome was henceforth defined as an *autoinflammatory/autoimmune syndrome induced by adjuvants* [7, 12].

The proposed criteria for the diagnosis of "ASIA" include a set of eight criteria (four major and four minor criteria, listed in Table 9.1). At least two major or one major and two minor criteria must be met [7].

The mechanism for the vaccines-induced autoimmunity is linked with three basic components of the vaccines: the infectious agents, the adjuvants, and the preservatives. Out of these, the adjuvant component seems to play a major role. In inducing autoimmunity, the infectious agent may act through the following specific mechanisms: molecular mimicry, epitope spreading, bystander activation, and/or polyclonal activation [13]. An adjuvant's main role is to provide physical protection to the antigens and assist the translocation of the antigen to the lymph node which would enhance the immune system response by mediating a longer and effective exposure of the antigen to the immune cells [7]. In the lymph nodes, adjuvants induce macrophages activation through toll-like receptor (TLR) binding and, by themselves, acting as *nonspecific (hyper)*stimulators of the immune system (see below).

Most adjuvants act by stimulating the immune system via two mechanisms. First, they carry the basic adjuvant/enhancer property on the immune system, and secondly, they may act as foreign substances capable to induce a foreign body reaction (FBR) through inflammasome activation [14]. The inflammasome's activation mechanism is shared between nonnative materials (e.g. metallic implants). Recent insights into the adverse mechanism of adjuvants showed that adjuvants can not only trigger autoimmunity but the effect of long-lasting exposure to adjuvants may go even further, resulting in hematologic malignancies of the immune system such as lymphomas [15–17]. The *lymphomagenesis* phenomenon has been linked to adjuvant's ability to maintain chronic, local, or systemic activation of the immune system and in particular to their ability to promote macrophage activation, thus impeding macrophage clearance [15, 17, 18]. Several cases of lymphoma were described mainly of diffuse large B-cell lymphoma type, related to chronic inflammation following metallic implants [19–22].

The adjuvant effect leading to ASIA syndrome is not universal but rather linked to a genetic predisposition determined by the human leukocyte antigen (HLA) complexes HLA-DRB1 and HLA-DQB1 [13]. However, these genetic barriers may be overcome by the co-exposure to multiple adjuvants or to other immunostimulant factors (incitants) such as infections [7].

Animal model as a proof of concept

In 2004, Madewell et al. [23] published a study describing six cases of cats developing lymphoma after vaccine injection. The tumor was characterized as disseminated malignant lymphoma without relation to the feline leukemia virus (FeLV) infection. The lymphoma emerged within 3–45 months after the histopathologic diagnosis of the "vaccine site-associated fibrosarcoma." In three cases, the immunohistochemistry for lymphocyte markers confirmed a T-cell phenotype of the tumor cells. One case was of the B-cell phenotype. Another case developed gastrointestinal lymphoma, and for the last case, the aspiration and cytopathology revealed lymphoma, but immunohistochemistry was not done. The typical features of "vaccine site-associated sarcomas" are peritumoral aggregates of lymphocytes, especially of T-cell type. The lymphoma development was not related to a specific type of vaccine [23].

Anderson and Potter [24, 25] have shown that the adjuvant pristane, which is known to induce arthritis [26] and lupus-related autoantibodies [27], induced IgA-secreting plasmacytomas (a B-cell lymphoproliferative disorder), "a unique form of carcinogenesis" in susceptible mouse strains, in particular the BALB/c.

Autoimmunity and lymphoma: role of immune chronic stimulation in lymphoma development

It has been emphasized that EBV-associated malignant lymphoma occurs particularly in patients who are treated with immunosuppressant therapies [2]. However, a Japanese study [28] reported that EBV-associated lymphoma occupied only a small fraction of all non-Hodgkin lymphomas in patients with rheumatoid arthritis (RA). Lymphomas associated with autoimmunity constitute a different spectrum of entities compared with lymphoma arising in patients without any known autoimmune or inflammatory conditions [29].

The dual relationship between autoimmunity and malignancies has long been accepted [30]. The risk of lymphoma is increased in patients with autoimmune diseases compared to the general population and vice versa. In particular, patients with lymphoma display high titers of autoimmune markers, indicating that the lymphoma and the autoimmune diseases are highly interconnected [31]. Different autoimmune diseases have different risk rates of lymphoma development. Patients with RA have a twofold increased risk of lymphoma, while systemic lupus erythematosus has a three- to fourfold risk [30]. Primary Sjögren's syndrome has a 16-fold risk [32]. The highest risk was seen in Hashimoto's thyroiditis where the patients exhibit a 60-fold increased risk of thyroid lymphoma [33]. The standardized incidence ratio (SIR), with a 95% confidence interval, for the more prevalent autoimmune diseases is listed in Table 9.2.

The most common type of lymphomas related to autoimmune diseases are the *non-Hodgkin lymphomas* (NHL). Among these, the mucosa-associated lymphoid tissue lymphomas (MALT) and the diffuse large B-cell lymphomas are the most prevalent [33, 41]. The MALT lymphomas are an indolent B-cell non-Hodgkin type of lymphoma occurring in a variety of organs including the stomach, salivary glands, intestine, and the thyroid gland. The gastric MALT lymphoma is an outstanding example of the close pathogenetic link between chronic inflammation and tumor development. Most patients (490%) with gastric MALT lymphoma are *H. pylori* positive [42]. MALT develops in the lymphoid aggregates induced by chronic antigenic stimulation and chronic

Table 9.2 Lymphoma in autoimmune diseases.

Disease	SIR	References
Primary Sjögren's syndrome	8.7–15.6	Kauppy et al. [34] and Theander et al. [32]
Secondary Sjögren's syndrome	4.5	Kauppy et al. [34]
Systemic lupus erythematosus	4.07–5.0	Bernatsky et al. [6] and Dreyer et al. [35]
Rheumatoid arthritis	2.08–3.1	Smitten et al. [36] and Mercer et al. [37]
Celiac disease	5.15–6.6	Grainge et al. [38] and Smedby et al. [39]
Systemic sclerosis	2.68	Zhang et al. [40]

SIR, *standardized incidence ratio, 95% confidence interval.*
Kauppy, Finnish population; Theander, Swedish population; Bernatsky, international; Dreyer, Danish population; Mercer, UK population; Smitten, international; Grainge, Scottish population; Smedby, Swedish population; Zhang, international.

inflammation [4, 42]. The multistep process of lymphomagenesis in MALT can go even further, undergoing transition to a higher-grade lymphoma: *the diffuse large B-cell lymphoma*. The latter represents a *blastic* version of the previous low-grade lymphoma, MALT [42].

Hodgkin's lymphomas were also associated with autoimmune diseases. Swedish data from 2009 have found an overall 2.7-fold increased risk of Hodgkin's lymphomas for all systemic autoimmune diseases combined [43]. RA severity (characterized by the presence of Felty's syndrome, high erythrocyte sedimentation rate, and/or secondary Sjögren's syndrome) and the cumulated disease activity (number of swollen and tender joints) appear to be strongly related to diffuse large B-cell lymphoma risk [29]. The immune cell activation in lymph nodes in patients with RA was seen in early arthritis and was associated with an increase in activated $CD19^+$ B cells and $CD69^+$ $CD8^+$ T cells compared with healthy individuals [44]. The diffuse large B-cell lymphoma in patients with RA has a worse outcome compared with de novo diffuse large B-cell lymphoma [31]. The role played by the B cells in RA is seen in the success of rituximab therapy (an anti-CD20 monoclonal antibody), which leads to an improvement in disease activity as evaluated through the *disease activity score* (DAS-28) [45]. Yet, the evidence that the risk of lymphoma is reduced in RA after biological therapy are inconclusive. Instead, after depleting the B cells with rituximab, another type of lymphoma, the T-cell lymphoma, has been reported [29, 46]. This behavior of immune system is compatible with the so-called *kaleidoscope phenomenon* [47, 48]. It stresses the fact that when one immune pathway is blocked (e.g. with a drug), the immune system may use alternative pathways to reach another outcome (or opens up in a different fashion) (i.e. the above cited example of T-cell lymphoma development after anti-B-cell therapy). On the other side, the aggressive diffuse large B-cell lymphoma is also the most common form of non-Hodgkin's lymphoma seen in SLE. The risk of lymphoma in SLE is not associated with the therapy nor does it seem to be related to the secondary Sjögren's syndrome (SS) [30].

As stated above, and except for the rituximab therapy (where in a recent (2021) study [49] was seen a declining tendency in lymphoma risk), the improvement in biological therapies did not change the overall risk of lymphoma in the past decades [29]. This fact may imply that the outer control of inflammation, when acting upon a late event in the inflammatory chain, is not sufficient to prevent lymphomagenesis. As in the case of celiac disease, only by removing the first step in its pathogenesis, represented by the antigen (gluten) exposure, the risk of lymphoma could decrease [29]. The persistent immunologic assault during long periods of exposure to an antigen ends in a continuous, dynamic adaptive immune activation. The *"fail to switch off"* mechanism seems to be the pathophysiologic basis of T/B lymphocytes' ongoing stimulation that contributes to the genesis of lymphoma [4, 50].

Hereunder are highlighted three aspects of the chronic/ongoing inflammation that could bridge the gap between autoimmunity and lymphoma development:

(i) *Breakdown of ROS homeostasis*

An adjusted and fine-tuned *redox balance* is essential for the regulation of inflammation and prevention of the development of overt autoimmunity. Reactive oxygen species (ROS) comprise a family of short-lived molecules including O_2^-, H_2O_2, and •OH, also known as free radicals. Physiological roles for ROS in cells span from aiding immunity (e.g. oxidative bursts in phagocytes to eliminate pathogens) to acting as signaling molecules (e.g. H_2O_2 regulating NF-kB or MAPK pathways) [51]. The main endogenous producers of ROS are mitochondria, NADPH oxidase (NOX), peroxisomes, and endoplasmic reticulum (in which H_2O_2 is a by-product of protein folding). Exogenously produced ROS is detected upon exposure to ionizing radiation, chemotherapeutic drugs, and many environmental insults that affect organelles and enzymes within the cells. Aluminum-based adjuvants are able to cause an oxidative (increased rate of ROS formation) and inflammatory response [52]. Moreover, irrespective of adjuvant composition, or tissue derivation of cells, a dose-dependent aluminum-based adjuvant would cause the *same degree* of necrosis that then leads to pro-inflammatory cytokine release [52].

ROS have long been recognized as mediators of DNA damage. ROS imbalance promotes the initiation, onset, and pathogenesis of several autoimmune diseases. In the chronic stages of autoimmune diseases, high ROS levels are often observed, causing cell and tissue damage such as total destruction of pancreas beta-cells or degradation of joints cartilage in RA. Chronic inflammation exposes body cells to cumulative ROS concentrations and can influence several signaling pathways that could drive to the rise of lymphoma. Prolonged high levels of ROS are essential for cellular transformation and tumorigenesis. ROS damage of DNA leads to the *genomic instability*. Lymphomas that are derived from sites of chronic inflammation appear to have a chemoresistant phenotype resulting from enhanced antioxidant defenses [53]. Unexpectedly, it was shown by Campbell et al. [54] and Becaria et al. [49] that prolonged exposure to low levels of aluminum, even as present in the drinking water, enhances oxidative and inflammatory markers, specifically, in mouse brains (which, according to the authors, may be involved in age-related neurological disorders) [54, 55].

(ii) *Transition from low Treg in autoimmune disorders to high Treg in lymphomas mediated by chronic inflammation*

Although autoimmune disorders and cancer are considered immunological opposites, both autoimmunity and *early* cancers are initiated and promoted within a *similar inflammatory setting* [56]. Regulatory T cells (Tregs) are highly immunosuppressive subsets of $CD4^+$ (or, recently, $CD8^+$ T) lymphocytes. During its course of growth, malignancy progresses from a pro-inflammatory, "low-Treg" disease (characteristic to autoimmune diseases too), to an anti-inflammatory, "high-Treg" disease [56]. Tregs cells are key players in tumor immune escape. A diversity of Tregs-mediating immunosuppression is seen in both NHL and classic Hodgkin lymphoma (cHL). Especially in NHL, the tumor cells appear to be powerful inducers of Treg cells (which may represent a new therapeutic target) [57, 58].

(iii) *PD-1 is upregulation in late/advanced autoimmune processes and incipient lymphoma*

Coinhibitory receptors such as programmed cell death protein-1 (PD-1), cytotoxic T lymphocyte antigen-4 (CTLA-4), and others were reported to be the main hallmark of T-cell exhaustion. T-cell exhaustion is a state of relatively reduced/arrested T-cell functionality caused by prolonged antigen exposure. It is shared among the spectrum of viral infection (viral persistence associated with poor clearance), autoimmune disease, and cancer (including Hodgkin's and non-Hodgkin's lymphomas [59]). Adjuvants that by their very nature activate chronically and nonspecifically the immune system (see sections titled Foreign body reaction (FBR) and lymphoma and Silicone versus aluminum compounds and lymphomagenesis association) may also join the list. Persistent antigen stimulation under *suboptimal* conditions appears

> to be the key to the induction of T-cell exhaustion [60]. Exhausted T cells have reduced (yet recoverable) functionality in which the cytolytic activity and cytokine secretion are impaired. The T-cell exhaustion is associated with ineffective control of persisting infections and tumors (as exhausted tumor-infiltrating lymphocytes fail to control tumor progression). In contrast to cancer or infection, T-cell exhaustion is associated with a favorable clinical outcome in autoimmune diseases (e.g. fewer relapses) as well as in organ transplantation (i.e. prevention of allograft rejection). This positive side to T-cell exhaustion, which, under physiological conditions, controls or limits autoimmunity (including T1D and SLE), serves as a mechanism to protect against tissue damage from an overwhelming CD8T cell response [61]. Even more, exhaustion functions as a brake by blocking T-cell proliferation under chronic antigenic stimulation, preserving the immunological reserve, preventing further use of resources, and allowing immune potential regeneration [62].

Exhausted T cells are not inert. T-cell exhaustion is not a terminal fate and, rather than leading inexorably to apoptotic death, constitutes a specific, stable, and heritable state of differentiation, a distinct epigenetic state of $CD8^+$ T and $CD4^+$ T cells that still *retains* some residual function [63, 64]. T-cell exhaustion represents a *continuous spectrum* of cellular "dysfunction," spanning from stem-like to terminally differentiated cell subsets [65, 66].

At the molecular level, exhaustion *preserves* T-cell clones repertoire [62], that is, assists with the retention of antigen-specific T cells within the repertoire under chronic antigenic stimulation (required for immunosurveillance), thus preventing the downward path toward oligo- and monoclonality (or *clone immunodominancy*).

When it comes to autoimmunity–lymphoma connection, the versatile, multifaceted nature of T-cell exhaustion may be better represented by the imagery of "a wheel within a wheel" [67]; so complicated in arrangement that at first sight they appeared to be in confusion, yet they move in perfect harmony. During the progression of the autoimmune processes, PD-1 upregulation with the subsequent T-cell exhaustion is more marked in the late/chronic stages of disease. PD-1 upregulation works as a barrier restraining disease progression and *preserving* the immunological reserve.

Cancer starts with T-cell exhaustion to progressively expand toward overt immune evasion of tumor. PD-1 remains upregulated on T cells as long as TCR engagement is sustained. However, PD-1 expression is driven not by a sole antigen but by a *diverse range* of oncoantigens (triggering TCR) that affect in an uneven manner T-cell responses determining degrees of "exhaustion severity" and creating (at least two classes of) *subdominant* $TCD8^+$ clones and *immunodominant clones*. The higher the titer of inhibitory molecules expressed by the exhausted T cells, the more severe the exhaustion. A recent (2018) and fascinating study [68] demonstrated that the success of immunotherapy using checkpoint inhibitors (i.e. [PD-L1]-blocking Abs.) consisted in alleviating clonal immunodominance, yet not by triggering down the immunodominant clone/s but by acting upon the subdominant clones (of severe exhaustion), relieving their immunosuppressive pressure, increasing their size, and invigorating the $TCD8^+$ responses. Overall, the anti-PD-1 therapy increased the *epitope breadth* of the $TCD8^+$ broadening the T-cell responses within the tumor.

The above study shows that although oligo- and monoclonality may characterize autoimmunity and neoplasia, respectively, the immunodominant clone/s may not be the direct cause of immunopathology in cancers (or autoimmunity), but rather it is the decrease in clonal diversity and the loss of lymphocytes connectivity the real culprits behind cancer poor recovery (see also Vaz and Carvalho [69]).

Triggering the immunodominant clones in cancer rather than invigorating/boosting the subdominant clones could explain the failure of traditional treatment approaches in cancer.

Of note, it should be mentioned that T-cell exhaustion is only in part reversible upon antigen removal [70, 71]. There are exhausted, conserved epigenetic states of T cells that persist independent and *in the absence* of antigen stimulation [64, 72].

Vaccination and acute lymphoma development

A vaccination event, acting upon a previously dysfunctional immune system, can push the immune system toward lymphomagenesis. Porto et al. [73] reported a typical case of a 61-year-old woman under treatment for RA who developed pseudolymphoma after varicella zoster virus vaccination. Another case was of a 31-year-old female with a history of pseudolymphoma on the left arm at the vaccination site. She received a second injection with the meningoencephalitis vaccine on the right upper arm four years after the first vaccination and developed a second pseudolymphoma at the new injection site [74]. The third case is represented by a 15-year-old girl with a history of urticaria since 2005, allergy to penicillin and obesity that after the second dose of papillomavirus vaccination in 2008 developed Hodgkin lymphoma [personal communication]. More cases of Hodgkin lymphoma related to vaccination are detailed (see ref. [16]). The above-documented cases show that a vaccination event may trigger lymphoma or pseudolymphoma in patients with a previous history of autoinflammatory disease or allergy. Manifestations such as myalgia, chronic fatigue, and vitiligo were also present in some of the patients who developed pseudolymphoma following vaccination [17]. It stresses the fact that lymphoma may be a part and seen as a new facet of the "ASIA" spectrum. Specific metal (Morin) stains, electronic microscopy, microanalysis, and immunologic cutaneous provocation tests have demonstrated the participation of adjuvants such as aluminum in these cutaneous reactions [74].

Foreign body reaction (FBR) and lymphoma

Nanomaterials such as silica and aluminum as well as large particles of synthetic polymers used in prosthesis, plastics, or glass all evoke within the body a *foreign body response* (FBR). The acute inflammatory response to foreign bodies has been identified as Nlrp3 inflammasome activation dependent. Foreign materials irrespective of their size can activate the inflammasome and induce an inflammatory infiltrate which is dependent on the inflammasome components NLRP3, Asc, and caspase 1 [14]. The activation of the NRLP3 inflammasome stimulates the release of IL-1b, IL-18, and IL-33 cytokines [14, 75]. These cytokines are responsible for the initiation and perpetuation of the inflammatory responses. Macrophage activation characterizes the initiation of the FBR with a giant cell formation, fibroblast activation, and collagen matrix deposition. The FBR consists of overlapping acute and persistent inflammatory phases coupled with collagenous encapsulation. It has further been observed that common anti-inflammatory drugs such as aspirin can inhibit the inflammasome pathway and significantly reduce the FBR to foreign materials [14]. The link between implant prosthesis and malignancy has not been established until recently. In 1994, Coleman et al. [76] stated that studies of human implants have revealed no malignant tumor production due to long-term polymeric implants. However, the malignancies associated with prosthesis implants are not epithelial cancers but *hematologic malignancies* [15, 20]. In fact, a reduction in breast cancer incidence was observed in silicone breast implants, especially in cases where subglandular implants were used relative to women with submuscular implants [77–79]. Nonetheless, a newly recognized Food and Drug Administration (FDA, 2019) type of hematologic malignancy was described related to silicone breast implants: the *anaplastic large-cell lymphoma* (ALCL) [80]. The FDA raises awareness about breast implants in its webpage, stating that ACLC arises in patients with silicone breast implants "regardless of filling or texture," and that "ALCL is (rather) a type of lymphoma and not a cancer of the breast tissue" [ibid].

Furthermore, there are documented reports of lymphoma arising in cases of joint implants prosthesis and other metallic implants [20, 21]. The spectrum of FBR is not limited to prosthesis/implants. The adjuvant property of the metals in vaccines becomes more complex when added to the foreign body characteristic of the metal itself. Irrespective of the origin, foreign bodies act as xenografts, thereby evoking an FBR with the potential risk for lymphoma [14, 20].

Lipophilicity is a common characteristic of many potent adjuvants.

Through their lipophilicity or by interacting with lipid moieties in the cell membranes forming *lipophilic complexes*, many potent adjuvants act by altering the cell barrier and triggering an immune response [81–87]. The oral administration or intramuscular injection of lipophilic compounds (e.g. drugs) targets preferentially the lymphatics to then gain access to the systemic circulation [81, 82]. The rate of absorption of an injected drug depends on its lipophilicity degree and the route of administration (i.e. intramuscular vs. subcutaneous). Following administration, a lipophilic drug, through the lymph draining, reaches the lymph nodes and acts on the lymphoid cells [81]. The fat-containing tissues act as *dispenser* for lipophilic substances [83], ensuring a low and sustained activation of the immune cells in the lymphatic nodes.

Derived from the Latin word *adjuvare* (help), the term adjuvant encompasses a broad spectrum of substances as aluminum salts, squalene, oil-based adjuvants, virosomes, TLR-related adjuvants, lipopolysaccharide (LPS), and others. All of them work by enhancing, prolonging, and accelerating the effect of other agents by triggering a Th1 and/or a Th2 type of cytokine response [84, 88]. Some adjuvants in vaccines can be used to stabilize the formulations of the antigens. The fact that activation of TLR leads to adaptive immune response to foreign entities (i.e. antigen presentation) explains why adjuvants are designed to mimic TLR ligands in order to trigger a Th1 response [84]. An adjuvant that enhances the innate immune response will also lead to an enhanced adaptive response.

Adjuvants are considered nonspecific stimulators of the immune system. They help to deposit and sequester the injected material, forcing an increase in the antibody response. Aluminum is the adjuvant most used in vaccines [89]. Nonetheless, there are several general toxicity issues associated with the use of aluminum in vaccines that have thus far been neglected. For example, in mice and rats, the injection of aluminum nanoparticles in vaccine-relevant exposures results in their depositions in distant organs such as spleen and brain where the nanomaterial can persist for more than a year after injection [89]. Nanoalumina was further shown to cause neurovascular injury and blood–brain barrier damage. It markedly reduces human brain microvascular endothelial cells viability, alters mitochondrial potential, increases cellular oxidation, and decreases tight junction protein expression as compared to control nanoparticles. The nanoalumina does so by inducing mitochondrial damage and autophagy of the endothelial cells [90]. Nanoalumina is one of the most abundantly manufactured engineered nanomaterials [91].

Many aluminum adjuvancy mechanisms were proposed. Both the extracellular host DNA released from dying cells and the uric acid induction (a catabolic product of nucleotides) act as endogenous adjuvants preferentially boosting the TH2-dependent humoral responses [92, 93]. Primarily, the mechanism of aluminum adjuvancy was thought to be through NLRP3 inflammasome signal-dependent (a mechanism compatible with the acute FBR) and leading to the secretion of pro-inflammatory cytokines IL-1b, IL-18, and IL-33 [75]. Recent insights (2014) into the mechanism of aluminum show that the NLRP3 pathway is neither unique nor indispensable for the adjuvant properties of aluminum. In particular, Flach et al. [85] have demonstrated that immune stimulation by aluminum is driven by its interactions with *lipids*, and this pathway does not depend on inflammasome activation. The aluminum–lipid interaction alters the structure of cholesterol and sphingomyelin in the plasma membrane of dendritic cells [ibid]. Aluminum-binding lipids on membrane cell form a *lipophilic complex* that was shown to disrupt the metabolism of membrane phospholipids altering key signal-transduction pathways [87]. Flach et al. [85] used the atomic force microscopy to reveal strong and selective binding between aluminum and dendritic cells. Crystalline aluminum binds lipid moieties on dendritic cell membrane and, without entering the cell, promotes lipid sorting in the cell membrane, leading to dendritic cell activation and inflammation [85, 86]. The alteration in the structure of dendritic cells lipid membrane points to the mechanism of citrullination in which alteration in the 3D molecule conformation leads to *neo*-epitopes formation and antibodies synthesis [94]. It should be noted that sphingomyelins are not lipid molecules specific to *sole* dendritic cells, but they are also present in the myelin sheath overlaying axons. As an example, the Guillain–Barre syndrome, part of autoinflammatory syndromes induced by adjuvants (ASIA), is an acute inflammatory demyelinating polyneuropathy. The disease is characterized by antibodies against sphingomyelin [95]. Guillain–Barre' is triggered by an infection or vaccination event [96].

Another adjuvant used in vaccines is *pristane*. It is a lipophilic branched alkane hydrocarbon obtained from shark liver oil. Pristane shares the adjuvant mechanism properties with other naturally occurring hydrocarbons. The incomplete Freund's adjuvant (IFA) is a water-in-oil emulsion, and the complete Freund's adjuvant (CFA) is IFA containing in addition the heat-killed mycobacteria. The mycolic acid of the mycobacteria wall is also a fatty acid. It has an alpha-alkylating group [97]. The MF59 adjuvant is a submicrometer oil-in-water emulsion of squalene and other compounds used in the influenza vaccines. Squalene is 30-carbon organic compound obtained from shark liver oil and plant sources (primarily vegetable oils). The AS03 adjuvant is also a squalene-based immunologic adjuvant. The AS04 adjuvant consists of aluminum phosphate and monophosphoryl lipid A (MPL). The AS02 adjuvant also contains MPL. The QS-21 is a product obtained from *Quillaja saponaria* tree as a collection of saponins. Saponaria is derived from the Latin *sapo* (stem sapon), meaning "soap" (fat mixed with alkali) [84]. Severe local reactions, granulomas and toxicity include severe hemolysis, were seen to be induced by the affinity of saponins for the cholesterol present in erythrocyte membranes, resulting in membrane solubilization and hemolysis [98]. The immunostimulatory complexes (ISCOMS) are virus-like particles of 30–40 nm with dodecahedric structure, mainly composed of *Quillaja* saponins, cholesterol, phospholipids, and the antigen [84, 98]. Lipopolysaccharides (LPS), also known as lipoglycans and endotoxins, are potent adjuvants in vaccines. They form the wall of Gram-negative bacteria. The adjuvant property of LPS is attributed to their lipidic component, the lipid A fraction [84]. Interestingly, there is a common feature in all of the abovementioned adjuvants: that is, their *lipophilic nature* (see Table 9.3). This fact is in accordance with Freund's observations made in 1956. When recounting Rabinovich's finding, Freund noted that by adding butter (lipid) to the injected *Mycobacterium butyricum* in the experiment animals, the type of immune response changed, namely a systemic cellular reaction was triggered rather than just a localized tubercle lesion at the site of injection [98]. Injection of mycobacteria within a fatty excipient was first used by Rabinovich in Koch's laboratory in 1897. Later, in 1925, Ramon demonstrated that it is also possible to artificially increase the diphtheria or tetanus antitoxin levels by adding lecithin or saponin to the vaccines [98]. In contrast, a nonfatty, pure protein molecule failed to elicit a primary response in immunization [100, 101]. For example,

Table 9.3 The lipophilic nature of adjuvants[a] (similar to lipophilic drugs) is fundamental for their pharmacokinetic properties.

Aluminum	Alum–lipid interaction
Pristane	Lipophilic branched alkane hydrocarbon
IFA	Water-in-oil emulsion
CFA	IFA + mycolic acid (fatty acid)
Squalene	Unsaturated oil from the liver shark/vegetable oils
MF59	Submicrometer oil-in-water emulsion of squalene
QS-21	A collection of saponins from *Quillaja tree*
AS03	Squalene-oil-based adjuvant
AS02	Monophosphoryl lipid A (MPL) + QS-21
AS04	Monophosphoryl lipid A (MPL) + aluminum phosphate
ISCOMs	*Quillaja* saponins, cholesterol, and phospholipid
LPS	Lipid A fraction
PDM[a]	Oily, sticky, and emulsifying substance

It is responsible for their abortion, distribution, deposit, toxicity, metabolism, and excretion.

[a] As an exception, silicone, an oily and sticky substance with adjuvant properties, is not a lipophilic molecule. Yet, it does have the strong ability to alter lipids. Silicone is an emulsifier [99].Source: Adapted from Supersaxo et al. [81], Charman [82], Kadir [83], Israeli et al. [84], Flach et al. [85], Mbow et al. [86], and Martínez-Estévez et al. [87].

the tetanus toxoid alone or diphtheria alone does not induce any immune responses. They require aluminum-binding lipids to trigger an efficient immune response [102]. Interesting enough, not only that adjuvants are capable of orchestrating a cellular immune response regardless of the presence of an immunogen, but it seems that the *sole* immunogen cannot trigger a long-lasting immune response without the aid of adjuvant components.

The *lipophilic* nature of adjuvants (similar to those of lipophilic drugs) is an essential precondition to their pharmacokinetic properties (Table 9.3). As an exception, silicone — an oily, sticky substance with adjuvant properties – is not a lipophilic molecule, but it does have the strong ability to alter lipids. Silicone affects lipid compounds by acting as an emulsifier [99].

Of note, lipophilic substances, which are sometimes illegally injected for cosmetic purposes, may have an immune adjuvant effect and have been reported as possible inducers of the ASIA syndrome [13, 103].

It is well known that the membranes of all body cells are constituted by a lipid bilayer barrier. To which extent the cells of the immune system, the nervous system, or other tissues may be a potential target for adjuvants remains yet to be investigated.

Oil-in-water emulsions are considered the most efficient human vaccine adjuvants inducing *earlier* and strong immunocompetent milieu [101], paving the way for an antigen to act. Subcutaneous injections of mineral oils produce sclerosing lipogranulomas [84]. When absorbed throughout the body, they cause lipogranulomas in the lymph nodes, spleen, and other organs where they are distributed. Granuloma formation is the hallmark of many autoimmune diseases including vasculitis granulomatosa or sarcoidosis, and the formation of granuloma is associated with the production of autoantibodies including antineutrophil cytoplasmic antibodies (ANCAs). In salmon fish, the intraperitoneal immunization with oil-adjuvant vaccines resulted in granulomatous disease and the production of antinuclear antibodies, anti-beta2GPI, and anti-ferritin. [9]. It is well known that the granuloma formation in infectious diseases as tuberculosis has the role to encapsulate and contain the foreign bacteria [104].

Silicone versus aluminum compounds and lymphomagenesis association

In silicone breast implants, the capsule formation is overlapped with the chronic process of the tissue repair. Healing involves inflammation. Silicone, similar to the aluminum adjuvant, is transported from the injection site and travel within macrophages until it reaches the lymph nodes. Blum et al. [105] published the case of a 50-year-old woman carrying a bilateral SBI for 10 years in which the lymph node biopsy showed that giant cells have created granulomatous structures encapsulating the silicone particles. Aluminum meets the same characteristics. In animal experiments, injected aluminum nanomaterials are taken up by monocytes in tissues (e.g. fluorescent aluminum surrogates). They first drain to lymph nodes to thereafter circulate in blood within phagocytes – subsequently reaching the spleen and other distant organs [50, 106].

Aluminum-containing vaccine is not the only source of aluminum. This metal may also be present in high amounts in dialysate and intravenous solutions, antacids, buffered aspirins, anti-diarrheal products, bone cement, and in cosmetic products [107, 108]. Aluminum compounds are able to form agglomerates. A granulomatous lesion called macrophagic myofasciitis (MMF) associated with symptoms such as myalgia, chronic fatigue, and cognitive dysfunction was first reported in 1998 in 200 cases [50]. MMF was associated with a long-term persistence of vaccine-derived aluminum hydroxide in muscle. Maubec et al. [17] have reported nine cases of aluminum-related pseudolymphoma development at the site of injection after hepatitis B vaccination in eight patients and following hepatitis A vaccination in one patient. Similar to aluminum, silicone implants (SBI) have also been associated with the lymphomagenesis process. In 2014, a review article by Miranda et al. [15] identifies 60 cases of ALCL, exclusively related with the SBI. ALCL arises adjacent to the breast implant site, and it is confined to the capsule. ALCL is a localized non-Hodgkin lymphoma characterized by its strong immunopositivity for CD30 along with a 100% negative expression of anaplastic lymphoma kinase. There is a good and poor prognosis associated with the presentation of the lymphomas in SBI; accordingly, presentations as an effusion-associated fibrous capsule surrounding the implant and as a mass were both seen, the latter being associated with a poor prognosis. In the Miranda et al. study, the patients who received chemotherapy did not show a better overall or progression-free survival. However, the patients who opted for "watchful waiting" after implant removal had much better outcome. The removal of the inciting agent (the silicone breast implant) led to complete remission. A complete remission of symptomatology was also seen for conditions such as the *silicone implant incompatibility syndrome* (SIIS) [71]. As one major criterion of the ASIA syndrome was fulfilled in both cases (SBI and SIIS) (that is the removal of inciting agent leading to the condition improvement), this makes lymphoma, when induced by silicone, part of the ASIA syndrome (Table 9.1). One of the widely used silicone types is the polydimethylsiloxane (PDMS), a *silicone oil* used in cosmetics. The versatility of silicone chemistry provides the material many unique properties. They function as emulsifiers, wetters, form films, alter foam [99], or as a penetrant surfactant–adjuvant for pesticides and fungicides [109]. Experiments performed by Nagase et al. [110] showed that silicone polymer molecules can act as methylating agents under the environmental conditions. The cellular behavior of the injected silicone in a mouse model in a time span of three days was characterized specifically by a locally mild inflammatory reaction consisting primarily of infiltration of polymorphonuclear leukocytes, plasma cells, and macrophages trying to contain the silicone [111]. Between the 4th and 10th days, the PMN cells decreased in number, and there was a definite predominance of lymphocytes, fibroblasts, and plasma cells. This last pattern of lymphocytic predominance was the pattern that remained unchanged during the following 18 months of observation. Chronic stimulation of the immune system through adjuvants leads to a delayed type response which when persists results in a downregulatory response [100] characterized by high levels of IL-10, a cytokine also expressed in mouse model of silicone implant [8] and in the model of chronic stress-induced immune suppression [112]. The IL-10 is a Th2 cytokine [113]. Silicone works by triggering a Th2 response, and so does the other adjuvant, the aluminum.

Lymphomagenesis in inflammatory diseases from a different perspective

Different autoimmune diseases are related and can be present concomitantly in the same individual [114]. Healthy individuals have clones of autoreactive T and B cells that have escaped from thymus deletion and circulate in the periphery, reaching lymph nodes, spleen, and other organs. Furthermore, the nonspecific stimulation of the immune system by adjuvants in vaccines could enhance the expansion of such self-reactive T-cell clones too. Such adjuvant-related effect could in turn lead to a significant and pathologically increment of the cellular and humoral-mediated inflammatory responses. Consistent with this hypothesis, Routsias et al. [42] state that in a portion of patients with Sjögren's syndrome, the initial stage of the disease is characterized by the presence of both polyclonal B-cell activation and also specific B-lymphocyte clones. Saadoun et al. [115] have observed that an unusual autoreactive B-cell population expansion is responsible for the lymphoma development in primary Sjögrens's syndrome.

Conclusions and future goals

Although it is commonly considered that an adjuvant does not have an antigenic effect by itself, the *ASIA syndrome* is gathering every day an increasing number of clinical reports indicating that a strong link between adjuvants and immunologic disorders does exist. The mechanisms by which various adjuvants may induce autoimmune manifestations are not necessarily linked to the induction of specific antibodies but rather to a multifaceted and sustained stimulation of immune responses. Moreover, the synergistic effect of adjuvant *coadministration*, part of the current adult and childhood vaccination schedules, may induce a cascade of events that could further lead to a prolonged lymphocyte activation, ultimately resulting in immune system dysregulation. Thus, doctors or any health care providers might want to keep an open eye to patients' symptoms and to look for the cause/s remembering that *everything is potentially autoimmune until proven otherwise* [116].

References

1. National Institutes of Health USA.gov 2012. Understanding autoimmune diseases. http://www.niams.nih.gov/HEALTH_INFO/Autoimmune/understanding_autoimmune.pdf (accessed 20 April 2022).
2. Kapatai, G. and Murray, P. (2007). Contribution of the Epstein–Barr virus to the molecular pathogenesis of Hodgkin lymphoma. *J. Clin. Pathol.* 60 (12): 1342–1349.
3. Shehab, T.M., Hsi, E.D., Poterucha, J.J. et al. (2001). *Helicobacter pylori*-associated gastric MALT lymphoma in liver transplant recipients. *Transplantation* 71: 1172–1175.
4. Sagaert, X., Van Cutsem, E., De Hertogh, G. et al. (2010). Gastric MALT lymphoma: a model of chronic inflammation induced tumor development. *Nat. Rev. Gastroenterol. Hepatol.* 7 (6): 336–346.
5. Mariette, X. (2001). Lymphomas complicating Sjögren's syndrome and hepatitis C virus infection may share a common pathogenesis: chronic stimulation of rheumatoid factor B cells. *Ann. Rheum. Dis.* 60: 1007–1010.
6. Bernatsky, S., Ramsey-Goldman, R., Labrecque, J. et al. (2013). Cancer risk in systemic lupus: an updated international multi-centre cohort study. *J. Autoimmun.* 42: 130–135.
7. Shoenfeld, Y. and Agmon-Levin, N. (2011). 'ASIA'—autoimmune/inflammatory syndrome induced by adjuvants. *J. Autoimmun.* 36 (1): 4–8.
8. Schaefer, C.J., Lawrence, W.D., and Wooley, P.H. (1999). Influence of long-term silicone implantation on type II collagen induced arthritis in mice. *Ann. Rheum. Dis.* 58: 503–509.
9. Koppang, E.O., Bjerkås, I., Haugarvoll, E. et al. (2008). Vaccination-induced systemic autoimmunity in farmed Atlantic salmon. *J. Immunol.* 181 (7): 4807–4814.
10. Schaefer, C.J. and Wooley, P.H. (1999). The influence of silicone implantation on murine lupus in MRL lpr/lpr mice. *J. Rheumatol.* 26 (10): 2215–2221.
11. Dimitrijević, L., Živković, I., Stojanović, M. et al. (2012). Vaccine model of antiphospholipid syndrome induced by tetanus vaccine. *Lupus* 21 (2): 195–202.
12. Agmon-Levin, N., Hughes, G.R., and Shoenfeld, Y. (2012). The spectrum of ASIA: 'Autoimmune (auto-inflammatory) syndrome induced by adjuvants'. *Lupus* 21 (2): 118–120.
13. Perricone, C., Colafrancesco, S., Mazor, R.D. et al. (2013). Autoimmune/inflammatory syndrome induced by adjuvants (ASIA) 2013: unveiling the pathogenic, clinical and diagnostic aspects. *J. Autoimmun.* 47: 1–16.
14. Malik, A.F., Hoque, R., and Ouyang, X. (2011). Inflammasome components Asc and caspase-1 mediate biomaterial-induced inflammation and foreign body response. *Proc. Natl Acad. Sci. USA* 108 (50): 20095–20100.
15. Miranda, R.N., Aladily, T.N., Prince, H.M. et al. (2014). Breast implantassociated anaplastic large-cell lymphoma: long-term follow-up of 60 patients. *J. Clin. Oncol.* 32: 114–120.
16. Bichel, L. (1976). Postvaccinial lymphadenitis developing into Hodgkin's disease. *Acta Med. Scand.* 199 (6): 523–525.
17. Maubec, E., Pinquier, L., Viguier, M. et al. (2005). Vaccination-induced cutaneous pseudolymphoma. *J. Am. Acad. Dermatol.* 52 (4): 623–629.
18. Hernández, I., Sanmartín, O., Cardá, C. et al. (2008). Pseudolinfoma B inducido por hidróxido de aluminio tras tratamiento hiposensibilizante [B-cell pseudolymphoma caused by aluminium hydroxide following hyposensitization therapy]. *Actas Dermosifiliogr.* 99 (3): 213–216.
19. Sanchez-Gonzalez, B., Garcia, M., Montserrat, F. et al. (2013). Diffuse large B-cell lymphoma associated with chronic inflammation in metallic implant. *J. Clin. Oncol.* 31 (10): e148–e151.
20. Chaudhry, M.S., Mather, H., Marks, A., and Naresh, K. (2011). Diffuse large B cell lymphoma complicating total knee arthroplasty: case report and literature review of the association of diffuse large B-cell lymphoma with joint replacement. *Acta Haematol.* 126 (3): 141–146.
21. Cheuk, W., Chan, A.C., Chan, J.K. et al. (2005). Metallic implant-associated lymphoma: a distinct subgroup of large B-cell lymphoma related to pyothorax-associated lymphoma? *Am. J. Surg. Pathol.* 29 (6): 832–836.
22. Lidgren, L. (2008). Chronic inflammation, joint replacement and malignant lymphoma. *J. Bone Joint Surg. (Br.)* 90 (1): 7–10.
23. Madewell, B.R., Gieger, T.L., Pesavento, P.A., and Kent, M.S. (2004). Vaccine site-associated sarcoma and malignant lymphoma in cats: a report of six cases (1997–2002). *J. Am. Anim. Hosp. Assoc.* 40: 47–50.
24. Anderson, P.N. and Potter, M. (1969). Induction of plasma cell tumours in BALB-c mice with 2,6,10,14-tetramethylpentadecane (pristane). *Nature* 222 (5197): 994–995.

25. Potter, M. (1968). A resume' of the current status of the development of plasma-cell tumors in mice. *Cancer Res.* 28: 1891–1896.
26. Wooley, P.H. and Whalen, J.D. (1991). Pristane-induced arthritis in mice. III. Lymphocyte phenotypic and functional abnormalities precede the development of pristane-induced arthritis. *Cell. Immunol.* 138 (1): 251–259.
27. Kuroda, Y., Nacionales, D.C., Akaogi, J. et al. (2004). Autoimmunity induced by adjuvant hydrocarbon oil components of vaccine. *Biomed. Pharmacother.* 58: 325–337.
28. Kojima, M., Itoh, H., Shimizu, K. et al. (2006). Malignant lymphoma in patients with systemic rheumatic disease (rheumatoid arthritis, systemic lupus erythematosus, systemic sclerosis, and dermatomyositis): a clinicopathologic study of 24 Japanese cases. *Int. J. Surg. Pathol.* 14 (1): 43–48.
29. Baecklund, E., Smedby, K.E., Sutton, L.A. et al. (2014). Lymphoma development in patients with autoimmune and inflammatory disorders—what are the driving forces? *Semin. Cancer Biol.* 24: 61–70.
30. Bichile, T. and Petri, M. (2014). Incidence of lymphoma associated with underlying lupus: lessons learned from observational studies. *Curr. Opin. Rheumatol.* 26 (2): 111–117.
31. Tarella, C., Gueli, A., Ruella, M., and Cignetti, A. (2013). Lymphocyte transformation and autoimmune disorders. *Autoimmun. Rev.* 12 (8): 802–813.
32. Theander, E., Henriksson, G., Ljungberg, O. et al. (2006). Lymphoma and other malignancies in primary Sjögren's syndrome: a cohort study on cancer incidence and lymphoma predictors. *Ann. Rheum. Dis.* 65 (6): 796–803.
33. Smedby, K.E., Baecklund, E., and Askling, J. (2006). Malignant lymphomas in autoimmunity and inflammation: a review of risks, risk factors, and lymphoma characteristics. *Cancer Epidemiol. Biomark. Prev.* 15 (11): 2069–2077.
34. Kauppi, M., Pukkala, E., and Isoma¨ki H. (1997). Elevated incidence of hematologic malignancies in patients with Sjögren's syndrome compared with patients with rheumatoid arthritis (Finland). *Cancer Causes Control* 8 (2): 201–204.
35. Dreyer, L., Faurschou, M., Mogensen, M., and Jacobsen, S. (2011). High incidence of potentially virus-induced malignancies in systemic lupus erythematosus: a long-term followup study in a Danish cohort. *Arthritis Rheum.* 63: 3032–3037.
36. Smitten, A.L., Simon, T.A., Hochberg, M.C., and Suissa, S. (2008). A meta-analysis of the incidence of malignancy in adult patients with rheumatoid arthritis. *Arthritis Res. Ther.* 10 (2): R45.
37. Mercer, L.K., Davies, R., Galloway, J. et al. (2013). Risk of cancer in patients receiving non-biologic disease-modifying therapy for rheumatoid arthritis compared with the UK general population. *Rheumatology (Oxford)* 52: 91–98.
38. Grainge, M.J., West, J., Solaymani-Dodaran, M. et al. (2012). The long-term risk of malignancy following a diagnosis of coeliac disease or dermatitis herpetiformis: a cohort study. *Aliment. Pharmacol. Ther.* 35 (6): 730–739.
39. Smedby, K.E., Åkerman, M., Hildebrand, H. et al. (2005). Malignant lymphomas in coeliac disease: evidence of increased risks for lymphoma types other than enteropathytype T cell lymphoma. *Gut* 54 (1): 54–59.
40. Zhang, J.Q., Wan, Y.N., Peng, W.J. et al. (2013). The risk of cancer development in systemic sclerosis: a meta-analysis. *Cancer Epidemiol.* 37 (5): 523–527.
41. Voulgarelis, M. and Skopouli, F.N. (2007). Clinical, immunologic, and molecular factors predicting lymphoma development in Sjogren's syndrome patients. *Clin. Rev. Allergy Immunol.* 32 (3): 265–274.
42. Routsias, J.G., Goules, J.D., Charalampakis, G. et al. (2013). Malignant lymphoma in primary Sjögren's syndrome: an update on the pathogenesis and treatment. *Semin. Arthritis Rheum.* 43 (2): 178–186.
43. Kristinsson, S.Y., Landgren, O., Sjöberg, J. et al. (2009). Autoimmunity and risk for Hodgkin's lymphoma by subtype. *Haematologica* 94 (10): 1468–1469.
44. Van Baarsen, L.G., de Hair, M.J., Ramwadhdoebe, T.H. et al. (2013). The cellular composition of lymph nodes in the earliest phase of inflammatory arthritis. *Ann. Rheum. Dis.* 72 (8): 1420–1424.
45. Volkmann, E.R., Agrawal, H., Maranian, P., and Furst, D.E. (2010). Rituximab for rheumatoid arthritis: a meta-analysis and systematic review. *Clin. Med. Insights Ther.* 2: 749–760.
46. Sluzevich, J.C., Hall, M.R., and Roy, V. (2012). Subcutaneous panniculitis-like T-cell lymphoma after rituximab. *J. Am. Acad. Dermatol.* 67 (5): e223–e225.
47. Blank, M. and Gershwin, M.E. (2008). Autoimmunity: from the mosaic to the kaleidoscope. *J. Autoimmun.* 30 (1–2): 1–4.

48. Anaya, J.M., Corena, R., Castiblanco, J. et al. (2007). The kaleidoscope of autoimmunity: multiple autoimmune syndromes and familial autoimmunity. *Expert. Rev. Clin. Immunol.* 3 (4): 623–635.
49. Hellgren, K., Di Giuseppe, D., Smedby, K.E. et al. (2021). Lymphoma risks in patients with rheumatoid arthritis treated with biological drugs-a Swedish cohort study of risks by time, drug and lymphoma subtype. *Rheumatology (Oxford, England)* 60 (2): 809–819. https://doi.org/10.1093/rheumatology/keaa330.
50. Gherardi, R.K. (2003). Lessons from macrophagic myofasciitis: towards definition of a vaccine adjuvant-related syndrome. *Rev. Neurol. (Paris)* 159 (2): 162–164.
51. Srinivas, U.S., Tan, B., Vellayappan, B.A., and Jeyasekharan, A.D. (2019). ROS and the DNA damage response in cancer. *Redox Biol.* 25: 101084. https://doi.org/10.1016/j.redox.2018.101084.
52. Nies, I., Hidalgo, K., Bondy, S.C., and Campbell, A. (2020). Distinctive cellular response to aluminum based adjuvants. *Environ. Toxicol. Pharmacol.* 78: 103404. https://doi.org/10.1016/j.etap.2020.103404.
53. Tome, M.E., Frye, J.B., Coyle, D. et al. (2012). Lymphoma cells with increased anti-oxidant defenses acquire chemoresistance. *Exp. Ther. Med.* 3 (5): 845–852. https://doi.org/10.3892/etm.2012.487.
54. Campbell, A., Becaria, A., Lahiri, D.K. et al. (2004). Chronic exposure to aluminum in drinking water increases inflammatory parameters selectively in the brain. *J. Neurosci. Res.* 75 (4): 565–572. https://doi.org/10.1002/jnr.10877.
55. Becaria, A., Lahiri, D.K., Bondy, S.C. et al. (2006). Aluminum and copper in drinking water enhance inflammatory or oxidative events specifically in the brain. *J. Neuroimmunol.* 176 (1–2): 16–23.
56. Elkoshi, Z. (2022). Cancer and autoimmune diseases: a tale of two immunological opposites? *Front. Immunol.* 13: 821598. https://doi.org/10.3389/fimmu.2022.821598.
57. Mittal, S., Marshall, N.A., Duncan, L. et al. (2008). Local and systemic induction of $CD4^+$ $CD25^+$ regulatory T-cell population by non-Hodgkin lymphoma. *Blood* 111 (11): 5359–5370. https://doi.org/10.1182/blood-2007-08-105395.
58. Wang, J. and Ke, X.Y. (2011). The four types of Tregs in malignant lymphomas. *J. Hematol. Oncol.* 4: 50. https://doi.org/10.1186/1756-8722-4-50.
59. Gravelle, P., Burroni, B., Péricart, S. et al. (2017). Mechanisms of PD-1/PD-L1 expression and prognostic relevance in non-Hodgkin lymphoma: a summary of immunohistochemical studies. *Oncotarget* 8 (27): 44960–44975. https://doi.org/10.18632/oncotarget.16680.
60. Miggelbrink, A.M., Jackson, J.D., Lorrey, S.J. et al. (2021). CD4 T-cell exhaustion: does it exist and what are its roles in cancer? *Clin. Cancer Res.* 27 (21): 5742–5752. https://doi.org/10.1158/1078-0432.CCR-21-0206.
61. Cornberg, M. et al. (2013). Clonal exhaustion as a mechanism to protect against severe immunopathology and death from an overwhelming CD8 T cell response. *Front. Immunol.* 4: 475.
62. Pawelec, G. (2019). Is there a positive side to T cell exhaustion? *Front. Immunol.* 10: 111. https://doi.org/10.3389/fimmu.2019.00111.
63. Wherry, E.J. and Kurachi, M. (2015). Molecular and cellular insights into T cell exhaustion. *Nat. Rev. Immunol.* 15 (8): 486–499. https://doi.org/10.1038/nri3862.
64. Utzschneider, D.T. et al. (2013). T cells maintain an exhausted phenotype after antigen withdrawal and population reexpansion. *Nat. Immunol.* 14: 603–610.
65. Dolina, J.S., Van Braeckel-Budimir, N., Thomas, G.D., and Salek-Ardakani, S. (2021). $CD8^+$ T cell exhaustion in cancer. *Front. Immunol.* 12: 715234. https://doi.org/10.3389/fimmu.2021.715234.
66. McKinney, E.F. and Smith, K.G. (2016). T cell exhaustion and immune-mediated disease-the potential for therapeutic exhaustion. *Curr. Opin. Immunol.* 43: 74–80. https://doi.org/10.1016/j.coi.2016.09.005.
67. Ezekiel 1:16. *English Standard Version (ESV) Bible*, 2007. Wheaton, IL: Crossway Books.
68. Memarnejadian, A., Meilleur, C.E., Shaler, C.R. et al. (2017). PD-1 blockade promotes epitope spreading in anticancer $CD8^+$ T cell responses by preventing fratricidal death of subdominant clones to relieve immunodomination. *J. Immunol.* 199 (9): 3348–3359. https://doi.org/10.4049/jimmunol.1700643.
69. Vaz, N.M. and Carvalho, C.R. (2015). On the origin of immunopathology. *J. Theor. Biol.* 375: 61–70. https://doi.org/10.1016/j.jtbi.2014.06.006.
70. Han, S., Asoyan, A., Rabenstein, H. et al. (2010). Role of antigen persistence and dose for CD4? T-cell exhaustion and recovery. *Proc. Natl Acad. Sci. USA* 107 (47): 20453–20458.
71. Kappel, R., Cohen Tervaert, J., and Pruijn, G. (2014). Autoimmune/inflammatory syndrome induced by adjuvants (ASIA) due to silicone implant incompatibility syndrome in three sisters. *Clin. Exp. Rheumatol.* 32 (2): 256–258.

72. Yates, K.B., Tonnerre, P., Martin, G.E. et al. (2021). Epigenetic scars of CD8⁺ T cell exhaustion persist after cure of chronic infection in humans. *Nat. Immunol.* 22 (8): 1020–1029. https://doi.org/10.1038/s41590-021-00979-1.
73. Porto, D.A., Comfere, N.I., Myers, L.M., and Abbott, J.J. (2010). Pseudolymphomatous reaction to varicella zoster virus vaccination: role of viral in situ hybridization. *J. Cutan. Pathol.* 37 (10): 1098–1102.
74. Cerroni, L., Borroni, R.G., Massone, C. et al. (2007). Cutaneous B-cell pseudolymphoma at the site of vaccination. *Am. J. Dermatopathol.* 29 (6): 538–542.
75. Eisenbarth, S.C., Colegio, O.R., O'Connor, W. et al. (2008). Crucial role for the Nalp3 inflammasome in the immunostimulatory properties of aluminium adjuvants. *Nature* 453: 1122–1126.
76. Coleman, D.L., King, R.N., and Andrade, J.D. (1974). The foreign body reaction: a chronic inflammatory response. *J. Biomed. Mater. Res.* 8 (5): 199–211.
77. Pan, S.Y., Lavigne, E., Holowaty, E.J. et al. (2012). Canadian breast implant cohort: extended follow-up of cancer incidence. *Int. J. Cancer* 131: E1148–E1157.
78. Friis, S., Hölmich, L.R., McLaughlin, J.K. et al. (2006). Cancer risk among Danish women with cosmetic breast implants. *Int. J. Cancer* 118: 998–1003.
79. Brisson, J., Holowaty, E.J., Villeneuve, P.J. et al. (2006). Cancer incidence in a cohort of Ontario and Quebec women having bilateral breast augmentation. *Int. J. Cancer* 118: 2854–2862.
80. US Food and Drug Administration 2019. Breast Implant Associated-Anaplastic Large Cell Lymphoma (BIA-ALCL) - Letter to Health Care Providers. https://www.fda.gov/medical-devices/letters-health-care-providers/breast-implant-associated-anaplastic-large-cell-lymphoma-bia-alcl-letter-health-care-providers (accessed on April 2022).
81. Supersaxo, A., Hein, W.R., and Steffen, H. (1991). Mixed micelles as a proliposomal, lymphotropic drug carrier. *Pharm. Res.* 8 (10): 1286–1291.
82. Charman, W.N. (2000). Lipids, lipophilic drugs, and oral drug deliverysome emerging concepts. *J. Pharm. Sci.* 89 (8): 967–978.
83. Kadir, F. (1993). Intramuscular and subcutaneous drug delivery: encapsulation in liposomes and other methods to manipulate drug availability. *Pharm. World Sci.* 15 (4): 173–175.
84. Israeli, E., Agmon-Levin, N., Blank, M., and Shoenfeld, Y. (2009). Adjuvants and autoimmunity. *Lupus* 18 (13): 1217–1225.
85. Flach, T.L., Ng, G., and Hari, A. (2011). Alum interaction with dendritic cell membrane lipids is essential for its adjuvanticity. *Nat. Med.* 17 (4): 479–487.
86. Mbow, M.L., de Gregorio, E., and Ulmer, J.B. (2011). Alum's adjuvant action:grease is the word. *Nat. Med.* 17: 415–416.
87. Martínez-Estévez, M., Racagni-Di Palma, G., Muñoz-Sánchez, J.A. et al. (2003). Aluminium differentially modifies lipid metabolism from the phosphoinositide pathway in Coffea arabica cells. *J. Plant Physiol.* 160 (11): 1297–1303. https://doi.org/10.1078/0176-1617-01168.
88. Petrovsky, N. (2006). Novel human polysaccharide adjuvants with dual Th1 and Th2 potentiating activity. *Vaccine* 24 (Suppl 2): S26–S29.
89. Tomljenovic, L. and Shaw, C.A. (2011). Aluminum vaccine adjuvants: are they safe? *Curr. Med. Chem.* 18 (17): 2630–2637.
90. Chen, L., Zhang, B., and Toborek, M. (2013). Autophagy is involved in nanoalumina-induced cerebrovascular toxicity. *Nanomedicine* 9 (2): 212–221.
91. Chen, L., Yokel, R.A., Hennig, B., and Toborek, M. (2008). Manufactured aluminum oxide nanoparticles decrease expression of tight junction proteins in brain vasculature. *J. NeuroImmune Pharmacol.* 3 (4): 286–295.
92. Marichal, T., Ohata, K., Bedoret, D. et al. (2011). DNA released from dying host cells mediates aluminum adjuvant activity. *Nat. Med.* 17 (8): 996–1002.
93. Marrack, P., McKee, A.S., and Munks, M.W. (2009). Towards an understanding of the adjuvant action of aluminium. *Nat. Rev. Immunol.* 9 (4): 287–293.
94. Robinson, W.H. and Sokolove, J. (2012). Citrullination of fibrinogen: generation of neoepitopes and enhancement of immunostimulatory properties. *Arthritis Res. Ther.* 14 (Suppl 1): O30.
95. Fredman, P. and Lekman, A. (1997). Glycosphingolipids as potential diagnostic markers and/or antigens in neurological disorders. *Neurochem. Res.* 22 (8): 1071–1083.

96. Israeli, E., Agmon-Levin, N., Blank, M. et al. (2012). Guillain–Barre' syndrome—a classical autoimmune disease triggered by infection or vaccination. *Clin. Rev. Allergy Immunol.* 42 (2): 121–130.
97. Takayama, K., Wang, C., and Besra, G.S. (2005). Pathway to synthesis and processing of mycolic acids in Mycobacterium tuberculosis. *Clin. Microbiol. Rev.* 18 (1): 81–101.
98. Petrovsky, N. and Aguilar, J.C. (2004). Vaccine adjuvants: current state and future trends. *Immunol. Cell Biol.* 82: 488–496.
99. O'Lenick, T. and O'Lenick, T. (2011). Altering organic oils with silicones. *H&PC Today* 6 (1): 72–75.
100. Billiau, A. and Matthys, P. (2001). Modes of action of Freund's adjuvants in experimental models of autoimmune diseases. *J. Leukoc. Biol.* 70 (6): 849–860.
101. Mosca, F., Tritto, E., Muzzi, A. et al. (2008). Molecular and cellular signatures of human vaccine adjuvants. *Proc. Natl Acad. Sci. USA* 105 (30): 10501–10506.
102. Butler, N.R., Voyce, M.A., Burland, W.L., and Hilton, M.L. (1969). Advantages of aluminium hydroxide adsorbed combined diphtheria, tetanus, and pertussis vaccines for the immunization of infants. *Br. Med. J.* 1 (5645): 663–666.
103. Vera-Lastra, O., Medina, G., del Pilar, C.-D.M. et al. (2012). Human adjuvant disease induced by foreign substances: a new model of ASIA (Shoenfeld's syndrome). *Lupus* 21: 128e35.
104. Ulrichs, T. and Kaufmann, S.H. (2006). New insights into the function of granulomas in human tuberculosis. *J. Pathol.* 208: 261–269.
105. Blum, A., Abboud, W., Shajrawi, I., and Tatour, I. (2007). Prolonged fever due to silicone granulomatosis. *Isr. Med. Assoc. J.* 9 (2): 121–122.
106. Gherardi, R.K., Coquet, M., Cherin, P. et al. (2001). Macrophagic myofasciitis lesions assess long-term persistence of vaccine-derived aluminium hydroxide in muscle. *Brain* 124 (Pt 9): 1821–1831.
107. Krewski, D., Yokel, R.A., Nieboer, E. et al. (2007). Human health risk assessment for aluminium, aluminium oxide, and aluminium hydroxide. *J. Toxicol. Environ. Health B Crit. Rev.* 10 (Suppl 1): 1–269.
108. Tomljenovic, L. (2011). Aluminum and Alzheimer's disease: after a century of controversy, is there a plausible link? *J. Alzheimers Dis.* 23 (4): 567–598.
109. Stevens, P.J.G. (1993). Organosilicone surfactants as adjuvants for agrochemicals. *Pesticide Sci.* 38: 103–122. doi: 10.1002/ps.2780380206. https://www.trianglecc.com/wp-content/uploads/2014/05/TRC-Silicone-100-sell-sheet.pdf
110. Nagase, H., Ose, Y., and Sato, T. (1988). Possible methylation of inorganic mercury by silicones in the environment. *Environ. Sci. Total Environ.* 73 (1–2): 29–38.
111. Andrews, J.M. (1966). Cellular behavior to injected silicone fluid: a preliminary report. *Plast. Reconstr. Surg.* 38 (6): 581–583.
112. Hu, D., Wan, L., Chen, M. et al. (2014). Essential role of IL-10/STAT3 in chronic stress-induced immune suppression. *Brain Behav. Immun.* 36: 118–127.
113. Kleinewietfeld, M. and Hafler, D.A. (2014). Regulatory T cells in autoimmune neuroinflammation. *Immunol. Rev.* 259 (1): 231–244.
114. Elefsiniotis, I.S., Papatsimpas, G., Liatsos, G.D. et al. (2008). Atypical autoimmune polyglandular syndrome type 3 overlapped by chronic HCV infection resulting in carcinogenesis and fatal infection. *South. Med. J.* 101 (7): 756–758.
115. Saadoun, D., Terrier, B., Bannock, J. et al. (2013). Expansion of autoreactive unresponsive CD21-/low B cells in Sjögren's syndrome—associated lymphoproliferation. *Arthritis Rheum.* 65: 1085–1096.
116. Shoenfeld, Y. (2013). Everything is autoimmune until proven otherwise. *Clin. Rev. Allergy Immunol.* 45 (2): 149–151. https://doi.org/10.1007/s12016-013-8385-8.

10 Chronic Fatigue Syndrome

Kassem Sharif
[1]Department of Gastroenterology, Sheba Medical Centre, Tel-Hashomer, Israel
[2]Zabludowicz Center for Autoimmune Diseases, Sheba Medical Center, Tel-Hashomer, Israel
[3]Sackler Faculty of Medicine, Tel Aviv University, Tel Aviv, Israel

Introduction

Chronic fatigue syndrome (CFS) is a heterogeneous complex disorder which is essentially characterized by profound debilitating fatigue limiting a patient's functional capability and negatively influence the quality of life. CFS is a clinical diagnosis of exclusion which is appointed when other etiologies for fatigues have been ruled out [1]. Over the course of the years, different criteria were proposed that described the various aspects of CFS. In 1988, the Centers for Disease Control and Prevention (CDC) devised a criterion that focused mainly on physical symptoms [1]. To emphasize the mental fatigue and neurological background of the disease, the Oxford criteria were developed in 1991 [2]. These criteria were replaced by the broader revised definition of CDC in 1994, which became the most acceptable criteria and identified CFS patients as sufferers of profound incapacitating fatigue longer than six months with at least four concomitant symptoms including headache, arthralgia, myalgia, postexceptional malaise, and tender lymph nodes, among others.

The burden of CFS is substantial and has a widespread significance. In the United States, an estimated 422 per 100,000 people suffer from CFS, many of whom are undiagnosed [3, 4]. The worldwide prevalence of CFS ranges from 0.2% to 2.7%, according to various epidemiological studies [5, 6]. Although ethical or racial differences were not noticed, women are four times more likely to be affected than men [7, 8]. CFS occurs most often in the 40–59 years age group and in the geriatric population, with increased incidence toward older ages [7, 9].

The etiology of CFS is unclear and is presumed to be multifactorial. Suspected pathogens include Epstein–Barr virus (EBV), cytomegalovirus (CMV), human herpes virus (HHV-6), and parvovirus B19 [10–12]. Although the exact mechanism is to be elucidated, molecular mimicry has been suggested as a plausible cause [13]. Hypothalamic–pituitary–adrenal axis (HPA) hypoactivity has been shown to play a possible influencer in the disease pathology. Decreased adrenocorticotropic hormones, serum dehydroepiandrosterone (DHEA) sulfate, and others have been shown to be biological markers for CFS [14, 15]. Other contributory etiologic factors have been proposed to play an integral role in the disease pathogenesis including genetic, immunologic, and neurologic factors [16, 17]. In other instances, CFS can be approached in a biopsychosocial framework, the trigger of the disease could be organic as indicated by a preceding viral infection, but perpetuated by a combination of certain personality traits (psychology) and social environmental factors

Autoimmune Disorders: Adjuvants and Other Risk Factors in Pathogenesis, First Edition.
Edited by Abdulla Watad, Nicola Luigi Bragazzi, and Yehuda Shoenfeld.

(sociology) [18]. This model was criticized because it encouraged physicians to disregard physical symptoms and view them as somatized rather than require medical intervention [19].

CFS is not a new disease, similar conditions have been observed across the previous centuries but with different names; in this review, we discuss the history of CFS, and how this disease could be explained through modern entities.

The evolutionary history of "chronic fatigue syndrome"

1750, Febricula

In 1750, an essay was published by Sir Richard Manningham, a renowned English physician and man-midwife. In his essay, Sir Manningham discusses the symptoms, nature, causes, and cure of a condition known as *Febricula* or little fever, a disease that was characterized by several symptoms yet lacked objectively measured findings. The following are brief excerpts from his vivid report:

"At the beginning patients feel merely languid or uneasy, with flying pain, dryness of the lips and tongue but no thirst; in a day or two they find themselves often giddy, dispirited and anxious without apparent reason, and passing pale urine. They have transient fits of chillness, a low, quick and unequal pulse, sometimes cold clammy sweats." He continues adding "A form of mania is a consequence of it, where it has been neglected, of late years this species of madness has been more than an ordinarily frequent, all sorts were liable to it, but mostly valetudinarians, delicate persons, and those in the decline of life" [20].

In this condition, Sir Manningham highlights that low-grade fever, lassitude, and cognitive dysfunction are the presenting features of this disease entity; while this description was provided, a concrete etiology or pathogenesis was lacking [20].

1879, Neurocirculatory asthenia

Around 1870s, George Miller Beard, an American psychiatrist and neurologist, shed the light on a newly identified entity, neurocirculatory asthenia (NCA). This term was synonymous to the British term, effort syndrome, which was characterized by symptoms of the cardiovascular system including palpitations, tachycardia, increased sweating, and cold clammy hands and feet that are not dependent on any known pathologic process of the heart or blood vessels but associated with functional nervous disturbance [21]. Of great frequency were the neurological symptoms including anxiety, depression, weakness, and excessive fatigability. Additional reported symptoms included nonspecific gastrointestinal symptoms which were decidedly common, including gastric discomfort distention and sudden diarrhea [21]. NCA is hallmarked by the hard-to-measure objective findings as compared to the prominent subjective findings; therefore, the associated asthenia and cardiovascular phenomena are thought to occur subsequent to functional disturbance of the nervous system and not secondary to organic disease [22]. NCA was more prominently identified in stressful conditions among soldiers during war time. It has been recognized in the Crimean War by the British, the American Civil War by DaCosta and Hartshorne, and after World war I [22].

During the years of the American Civil War, Jacob Mendes Da Costa observed the prevalence of cardiovascular disease symptoms in the absence of findings on physical examination, which included fatigue upon exertion, dyspnea, and chest pain, among others. The term Da Costa's syndrome or soldier's heart was then replaced by various names including cardiac neurosis and NCA. Among investigated soldiers, Da Costa reported interesting finding of a pulse that is greatly and rapidly influenced by position [23]. This phenomenon is known as orthostatic intolerance. Such incidences prevented soldiers from keeping up with exertions during training or war. This condition that forms the bases of modern concept is known as postural orthostatic tachycardia syndrome (POTS) [24].

The concept of NCA was further emphasized by the cardiologist Thomas Lewis who expanded the topic by dividing NCA patients into six distinct groups. This subcategorization aimed to show that this clinical entity develops under various conditions. The first and largest group included patients with inherent nervous instability and constitutional weakness or have a decreased standpoint from a nervous or emotional standpoint. The second group included patients who developed the disease post fatigue due to hard work and lack of rest. The third and fourth groups included patients who developed the disease postinfections, acute or chronic, respectively. The fifth group pertains to patients who developed the disease as a result of gas poisoning. The final group includes patients with incipient but unrecognizable heart disease [25].

1934, Atypical poliomyelitis

In Los Angeles County general hospital, in 1934, an outbreak of muscle pain of long duration, tenderness, weakness, memory problems, concentration difficulties, sleep disturbance, emotional liability, and profound postexceptional fatigue were witnessed among close to 200 hospital staff members. The inflicted group were incapable of engaging in their premorbid occupational duties even six months after the disease onset. The clinical presentation with which these patients presented was suspicious of polio virus. In contrast to patients infected with typical polio virus, this subgroup did not develop muscle wasting as expected in typical poliomyelitis patients. Alexander Gilliam, a professor in the field of epidemiology in Johns Hopkins medical school, documented this epidemic and coined the term atypical poliomyelitis due to the fact that mortality was very low [26].

Several similar outbreaks were reported in the years close to the Los Angeles County general hospital event; similar clinical presentation was observed among administrative candidates in Wisconsin in 1936; citizens of two rural towns in 1937 in Switzerland; and among 70 Swiss soldiers in 1937 [27].

1948, Akureyri disease (Iceland disease)

In the winter of 1948–1949, an outbreak of fatigue and muscular weakness, a description that was similar to the event that happened in the general hospital, was witnessed in the capital of northern Iceland, Akureyri. This epidemic affected close to 500 of the inhabitants, and patients suffered from pronounced fatigue and muscular weakness that comes during the day and is more profound postexercise [28]. Accompanying symptoms included autonomic disturbances such as orthostatic tachycardia, vasomotor instability, emotional liability, depression, and impaired concentration [29]. This epidemic lasted for three months, and it became apparent that it is not poliomyelitis.

1955, Royal Free disease

During the spring of 1955 in the Royal Free Hospital in the United Kingdom, an outbreak was documented when numerous number of patients were admitted to the hospital with nonspecific symptoms. Patients complained initially from a flu-like malaise, which became more prominent with extreme muscle fatigue after minimal exertion. Moreover, patients complained of cognitive problems including short-term memory problems and concentration problems as well as blurred vision, headaches, and unusual skin sensations [30]. This specific outbreak was significant due to the fact that in July of the same year, 300 staff members had similar symptoms. As a result, the hospital was forced to be closed due to lack of manpower [30]. This syndrome was termed Royal Free disease, and it was not until Donald Acheson, a British physician and epidemiologist who later severed as chief medical officer of the United Kingdom, devised the term benign myalgic encephalomyelitis in an editorial published in The Lancet in 1956 [31]. Dr. Melvin Ramsay, a consultant physician in infectious diseases at the Royal Free Hospital at that time, later officially coined the term and added to the description, drawing on his extensive first-hand experience of the Royal Free Hospital outbreak [32]. There were several similar yet smaller outbreaks in the United Kingdom including Middlesex, Newcastle, and London in the years spanning between 1952 and 1970.

1955–1986, Myalgic encephalomyelitis

In 1986, Dr. Melvin Ramsey provided a description of myalgic encephalomyelitis based on clinical observations from Royal Free hospital outbreak, The Ramsay Definition for myalgic encephalomyelitis (1968):

"A syndrome initiated by a virus infection, commonly in the form of a respiratory or gastrointestinal illness with significant headache, malaise and dizziness sometimes accompanied by lymphadenopathy or rash." . . . "characteristic findings include: neurological disturbance - unpredictable state of central nervous system exhaustion following mental of physical exertion which may be delayed and require several days for recovery" . . . . "dysfunction of autonomic and sensory nervous system (orthostatic)" . . . "cognitive problems" . . . "musculo-skeletal dysfunction in a proportion of patients."

1984, Tapanui outbreak

In the small town of Tapanui in New Zealand's south island, during 1984, Dr. Peter Grahame Snow described a flu-like malaise and prolonged fatigue. This outbreak was studied by two additional doctors who together with Dr. Snow published an article that aimed to describe the unexplained illness among 28 patients who presented with nonspecific tiredness, mood and sleep disturbances, headaches, and joints and muscle pain. In their communication, they suggested an unidentified virus to be the most likely cause, and this outbreak may resemble other outbreaks of NCA [33]. In a 10-year follow-up study conducted on 21 of the original patients, Levine et al. [34] demonstrated that 50% of the patients met the current criteria for CDC definition for CFS, and 11 had prolonged idiopathic fatigue; moreover, among those CFS criteria, a female preponderance was noted [34].

1984, Chronic Epstein–Barr virus syndrome

In 1984, an outbreak near Nevada gained significant attention. A group of otherwise healthy adults displayed symptoms of lassitude, profound fatigue, malaise, sore throat, tender lymph nodes, and signs of cognitive impairment including confusion, depression, and decreased memory, with lack of objective findings on examination or laboratory abnormalities expect for elevated titers to EBV antigens [35–37]. Therefore, physicians and scientists pondered whether this phenomenon was related to the reactivation of a latent infection by Epstein–Barr virus, and hence the name chronic EBV syndrome. Although a case definition was absent, the diagnosis of chronic EBV syndrome was given by physicians on the basis of detectable EBV titers. Subsequent to these observations, in 1985–1986, several studies questioned the diagnostic value of positive EBV serologic finding and the proposed relationship between the virus and the condition [38, 39]. This was based on several reports that documented similar associations between several other viruses including cytomegalovirus and herpes virus type 1 and 2 and the fact that at that time serological results were poorly reproducible, both within or among laboratories [38, 39].

In 1987, the Division of Viral Disease of the CDC conducted a focused group meeting for physicians, public health epidemiologists, and academic researchers who due to the lack of concrete relationship between EBV and these symptoms rendered it premature to focus research only on EBV. The group devised an operational concept that recognizes the condition as a syndrome and coined the term chronic fatigue syndrome to include and reflect the most eminent symptoms.

1987, Chronic fatigue syndrome

In the 1987 meeting held by the CDC, a working case definition for chronic fatigue syndrome was devised. For a case to be defined, two major criteria are required, in addition to the minor criteria, as follows: 6 or more of the 11 symptoms criteria and 2 or more of the 3 physical criteria; or 8 or more of the 11 symptoms criteria. The major criteria included (i) debilitating fatigue that does not resolve with bed rest for a period of at least six months, severe enough to cause reduction in daily activity below 50% of the patient's premorbid activity (ii) exclusion of other medical conditions including malignancy, autoimmune disease, chronic infections, fungal infections, chronic psychiatric diseases, endocrine diseases, or drug dependency, among others. Symptoms criteria included mild fever, fatigue post mild exertion, sore throat, painful lymph nodes, myalgia, muscle weakness, generalized headache, arthralgia, sleep disturbance, and neuropsychological complaints. Physical criteria included documented twice at least in one month, low-grade fever, palpable lymph nodes, and nonexudative pharyngitis [40].

The definition proposed by Holmes et al. [40] was descriptive and free from etiological implications; furthermore, it proposed an operational definition and showed inadequate and poorly described sampling procedures, choice of comparison groups, and measure of reliability, and thus, it was proven to be unsatisfactory in practice [41, 42]. Hence, in 1990, a meeting was held in Green College and included British psychosocial psychiatrics and devised the Oxford 1991 definition, which entailed two distinct disorders, chronic fatigue syndrome of unknown etiology (CFS) and another subset known as postinfectious fatigue syndrome (PIFS). According to their definition, fatigue is a principal symptom that does not have a lifelong onset but is severe, disabling, and affects the physical and mental functioning for a minimum of six months with other concomitant symptoms including myalgia and mood and sleep disturbances, among others. Patients with organic causes such as anemia or established psychiatric condition should be excluded. PIFS follows similar diagnostic guidelines for CFS but with additional evidence of infection at onset or presentation of the disease, with the symptoms of fatigue present for a minimum of six months after disease onset with a laboratory corroborated evidence for the presence of infection [2].

Currently, the most widely accepted and favored definition for CFS is the CDC 1994 definition known as Fukuda definition [43], which requires the patient to have chronic fatigue for more than six months with minimal exertion that interferes with daily activity and only four of eight symptoms such as postexertion malaise, unrefreshing sleep, impaired memory, arthralgia, headache, tender lymph nodes, or sore throat. According to this criteria, CSF is diagnosed only after the exclusion of psychiatric and medical conditions that can explain chronic fatigue. Due to the fact that Fukuda definition necessitates four out of eight symptoms, it stands to reason that a diagnosis could be made without certain critical elements such as postexertion malaise and cognitive impairment [43]. Therefore, Fukuda criteria are regarded as less specific than homes criteria. Moreover, Fukuda definition was criticized because it lacked specific operational definitions and guidelines and instead contained vaguely worded criteria; therefore, its use in clinical setting as diagnostic tool is limited [4, 44].

In 2003, the Canadian consensus criteria were devised, which differed from Fukuda definition by destressing fatigue as the only major criteria; therefore, for CSF case, it is defined as fatigue, postexertion malaise, sleep dysfunction, and myalgia/arthralgia for more than six months with at least two cognitive manifestations including impaired concentration, information processing, and sensory disturbances, among others, and at least one or more of the symptoms from these categories, including (i) autonomic manifestations such as orthostatic intolerance – neutrally mediated hypotension, POTS, irritable bowel syndrome, urinary frequency and bladder dysfunction, and palpitation, (ii) neuroendocrine manifestations such as thermostatic stability, sweating episodes, and cold clammy hands and feet. (iii) Immune manifestation including tender lymph nodes, recurrent sore throat, recurrent flu-like symptoms, and general malaise [45].

Over the course of the years, various criteria have been suggested until 2015, when under the request of the Department of Health and Human Services, the National Academy of Medicine proposed the redefinition of ME/CFS and change of its name to systemic exertion intolerance disease. According to the committee, "This name captures a central characteristic of the disease: the fact that exertion of any sort – physical, cognitive, or emotional – can adversely affect patients in many organ systems and in many aspects of their lives. The committee believes systemic exertion intolerance disease appropriately captures the complexity and severity of the illness" [46].

In their criteria, three symptoms are mandatory, including substantial reduction in engagement in preillness levels of occupation in social and personal activities for more than six months accompanied by profound fatigue that is not alleviated by stress, postexertion malaise, unrefreshing sleep, and at least one of the two manifestations, cognitive impairment and/or orthostatic intolerance.

The newly devised criteria selected more patients who have less impairment and fewer symptoms than other criteria; in addition, it included more individuals with psychiatric conditions such as depression. Furthermore, SEID increased the [47] prevalence as compared to Fukuda definition by 2.8 times [48].

CFS syndrome through modern concepts

CFS belongs to a larger group of diseases known as central sensitivity syndrome. Central sensitization includes the state where central nervous system amplifies sensory input. In the wide spectrum of these disease are fibromyalgia, irritable bowel syndrome, and POTS, among others [49].

CFS and fibromyalgia share several clinical manifestations including fatigue, headache, impaired memory, sleep disturbance, and decreased concentration [50]. The diagnosis of both conditions poses a diagnostic enigma due to the nonspecific nature of patient's complaints and the high overlap in symptomatology and the lack of sufficient explanation despite decades of research [51]. In the literature, there is a strong debate on whether CFS and FM belong or do not belong to the same disease entity despite sharing resembling symptoms, and therefore, the relationship between these disorders remains uncertain [52, 53].

POTS disease is a heterogeneous disorder of the autonomic system that results in substantial increase in heart rate with position changes that leads to decrease in blood flow to the brain and cerebral hypoperfusion [54]. POTS disease has been shown to be closely related with CFS, and it is estimated that 40% of CFS patients suffer from POTS [55]. Correspondingly, it has been shown that the large majority of patients with diagnosed POTS satisfy the criteria for CFS [56]. CFS symptoms that are more pronounced in POTS patients include profound fatigue, unrefreshing sleep, and impaired cognitive capabilities. Other symptoms including sore throat, tender lymph nodes, and arthralgia are found in POTS, albeit in a decreased prevalence. Therefore, these findings support the great overlap between these conditions [56, 57].

Autoimmune/inflammatory syndrome induced by adjuvants (ASIA), also known as Shoenfeld's syndrome, is a disease entity introduced by Shoenfeld et al. [58] in 2011, which comprises closely related immune diseases that share a history of exposure to an adjuvant material [58]. To aid the diagnosis, Shoenfeld et al. [58] proposed a suggested criteria for the diagnosis of ASIA including four major and four minor criteria; fulfillment of either two major or one major and two minor criteria is required for establishing the diagnosis. The major criteria include exposure to external stimulus (infection, vaccine, silicone, and adjuvant) and appearance of typical manifestations including arthralgia, myalgia, chronic fatigue, cognitive impairment, pyrexia, dry mouth, and neurologic manifestations. The minor criteria include the development of autoantibodies against the suspected adjuvant, other clinical manifestations including irritable bowel syndrome, and specific HLA types including HLA DRB1 and HLA DQB1. On closer inspection of this criteria, it is highly evident that both CFS and ASIA share multiple aspects, and they cannot be looked at as two separate entities. By definition, ASIA syndrome necessitates the exposure to a triggering event in a genetically susceptible individual, for example viral antigens or adjuvants in vaccinations. Although not part of a standard criteria, vaccine administration has been reported to precede the development of the clinical picture of CFS and fibromyalgia. Several cases of POTS and CFS were reported postvaccinations with qHPV vaccine Gardasil [59]. Moreover, novel H1N1 influenza vaccination was also shown to be involved in the development of this immune response [60]. In a study conducted by Agmon-Levin et al. [59], all 19 patients who developed fibromyalgia or CFS following hepatitis B vaccine fulfilled the suggested criteria for ASIA. This suggests that in cases of CFS and fibromyalgia, there might exist a temporal relationship to immunization as part of ASIA syndrome.

Furthermore, it has been postulated that autoimmune disease would manifest early with ill-defined symptoms (arthralgia, weakness, and myalgia – typical of ASIA and CFS) and would be ignored and deemed insignificant. Such symptoms are perceived as a bridge between the early stage and the full-blown autoimmune disease picture. The bridging symptoms typically progress slowly and insidiously. Upon exposure to a secondary immune stimulus (i.e. antigen and adjuvant), the acute clinical manifestation of the disease is triggered [61].

Looking from another angle, in the preliminary report published by Calabrese et al. [62], an observation of a large number of patients with conditions resembling primary Sjögren's syndrome (SS) among patients presenting with CFS specialized clinic was reported. This cultivated a possible ideation that within patients with CFS, there might be a population presenting with occult SS. Of a randomly selected 27 patients with severe dominating fatigues and complaints of myalgia, 20 met the criteria of fibromyalgia, and 16 had abnormal Shrimmer test. On minor salivary gland biopsy, an abnormality was detected in 20 cases. Antibodies to nuclear antigen were present in 16 of 28, but anti-Ro was present in only one case. In this group, 13 patients had eight or more CDC minor criteria, and 18 met six or more of the criteria. Such findings highlighted the possible existence of a common and overlooked clinical subset of CFS with symptoms such as SS, and therefore, more extensive work is needed to evaluate and define these symptoms [62]. Of note, symptoms of SS are apparent in various diagnostic criteria including ASIA and in the earliest description of this disease entity, for instance Ferbricula in the 1750s. Additional work by Nishikai et al. [63] demonstrated that one-third of the CFS patients with Sicca syndrome fulfilled the diagnostic criteria for seronegative SS [63].

Conclusion

The entity CFS is not a novelty. As early as the 1750s, a confusing constellation of symptoms have been attributed to the same disease, albeit with various different names. Whether CFS has autoimmune component or is a condition that precedes a full-blown autoimmune disease remains to be elucidated. Emerging evidence highlight the heterogeneity and the wide spectrum of this syndrome, and accumulated evidence show the relationship of this entity to various other conditions. More in-depth research is required to better understand the etiologic factors and putatively uncover the objective findings that could aid in disease diagnosis.

References

1. Reyes, M., Gary, H.E. Jr., Dobbins, J.G. et al. (1997). Surveillance for chronic fatigue syndrome--four U.S. cities, September 1989 through August 1993. *MMWR CDC Surveill. Summ.* 46 (2): 1–13.
2. Sharpe, M.C., Archard, L.C., Banatvala, J.E. et al. (1991). A report--chronic fatigue syndrome: guidelines for research. *J. R. Soc. Med.* 84 (2): 118–121.
3. Maquet, D., Demoulin, C., and Crielaard, J.M. (2006). Chronic fatigue syndrome: a systematic review. Annales de readaptation et de medecine physique: revue scientifique de la Societe francaise de reeducation fonctionnelle de readaptation et de medecine physique. *Arch. Intern. Med.* 49 (6): 337–47, 418–27.
4. Jason, L.A., Richman, J.A., Rademaker, A.W. et al. (1999). A community-based study of chronic fatigue syndrome. *Arch. Intern. Med.* 159 (18): 2129–2137.
5. Lawrie, S.M., Manders, D.N., Geddes, J.R., and Pelosi, A.J. (1997). A population-based incidence study of chronic fatigue. *Psychol. Med.* 27 (2): 343–353.
6. Jason, L.A., Taylor, R., Wagner, L. et al. (1995). Estimating rates of chronic fatigue syndrome from a community-based sample: a pilot study. *Am. J. Community Psychol.* 23 (4): 557–568.
7. Griffith, J.P. and Zarrouf, F.A. (2008). A systematic review of chronic fatigue syndrome: don't assume it's depression. *Prim. Care Companion J. Clin. Psychiatry* 10 (2): 120–128.
8. Centers for Disease Control and Prevention. (2017). Chronic fatigue syndrome.
9. Lee, S., Yu, H., Wing, Y. et al. (2000). Psychiatric morbidity and illness experience of primary care patients with chronic fatigue in Hong Kong. *Am. J. Psychiatry* 157 (3): 380–384.
10. Ablashi, D.V., Eastman, H.B., Owen, C.B. et al. (2000). Frequent HHV-6 reactivation in multiple sclerosis (MS) and chronic fatigue syndrome (CFS) patients. *J. Clin. Virol.* 16 (3): 179–191.
11. Kerr, J.R. and Mattey, D.L. (2008). Preexisting psychological stress predicts acute and chronic fatigue and arthritis following symptomatic parvovirus B19 infection. *Clin. Infect. Dis.* 46 (9): e83–e87.

12. Lerner, A.M., Beqaj, S.H., Deeter, R.G., and Fitzgerald, J.T. (2004). IgM serum antibodies to Epstein-Barr virus are uniquely present in a subset of patients with the chronic fatigue syndrome. *In vivo (Athens, Greece)* 18 (2): 101–106.
13. Mahagna, H., Mahroum, N., and Amital, H. (2015). *Infections, Vaccinations, and Chronic Fatigue Syndrome. Vaccines and Autoimmunity*, 345–348. Wiley.
14. Wheatland, R. (2005). Chronic ACTH autoantibodies are a significant pathological factor in the disruption of the hypothalamic-pituitary-adrenal axis in chronic fatigue syndrome, anorexia nervosa and major depression. *Med. Hypotheses* 65 (2): 287–295.
15. Kuratsune, H., Yamaguti, K., Sawada, M. et al. (1998). Dehydroepiandrosterone sulfate deficiency in chronic fatigue syndrome. *Int. J. Mol. Med.* 1 (1): 143–146.
16. Byrne, E. (1991). The chronic fatigue syndrome: a reappraisal and unifying hypothesis. *Clin. Exp. Neurol.* 28: 128–138.
17. Klimas, N.G., Salvato, F.R., Morgan, R., and Fletcher, M.A. (1990). Immunologic abnormalities in chronic fatigue syndrome. *J. Clin. Microbiol.* 28 (6): 1403–1410.
18. Geraghty, K.J. and Esmail, A. (2016). Chronic fatigue syndrome: is the biopsychosocial model responsible for patient dissatisfaction and harm? *Br. J. Gen. Pract.* 66 (649): 437–438.
19. Raine, R., Carter, S., Sensky, T., and Black, N. (2004). General practitioners' perceptions of chronic fatigue syndrome and beliefs about its management, compared with irritable bowel syndrome: qualitative study. *BMJ* 328 (7452): 1354–1357.
20. Manningham, R. (1760). *The Symptoms, Nature, Causes, and Cure of the Febricula, or, Little Fever: Commonly called the Nervous or Hysteric Fever; The Fever on the Spirits; Vapours, Hypo, or Spleen.* By Sir Richard Manningham, Knt. M. D. F. R. S. and of the College of Physicians, London., 4e. London: Printed for G. Kearsly, at the Golden-Lion in Ludgate-Street.
21. Harvey, S.B., Wessely, S., Kuh, D., and Hotopf, M. (2009). The relationship between fatigue and psychiatric disorders: evidence for the concept of neurasthenia. *J. Psychosom. Res.* 66 (5): 445–454.
22. Oppenheimer, B.S. (1942). Neurocirculatory asthenia and related problems in military medicine. *Bull. N. Y. Acad. Med.* 18 (6): 367–382.
23. Da Costa, J.M. (1951). On irritable heart. *Am. J. Med.* 11 (5): 559–567.
24. Da, P.O. (1987). Costa's syndrome or neurocirculatory asthenia. *Br. Heart J.* 58 (4): 306–315.
25. Robey, W.H. Jr. and Boas, E.P. (1918). Neurocirculatory asthenia. *J. Am. Med. Assoc.* 71 (7): 525–529.
26. Patarca-Montero, R. (2004). *Medical Etiology, Assessment, and Treatment of Chronic Fatigue and Malaise*, 6–7. Haworth Press.
27. Shorter, E. (1993). Chronic fatigue in historical perspective. *Ciba Found. Symp.* 173: 6–16; discussion -22.
28. Sigurdsson, B., Sigurjónsson, J., Sigurdsson, J.H.J. et al. (1950). A disease epidemic in Iceland simulating poliomyelitis. *Am. J. Epidemiol.* 52 (2): 222–238.
29. Ramsay, A.M., Dowsett, E.G., Dadswell, J.V. et al. (1977). Icelandic disease (benign myalgic encephalomyelitis or Royal Free disease). *Br. Med. J.* 1 (6072): 1350.
30. Dawson, J. (1987). Royal free disease: perplexity continues. *Br. Med. J. (Clin. Res. Ed.)* 294 (6568): 327–328.
31. Ali, N. (2015). *Understanding Chronic Fatigue Syndrome*. Rowman & Littlefield.
32. Ramsay, A.M. (1965). Hysteria and "Royal Free Disease". *Br. Med. J.* 2 (5469): 1062.
33. Poore, M., Snow, P., and Paul, C. (1984). An unexplained illness in West Otago. *N. Z. Med. J.* 97 (757): 351–354.
34. Levine, P.H., Snow, P.G., Ranum, B.A. et al. (1997). Epidemic neuromyasthenia and chronic fatigue syndrome in West Otago, New Zealand: a 10-year follow-up. *Arch. Intern. Med.* 157: 750.
35. Tobi, M., Morag, A., Ravid, Z. et al. (1982). Prolonged atypical illness associated with serological evidence of persistent Epstein-Barr virus infection. *Lancet (London, England)* 1 (8263): 61–64.
36. DuBois, R.E., Seeley, J.K., Brus, I. et al. (1984). Chronic mononucleosis syndrome. *South. Med. J.* 77 (11): 1376–1382.
37. Jones, J.F., Ray, C.G., Minnich, L.L. et al. (1985). Evidence for active Epstein-Barr virus infection in patients with persistent, unexplained illnesses: elevated anti-early antigen antibodies. *Ann. Intern. Med.* 102 (1): 1–7.
38. Holmes, G.P., Kaplan, J.E., Stewart, J.A. et al. (1987). A cluster of patients with a chronic mononucleosis-like syndrome: is epstein-barr virus the cause? *JAMA* 257 (17): 2297–2302.
39. Buchwald, D., Sullivan, J.L., and Komaroff, A.L. (1987). Frequency of 'chronic active epstein-barr virus infection' in a general medical practice. *JAMA* 257 (17): 2303–2307.

40. Holmes, G.P., Kaplan, J.E., Gantz, N.M. et al. (1988). Chronic fatigue syndrome: a working case definition. *Ann. Intern. Med.* 108 (3): 387–389.
41. Manu, P., Lane, T.J., and Matthews, D.A. (1988). The frequency of the chronic fatigue syndrome in patients with symptoms of persistent fatigue. *Ann. Intern. Med.* 109 (7): 554–556.
42. David, A.S., Wessely, S., and Pelosi, A.J. (1988). Postviral fatigue syndrome: time for a new approach. *Br. Med. J. (Clin. Res. Ed.)* 296 (6623): 696–699.
43. Fukuda, K., Straus, S.E., Hickie, I. et al. (1994). The chronic fatigue syndrome: a comprehensive approach to its definition and study. International Chronic Fatigue Syndrome Study Group. *Ann. Intern. Med.* 121 (12): 953–959.
44. Jason, L.A., Torres-Harding, S.R., Taylor, R.R., and Carrico, A.W. (2001). A comparison of the 1988 and 1994 diagnostic criteria for chronic fatigue syndrome. *J. Clin. Psychol. Med. Settings* 8 (4): 337–343.
45. Carruthers, B.M., Jain, A.K., De Meirleir, K.L. et al. (2003). Myalgic encephalomyelitis/chronic fatigue syndrome. *J. Chronic Fatigue Syndr.* 11 (1): 7–115.
46. Institute of Medicine (2015). *Beyond Myalgic Encephalomyelitis/Chronic Fatigue Syndrome: Redefining an Illness.* Washington, DC: The National Academies.
47. Jason, L.A., Sunnquist, M., Brown, A. et al. (2015). Reflections on the Institute of Medicine's systemic exertion intolerance disease. *Pol. Arch. Med. Wewn.* 125 (7–8): 576–581.
48. Jason, L.A., Sunnquist, M., Kot, B., and Brown, A. (2015). Unintended consequences of not specifying exclusionary illnesses for systemic exertion intolerance disease. *Diagnostics* 5 (2): 272–286.
49. Fleming, K.C. and Volcheck, M.M. (2015). Central sensitization syndrome and the initial evaluation of a patient with fibromyalgia: a review. *Rambam Maimonides Med. J.* 6 (2): e0020.
50. McKay, P.G., Duffy, T., and Martin, C.R. (2009). Are chronic fatigue syndrome and fibromyalgia the same? Implications for the provision of appropriate mental health intervention. *J. Psychiatr. Ment. Health Nurs.* 16 (10): 884–894.
51. Abbi, B. and Natelson, B.H. (2013). Is chronic fatigue syndrome the same illness as fibromyalgia: evaluating the 'single syndrome' hypothesis. *QJM Int. J. Med.* 106 (1): 3–9.
52. Aaron, L.A. and Buchwald, D. (2001). A review of the evidence for overlap among unexplained clinical conditions. *Ann. Intern. Med.* 134 (9 Pt 2): 868–881.
53. Clauw, D.J. and Chrousos, G.P. (1997). Chronic pain and fatigue syndromes: overlapping clinical and neuroendocrine features and potential pathogenic mechanisms. *Neuroimmunomodulation* 4 (3): 134–153.
54. Grubb, B.P., Kanjwal, Y., and Kosinski, D.J. (2006). The postural tachycardia syndrome: a concise guide to diagnosis and management. *J. Cardiovasc. Electrophysiol.* 17 (1): 108–112.
55. Schondorf, R., Benoit, J., Wein, T., and Phaneuf, D. (1999). Orthostatic intolerance in the chronic fatigue syndrome. *J. Auton. Nerv. Syst.* 75 (2–3): 192–201.
56. Okamoto, L.E., Raj, S.R., Peltier, A. et al. (2012). Neurohumoral and haemodynamic profile in postural tachycardia and chronic fatigue syndromes. *Clin. Sci.* 122 (4): 183–192.
57. Stewart, J.M., Gewitz, M.H., Weldon, A., and Munoz, J. (1999). Patterns of orthostatic intolerance: the orthostatic tachycardia syndrome and adolescent chronic fatigue. *J. Pediatr.* 135 (2 Pt 1): 218–225.
58. Shoenfeld, Y. and Agmon-Levin, N. (2011). 'ASIA' – autoimmune/inflammatory syndrome induced by adjuvants. *J. Autoimmun.* 36 (1): 4–8.
59. Agmon-Levin, N., Zafrir, Y., Kivity, S. et al. (2014). Chronic fatigue syndrome and fibromyalgia following immunization with the hepatitis B vaccine: another angle of the 'autoimmune (auto-inflammatory) syndrome induced by adjuvants' (ASIA). *Immunol. Res.* 60 (2–3): 376–383.
60. Tsai, C.K., Chu, H., and Cheng, C.A. (2011). Novel H1N1 infl uenza vaccine the cause of postural orthostatic tachycardia syndrome followed by cerebral hypoperfusion. *J. Med. Sci.* 31 (2): 91–93.
61. Poser, C.M. and Behan, P.O. (1982). Late onset of Guillain-Barre syndrome. *J. Neuroimmunol.* 3 (1): 27–41.
62. Calabrese, L.H., Davis, M.E., and Wilke, W.S. (1994). Chronic fatigue syndrome and a disorder resembling Sjogren's syndrome: preliminary report. *Clin. Infect. Dis.* 18 (Suppl 1): S28–S31.
63. Nishikai, M., Akiya, K., Tojo, T. et al. (1996). 'Seronegative' Sjogren's syndrome manifested as a subset of chronic fatigue syndrome. *Br. J. Rheumatol.* 35 (5): 471–474.

11 Autoantibodies and Autonomic Nervous System

Iana Leineman[1], Varvara Ryabkova[2,3], and Natalia Gavrilova[4,5]

[1]Department of Therapy, Rheumatology, Examination of Temporary Disability and Quality of Medical Care Named After E.E. Eichwald, North-Western State Medical University Named After I.I.Mechnikov, Saint Petersburg, Russia
[2]Laboratory of the Mosaic of Autoimmunity, Department of Pathology, Saint Petersburg State University, Saint Petersburg, Russia
[3]Department of Hospital Therapy Named after Academician M.V. Chernorutskii, Research Institute of Rheumatology and Allergology, Pavlov First Saint Petersburg State Medical University, Saint Petersburg, Russia
[4]Federal State Budget Educational Institution of Higher Education "St. Petersburg State University", University Emb., 7-9, Saint Petersburg, Russia
[5]St Petersburg State University Hospital, Saint Petersburg, Russia

G-protein-coupled receptor antibodies: basic facts and historical perspective

G-protein-coupled receptors (GPCRs) located on the eukaryotic cell surface play an important role in mediating responses to the majority of neurotransmitters and hormones in humans and other vertebrates. They represent the largest group of the membrane proteins and take part in the response to a large number of endogenous (biogenic amines, cations, lipids, peptides, and glycoproteins) and exogenous (medications, photons, tastants, and odorants) ligands and stimuli. Impairment of the GPCR signaling pathways is evaluated in various pathologies, including metabolic, immunological, and neurodegenerative disorders, as well as in cancer and infectious diseases [1]. High titers of the anti-GPCR antibodies (anti-GPCR autoantibodies) have been described in the past 20 years in various medical conditions, including rheumatic, neurological, and cardiovascular diseases and acute vascular rejection [2]. The fundamental characteristic of these autoantibodies is their ability to bind cell receptors and activate or inhibit intracellular signaling pathways mainly in the allosteric mode of action [3]. Therefore, Fcγ-mediated functions of autoantibodies that lead to the tissue inflammation in many autoimmune diseases are not typical for anti-GPCR autoantibodies, which may be an important observation helping to understand the pathogenesis in the abovementioned conditions.

Graves' disease was the first described example of an autoimmune disease caused by agonistic autoantibodies that activate GPCRs, resulting in thyroid hormone production and proliferation of

Autoimmune Disorders: Adjuvants and Other Risk Factors in Pathogenesis, First Edition.
Edited by Abdulla Watad, Nicola Luigi Bragazzi, and Yehuda Shoenfeld.

the thyroid cells. In this case, the "thyroid stimulator" was evaluated, which interacted with the thyroid-stimulating hormone receptor. This "stimulator" was further proved to be an autoantibody [4]. Later, antagonistic and neutral antibodies to the thyroid cells have also been described [5], showing a wide variety of possible clinical effects of autoimmune conditions.

Studying the role of GPCRs of the autonomic nervous system (ANS), in particular, adrenergic and muscarinic receptors, may be an important aim in the understanding of pathophysiological processes in various somatic diseases. Knowing the possible stimulating and inhibitory roles of such autoantibodies, one cannot exclude their influence on both central and peripheral nervous systems. One of the most important roles may be played by autoantibodies against β1-adrenergic receptors (β1AdR), which are expressed in cardiomyocytes and, therefore, described mainly in cardiovascular diseases [6]. Anti-β1AdR autoantibodies are able to activate adenylate cyclase, which leads to the accumulation of cyclic adenosine monophosphate and activation of protein kinase A, developing a wide range of metabolic and neuroendocrine disorders. As a result, the contractility of the heart increases, which may cause the development of systolic dysfunction, myocardial remodeling, and development of heart failure and tachyarrhythmias [7].

Autoantibodies against β2-adrenergic receptors (β2AdR) are more difficult to study, possibly due to the wider distribution of β2AdR in the body. However, several independent scientific groups have described their possible roles in the pathogenesis of bronchial asthma, glaucoma, autoimmune/inflammatory syndrome induced by adjuvants (ASIA), fibromyalgia (FM), chronic fatigue syndrome, and dementia [8, 9]. It is currently accepted that functional autoantibodies may be present in diseases without known autoimmune origins. This idea was first described in 1980 in patients with rhinitis and asthma, where autoantibodies to β2AdR were shown to desensitize receptors by impairing ligand binding [10]. Such a variety of pathologies can be explained due to the expression of β2AdR on innate and adaptive immune cells, establishing an important link between the nervous and immune systems [11]. When β2AR is activated, immunosuppression is expected, but in a certain situation, the development of pro-inflammatory effects can also be evaluated [11, 12].

α1-adrenergic receptors (α1AdR) mediate smooth muscle contraction and play an important role in neurotransmission and cognition [13]. Autoantibodies to α1-AR have been mainly described in vascular pathology, including hypertension, postural orthostatic tachycardia syndrome (POTS), and in dementia and other cognitive diseases [14, 15].

Five AAb against G-protein-coupled muscarinic acetylcholine receptors (mAChR) were described (M1–M5) that are involved in heart rate regulation, smooth muscle contraction, glandular secretion, and central nervous system function [16]. Autoantibodies to M1 mAChR have been evaluated in a number of neurophysiological diseases, and M2 mAChR in cardiovascular diseases [17, 18]. Autoantibodies that are widely described in autoimmune diseases, for example in Sjögren's syndrome, are autoantibodies to M3 mAChR [19–21].

Associations between anti-GPCR antibodies and clinical manifestations of dysautonomia

Balancing sympathetic and parasympathetic effects, ANS plays a main role in the maintenance of homeostasis and resistance to environmental factors. GPCRs are present in ANS in different organs and tissues. They are responsible for a wide range of functions such as digestion (from salivation to intestinal motility), regulation of cardiovascular and respiratory systems, cognitive functions, and even regulation of the immune system [22]. Changes in ANS balance lead to the development of dysautonomia, which can include symptoms such as chronic fatigue, widespread pain, myalgia and arthralgia, cognitive dysfunction, and ophthalmic, cardiovascular, gastrointestinal, and urinary impairments (Figure 11.1). This common cluster is described in patients with chronic fatigue syndrome/myalgic encephalomyelitis (CFS/ME), fibromyalgia (FM), postvaccination conditions, manifestations associated with silicone breast implants (SBI), postinfection

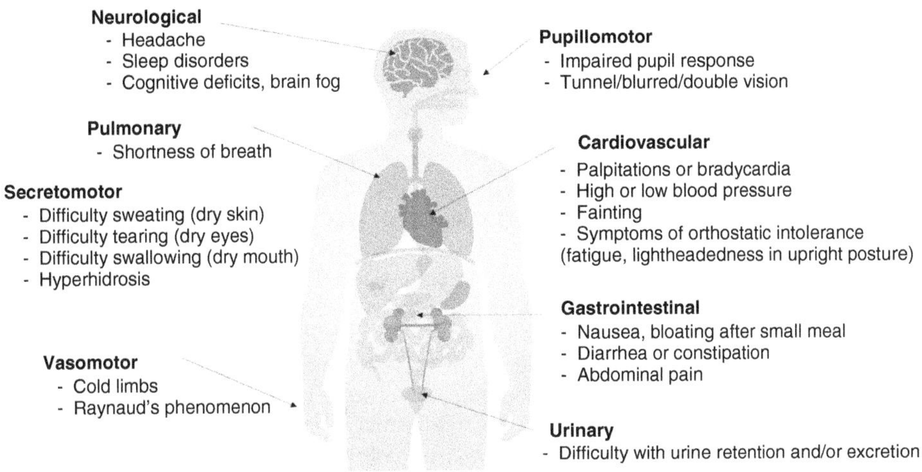

Figure 11.1 Clinical manifestations of dysautonomia.

conditions (Epstein–Barr virus, COVID-19, etc.), and several rheumatic diseases [23]. This observation alludes to the possible presence of a common pathological pathway in the autoimmune dysautonomia development [23, 24]. This hypothesis is also supported by the described correlations between autonomic manifestations and the titers of anti-GPCR autoantibodies.

Tanaka et al. showed that the presence of anti-M1 mAChR antibodies was associated with clinical symptoms such as muscle weakness in patients with CFS/ME [17]. Knowing that M1 mAChR are expressed in the cortex and hippocampus, cognitive impairment in this group of patients may be explained with the presence of anti-mAChR antibodies and symptoms such as forgetfulness and difficulty in thinking [17]. Later, Freitag et al. demonstrated the correlation between anti-GPCR antibodies and the severity of key clinical symptoms in CFS/ME. Interestingly, the titers of antibodies against α1,2 AdR, α1,2,3 AdR, and M3,4 mAChR were linked with the severity of fatigue, muscle pain, and cognitive symptoms only in patients with infection-triggered CFS/ME [24]. The correlation between anti-α1,2 AdR antibodies and the gastrointestinal symptoms was described as well as between anti-α1, β2 AdR and M4 mAChR antibodies and the pupillomotor symptoms [24]. In contrast, the non-infection-triggered CFS group showed only strong correlations of anti-α1,2 AdR and β1,2 AdR antibodies with the orthostatic dysfunction as in patients with POTS [14]. POTS is characterized by impaired balance and posture functions where the adrenergic and renin angiotensin systems play a major role. The high titers of autoantibodies to the α1 AdR, β1,2 AdR [25], anti-M4 mAChR [14], and angiotensin II type 1 receptor (AT1R) [26] in sera from patients with POTS also support the theory of autoimmune pathophysiological mechanisms for this condition.

Eighty percent of patients with post-COVID-19 syndrome have more than one dysautonomia symptom, including chronic fatigue, breathlessness, palpitations, POTS, chest pain, and presyncope or syncope episodes [27]. The majority of these symptoms can be considered to be linked with the presence of up to 20 anti-GPCR autoantibodies, which were demonstrated by Cabral-Marques et al. [28]. SARS-CoV-2 is definitely not the only one virus that may trigger autoimmune diseases/disorders development. Other possible viruses include parvovirus B19, Epstein–Barr virus, cytomegalovirus, herpes virus-6, human T-cell lymphotropic virus type 1, hepatitis A and C, and rubella virus [22]. Human papillomavirus and its vaccination can also lead to dysautonomia, probably due to the development of autoimmune disorders. Anti-GPCRs were identified in young Japanese women with symptoms of POTS, fatigue, chronic regional pain syndrome, and cognitive dysfunction [29]. A significant increase in the titer of antibodies to both adreno- and cholinergic receptors was shown in comparison with the control group [29].

Women with SBIs were described to have autonomic-related symptoms such as severe chronic fatigue, cognitive impairment, widespread pain, memory loss, sleep disorders, palpitations, depression, and hearing abnormalities [30]. For the first time, Halpert et al. demonstrated a significant reduction in the titers of anti-β1 AdR, anti-AT1R, and anti-endothelin receptor type A (anti-ETAR) autoantibodies in women with silicone implants [30]. And especially anti-β1 AdR autoantibodies were found to correlate with sleep disorders and depression [30]. The improvement of symptoms in up to 80% of the patients after the explantation of the silicone implants [31] with a good clinical response to steroids, cytostatic drugs, and plasmapheresis [32] alluded to the possible presence of autoimmune disorder within the conception of ASIA syndrome.

Patients with rheumatic diseases such as systemic sclerosis, systemic lupus erythematosus, rheumatoid arthritis, and primary Sjögren's syndrome were also found to have high anti-GPCR antibodies titers [2, 33–35]. Sjögren's syndrome is one of the most studied diseases in which both manifestations of dysautonomia and an increase in the titers of antagonistic functional autoantibodies, in particular, to the M3 receptor, are observed. Autoantibodies against M3 disrupt cholinergic neurotransmission in the gastrointestinal tract, which is associated with autonomic dysregulation, such as decreased motor function of the esophagus, sense of "fullness" after a meal, and impaired intestinal motility in patients with Sjögren's syndrome [36]. It is important to note that the salivary and lacrimal glands also express the M3 receptor, which may be an important factor in the pathogenesis of autoimmune exocrinopathy, leading to the development of xerophthalmia and xerostomia [19]. So, the anti-M3 mAChR antibodies potentially could be a new biomarker to differentiate dry eyes due to Sjögren's syndrome from dry eyes of any other reasons [19].

Gastrointestinal dysmotility in systemic sclerosis is also considered to be associated with circulating autoantibodies against the M3 mAChR [37]. Also, anti-AT1R and anti-ETAR antibodies could be used as important biomarkers of disease progression [34]. The associations were found between anti-AT1R and anti-ETAR antibodies and vascular complications such as pulmonary arterial hypertension as well as mortality and therapy response [34, 35]. Avouac et al. showed that anti-ETAR antibodies were strong predictors for digital ulcers in patients with systemic sclerosis [38] (Table 11.1).

The autoimmune concept for dysautonomia

The hypothesis of autoimmune autonomic disbalance needs further proof and can be supported by several observations. Patients with clinically significant anti-GPCR antibody titers may manifest with the symptoms of autoimmune disease, such as arthralgia, myalgia, flu-like condition, and brain fog. A genetic predisposition and a family history of autoimmune diseases can be frequently identified. Even for fibromyalgia, there are signs of chronic pain syndrome in the patients' family. An important factor for an autoimmune condition is the predominance in women and in young people without other proven somatic diseases. Many studies alluded to the provoking role of a trigger (stress, adjuvants, and bacterial or viral agents), which leads to an overstimulation of the immune system. Viruses, among which *Herpesviridae* spp. [57] and COVID-19 [58], in addition to direct damage of the nervous system, can cause autoimmune phenomenon due to immunological mimicry described in many rheumatic diseases and autoimmune conditions. Due to the fact that anti-GPCR antibodies are functional, probably the overstimulation of the immune system can lead to higher levels of autoantibodies, which cause disbalance in ANS [22].

Animal studies provide valuable information and support the idea of autoimmune involvement of ANS. Li et al. demonstrated in vivo the role of adrenergic autoantibodies in the pathophysiology of POTS [59]. In their study, immunization of laboratory rabbits with α1 and β1 AdR peptides resulted in the production of functional α1 AdR and β1 AdR autoantibodies, as well as changes in the cardiovascular response to catecholamines, contributing to postural tachycardia without affecting the blood pressure [59].

Table 11.1 The autoantibodies directed against G-protein-coupled receptors in various diseases.

GPCR	Disease	References
α_1-AdR	Preeclampsia	[39]
	Prostate cancer	[40]
	Dementia	[41]
	POTS	[14, 25, 26]
	Arterial hypertension	[42]
β1 AdR	Dilated cardiomyopathy	[42]
	Ischemic cardiomyopathy	[42]
	Heart failure	[42]
	Myocarditis	[42]
	Atrial fibrillation	[42]
	Chagas disease	[42]
	POTS	[14, 25, 26]
	Women with silicone breast implants	[30]
	Diabetes type 2	[43]
β2 AdR	Heart failure	[42]
	Bronchial asthma	[10, 44]
	Chronic fatigue syndrome	[45]
	POTS	[14, 25, 26]
	Dementia	[41]
	Diabetes type 2	[46]
	Complex regional pain	[47]
M1 mAChR	Schizophrenia	[48]
	Mood disorders	[17]
	Chronic fatigue syndrome	[45]
	POTS	[14, 25, 26]
M2 mAChR	Heart failure	[42]
	Atrial fibrillation	[42]
	Myocarditis	[42]
	Chagas disease	[42]
	Dilated cardiomyopathy	[42]
	POTS	[14, 25, 26]
	Chronic fatigue syndrome	[45]
	Complex regional pain	[47]
M3 mAChR	Sjögren's syndrome	[19, 20]
	Systemic sclerosis	[33]
	POTS	[14, 25, 26]
	Chronic fatigue syndrome	[45]
M4 mAChR	POTS	[14, 25, 26]
M5 mAChR	POTS	[14, 25, 26]
Type 1 angiotensin II receptor	Hypertension	[49]
	Systemic sclerosis	[33]
	Systemic lupus erythematosus	[50]
	Women with silicone breast implants	[30]
	Diabetes type 2	[43]
Endothelin 1 receptor	Systemic sclerosis	[33–35, 51]
	Systemic lupus erythematosus	[52]
	Women with silicone breast implants	[30]
	Prostate cancer	[40]
	Dementia	[41]
Thyrotropin receptor	Graves' disease	[53]
Extracellular calcium-sensing receptor	Hypoparathyroidism	[54, 55]
	Primary Sjögren's syndrome	[56]

Passive transfer from the Sjögren's syndrome patients of IgG with an inhibitory anti-M3 mAChR activity [60] or monoclonal anti-M3 mAChR autoantibodies [61] to mice reproduced the signs of an overactive bladder and decreased salivation.

Another animal model demonstrated that IgG from the patients with systemic sclerosis binds to the M3-AChR on rat colonic smooth muscles and mesenteric plexus and attenuates smooth muscle contraction [62].

In a pioneering study, Goebel et al. passively transferred IgG from a patient with fibromyalgia to mice, which led to the development of autonomic dysregulation, which is one of the most important criteria for proving the autoimmune genesis of a disease [63]. Fibromyalgia IgG does not cause a single symptom but polymodal disturbances of mechanical and cold hypersensitivity and locomotor activity in mice. It has also been shown that no damage to the brain structures occurred. The symptoms were associated with the accumulation of IgG in the dorsal root ganglia (DRG) [63]. This fact supports the hypothesis of prof. Manuel Martínez-Lavín, who proposed the DRG as a key structure where psychological distress, physical trauma, or autoimmune diseases are transformed into a neuropathic pain [64]. In several studies on mice, the development of a sterile inflammation in the DRG and disruption of the normal connection between the sympathetic nervous system (SNS) and the nociceptive system were demonstrated after a mechanical trauma [65] and significant stress exposure [66]. Chronic or acute stress may also trigger a neurological dysfunction and the new antigenic potential in tissues with the development of immune-induced localized inflammation. Knowing that glial cells cover not only the bodies of neurons of DRG but also neurons of sympathetic and parasympathetic ganglia, one can expect the development of dysautonomia in such patients [67]. Thus, fibromyalgia is not only a widespread pain syndrome but also a complex of symptoms associated with an autonomic dysfunction, manifested by symptoms of autonomic dysregulation, primarily in the cardiovascular system [64, 68]. Neurovascular disorders of blood flow autoregulation with tissue hypoxia and secondary metabolic and autonomic adaptations suggest a pathological pathway in patients with ME/CSF in accordance with the concept of Fluge et al. [69]. The authors also considered that anti-GPCR autoantibodies play the main role in dysautonomia by affecting the endothelium and small nerve fibers [42, 69] (Figure 11.2).

Potential treatment strategy of dysautonomia

Due to the functional role of antibodies, normalizing the titers of the anti-GPCR autoantibodies in patients with autoimmune conditions to levels observed in healthy subjects with autonomic balance is a challenging therapeutic approach.

In several studies, the hypothesis of autoimmune dysautonomia appeared after an observation of the beneficial treatment regimens widely used in patients with oncology and rheumatology. Removal of anti-β2 AdR and anti-M3/M4 mAChR autoantibodies from the blood of patients with ME/CFS with immunoadsorption methods can also be an important factor confirming the autoimmune pathogenesis of this disease [9]. A reduction in antibody titers against β-2 AdR has been demonstrated in patients with a clinical response to B-cell depletion therapy with rituximab [45], resulting in a reduction in clinical symptoms of fatigue, POTS, and myalgia. A similar beneficial effect has been noted with ME/CFS treatment with cyclophosphamide [70].

Kumar et al. demonstrated that dysmotility in systemic sclerosis progresses from IgG-induced blockage of cholinergic neurotransmission (neuropathy) to inhibition of acetylcholine action at the smooth muscle cell (myopathy) and suggested that systemic sclerosis-associated intestinal dysfunction may be potentially reversible with anti-idiotypic antibodies in intravenous immunoglobulin (IVIG) that block the activity of pathogenic systemic sclerosis IgG [62, 71]. The efficacy of IVIG on the overall gastrointestinal symptoms (and in particular on gastroesophageal reflux disease symptoms) was recently demonstrated in two cohorts of patients with systemic sclerosis [72]. A retrospective review of four patients with Sjögren's syndrome and dysautonomia who received

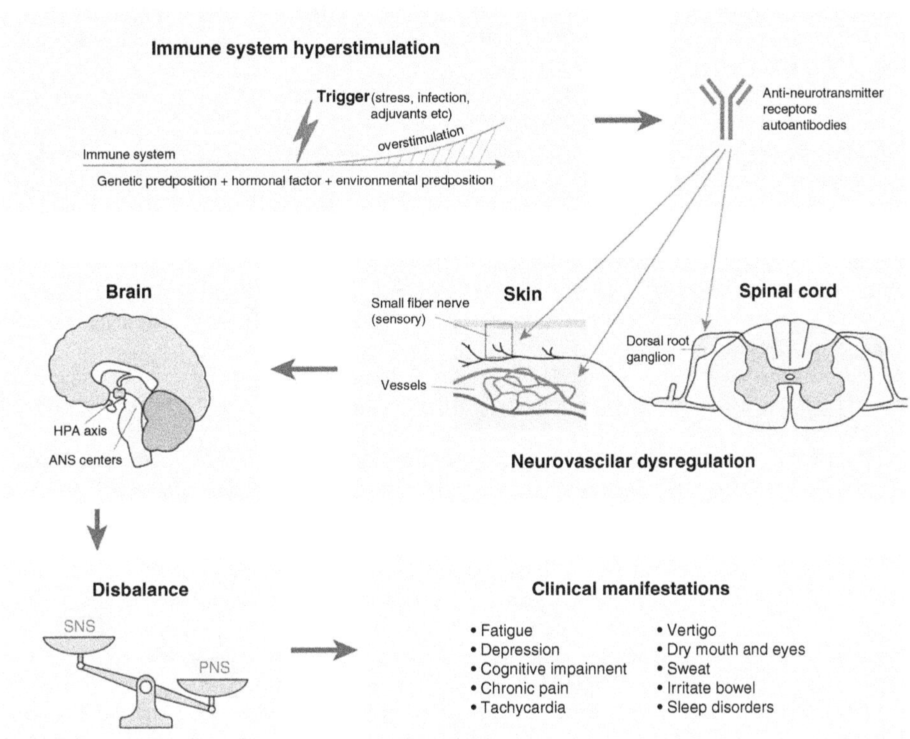

Figure 11.2 In genetically predisposed patients, triggers such as infection, stress, adjuvants, and silicone with the specific hormonal background could stimulate higher titers of antineurotransmitter receptor autoantibodies, which leads to the development of neurovascular dysregulation. Then, activation of autonomic nervous system (ANS) centers and hypothalamic–pituitary–adrenal axis (HPA) changes the balance between parasympathetic (PNS) and sympathetic nervous system (SNS) and contributes to the appearance of clinical manifestations of dysautonomia.

IVIG demonstrated the marked clinical and functional improvements in autonomic testing in all four patients [73]. Such promising results of IVIG were shown in improving small-fiber neuropathy on both the clinical and the pathophysiologic levels in patients with fibromyalgia [74]. So, IVIG could be potentially used in patients with autoimmune dysautonomia.

Not only the normalization of the levels of anti-GPCR autoantibodies but also the use of physical exercises as a therapeutic method can improve the condition of patients by balancing the activity between the SNS and the parasympathetic nervous system (PNS). Regular exercises and physical activity also should be added to the patients' daily routine.

References

1. Heng, B.C., Aubel, D., and Fussenegger, M. (2013). An overview of the diverse roles of G-protein coupled receptors (GPCRs) in the pathophysiology of various human diseases. *Biotechnol. Adv.* 31 (8): 1676–1694. https://doi.org/10.1016/j.biotechadv.2013.08.017.
2. Meyer, C. and Heidecke, H. (2018). Antibodies against GPCR. *Front. Biosci. (Landmark Ed).* 23 (11): 2177–2194. https://doi.org/10.2741/4698.
3. Skiba, M.A. and Kruse, A.C. (2021). Autoantibodies as endogenous modulators of GPCR signaling. *Trends Pharmacol. Sci.* 42 (3): 135–150. https://doi.org/10.1016/j.tips.2020.11.013.

4. Meek, J.C., Jones, A.E., Lewis, U.J., and Vanderlaan, W.P. (1964). Characterization of the long-acting thyroid stimulator of Graves' disease. *Proc. Natl. Acad. Sci. U. S. A.* 52 (2): 342–349. https://doi.org/10.1073/pnas.52.2.342.
5. Rees Smith, B., McLachlan, S.M., and Furmaniak, J. (1988). Autoantibodies to the thyrotropin receptor. *Endocr. Rev.* 9 (1): 106–121. https://doi.org/10.1210/edrv-9-1-106.
6. Bornholz, B., Roggenbuck, D., Jahns, R., and Boege, F. (2014). Diagnostic and therapeutic aspects of β1-adrenergic receptor autoantibodies in human heart disease. *Autoimmun. Rev.* 13 (9): 954–962. https://doi.org/10.1016/j.autrev.2014.08.021.
7. Ali, D.C., Naveed, M., Gordon, A. et al. (2020). β-Adrenergic receptor, an essential target in cardiovascular diseases. *Heart Fail. Rev.* 25 (2): 343–354. https://doi.org/10.1007/s10741-019-09825-x.
8. Jünemann, A., Hohberger, B., Rech, J. et al. (2018). Agonistic autoantibodies to the β2-adrenergic receptor involved in the pathogenesis of open-angle glaucoma. *Front. Immunol.* 12 (9): 145. https://doi.org/10.3389/fimmu.2018.00145.
9. Scheibenbogen, C., Loebel, M., Freitag, H. et al. (2018). Immunoadsorption to remove ß2 adrenergic receptor antibodies in chronic fatigue syndrome CFS/ME. *PLoS One* 13 (3): e0193672. https://doi.org/10.1371/journal.pone.0193672.
10. Venter, J.C., Fraser, C.M., and Harrison, L.C. (1980). Autoantibodies to beta 2-adrenergic receptors: a possible cause of adrenergic hyporesponsiveness in allergic rhinitis and asthma. *Science* 207 (4437): 1361–1363. https://doi.org/10.1126/science.6153472.
11. Chhatar, S. and Lal, G. (2021). Role of adrenergic receptor signalling in neuroimmune communication. *Curr. Res. Immunol.*. 2: 202–217. https://doi.org/10.1016/j.crimmu.2021.11.001.
12. Wu, L., Tai, Y., Hu, S. et al. (2018). Bidirectional role of β2-adrenergic receptor in autoimmune diseases. *Front. Pharmacol.* 9: 1313. https://doi.org/10.3389/fphar.2018.01313.
13. Perez, D.M. (2021). Current developments on the role of α_1-adrenergic receptors in cognition, cardioprotection, and metabolism. *Front. Cell Dev. Biol.* 9: 652152. https://doi.org/10.3389/fcell.2021.652152.
14. Gunning, W.T. 3rd, Kvale, H., Kramer, P.M. et al. (2019). Postural orthostatic tachycardia syndrome is associated with elevated G-protein coupled receptor autoantibodies. *J. Am. Heart Assoc.* 8 (18): e013602. https://doi.org/10.1161/JAHA.119.013602.
15. Karczewski, P., Pohlmann, A., Wagenhaus, B. et al. (2012). Antibodies to the α1-adrenergic receptor cause vascular impairments in rat brain as demonstrated by magnetic resonance angiography. *PLoS One* 7 (7): e41602. https://doi.org/10.1371/journal.pone.0041602.
16. Kruse, A.C., Kobilka, B.K., Gautam, D. et al. (2014). Muscarinic acetylcholine receptors: novel opportunities for drug development. *Nat. Rev. Drug Discov.* 13 (7): 549–560. https://doi.org/10.1038/nrd4295.
17. Tanaka, S., Matsunaga, H., Kimura, M. et al. (2003). Autoantibodies against four kinds of neurotransmitter receptors in psychiatric disorders. *J. Neuroimmunol.* 141 (1–2): 155–164. https://doi.org/10.1016/s0165-5728(03)00252-2. Erratum in: (2003). J. Neuroimmunol. 144(1–2): 148.
18. Nussinovitch, U. and Shoenfeld, Y. (2012). The diagnostic and clinical significance of anti-muscarinic receptor autoantibodies. *Clin. Rev. Allergy Immunol.* 42 (3): 298–308. https://doi.org/10.1007/s12016-010-8235-x.
19. Bacman, S., Berra, A., Sterin-Borda, L., and Borda, E. (2001). Muscarinic acetylcholine receptor antibodies as a new marker of dry eye Sjögren syndrome. *Invest. Ophthalmol. Vis. Sci.* 42 (2): 321–327.
20. Mona, M., Mondello, S., Hyon, J.Y. et al. (2021). Clinical usefulness of anti-muscarinic type 3 receptor autoantibodies in patients with primary Sjögren's syndrome. *Clin. Exp. Rheumatol.* 39 (4): 795–803.
21. Riemekasten, G., Petersen, F., and Heidecke, H. (2020). What makes antibodies against G protein-coupled receptors so special? A novel concept to understand chronic diseases. *Front. Immunol.* 11: 564526. https://doi.org/10.3389/fimmu.2020.564526.
22. Halpert, G. and Shoenfeld, Y. (2020). SARS-CoV-2, the autoimmune virus. *Autoimmun. Rev.* 19 (12): 102695. https://doi.org/10.1016/j.autrev.2020.102695.
23. Shoenfeld, Y., Ryabkova, V.A., Scheibenbogen, C. et al. (2020). Complex syndromes of chronic pain, fatigue and cognitive impairment linked to autoimmune dysautonomia and small fiber neuropathy. *Clin. Immunol.* 214: 108384. https://doi.org/10.1016/j.clim.2020.108384.
24. Freitag, H., Szklarski, M., Lorenz, S. et al. (2021). Autoantibodies to vasoregulative G-protein-coupled receptors correlate with symptom severity, autonomic dysfunction and disability in myalgic encephalomyelitis/chronic fatigue syndrome. *J. Clin. Med.* 10 (16): 3675. https://doi.org/10.3390/jcm10163675.

25. Li, H., Yu, X., Liles, C. et al. (2014). Autoimmune basis for postural tachycardia syndrome. *J. Am. Heart Assoc.* 3: e000755. https://doi.org/10.1161/JAHA.113.000755.
26. Yu, X., Li, H., Murphy, T.A. et al. (2018). Angiotensin II type 1 receptor autoantibodies in postural tachycardia syndrome. *J. Am. Heart Assoc.* 7 (8): e008351. https://doi.org/10.1161/JAHA.117.008351.
27. Lopez-Leon, S., Wegman-Ostrosky, T., Perelman, C. et al. (2021). More than 50 long-term effects of COVID-19: a systematic review and meta-analysis. *Sci. Rep.* 11 (1): 16144. https://doi.org/10.1038/s41598-021-95565-8.
28. Cabral-Marques, O., Halpert, G., Schimke, L.F. et al. (2022). Autoantibodies targeting GPCRs and RAS-related molecules associate with COVID-19 severity. *Nat. Commun.* 13 (1): 1220. https://doi.org/10.1038/s41467-022-28905-5.
29. Ikeda, S.-I., Hineno, A., Scheibenbogen, C. et al. (2019). Autoantibodies against autonomic nerve receptors in adolescent Japanese girls after immunization with human papillomavirus vaccine. *Ann. Arthritis Clin. Rheumatol.* 2: 1014.
30. Halpert, G., Watad, A., Tsur, A.M. et al. (2021). Autoimmune dysautonomia in women with silicone breast implants. *J. Autoimmun.* 120: 102631. https://doi.org/10.1016/j.jaut.2021.102631.
31. Tervaert, J.W.C., Colaris, M.J., and van der Hulst, R.R. (2017). Silicone breast implants and autoimmune rheumatic diseases: myth or reality. *Curr. Opin. Rheumatol.* 29 (4): 348–354. https://doi.org/10.1097/BOR.0000000000000391.
32. Fuzzard, S.K., Teixeira, R., and Zinn, R. (2019). A review of the literature on the management of silicone implant incompatibility syndrome. *Aesthet. Plast. Surg.* 43 (5): 1145–1149. https://doi.org/10.1007/s00266-019-01407-4.
33. Cabral-Marques, O. and Riemekasten, G. (2016). Vascular hypothesis revisited: role of stimulating antibodies against angiotensin and endothelin receptors in the pathogenesis of systemic sclerosis. *Autoimmun. Rev.* 15 (7): 690–694. https://doi.org/10.1016/j.autrev.2016.03.005.
34. Riemekasten, G., Philippe, A., Näther, M. et al. (2011). Involvement of functional autoantibodies against vascular receptors in systemic sclerosis. *Ann. Rheum. Dis.* 70 (3): 530–536. https://doi.org/10.1136/ard.2010.135772.
35. Günther, J., Kill, A., Becker, M.O. et al. (2014). Angiotensin receptor type 1 and endothelin receptor type A on immune cells mediate migration and the expression of IL-8 and CCL18 when stimulated by autoantibodies from systemic sclerosis patients. *Arthritis Res. Ther.* 16 (2): R65. https://doi.org/10.1186/ar4503.
36. Cavill, D., Waterman, S.A., and Gordon, T.P. (2004). Antibodies raised against the second extracellular loop of the human muscarinic M3 receptor mimic functional autoantibodies in Sjögren's syndrome. *Scand. J. Immunol.* 59 (3): 261–266. https://doi.org/10.1111/j.0300-9475.2004.01395.x.
37. Singh, J., Cohen, S., Mehendiratta, V. et al. (2012). Effects of scleroderma antibodies and pooled human immunoglobulin on anal sphincter and colonic smooth muscle function. *Gastroenterology* 143 (5): 1308–1318. https://doi.org/10.1053/j.gastro.2012.07.109.
38. Avouac, J., Riemekasten, G., Meune, C. et al. (2015). Autoantibodies against endothelin 1 type A receptor are strong predictors of digital ulcers in systemic sclerosis. *J. Rheumatol.* 42 (10): 1801–1807. https://doi.org/10.3899/jrheum.150061.
39. Ma, G., Li, Y., Zhang, J. et al. (2013). Association between the presence of autoantibodies against adrenoreceptors and severe pre-eclampsia: a pilot study. *PLoS One* 8 (3): e57983. https://doi.org/10.1371/journal.pone.0057983.
40. Wallukat, G., Jandrig, B., Becker, N.P. et al. (2020). Autoantibodies directed against α1-adrenergic receptor and endothelin receptor A in patients with prostate cancer. *Auto Immun. Highlights* 11 (1): 13. https://doi.org/10.1186/s13317-020-00136-y.
41. Wallukat, G., Prüss, H., Müller, J., and Schimke, I. (2018). Functional autoantibodies in patients with different forms of dementia. *PLoS One* 13 (3): e0192778. https://doi.org/10.1371/journal.pone.0192778. Erratum in: (2018). *PLoS One* 13(8): e0203253.
42. Ryabkova, V.A., Shubik, Y.V., Erman, M.V. et al. (2019). Lethal immunoglobulins: autoantibodies and sudden cardiac death. *Autoimmun. Rev.* 18 (4): 415–425. https://doi.org/10.1016/j.autrev.2018.12.005.
43. Zhao, L.S., Liao, Y.H., Xiang, G.D. et al. (2010). Positive rate of autoantibodies against adrenergic receptors beta1 and angiotensin II type 1 receptors in the type 2 diabetes mellitus with or without hypertension. *Zhonghua Xin Xue Guan Bing Za Zhi* 38 (2): 139–142.

44. Turki, J. and Liggett, S.B. (1995). Receptor-specific functional properties of beta 2-adrenergic receptor autoantibodies in asthma. *Am. J. Respir. Cell Mol. Biol.* 12 (5): 531–539. https://doi.org/10.1165/ajrcmb.12.5.7742016.
45. Loebel, M., Grabowski, P., Heidecke, H. et al. (2016). Antibodies to β adrenergic and muscarinic cholinergic receptors in patients with chronic fatigue syndrome. *Brain Behav. Immun.* 52: 32–39. https://doi.org/10.1016/j.bbi.2015.09.013.
46. Werner, C., Müller, N., and Müller, U.A. (2019). Agonistic autoantibodies against B2-adrenergic receptors correlating with macrovascular disease in longstanding diabetes type 2. *Acta Diabetol.* 56 (6): 659–665. https://doi.org/10.1007/s00592-019-01296-8.
47. Kohr, D., Singh, P., Tschernatsch, M. et al. (2011). Autoimmunity against the $\beta 2$ adrenergic receptor and muscarinic-2 receptor in complex regional pain syndrome. *Pain* 152 (12): 2690–2700. https://doi.org/10.1016/j.pain.2011.06.012.
48. Ryan, A.E., Mowry, B.J., Kesby, J.P. et al. (2019). Is there a role for antibodies targeting muscarinic acetylcholine receptors in the pathogenesis of schizophrenia? *Aust. N. Z. J. Psychiatry* 53 (11): 1059–1069. https://doi.org/10.1177/0004867419864438.
49. Civieri, G., Iop, L., and Tona, F. (2022). Antibodies against angiotensin II type 1 and endothelin 1 type A receptors in cardiovascular pathologies. *Int. J. Mol. Sci.* 23 (2): 927. https://doi.org/10.3390/ijms23020927.
50. Xiong, J., Liang, Y., Yang, H. et al. (2013). The role of angiotensin II type 1 receptor-activating antibodies in patients with lupus nephritis. *Int. J. Clin. Pract.* 67 (10): 1066–1067. https://doi.org/10.1111/ijcp.12242.
51. Kawaguchi, Y., Takagi, K., Hara, M. et al. (2004). Angiotensin II in the lesional skin of systemic sclerosis patients contributes to tissue fibrosis via angiotensin II type 1 receptors. *Arthritis Rheum.* 50 (1): 216–226. https://doi.org/10.1002/art.11364.
52. Guo, L., Li, M., Chen, Y. et al. (2015). Anti-endothelin receptor type A autoantibodies in systemic lupus erythematosus-associated pulmonary arterial hypertension. *Arthritis Rheumatol.* 67 (9): 2394–2402. https://doi.org/10.1002/art.39212.
53. Minich, W.B., Lenzner, C., and Morgenthaler, N.G. (2004). Antibodies to TSH-receptor in thyroid autoimmune disease interact with monoclonal antibodies whose epitopes are broadly distributed on the receptor. *Clin. Exp. Immunol.* 136 (1): 129–136. https://doi.org/10.1111/j.1365-2249.2004.02417.x.
54. Tomar, N., Gupta, N., and Goswami, R. (2013). Calcium-sensing receptor autoantibodies and idiopathic hypoparathyroidism. *J. Clin. Endocrinol. Metab.* 98 (9): 3884–3891. https://doi.org/10.1210/jc.2013-2158.
55. Kifor, O., McElduff, A., LeBoff, M.S. et al. (2004). Activating antibodies to the calcium-sensing receptor in two patients with autoimmune hypoparathyroidism. *J. Clin. Endocrinol. Metab.* 89 (2): 548–556. https://doi.org/10.1210/jc.2003-031054.
56. Harris, H.E., Kemp, E.H., Brown, E.M. et al. (2011). First report of anti-calcium-sensing receptor antibodies in a patient with Sjogren's syndrome and primary hypoparathyroidism. *Rheumatology* 50 (6): 1173–1175. https://doi.org/10.1093/rheumatology/ker128.
57. Duarte, L.F., Altamirano-Lagos, M.J., Tabares-Guevara, J.H. et al. (2021). Asymptomatic herpes simplex virus type 1 infection causes an earlier onset and more severe experimental autoimmune encephalomyelitis. *Front. Immunol.* 12: 635257. https://doi.org/10.3389/fimmu.2021.635257.
58. Dotan, A., Muller, S., Kanduc, D. et al. (2021). The SARS-CoV-2 as an instrumental trigger of autoimmunity. *Autoimmun. Rev.* 20 (4): 102792. https://doi.org/10.1016/j.autrev.2021.102792.
59. Li, H., Scherlag, B.J., Kem, D.C. et al. (2014). Atrial tachyarrhythmias induced by the combined effects of $\beta 1/2$-adrenergic autoantibodies and thyroid hormone in the rabbit. *J. Cardiovasc. Transl. Res.* 7 (6): 581–589. https://doi.org/10.1007/s12265-014-9573-5.
60. Wang, F., Jackson, M.W., Maughan, V. et al. (2004). Passive transfer of Sjogren's syndrome IgG produces the pathophysiology of overactive bladder. *Arthritis Rheum.* 50 (11): 3637–3645. https://doi.org/10.1002/art.20625.
61. Nguyen, K.H., Brayer, J., Cha, S. et al. (2000). Evidence for antimuscarinic acetylcholine receptor antibody-mediated secretory dysfunction in nod mice. *Arthritis Rheum.* 43 (10): 2297–2306. https://doi.org/10.1002/1529-0131(200010)43:10<2297::AID-ANR18>3.0.CO;2-X.
62. Kumar, S., Singh, J., Kedika, R. et al. (2016). Role of muscarinic-3 receptor antibody in systemic sclerosis: correlation with disease duration and effects of IVIG. *Am. J. Physiol. Gastrointest. Liver Physiol.* 310 (11): G1052–G1060. https://doi.org/10.1152/ajpgi.00034.2016.

63. Goebel, A., Krock, E., Gentry, C. et al. (2021). Passive transfer of fibromyalgia symptoms from patients to mice. *J. Clin. Invest.* 131 (13): e144201. https://doi.org/10.1172/JCI144201.
64. Martínez-Lavín, M. (2021). Dorsal root ganglia: fibromyalgia pain factory? *Clin. Rheumatol.* 40 (2): 783–787. https://doi.org/10.1007/s10067-020-05528-z.
65. McLachlan, E.M. and Hu, P. (2014). Inflammation in dorsal root ganglia after peripheral nerve injury: effects of the sympathetic innervation. *Auton. Neurosci.* 182: 108–117. https://doi.org/10.1016/j.autneu.2013.12.009.
66. Hung, C.H., Lee, C.H., Tsai, M.H. et al. Activation of acid-sensing ion channel 3 by lysophosphatidylcholine 16:0 mediates psychological stressinduced fibromyalgia-like pain. *Ann. Rheum. Dis.* 79: 1644–1656. https://doi.org/10.1136/annrheumdis-2020-218329.
67. Hanani, M. and Spray, D.C. (2020). Emerging importance of satellite glia in nervous system function and dysfunction. *Nat. Rev. Neurosci.* 21 (9): 485–498. https://doi.org/10.1038/s41583-020-0333-z. Erratum in: (2020). *Nat. Rev. Neurosci.*
68. Morelli, C., Castaldi, L., Brown, S.J. et al. (2021). Identification of a population of peripheral sensory neurons that regulates blood pressure. *Cell Rep.* 35 (9): 109191. https://doi.org/10.1016/j.celrep.2021.109191.
69. Fluge, Ø., Tronstad, K.J., and Mella, O. (2021). Pathomechanisms and possible interventions in myalgic encephalomyelitis/chronic fatigue syndrome (ME/CFS). *J. Clin. Invest.* 131 (14): e150377. https://doi.org/10.1172/JCI150377.
70. Rekeland, I.G., Fosså, A., Lande, A. et al. (2020). Intravenous cyclophosphamide in myalgic encephalomyelitis/chronic fatigue syndrome. An open-label phase II study. *Front. Med.* 7: 162. https://doi.org/10.3389/fmed.2020.00162.
71. Berger, M., McCallus, D.E., and Lin, C.S. (2013). Rapid and reversible responses to IVIG in autoimmune neuromuscular diseases suggest mechanisms of action involving competition with functionally important autoantibodies. *J. Peripher. Nerv. Syst.* 18 (4): 275–296. https://doi.org/10.1111/jns5.12048.
72. Gomes, J.P., Santos, L., and Shoenfeld, Y. (2019). Intravenous immunoglobulin (IVIG) in the vanguard therapy of Systemic Sclerosis. *Clin. Immunol.* 199: 25–28. https://doi.org/10.1016/j.clim.2018.12.006.
73. Goodman, B.P. (2019). Immunoresponsive autonomic neuropathy in Sjögren syndrome-case series and literature review. *Am. J. Ther.* 26 (1): e66–e71. https://doi.org/10.1097/MJT.0000000000000583.
74. Metyas, S., Youssef, H., Che, C. et al. (2018). Improvement in fibromyalgia symptoms and skin biopsy results in patients with fibromyalgia and small fiber neuropathy treated with intravenous immune globulin infusion (IVIG). In: *Arthritis Rheumatology*. New Jersey, NJ, USA: Wiley.

12 Postural Orthostatic Tachycardia Syndrome (POTS) as a Part of ASIA Syndrome

Paula David
Department of Internal Medicine 'B', Sheba Medical Center, Tel-Hashomer, Israel

Introduction

Postural Orthostatic Tachycardia Syndrome (POTS) is a clinical condition in which patients present with tachycardia and discomfort symptoms when assuming the orthostatic position without hypotension. Orthostatic tachycardia is described as an elevation of 30 bpm from the heart rate measured before standing or maintenance of the heart rate, within 10 minutes of standing, or superior of 120 bpm [1]. The symptoms include palpitations, lightheadedness, blurred vision, generalized weakness, and fatigue, among others. The syndrome is more common in women than in men, particularly among young women in the fertile age [1]. The physiopathology of POTS combines multiple and coexistent mechanisms, such as autonomic denervation, hypovolemia, and hyperadrenergic stimulation [2]. Although its etiology remains unclear, many studies had recently supported the hypothesis of it being an autoimmune disease. Most of them based their claims on laboratory findings of autoantibodies in patients with POTS as well as on its association with other autoimmune diseases [3–8].

Autoimmune/inflammatory syndrome induced by adjuvants (ASIA) consists of a cluster of related immune-mediated entities with a common clinical picture that flourished after exposure to adjuvants in genetically predisposed individuals. The most described adjuvants are silicone, aluminum salts and other metals, and vaccines. Usually, when the trigger is removed, the symptoms get better [9].

ASIA shares similarities with well-established syndromes such as macrophagic myofasciitis syndrome, gulf war syndrome, silicone implants incompatibility syndrome, sarcoidosis, Sjögren's syndrome, and undifferentiated connective tissue diseases as well as more general symptoms, such as fatigue, myalgia, arthralgia, generalize pain, sleep disturbances, hair loss, and neurologic manifestations, among others [9, 10].

Recently, those symptoms were related to an autoimmune neurosensory dysautonomia, involving autoantibodies against G-protein-coupled receptors of the autonomic nervous system and resulting in small-fiber neuropathy [8]. These autoantibodies have been described in several autoimmune diseases associated with both autonomic disorders and ASIA, such as Sjögren's syndrome,

Autoimmune Disorders: Adjuvants and Other Risk Factors in Pathogenesis, First Edition.
Edited by Abdulla Watad, Nicola Luigi Bragazzi, and Yehuda Shoenfeld.

multiple sclerosis (MS), and myasthenia gravis [11–17], and shown to be dysregulated in women with silicone incompatibility syndrome [18].

POTS was previously described in individuals suffering from ASIA, being present in 2.6–4.3% of the patients [19, 20].

This chapter discusses why POTS should be considered part of ASIA syndrome, including its association with antibodies against target G-coupled proteins, small-fiber neuropathy, chronic inflammation, and other autoimmune diseases.

POTS and autoantibodies

In the past decades, possibility of POTS being an autoimmune disease has been investigated worldwide. The central argument for this hypothesis is the finding of autoantibodies in POTS patients' sera. These antibodies mainly target G-coupled proteins, including muscarinic, nicotinic, and adrenergic receptors [3, 4, 7, 21]. Nicotinic acetylcholine receptors (nAchR) are inotropic receptors found in the central nervous system (CNS) and peripheral nervous system (PNS) and in the motor endplate of skeletal muscles [22, 23]. Muscarinic receptors are part of the parasympathetic nervous system, in both CNS and PNS. There are five subtypes of muscarinic cholinergic receptors(mAchR) nominated from M_1 to M_5. M_1 and M_3 are stimulatory receptors leading to vasoconstriction and dilation in the vasculature, while M_2 is an inhibitory receptor located in the heart and the smooth muscle. M_4 also has a negative inotropic effect in the heart by releasing neurotransmitters in the atrial area. The function of M_5 is still unclear [24, 25]. The adrenergic receptors are classified into four subtypes (α1, α2, β1, and β2) and are widely distributed among the human body, but essentially, the α receptors promote smooth muscle contraction, and the β receptors when stimulated lead to smooth cell relaxation, heart muscle contraction, and glycogenolysis [26]. Thus, considering the receptors' functions and significance toward the vascular system, autoantibodies with the antagonist and/or agonist activity could be related to POTS and indicate a possible autoimmune etiology. Autoantibodies against G-protein-coupled receptors have been previously correlated with other cardiovascular diseases (Chagas' disease, idiopathic dilated cardiomyopathy, and ischemic heart disease) and suggested as biomarkers of inflammation and myocardial damage [27, 28]. Furthermore, the same antibodies were found to be positive in autoimmune diseases such as Sjögren's syndrome and systemic sclerosis [29, 30].

In Spain [3], researchers scanned 55 POTS patients' sera looking for nine types of G-protein-coupled receptors autoantibodies. They found that 89% of their subjects tested positive for antibodies against α1 adrenergic receptors (α1AR), and 51% showed concurrent elevation of antibodies against the mAchR M_4. Most likely the second is dependent on the existence of the first. Likewise, antibodies against β1 and β2 adrenergic receptors (β1AR and β2AR) and α2 adrenergic receptor (α2AR) were detected in the subjects with their presence also appearing to be dependent on the presence of α1AR antibodies. When compared to controls, POTS patients have also be shown to have significantly higher positivity antibodies against M_1 and M_2 receptors, also suggesting a possible role of autoimmunity in the syndrome etiology [21].

The increased levels of α1AR autoantibodies in POTS patients in comparison to controls were proposed to be responsible for a compensatory sympathoneural activation of these receptors leading to peripheral vasoconstriction, while the higher levels of β1AR and β2AR agonistic antibodies could explain the tachycardia and increased plasma norepinephrine measures often presented in this disorder [4].

Indeed, the immunoglobulin G of POTS patients was shown to bind to adrenergic receptors, specifically the α1AR, the β1AR, and the β2AR, and activate them. This activation was blocked when pharmacologic adrenergic antagonist drugs were administered [7].

The potential mechanism of molecular mimicry leading to anti-G-protein-coupled receptors antibodies release has been proposed [3]. Many POTS patients have a history of Epstein-Barr Virus infection and gastrointestinal pain possibly related to enteric viral infection before starting POTS symptoms and/or antecedent to the diagnosis. That way, similar to other autoimmune diseases [6, 31], a viral infection could be one of the triggers to the autoimmune response and POTS development. Because other infections – mostly respiratory, gastrointestinal, and dermatological – preceding POTS were also described in the literature, instead of molecular mimicry, they could also represent a nonspecific trigger to develop the disease in predisposed patients [29]. Recently, POTS was also described following the COVID-19 infection [32].

In Japan, it was also reported that female patients presented with POTS symptoms after receiving human papillomavirus (HPV) vaccination, and that those subjects had higher levels of anti-G-coupled proteins than nonvaccinated controls, suggesting that vaccination could also play a role in inducing autoimmunity and consequently clinical features on these patients [33]. Vaccination has previously been widely described as one of the most common adjuvants in Autoimmune Syndrome Induced by Adjuvants (ASIA) [34–37].

POTS and chronic inflammation

On chronic inflammation processes, pro-inflammatory cytokines such as interleukins (IL) 1 and 6 and tumor necrosis factor (TNF) are released. Those molecules are responsible for many symptoms presented in these situations, including malaise, nausea, temperature changes, and tachycardia. Those pro-inflammatory citokynes also lead to vasodilation and enhance vascular permeability, having a role in volume dysregulation, and hyperadrenergic state also seen in those conditions [38]. POTS patients were shown to present, in addition to the autoantibodies previously mentioned, signs of chronic immune activation, such as high measurements of IL-6, a pro-inflammatory cytokine. [39]. There is an exacerbated sympathetic activity in POTS patients that one could claim to be associated with chronic inflammation or autoimmunity since the immune system and the autonomic nervous system are known to influence each other. The vagus nerve, for example, regulates the heart frequency and gastrointestinal movements among other visceral functions and also takes part in a neuroinflammatory reflex, through which it reduces pro-inflammatory cytokine levels by cholinergic enervating the spleen and other immune organs. Adrenergic stimulation, on the other hand, can increase the IL-6 and other inflammatory molecules release [38].

POTS and other autoimmune diseases

Many autoimmune disorders, including MS, Systemic Lupus Erythematosus (SLE), Sjögren's Syndrome (SS), and Celiac Disease (CD), had been described as correlated to POTS [5, 6, 40–43]. In one study, medical records of 100 patients with POTS were analyzed, and it was found that 20% of their patients were found to be diagnosed with another autoimmune disorder [6]. They also found an increased prevalence of markers of autoimmunity, such as antinuclear antibody (ANA) and antiphospholipid antibodies. Almost one-third of the patients were positive to at least one of the tested autoimmune markers, 25% of the patients being positive to ANA. In another research, when compared to the general population, POTS patients were shown to more commonly refer to themselves as being sensitive to gluten (42% versus 19%, $p < 0.0001$), and more than that, they have a higher prevalence of biopsy-confirmed CD (4% versus 1%, $p = 0.03$) [41]. Thyroid disease has also been described as more prevalent among those patients [6, 40]. From all the autoimmune conditions associated with POTS, SS deserves a highlight. SS and POTS have many symptoms in common – dry eyes, dry mouth, lightheadedness, GI motility dysfunction, and others – and are more common in women and may be accompanied by extreme fatigue and small-fiber neuropathy. It has been suggested that those complex syndromes may compose a new group of autoimmune conditions with antibodies targeting G-coupled proteins being part of their pathogenesis [8]. Furthermore, in a clinical analysis of 13 cases of SS patients with autonomic dysfunction, approximately 60% of them were found to fulfill the criteria for POTS [44]. It has been suggested that patients with POTS present with SS symptoms (especially dry mouth and dry eyes) should be tested for SS [45].

POTS and small-fiber neuropathy (SFN)

Small-Fiber Neuropathy (SFN) is a recently described medical condition that derives from distal impairment of small A-delta and C nerve fibers, leading to autonomic dysfunction and neuropathic pain. The confirmation of SFN usually requires a skin biopsy showing intraepidermal nerve fibers' decreased density, since the routine neuropathy diagnostic tests, such as electromyography and nerve conduction studies, appear to be normal in those patients, as long as their clinical and neurologic examinations [46–48]. SFN etiology remains unclear. However, immune-mediated, metabolic, hereditary, and other mechanisms have been suggested to be involved [49]. SFN has been shown to be related to many autoimmune conditions including SS, SLE, and CD [47]. Furthermore, it had also been described in POTS patients. In Germany, C fiber involvement was observed in 45% of the 84 patients with POTS analyzed – and the reduced density of those fibers was correlated to decreased adrenergic cardiac ^{123}I-metaiodobenzylguanadine (MIBG) uptake – suggesting an association between the small-fiber neuropathy and the reduced myocardial postganglionic sympathetic innervation that could explain the abnormal tachycardia in those patients [50]. Moreover, when looking into skin biopsies, 20% of POTS patients showed signs of SFN [51]. The association between POTS and SFN has also been related to more difficult resting, worse tachycardia, and reduced parasympathetic functions when compared to the ones that had no neuropathic signs [52].

Targeting autoimmunity for POTS treatment

The autoimmunity aspect of POTS pathogenesis opened the door for new therapeutic options for the disorder. To the best of our knowledge, there are no published clinical trials to date testing immunotherapies for POTS. However, the effective use of intravenous immunoglobulin (IVIG), subcutaneous immunoglobulin, and plasmapheresis has been reported in case reports and retrospective studies for POTS patients who did not respond well to conventional therapy (lifestyle changes and pharmacological treatment) [5, 8, 53–58]. In fact, the treatment responsiveness has been associated with the seropositivity for one or more autoantibodies [53].

POTS being one of the many arms of ASIA syndrome

The association among POTS, autoimmune conditions, and chronic inflammation: the higher prevalence of autoantibodies in those patients' sera, especially those targeting G-coupled proteins, and its correlation to small-fiber neuropathy support the hypothesis of POTS being an autoimmune disease and part of ASIA syndrome. The levels of muscarinic and adrenergic autoantibodies have been previously suggested to be used as biomarkers of other autoimmune conditions that present with dysautonomias, such as fibromyalgia, chronic fatigue syndrome, and ASIA syndrome, following silicone breast implants [30]. Moreover, de novo POTS was described previously following vaccination with aluminum as well as silicone implants [18, 57, 59, 60].

References

1. Sheldon, R.S., Grubb, B.P. 2nd, Olshansky, B. et al. (2015). 2015 heart rhythm society expert consensus statement on the diagnosis and treatment of postural tachycardia syndrome, inappropriate sinus tachycardia, and vasovagal syncope. *Hear Rhythm.* 12 (6): e41–e63.
2. Benarroch, E.E. (2012). Postural tachycardia syndrome: a heterogeneous and multifactorial disorder. *Mayo Clin. Proc.* 87 (12): 1214–1225. https://pubmed.ncbi.nlm.nih.gov/23122672.

3. Gunning, W.T. 3rd, Kvale, H., Kramer, P.M. et al. (2019). Postural orthostatic tachycardia syndrome is associated with elevated G-protein coupled receptor autoantibodies. *J. Am. Heart Assoc.* 8 (18): e013602–e013602. https://pubmed.ncbi.nlm.nih.gov/31495251.
4. Li, H., Yu, X., Liles, C. et al. (2014). Autoimmune basis for postural tachycardia syndrome. *J. Am. Heart Assoc.* 3 (1): e000755.
5. Schofield, J.R., Blitshteyn, S., Shoenfeld, Y., and Hughes, G.R.V. (2014). Postural tachycardia syndrome (POTS) and other autonomic disorders in antiphospholipid (Hughes) syndrome (APS). *Lupus* 23 (7): 697–702. https://pubmed.ncbi.nlm.nih.gov/24569396.
6. Blitshteyn, S. (2015). Autoimmune markers and autoimmune disorders in patients with postural tachycardia syndrome (POTS). *Lupus* 24 (13): 1364–1369. https://pubmed.ncbi.nlm.nih.gov/26038344.
7. Fedorowski, A., Li, H., Yu, X. et al. (2017). Antiadrenergic autoimmunity in postural tachycardia syndrome. *Europace* 19 (7): 1211–1219. https://pubmed.ncbi.nlm.nih.gov/27702852.
8. Shoenfeld, Y., Ryabkova, V.A., Scheibenbogen, C. et al. (2020). Complex syndromes of chronic pain, fatigue and cognitive impairment linked to autoimmune dysautonomia and small fiber neuropathy. *Clin. Immunol.* 214: 108384.
9. Watad, A., Sharif, K., and Shoenfeld, Y. (2017). The ASIA syndrome: basic concepts. *Mediterr. J. Rheumatol.* 28 (2): 64–69.
10. Borba, V., Malkova, A., Basantsova, N. et al. (2020). Classical examples of the concept of the ASIA syndrome. *Biomolecules* 10 (10): 1436. https://www.mdpi.com/2218-273X/10/10/1436.
11. Park, K., Haberberger, R.V., Gordon, T.P., and Jackson, M.W. (2011). Antibodies interfering with the type 3 muscarinic receptor pathway inhibit gastrointestinal motility and cholinergic neurotransmission in Sjögren's syndrome. *Arthritis Rheum.* 63 (5): 1426–1434.
12. Malysheva, O., Pierer, M., Wagner, U. et al. (2008). Association between β2 adrenergic receptor polymorphisms and rheumatoid arthritis in conjunction with human leukocyte antigen (HLA)-DRB1 shared epitope. *Ann. Rheum. Dis.* 67 (12): 1759–1764.
13. Jazdzewski, K., Bednarczuk, T., Stepnowska, M. et al. (2007). β-2-Adrenergic receptor gene polymorphism confers susceptibility to Graves disease. *Int. J. Mol. Med.* 19 (1): 181–186.
14. Metcalf, J.V., Bhopal, R.S., Gray, J. et al. (1997). Incidence and prevalence of primary biliary cirrhosis in the city of Newcastle upon Tyne, England. *Int. J. Epidemiol.* 26 (4): 830–836.
15. Cabral-Marques, O., Marques, A., Giil, L.M. et al. (2018). GPCR-specific autoantibody signatures are associated with physiological and pathological immune homeostasis. *Nat. Commun.* 9 (1): 5224.
16. Xu, B.Y., Huang, D., Pirskanen, R., and Lefvert, A.K. (2000). β2-adrenergic receptor gene polymorphisms in myasthenia gravis (MG). *Clin. Exp. Immunol.* 119 (1): 156–160.
17. Smith, A.J., Jackson, M.W., Wang, F. et al. (2005). Neutralization of muscarinic receptor autoantibodies by intravenous immunoglobulin in Sjögren syndrome. *Hum. Immunol.* 66 (4): 411–416.
18. Halpert, G., Watad, A., Tsur, A.M. et al. (2021). Autoimmune dysautonomia in women with silicone breast implants. *J. Autoimmun.* 120: 102631. https://www.sciencedirect.com/science/article/pii/S0896841121000391.
19. Watad, A., Bragazzi, N.L., McGonagle, D. et al. (2019). Autoimmune/inflammatory syndrome induced by adjuvants (ASIA) demonstrates distinct autoimmune and autoinflammatory disease associations according to the adjuvant subtype: insights from an analysis of 500 cases. *Clin. Immunol.* 203: 1–8.
20. Watad, A., Quaresma, M., Bragazzi, N.L. et al. (2018). The autoimmune/inflammatory syndrome induced by adjuvants (ASIA)/Shoenfeld's syndrome: descriptive analysis of 300 patients from the international ASIA syndrome registry. *Clin. Rheumatol.* 37 (2): 483–493.
21. Dubey, D., Hopkins, S., and Vernino, S. (2016). M1 and M2 muscarinic receptor antibodies among patients with postural orthostatic tachycardia syndrome: potential disease biomarker. *J. Clin. Neuromuscul. Dis.* 17 (3): 179S.
22. Galloway, A., Li, H., Vanderlinde-Wood, M. et al. (2015). Activating autoantibodies to the β1/2-adrenergic and M2 muscarinic receptors associate with atrial tachyarrhythmias in patients with hyperthyroidism. *Endocrine* 49 (2): 457–463. https://pubmed.ncbi.nlm.nih.gov/25500789.
23. Brimijoin, S. and Lennon, V.A. (1990). Autoimmune preganglionic sympathectomy induced by acetylcholinesterase antibodies. *Proc. Natl. Acad. Sci. U. S. A.* 87 (24): 9630–9634. https://pubmed.ncbi.nlm.nih.gov/2175909.
24. Haga, T. (2013). Molecular properties of muscarinic acetylcholine receptors. *Proc. Jpn Acad. Ser. B Phys. Biol. Sci.* 89 (6): 226–256. https://pubmed.ncbi.nlm.nih.gov/23759942.

25. Hurst, R., Rollema, H., and Bertrand, D. (2013). Nicotinic acetylcholine receptors: from basic science to therapeutics. *Pharmacol. Ther.* 137 (1): 22–54. https://pubmed.ncbi.nlm.nih.gov/22925690.
26. Schmidt, B. (2006). *The Adrenergic Receptors in the 21st Century* (ed. D.M. Perez). Totowa, NJ: Humana Press ChemMedChem [Internet]. 1(8):904. . https://doi.org/10.1002/cmdc.200600132.
27. Lund, A., Giil, L.M., Slettom, G. et al. (2018). Antibodies to receptors are associated with biomarkers of inflammation and myocardial damage in heart failure. *Int. J. Cardiol.* 250: 253–259. https://pubmed.ncbi.nlm.nih.gov/29046223.
28. Meyer, C. and Heidecke, H. (2018). Antibodies against GPCR. *Front. Biosci. Landmark* 23: 2177–2194. https://pubmed.ncbi.nlm.nih.gov/29772554.
29. Vernino, S. and Stiles, L.E. (2018). Autoimmunity in postural orthostatic tachycardia syndrome: current understanding. *Auton. Neurosci.* 215: 78–82. https://pubmed.ncbi.nlm.nih.gov/29909990.
30. Halpert, G., Amital, H., and Shoenfeld, Y. (2020). Dysregulation of G protein-coupled receptors of the autonomic nervous system, adrenergic and muscarinic acetylcholine receptors, in patients with autoimmune dysautonomic-related disorders. *Brain, Behav Immun. Health* 4: 100056.
31. Molina, V. and Shoenfeld, Y. (2005). Infection, vaccines and other environmental triggers of autoimmunity. *Autoimmunity* 38 (3): 235–245. https://pubmed.ncbi.nlm.nih.gov/16126512.
32. Miglis, M.G., Prieto, T., Shaik, R. et al. (2020). A case report of postural tachycardia syndrome after COVID-19. *Clin. Auton. Res.* 30 (5): 449–451. https://pubmed.ncbi.nlm.nih.gov/32880754.
33. Hineno, A., Ikeda, S.-I., Scheibenbogen, C. et al. (2019). Autoantibodies against autonomic nerve receptors in adolescent Japanese girls after immunization with human papillomavirus vaccine. *Ann. Arthritis Clin. Rheumatol.* 2 (2): 1014.
34. Guimarães, L.E., Baker, B., Perricone, C., and Shoenfeld, Y. (2015). Vaccines, adjuvants and autoimmunity. *Pharmacol. Res.* 100: 190–209.
35. Soriano, A., Nesher, G., and Shoenfeld, Y. (2015). Predicting post-vaccination autoimmunity: who might be at risk? *Pharmacol. Res.* 92: 18–22.
36. Watad, A., Quaresma, M., Brown, S. et al. (2017). Autoimmune/inflammatory syndrome induced by adjuvants (Shoenfeld's syndrome) - an update. *Lupus* 26 (7): 675–681.
37. Pellegrino, P., Clementi, E., and Radice, S. (2015). On vaccine's adjuvants and autoimmunity: current evidence and future perspectives. *Autoimmun. Rev.* 14 (10): 880–888.
38. Pavlov, V.A. and Tracey, K.J. (2012). The vagus nerve and the inflammatory reflex--linking immunity and metabolism. *Nat. Rev. Endocrinol.* 8 (12): 743–754. https://pubmed.ncbi.nlm.nih.gov/23169440.
39. Okamoto, L.E., Raj, S.R., Gamboa, A. et al. (2015). Sympathetic activation is associated with increased IL-6, but not CRP in the absence of obesity: lessons from postural tachycardia syndrome and obesity. *Am. J. Physiol. Heart Circ. Physiol.* 309 (12): H2098–H2107. https://pubmed.ncbi.nlm.nih.gov/26453329.
40. Shaw, B.H., Stiles, L.E., Bourne, K. et al. (2019). The face of postural tachycardia syndrome - insights from a large cross-sectional online community-based survey. *J. Intern. Med.* 286 (4): 438–448. https://pubmed.ncbi.nlm.nih.gov/30861229.
41. Penny, H.A., Aziz, I., Ferrar, M. et al. (2016). Is there a relationship between gluten sensitivity and postural tachycardia syndrome? *Eur. J. Gastroenterol. Hepatol.* 28 (12): 1383–1387. https://pubmed.ncbi.nlm.nih.gov/27606948.
42. Kanjwal, K., Karabin, B., Kanjwal, Y., and Grubb, B.P. (2010). Autonomic dysfunction presenting as postural orthostatic tachycardia syndrome in patients with multiple sclerosis. *Int. J. Med. Sci.* 7 (2): 62–67. http://www.medsci.org/v07p0062.htm.
43. Goodman, B.P. (2019). Immunoresponsive autonomic neuropathy in sjögren syndrome–case series and literature review. *Am. J. Ther.* 26 (1): e66–e71. https://pubmed.ncbi.nlm.nih.gov/28379880.
44. Goodman, B.P., Crepeau, A., Dhawan, P.S. et al. (2017). Spectrum of autonomic nervous system impairment in sjögren syndrome. *Neurologist* 22 (4): https://journals.lww.com/theneurologist/Fulltext/2017/07000/Spectrum_of_Autonomic_Nervous_System_Impairment_in.5.aspx.
45. Shiboski, C.H., Shiboski, S.C., Seror, R. et al. (2017). 2016 American College of Rheumatology/European League Against Rheumatism Classification Criteria for Primary Sjögren's Syndrome: A Consensus and Data-Driven Methodology Involving Three International Patient Cohorts. *Arthritis Rheumatol.* 69 (1): 35–45. https://pubmed.ncbi.nlm.nih.gov/27785888.
46. Lauria, G., Merkies, I.S.J., and Faber, C.G. (2012). Small fibre neuropathy. *Curr. Opin. Neurol.* 25 (5): 542–549.

47. Basantsova, N.Y., Starshinova, A.A., Dori, A. et al. (2019). Small-fiber neuropathy definition, diagnosis, and treatment. *Neurol. Sci. Off. J. Ital. Neurol. Soc. Ital. Soc. Clin. Neurophysiol.* 40 (7): 1343–1350.
48. Sene, D. (2018). Small fiber neuropathy: diagnosis, causes, and treatment. *Joint, Bone, Spine* 85 (5): 553–559.
49. Levine, T.D. (2018). Small fiber neuropathy: disease classification beyond pain and burning. *J. Cent. Nerv. Syst. Dis.* 10: 1179573518771703.
50. Haensch, C.-A., Tosch, M., Katona, I. et al. (2014). Small-fiber neuropathy with cardiac denervation in postural tachycardia syndrome. *Muscle Nerve.* 50 (6): 956–961.
51. Iodice, V., Low, D.A., Mathias, C.J. et al. (2015). Small fibre neuropathy and collagen IV reduction in postural tachycardia syndrome and joint hypermobility syndrome. *Auton. Neurosci.* 192: 125.
52. Gibbons, C.H., Bonyhay, I., Benson, A. et al. (2013). Structural and functional small fiber abnormalities in the neuropathic postural tachycardia syndrome. *PLoS One* 8: e84716.
53. Schofield, J.R. and Chemali, K.R. (2019). Intravenous immunoglobulin therapy in refractory autoimmune dysautonomias: a retrospective analysis of 38 patients. *Am. J. Ther.* 26 (5): e570–e582. https://journals.lww.com/americantherapeutics/Fulltext/2019/10000/Intravenous_Immunoglobulin_Therapy_in_Refractory.2.aspx.
54. Goto, Y., Sunami, Y., Sugaya, K. et al. (2021). A case of chronic postural tachycardia syndrome with positive anti-ganglionic acetylcholine receptor (gAChR) antibody. *Rinshō Shinkeigaku* 61 (8): 547–551.
55. Rodriguez, B., Hoepner, R., Salmen, A. et al. (2021). Immunomodulatory treatment in postural tachycardia syndrome: a case series. *Eur. J. Neurol.* 28 (5): 1692–1697.
56. Hendrickson, J.E., Hendrickson, E.T., Gehrie, E.A. et al. (2016). Complex regional pain syndrome and dysautonomia in a 14-year-old girl responsive to therapeutic plasma exchange. *J. Clin. Apher.* 31 (4): 368–374. https://doi.org/10.1002/jca.21407.
57. Blitshteyn, S. and Brook, J. (2017). Postural tachycardia syndrome (POTS) with anti-NMDA receptor antibodies after human papillomavirus vaccination. *Immunol. Res.* 65 (1): 282–284. https://doi.org/10.1007/s12026-016-8855-1.
58. Weinstock, L.B., Brook, J.B., Myers, T.L., and Goodman, B. (2018). Successful treatment of postural orthostatic tachycardia and mast cell activation syndromes using naltrexone, immunoglobulin and antibiotic treatment. *BMJ Case Rep.* 2018: bcr-2017–bcr-221405. http://casereports.bmj.com/content/2018/bcr-2017-221405.abstract.
59. Blitshteyn, S. (2014). Postural tachycardia syndrome following human papillomavirus vaccination. *Eur. J. Neurol.* 21 (1): 135–139.
60. Brinth, L., Theibel, A.C., Pors, K., and Mehlsen, J. (2015). Suspected side effects to the quadrivalent human papilloma vaccine. *Dan. Med. J.* 62 (4): A5064.

13 Role of the Small-fiber Neuropathy in the Pathogenesis of ASIA Syndrome

Natalia Gavrilova[1,2], E. Kamaeva[1], M. Lukashenko[1], and L. Soprun[1,2]

[1]Federal State Budget Educational Institution of Higher Education "St. Petersburg State University", University Emb., 7-9, Saint Petersburg, Russia
[2]St Petersburg State University Hospital, Saint Petersburg, Russia

Small-fiber neuropathy: definition and principles of diagnostics

Small-fiber neuropathy (SFN) is a disease of the peripheral nervous system that affects A-delta and C-type somatic and autonomic fibers, manifesting with sensory complications and dysautonomia [1–3].

Etiology and pathogenesis

The most common cause of SFN is considered to be metabolic dysfunction, including impaired glucose tolerance and type 2 diabetes mellitus ([1], Table 13.1). The intensity of clinical manifestations directly depends on the severity of the underlying disease and its associated conditions, microcirculatory dysfunction and dyslipidemia. Other metabolic disorders leading to the development of SFN include hypothyroidism, deficiency of vitamins B1 and B12, excess vitamin B6, and severe liver and kidney failure [1, 2].

Among infectious causes, human immunodeficiency virus (HIV) infection is the greatest contributor to the development of SFN. In rarer cases, neuropathy appears in connection with hepatitis C, Lyme disease, and leprosy. Cases of polyneuropathy resulting from toxic effects, including medications, are also described. Genetic causes of neuropathy include hereditary and familial amyloid neuropathies, and cases of neuroma have been described in patients with Fabry, Pompe, and Ehlers–Danlos diseases [1–3].

Nowadays, close attention is paid to the autoimmune causes of the neuropathy of smallest fibers, due to the huge amount of data confirming SFN in disease such as sarcoidosis [4], vasculitis [5], celiac disease [6, 7], Sjögren's syndrome (SjS, [8, 9]), and in diseases that are presumed to be immune mediated, such as fibromyalgia and chronic fatigue syndrome [2]. Many similarities are described between autoimmune SFN and autoimmune/inflammatory syndrome induced by

Autoimmune Disorders: Adjuvants and Other Risk Factors in Pathogenesis, First Edition.
Edited by Abdulla Watad, Nicola Luigi Bragazzi, and Yehuda Shoenfeld.

Table 13.1 Main known causes of the small-fiber neuropathy.

Metabolic diseases
Diabetes mellitus, impaired glucose tolerance
Hyperlipidemia
Hypothyroidism
Vitamin B1 and B12 deficiency
Excess of vitamin B6
Severe hepatic and renal failure
Immune-mediated and autoimmune causes
Guillain–Barré syndrome
Sjögren's syndrome
Systemic vasculitis
Sarcoidosis
Systemic lupus erythematosus
Celiac disease
Monoclonal gammopathy of unspecified origin
Amyloidosis
Paraneoplastic neuropathies
Inflammatory bowel diseases
Drugs and toxic substances
Antiretroviral therapy
Statins
Metronidazole
Industrial, environmental, and marine toxins
Alcohol abuse
Infectious causes
HIV
Epstein–Barr virus
Leprosy
Diphtheria
Chagas disease
Tangier disease
Botulism
Idiopathic causes
Family burning foot syndrome
Burning mouth syndrome
Erythromelalgia
Impulsive urges to defecation and rectal hypersensitivity
Hereditary causes
Fabry disease
Congenital sensory autonomic neuropathies
Charcot–Marie–Tooth pain type 2 syndrome
Generalized anhidrosis
Complex regional pain syndrome
Ross syndrome
Systemic amyloidosis
Pompe's disease
Ehlers–Danlos disease

Source: Adapted from Basantsova et al. [1], Ryabkova et al. [2], Shoenfeld et al. [3], Gavrilova et al. [4], Lacomis et al. [5], and Brannagan et al. [6].

adjuvants (ASIA) syndrome, which may allude to the common pathological processes in these conditions. Markers of inflammation, such as increased level of C-reactive protein, decreased level of components of the complement, and autoantibodies are often evaluated in patients with SFN, which suggests that autoimmune process may be one of the main causes of its development as well as in ASIA syndrome [10–12].

Much attention is paid to the role of pro-inflammatory cytokines. The expression levels of interleukin 2 (IL-2), IL-10, and transforming growth factor-beta-1 genes in peripheral blood were two times higher in patients with SNF [13]. In addition to the elevated expression levels in peripheral blood, increased expression levels in skin samples from affected areas of IL-6 (sevenfold) and IL-8 (fivefold) were also described in comparison with healthy controls. Local cytokine expression may explain mechanisms of neuropathic pain onset and maintenance as well as decrease in the number of cutaneous nerve fibers. In addition, histological examination often reveals infiltration of the patients' skin by immune cells such as T lymphocytes and macrophages [1]. However, cytokine expression levels and number of these cells do not correlate, suggesting the presence of other sources of cutaneous cytokine production, such as keratinocytes or fibroblasts [13].

In addition to the impact of cytokine-mediated dysfunction in the small-nerve fiber damage, the role of autoantibodies is also discussed. Sufficient number of studies are describing autoantibodies to the trisulfated heparin disaccharide (TS-HDS) and the fibroblast growth factor-3 (FGFR-3), which are evaluated in predominantly sensory neuropathies [14]. IgM and complement C5b-9 deposits around mid-caliber vessels and capillaries associated with loss of sensory axons are observed in patients along with the presence of the anti-TS-HDS IgM. FGFR-3 is a secreted cell surface receptor, and IgG antibodies to FGFR-3 have been described in sensory neuropathies. Autoantibodies to either TS-HDS-IgM (37%) or FGFR-3-IgG (15%) were mentioned in 48% of patients (74 of 155) with idiopathic SFN. It was also reported that female patients are prevailing among antibody-positive patients, and non-length-dependent patterns of SFN axon loss were more common [14, 15]. In addition to neuropathic manifestations of SFN, TS-HDS/FGFR3 antibodies were also present in patients with signs of generalized autonomic dysfunction [14]. The question of the pathogenetic role of autoantibodies in SFN remains unclear, but it may be valuable for identifying subgroups of "immune" SFN that might respond to immunomodulatory therapy.

Clinical manifestations

As was previously mentioned, dysfunction of the myelinated A-delta and the unmyelinated C-type nerve fibers results in sensory and autonomic complaints. The most frequent clinical manifestations include sensory dysfunction mainly in the form of pain and temperature hyper- or hyposensitivity as well as dysautonomic manifestations with the involvement of the exocrine glands (sweat, lacrimal, and salivary) and smooth muscles (in the vessels, gastrointestinal tract, bladder, and iris, [1–3], Table 13.2).

Table 13.2 Main symptoms of the small-fiber neuropathy.

Sensory symptoms	Dysautonomia symptoms
• Pain (burning, tingling) • Discomfort at night and sleep disturbance • Restless legs syndrome • Crampy • Allodynia • Hyperalgesia • Decreased pain sensitivity • Decreased temperature sensitivity	• Sweating disorders (absence or increase) • Dry eyes and/or mouth • Discoloration of the skin • Orthostatic intolerance • Hypersensitivity to the bright light, blurred vision, loss of fields of vision, tunnel vision • Gastrointestinal disorders (bloating, diarrhea, constipation) • Urinary disorder • Erectile dysfunction

Patient's examination reveals allodynia (perception of painless stimuli as painful), hyperalgesia (excessive perception of painful stimuli not corresponding to the strength of the stimulus causing it), decreased sensation of pain, and temperature sensitivity in the affected areas. In addition, there may be decreased vibration sensitivity, especially in the distal parts of the legs. Muscle strength, tendon reflexes, and proprioceptive sensitivity should remain normal, since such kind of dysfunction is a result of larger peripheral nerves damage [1]. Among the autonomic symptoms, there is a change in the color of the skin due to distal autonomic vasomotor regulation, and the skin over the affected area also may be dry, shiny, or atrophied. Dysfunction of the cardiovascular system may be described mainly in the form of orthostatic intolerance, especially postural orthostatic tachycardia syndrome [3, 16].

Two main clinical variants of SFN are described. More often can be seen polyneuropathic pattern, where the symptoms start with the most distant parts of the upper and low extremities (glove- or sock-like lesions) and then gradually spread up to the trunk. That type is called the length-dependent pattern (LD-SFN) and more often seen in metabolic SNF. The second option is less common. Non-length-dependent SFN (NLD-SFN) is characterized with mosaic distribution and usually alludes to the development of the ganglionopathy. Clinically, this type is manifested with severe sensory disturbances that first appear in the trunk, face, or more proximal limbs and then spread to other areas [17, 18]. There is evidence that NLD-SFN is more common in women, begins at a younger age, and is more likely to be associated with immune-mediated conditions than LD-SFN. Such conditions may include sarcoidosis, rheumatoid arthritis, SLE, Sjögren's syndrome, and mixed connective tissue disease. The systemic nature of the nerve fibers dysfunction and the possible presence of the undiagnosed autoimmune diseases undoubtedly add additional complexity to the process of NLD-SFN diagnostic process.

Diagnostic methods

For a long time, the symptoms of SFN remained unexplained, leaving the disease undiagnosed. Nowadays, the amount of scientific data has been growing and continues to accumulate, which became possible due to the development of specific diagnostic methods.

Clarification of clinical symptoms, assessment of their intensity, and dynamic observation are of great importance in the diagnosis of SFN. Pain syndrome, the leading one in the clinic, can be evaluated using different techniques. Visual analogue scale is recommended for pain intensity estimation [19–21]. The Rasch -built overall Disability Scale (SFN-RODS) and the Douleur Neuropathique 4 (DN4) questionnaire are used to diagnose neuropathic pain of any etiology [1]. Special questionnaires were also developed. One of the most frequently used questionnaires is the small-fiber neuropathy-symptoms inventory questionnaire (SFN-SIQ). Its basic limitation is the absence of quantitative gradation of symptom manifestation, which excludes the possibility of dynamic assessing of complaints [22]. The Autonomic Symptom Profile and the Composite Autonomic Symptom Score-31 (COMPASS-31) are used to assess autonomic symptoms [23].

The gold standard for instrumental examination of SFN is a skin biopsy followed by enzyme immunoassay or immunohistochemical analysis to assess the density of small nerve fibers in the epidermis of the skin. The European Federation of Neurological Societies has recommended a skin biopsy with PGP 9.5 staining as the class A standard. It is possible to perform biopsies in different localizations, which allows to estimate the density of epidermal nerve fibers in the proximal–distal direction, the sharp decrease of which in the shins and feet leads to the LD-SFN diagnosis [24]. The specificity and sensitivity of the method are about 88–92% [24].

Another method that can be applied for SFN diagnostics is the confocal microscopy (CM) of the cornea ([25], Figure 13.1). Automated sample analysis and standard evaluation criteria make the method suitable for the wide clinical use. Corneal CM is a painless, noninvasive method, so it has great advantages in pediatrics, gerontology, and in patients with chronic diseases. Also, this technique allows repeated analysis of the same area of the cornea, which is important for evaluation of therapy effectiveness and disease progression. Thus, this method can be considered as an additional diagnostic tool for the evaluation of SFN [25, 26].

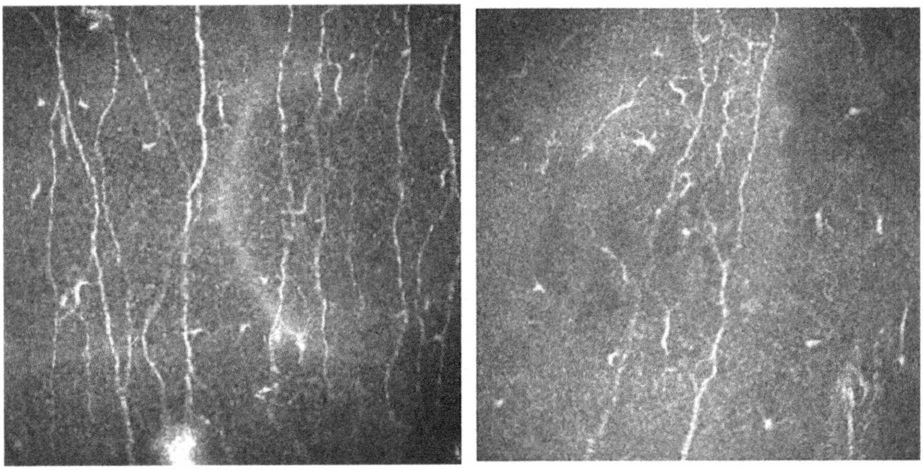

Figure 13.1 Small-fiber neuropathy in patients with post-COVID-19 syndrome, that is possibly have immune-mediated pathogenesis.

Table 13.3 Additional instrumental methods of small-fiber neuropathy diagnostics.

Method	Description of the methodology	Notes
Quantitative ship motor axon reflex testing (QSART)	A study of sweating in four areas of the body (forearm, thigh, lower leg, and foot) with assessment of postganglionic cholinergic nonmyelinated C-fiber function by acetylcholine ion electrophoresis. The test results are described in sweat volumes in nl/min, taking into account age and sex norms.	The sensitivity is 59–80%. Used to validate SFN questionnaires instead of counting nerve fiber density
Quantitative sensory testing (QST)	Measurement of heat, cold, and pain stimuli with noninvasive psychophysiological tests in a quiet room at a constant comfortable temperature. Study vibration, cold, heat, and pain sensitivity in selected areas of the body.	The overall sensitivity of the method is 65–80%, and its specificity is 37–94%. It is used to objectify the subjective results of a patient's sensitivity examination
Laser evoked potentials	Study of the function of A-delta and possibly C-type fibers in peripheral tissues and in the spinothalamic tract in response to laser stimulation	Sensitivity, 70–80% Application is limited by the availability of the necessary equipment and specialists with the appropriate qualifications
Assessment of heart rate variability (HRV)	Detection of abnormal regulation of the cardiovascular system due to autonomic dysfunction. Deep breathing tests, Valsalva test, and Tiltest are performed	

Other methods of SFN verification that are not widespread but are recommended for application in addition to the basic diagnostic methods include quantitative sudomotor axon reflex testing, quantitative sensory testing, laser-evoked potentials, and others (Table 13.3).

Blackmore et al. of the University of Alberta Hospital (Edmonton, Canada) proposed the following criteria for the diagnosis of SFN [27]:

- Valid SFN: pathology detected on neurological examination (pain/temperature sensitivity disorder) combined with changes detected on two of three – quantitative ship motor axon reflex testing (QSART), quantitative sensory testing (QST), or heart rate variability (HRV) – tests.
- Probable neuropathy – abnormalities on neurological examination and on one of three studies – QSART, QST, or HRV.
- Possible neuropathy – abnormalities on neurologic examination or on one of two tests – QSART or QST.

Small-fiber neuropathy treatment

Treatment of SFN should focus on treating the underlying cause of the disease and symptomatic treatment of neuropathic pain. In cases of metabolic SFN, lifestyle modification with control of diet and weight, availability of regular exercise, and adherence to strict glycemic control are of paramount importance for this category of patients and show significant improvement in SFN symptoms. Treatment of sarcoidosis, celiac disease, and other autoimmune conditions can also improve the course of SNF in these diseases but in some cases requires additional symptomatic treatment [1, 13, 21].

SFN as part of ASIA syndrome

In the concept of ASIA syndrome there are several diseases whose pathogenesis may include SFN. These conditions include sarcoidosis, SS, and silicone implant incompatibility syndrome (SIIS).

Sarcoidosis

Sarcoidosis is a systemic granulomatous disease of unclear etiology, characterized by the formation of immune granulomas in various organs, mainly in the lungs and lymphatic system [28]. It has been suggested that sarcoidosis may result from exposure to an unidentified antigen in individuals with a genetic predisposition, which triggers a Th1-type immune response with the formation of a granulomatous reaction [29].

There is a wide range of somatic symptoms, determined by the localization of the granulomatous process and its severity. However, no less important influence on the course of the disease and the patient's quality of life is caused by nonspecific systemic symptoms, which include fatigue, widespread pain, and cognitive impairment. From 30% to 60% of patients with sarcoidosis note individual symptoms typical for SFN, such as sensory and autonomic disorders [30, 31].

Chronic pain is one of the most common symptoms in patients with sarcoidosis [32]. These complaints usually include muscle pain, chest pain, abdominal pain, arthralgia, and headache. Symptoms may suggest neuropathic nature of the pain, which include sensory symptoms such as burning, numbness, paresthesia, or allodynia. More typical is the beginning of intermittent symptoms with migratory localization, which later become permanent and slowly progress over time. This peculiarity of the course of SFN in sarcoidosis can undoubtedly lead to additional difficulties in the differential diagnosis.

Another group of symptoms described in sarcoidosis patients include autonomic disorders, such as sweating dysfunction (hyperhidrosis or hypohidrosis); orthostatic intolerance; gastrointestinal motility disorders with nausea, constipation, or diarrhea; palpitations; and sexual and genitourinary tract dysfunction. Autonomic manifestations are rarely described separately; more often, they are observed with sensory disorders [33]. Many patients with sarcoidosis often report the symptoms of SFN as the most influencing their quality of life [31–33].

While there is a large amount of data on the pathological processes underlying sarcoidosis neuropathy affecting large nerve fibers, the mechanisms of SFN development remain unclear. In biopsies of distal parts of large nerves, noncaseous granulomas of the nerve fibers with necrotizing vasculitic changes as well as nerve infiltration with T cells and macrophages are described [34].

The exact causes of Aδ nerve fiber pathology are unknown. In contrast to the lesion of large nerves, the key point of pathogenesis in this case is not considered to be the formation of granulomas but systemic cytokine-mediated lesion. Other immune-mediated neuropathies are known to have increased cytokines such as IL-1β, IL-6, IL-8, and FNO-α. This assumption is confirmed by the detection of higher concentrations of these cytokines in the distal limbs of patients with SFN compared with the results of proximal biopsies. There is evidence for a role of genetic predisposition in the development of SFN in sarcoidosis patients, where the HLA-DQB1*0602 allele may play an important role in the pain progression and development [35].

The Small-Fiber Neuropathy Screening List (SFN-SL) is the most well-known and generally accepted questionnaire for detecting SFN in sarcoidosis. The questionnaire consists of two parts in which the frequency of symptoms and their intensity are assessed. The scores include symptoms such as limb and chest pain; coldness; hypersensitivity or tingling in the extremities; muscle spasms; palpitations; swallowing, digestion, and urination disorders; dry eyes; blurred vision; and dizziness. The score allows to rate the likelihood of SFN as moderate (>22 points) or very high (>48 points). This questionnaire allows a dynamic assessment of the patient's condition and may be useful in clinical studies; however, its use is valid only in pulmonary sarcoidosis. The skin biopsy, certainly the gold standard of diagnosis, can be particularly useful in the absence of a typically proximal–distal pattern and the presence of multiple areas of sensory impairment [36].

Sjögren's syndrome

Sjögren's syndrome (SS) is a chronic autoimmune disease characterized by mononuclear cell infiltration and progressive exocrine gland involvement. SS is usually manifested by dry mouth and eyes but can affect any exocrine gland as well as be accompanied by a variety of extraglandular manifestations [37]. SS, among the most common rheumatic diseases, can manifest as a primary condition or in combination with other autoimmune diseases such as rheumatoid arthritis, systemic lupus erythematosus, systemic sclerosis, and primary biliary cirrhosis and is a classic example of ASIA syndrome [38].

SS can have a variety of manifestations that are not limited to exocrine gland dysfunction and lymphocytic infiltration of other organs, which is explained by hyperactivation of immunity and dysregulation of the adaptive and innate immune systems. Neurological manifestations, according to various estimates, occur in 5–70% of patients with SS and include autonomic, sensory, and cognitive symptoms. The presence of a neuropathic and autonomic component is associated with SFN. Basically, SS is the most common systemic autoimmune disease associated with SFN [39]. Most commonly, patients with SFN report complaints of severe burning pain arising in the trunk, face, and proximal limbs. About 40% of patients with SFN report symptoms of this complication before the appearance of sicca syndrome, on average, five years before the diagnosis of SFN [40].

Silicone implant incompatibility syndrome

Adjuvant disease, siliconosis, or silicone implant incompatibility syndrome (SIIS) is a clinical syndrome associated with silicone implants that leads to the development of the autoimmune/inflammatory syndrome induced by adjuvants. The combination of these symptoms with generalized fatigue and affective and cognitive impairment in patients with SIIS meets the criteria for the diagnosis of CFS/ME, fibromyalgia, sarcoidosis, and/or undifferentiated connective tissue disease.

To answer the question about the presence or absence of SFN in SIIS, there is currently not enough conclusive clinical or theoretical data. The effect of silicone on peripheral nerve fibers has not been studied. To date, the evidence is limited to one study in which extraneural and direct injection of silicone into the sciatic nerve of mice was performed. A transient inflammatory response was observed, changing to fibrosis formation at 20 weeks [41]. The clinical picture of SIIS includes complaints of autonomic (orthostatic intolerance, gastrointestinal motility disorders, and sicca symptoms) and sensory (chest pain, paresthesias, myalgias, and arthralgias) disorders, suggesting SFN. Considering that in SFN cases the ENMG results are usually normal, one can make an assumption about the presence of SFN in these patients. However, additional studies with skin biopsy and quantitative sensory testing are needed to confirm these findings.

Conclusion

Neuropathy of small fibers is currently an understudied disease, where symptoms of the sensitive and autonomic nervous system dysfunction are observed. ASIA syndrome, at the same time, has a large number of clinical manifestations similar to neuropathy of small fibers, which can be detected in patients suffering from sarcoidosis, silicone implant incompatibility syndrome, and Sjögren's syndrome. Further study of this neurological complication can help in understanding clinical and pathogenetic processes and improving the quality of life of these patients.

References

1. Basantsova, N.Y., Starshinova, A.A., Dori, A. et al. (2019). Small-fiber neuropathy definition, diagnosis, and treatment. *Neurol. Sci.* 40 (7): 1343–1350. https://doi.org/10.1007/s10072-019-03871-x.
2. Ryabkova, V.A., Churilov, L.P., and Shoenfeld, Y. (2019). Neuroimmunology: what role for autoimmunity, neuroinflammation, and small fiber neuropathy in fibromyalgia, chronic fatigue syndrome, and adverse events after human papillomavirus vaccination? *Int. J. Mol. Sci.* 20 (20): 5164. https://doi.org/10.3390/ijms20205164.
3. Shoenfeld, Y., Ryabkova, V.A., Scheibenbogen, C. et al. (2020). Complex syndromes of chronic pain, fatigue and cognitive impairment linked to autoimmune dysautonomia and small fiber neuropathy. *Clin. Immunol.* 214: 108384. https://doi.org/10.1016/j.clim.2020.108384.
4. Gavrilova, N., Starshinova, A., Zinchenko, Y. et al. (2021). Small fiber neuropathy in sarcoidosis. *Pathophysiology.* 28 (4): 544–550. https://doi.org/10.3390/pathophysiology28040035.
5. Lacomis, D., Giuliani, M.J., Steen, V., and Powell, H.C. (1997). Small fiber neuropathy and vasculitis. *Arthritis Rheum.* 40 (6): 1173–1177. https://doi.org/10.1002/art.1780400624.
6. Brannagan, T.H. 3rd, Hays, A.P., Chin, S.S. et al. (2005). Small-fiber neuropathy/neuronopathy associated with celiac disease: skin biopsy findings. *Arch. Neurol.* 62 (10): 1574–1578. https://doi.org/10.1001/archneur.62.10.1574.
7. Zis, P., Sarrigiannis, P.G., Rao, D.G. et al. (2019). Small fiber neuropathy in coeliac disease and gluten sensitivity. *Postgrad. Med.* 131 (7): 496–500. https://doi.org/10.1080/00325481.2019.1650609.
8. Pindi Sala, T., Villedieu, M., Damian, L. et al. (2020). Long-term efficacy of immunoglobulins in small fiber neuropathy related to Sjögren's syndrome. *J. Neurol.* 267 (12): 3499–3507. https://doi.org/10.1007/s00415-020-10033-z.
9. Descamps, E., Henry, J., Labeyrie, C. et al. (2020). Small fiber neuropathy in Sjögren syndrome: comparison with other small fiber neuropathies. *Muscle Nerve.* 61 (4): 515–520. https://doi.org/10.1002/mus.26824.
10. Trevino, J.A. and Novak, P. (2021). TS-HDS and FGFR3 antibodies in small fiber neuropathy and Dysautonomia. *Muscle Nerve.* 64 (1): 70–76. https://doi.org/10.1002/mus.27245.
11. Chan, A.C.Y., Wong, H.Y., Chong, Y.F. et al. (2022). Novel autoantibodies in idiopathic small fiber neuropathy. *Ann. Neurol.* 91 (1): 66–77. https://doi.org/10.1002/ana.26268.
12. Borba, V., Malkova, A., Basantsova, N. et al. (2020). Classical examples of the concept of the ASIA syndrome. *Biomolecules.* 10 (10): 1436. https://doi.org/10.3390/biom10101436.
13. Uceyler, N., Kafke, W., Riediger, N. et al. (2010). Elevated proinflammatory cytokine expression in affected skin in small fiber neuropathy. *Neurology* 74 (22): 1806–1813.
14. Trevino, J.A. and Novak, P. (2021). TS-HDS and FGFR3 antibodies in small fiber neuropathy and Dysautonomia. *Muscle Nerve.* 64 (1): 70–76. https://doi.org/10.1002/mus.27245.
15. Levine, T.D., Kafaie, J., Zeidman, L.A. et al. (2020). Cryptogenic small-fiber neuropathies: serum autoantibody binding to trisulfated heparan disaccharide and fibroblast growth factor receptor-3. *Muscle Nerve.* 61 (4): 512–515.

16. Novak, P. (2020). Post COVID-19 syndrome associated with orthostatic cerebral hypoperfusion syndrome, small fiber neuropathy and benefit of immunotherapy: a case report. *eNeurologicalSci* 21: 100276. https://doi.org/10.1016/j.ensci.2020.100276.
17. Sopacua, M., Hoeijmakers, J.G.J., Merkies, I.S.J. et al. (2019). Small-fiber neuropathy: expanding the clinical pain universe. *J. Peripher. Nerv. Syst.* 24 (1): 19–33. https://doi.org/10.1111/jns.12298.
18. Sène, D. (2018). Small fiber neuropathy: diagnosis, causes, and treatment. *Joint Bone Spine.* 85 (5): 553–559. https://doi.org/10.1016/j.jbspin.2017.11.002.
19. Terkelsen, A.J., Karlsson, P., Lauria, G. et al. (2017). The diagnostic challenge of small fibre neuropathy: clinical presentations, evaluations, and causes. *Lancet Neurol.* 16 (11): 934–944. https://doi.org/10.1016/S1474-4422(17)30329-0. Erratum in: Lancet Neurol. 2017 Dec;16(12):954. PMID: 29029847.
20. Farhad, K. (2019). Current diagnosis and treatment of painful small fiber neuropathy. *Curr. Neurol. Neurosci. Rep.* 19 (12): 103. https://doi.org/10.1007/s11910-019-1020-1.
21. Zeidman, L.A. (2021). Advances in the management of small fiber neuropathy. *Neurol. Clin.* 39 (1): 113–131. https://doi.org/10.1016/j.ncl.2020.09.006.
22. Sun, B., Li, Y., Liu, L. et al. (2018). SFN-SIQ, SFNSL and skin biopsy of 55 cases with small fibre involvement. *Int. J. Neurosci.* 128 (5): 442–448. https://doi.org/10.1080/00207454.2017.1398152.
23. Ramírez, M., Guerra-Juárez, A., Miyake, D.Y. et al. (2021). Correlation between corneal nerve density and symptoms of small fiber neuropathy in patients with fibromyalgia: the confounding role of severe anxiety or depression. *J. Clin. Rheumatol.* 27 (8): e606–e608. https://doi.org/10.1097/RHU.0000000000001592.
24. Lauria, G., Hsieh, S.T., Johansson, O. et al. (2010). European Federation of Neurological Societies/Peripheral Nerve Society Guideline on the use of skin biopsy in the diagnosis of small fiber neuropathy. Report of a joint task force of the European Federation of Neurological Societies and the Peripheral Nerve Society. *Eur. J. Neurol.* 17 (7): 903–912, e44-9. https://doi.org/10.1111/j.1468-1331.2010.03023.x.
25. Egenolf, N., Zu Altenschildesche, C.M., Kreß, L. et al. (2021). Diagnosing small fiber neuropathy in clinical practice: a deep phenotyping study. *Ther. Adv. Neurol. Disord.* 14: 17562864211004318. https://doi.org/10.1177/17562864211004318.
26. Lukashenko, M.V., Gavrilova, N.Y., Bregovskaya, A.V. et al. (2021). Corneal confocal microscopy in the diagnosis of small fiber neuropathy: faster, easier, and more efficient than skin biopsy? *Pathophysiology.* 29 (1): 1–8. https://doi.org/10.3390/pathophysiology29010001.
27. Blackmore, D. and Siddiqi, Z.A. (2017). Diagnostic Criteria for Small Fiber Neuropathy. *J. Clin. Neuromuscul. Dis.* 18 (3): 125–131. https://doi.org/10.1097/CND.0000000000000154.
28. Heinle, R. and Chang, C. (2014). Diagnostic criteria for sarcoidosis. *Autoimmun. Rev.* 13 (4–5): 383–387.
29. Bindoli, S., Dagon, A., Torres-Ruiz, J.J. et al. (2016). Sarcoidosis and autoimmunity: From genetic background to environmental factors. *Isr. Med. Assoc. J.* 18: 197–202.
30. Hoitsma, E., De Vries, J., and Drent, M. (2011). The small fiber neuropathy screening list: construction and cross-validation in sarcoidosis. *Respir. Med.* 105 (1): 95–100.
31. Oudejans, L.C., Niesters, M., Brines, M. et al. (2017). Quantification of small fiber pathology in patients with sarcoidosis and chronic pain using cornea confocal microscopy and skin biopsies. *J. Pain Res.* 10: 2057–2065. https://doi.org/10.2147/JPR.S142683. PMID: 28894389; PMCID: PMC5584894.
32. Judson, M.A. (2010). Small fiber neuropathy in sarcoidosis: something beneath the surface. *Rep. Med.* 105: 1–2. Bakkers M, Faber CG, Drent M, Hermans MC, van Nes SI, Lauria G, De Baets M, Merkies IS. Pain and autonomic dysfunction in patients with sarcoidosis and small fibre neuropathy. *J. Neurol.* 2010; 257(12):2086-90. https://doi.org/10.1007/s00415-010-5664-7.
33. Said, G., Lacroix, C., Plante-Bordeneuve, V. et al. (2002). Nerve granulomas and vasculitis in sarcoid peripheral neuropathy: a clinicopathological study of 11 patients. *Brain* 125: 264–275.
34. Voorter, C.E., Drent, M., Hoitsma, E. et al. (2005). Association of HLA DQB1 0602 in sarcoidosis patients with small fiber neuropathy. *Sarcoidosis Vasc Diffuse Lung Dis.* 22 (2): 129–132. https://doi.org/10.1007/s11083-005-9013-x.
35. Hautsima, E., Faber, S., Roylyan, J.P. et al. (2002). Neuropathy of small fibers in sarcoidosis. *Lancet.* 359: 2085–2086.
36. Peri, Y., Agnon-Levin, N., Theodor, E., and Schoenfeld, Y. (2012). Sjogren's syndrome, old and new. *Best Pract. Res. Clin. Rheumatol.* 26 (1): 105–117.
37. Colafrancesco, S., Perricone, C., Priori, R. et al. (2014). Sjögren's syndrome: another facet of the autoimmune/inflammatory syndrome induced by adjuvants (ASIA). *J. Autoimmun.* 51: 10–16. https://doi.org/10.1016/j. jaut.2014.03.003.

38. Liu, X., Treister, R., Lang, M., and Oaklander, A.L. (2018). IVIg for apparently autoimmune small-fiber polyneuropathy: first analysis of efficacy and safety. *Ther. Adv. Neurol. Disord.* 11: 175628561774448. https://doi.org/10.1177/1756285617744484.
39. Birnbaum, J., Lalji, A., Saed, A., and Baer, A.N. (2019). Biopsy-proven small-fiber neuropathy in primary Sjögren's syndrome: neuropathic pain characteristics, autoantibody findings, and histopathologic features. *Arthritis Care Res.* 71 (7): 936–948.
40. Sanger, J.R., Kolachalam, R., Komorowski, R.A. et al. (1992). Shortterm effect of silicone gel on peripheral nerves: a histologic study. *Plast. Reconstr. Surg.* 89: 931-940 discussion 941-2http://www.ncbi.nlm.nih.gov/pubmed/1561264 (accessed 18 September 2019).
41. Shoaib, B.O., Patten, B.M., and Calkins, D.S. (1994). Adjuvant breast disease: an evaluation of 100 symptomatic women with breast implants or silicone fluid injections. *Keio J. Med.* 43: 79–87. http://www.ncbi.nlm.nih.gov/pubmed/8089958 (accessed 18 September 2019).

14 Tattoo as a Possible Trigger for Autoimmune Syndrome Induced by Adjuvants

Paula David

Department of Internal Medicine 'B', Sheba Medical Center, Tel-Hashomer, Israel

Introduction

Autoimmune/Inflammatory Syndrome Induced by Adjuvants (ASIA syndrome) is a group of immune conditions triggered by the exposure to adjuvants in genetically predisposed individuals [1]. Since its definition, many adjuvants have been described – the most reported being silicone implants, aluminum salts, and other metals and vaccines [2–6]. It has been shown that cessation of the exposure to those agents may relieve the symptoms and/or reduce autoantibodies levels [5–7]. Several disorders were considered to be classical examples of ASIA syndrome, such as Sarcoidosis, Sjögren's syndrome, silicone implant incompatibility, and undifferentiated connective tissue disease (UCTD) – in these disorders, genetic predisposition to autoimmunity, like the presence of HLADRB1 or PTPN22 genes, in addition to environmental factors may lead to the disease [8–10].

The so-called adjuvants are responsible for stimulating both the innate and the adaptive immune systems and for activating pattern recognition receptors, increasing the immune response to non-pathological stimuli in a genetically prone subject [11].

Recently, we described a case of classical ASIA syndrome in a 32-year-old woman who presented with arthralgia, sicca syndrome, dysautonomia including postural orthostatic tachycardia syndrome (POTS), and generalized fatigue after getting extensive tattoos (Figure 14.1). Her routine and autoimmune lab exams were unremarkable, but when looking for circulating autoantibodies against G-coupled-protein receptors of the autonomic nervous system, she had high levels of antibodies against beta-1 adrenergic receptor, beta-2 adrenergic receptor, and M3 acetylcholine receptor. Her electromyogram (EMG) was compatible to small-fiber neuropathy as well as her skin biopsy [12]. Other than the tattoos, she had no triggers.

Thus, we raised the question whether tattoo ink could also be a trigger to ASIA syndrome, and in this chapter, we discuss why.

Autoimmune Disorders: Adjuvants and Other Risk Factors in Pathogenesis, First Edition.
Edited by Abdulla Watad, Nicola Luigi Bragazzi, and Yehuda Shoenfeld.

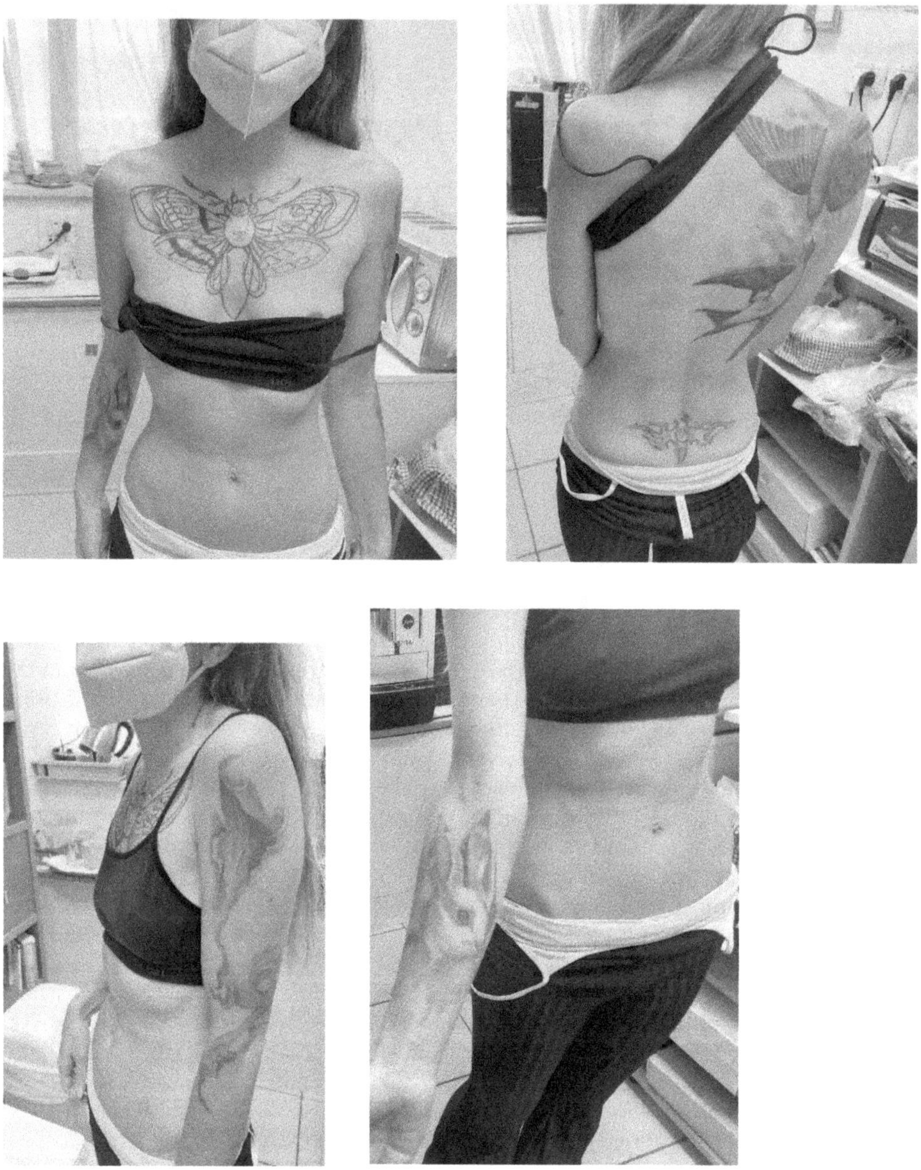

Figure 14.1 Images from our patient's extensive tattoos.

Tattoo and its components

Although tattoo has become more common in the past decades, it has been used for thousands of years in some cultures, usually with religion meanings [13]. Tattoos are made by injecting colorants in the human skin. After injection, those colorants may follow three different pathways: excretion from the skin during the wound process, accommodation in the dermis as solid pigment particles that creates the tattoo color by light absorption, and removal by lymphatic or blood circulation, arriving to local lymph nodes [14].

Tattoo colorants are composed of a group of chemical substances in which the coloring component is the most important element. The coloring in black tattoos is obtained by amorphous carbon particles, while more colorful tattoos are based on azo and polycyclic pigments [15]. Transforming tattoo ink into a specific color depends on a complex chemical process that involves by-products and impurities. In addition to the organic or inorganic pigment, the ink contains solvents and additives, preservatives, and *metals* [15].

The type of metal depends on the ink color and includes nickel, cobalt, chromium, lead, and aluminum salts [15, 16]. Specifically, the aluminum salts were described as ingredients of the violet ink [16]. Asia syndrome has been described as previously mentioned not only after aluminum but also following nickel and chromium exposure [17–19].

Our model patient, who had no symptoms previous to her fist tattoo, has various and extensive tattoos, including some with violet ink (that contains aluminum) (Figure 14.1). The presence of aluminum and other metals in ink may explain the mechanism through which tattoo may lead to ASIA syndrome, as observed in the described patient.

Sjögren's syndrome and tattoo

Sjögren's syndrome (SS) is an autoimmune condition in which salivary and lacrimal glands suffer inflammatory dysfunction, clinically expressed by sicca syndrome (dry eyes and mouth) and some extraglandular manifestations, such as arthralgia [20]. It can be idiopathic (primary) or in association to other autoimmune conditions (secondary) [20]. Our model patient presented to us with generalized arthralgia as well as dry mouth and eyes with a positive Schirmer test. Even though SS is considered one of the classic examples of ASIA syndrome [8], there are no reports in the literature that associate those symptoms with the presence of tattoo pigments. However, sicca syndrome has been described to be more incident after nickel and chromium exposure, which are components of many tattoo inks [17]. Sarcoidosis, on the other hand, another classic manifestation of ASIA syndrome, had been previously linked to tattoos [21–23].

Sarcoidosis and tattoo

Sarcoidosis is a systematic granulomatous disease that involves mainly the lungs and lymph nodes but may be found in different organs. Its pathogenesis is still unclear, but it involves a genetically prone individual that creates a TH1 immune response to an external antigen, leading to granuloma formation [24]. Many triggers were described, among them infections, autoantigens, and inorganic compounds [25]. Lung and skin sarcoidosis have been described after tattoo exposure, and interesting, in skin biopsy, noncaseating granulomas with black tattoo pigments were shown [23]. Both systemic sarcoidosis and granulomatous reaction without sarcoidosis have been observed following tattoo, with and without uveitis [21].

The fact that sarcoidosis granulomas usually occur in previous scar sites may explain their finding in tattoo areas, but it does not explain the finding of isolated eye inflammation, including posterior uveitis, panuveitis, and retinal vasculitis, consistent with sarcoidosis without skin manifestations [23, 26–28].

A possible explanation is that tattoo ink may induce immune responses, locally seen by granuloma formation in the tattoo area and systemically represented by other inflammatory manifestations, such as uveitis. Indeed, vitreous biopsy was performed in one of those patients showing no tattoo pigment and no granulomas, but a T-cell infiltration with atypia, validating the possibility of an autoimmune response to tattoos [29].

Postural orthostatic tachycardia syndrome, ASIA syndrome, and tattoo

Our model patient suffered from POTS. POTS is an autonomic disorder in which standing up provokes tachycardia and other autonomic symptoms without interfering on the blood pressure [30]. The most described autonomic symptoms are generalized fatigue, lightheadedness, palpitations, and blurred vision. POTS etiology is not well established, but in the past decades, evidences support the hypothesis of it being an autoimmune disease [31]. POTS patients were shown to commonly have autoantibodies targeting G-coupled proteins, such as the autonomic receptors (muscarinic, nicotinic, and adrenergic) [31–34]. In addition, an association between POTS and small-fiber neuropathy has been reported [35, 36], and moreover, Small Fiber Neuropathy (SFN) in POTS patients has been recently proposed as part of the mechanism through which abnormal tachycardia is seen in those subjects [36]. Interestingly, the EMG and skin biopsy of our model patients were consistent with SFN.

Similarities between silicone incompatibility syndrome (SIS) and ASIA syndrome following tattoo

SIS is a recently described condition in which general symptoms, such as sleep disturbances, general fatigue, generalized pain, depression, and hair loss, flourish following silicone breast implantation [8]. The past researches point to an autoimmune neurosensory dysautonomia that involves autoantibodies against autonomic nervous system receptors and that may result in small-fiber neuropathy in those individuals [37].

It is very similar to the clinical presentation of our model patient: she had depression, anxiety, and multiple neurologic complaints, with an Nerve Conduction Study (NCS)-EMG showing decreased sympathetic response on her right foot, with no signs of large-fiber polyneuropathy. This similarity led us to question whether these autoantibodies against G-protein-coupled receptors could be involved in the finding of POTS, sicca syndrome, paresthesia, and other signs of small-fiber neuropathy that were seen in our model patient after she got her tattoos. They have been described as part of the development of autoimmune disorders and dysautonomic conditions that are believed to have an immune etiology, including Sjögren's syndrome, rheumatoid arthritis, systemic lupus erythematosus, multiple sclerosis, myasthenia gravis, and POTS [38–44]. Indeed, our model patient was found to have increased circulation levels of anti-beta-1, anti-beta-2, and anti-M3 AAbs in comparison to the normal ranges in healthy women.

Potential therapies for ASIA syndrome following tattoo

ASIA syndrome has been described following injection of subcutaneous methyl methacrylate that has been used with esthetic goals in various body areas [45–47]. One of the proposed treatments is intralesional neodymium laser technique for removal of the substance [48]. The same technique has been largely used for tattoo removal mainly with esthetic goals [49, 50]. However, it could be a potential treatment for ASIA syndrome following tattoo as well. The removal of the adjuvant exposure, for example silicone implants extraction, in some cases of ASIA syndrome was shown to ameliorate the signs and symptom of the disease [51].

Conclusion

In this chapter, we propose that tattoo pigment should be considered as one of the adjuvants that trigger ASIA syndrome and question its safety in individuals genetically prone to develop autoimmunity. To reinforce our proposal, we described a model patient who has autoimmune condition in her background and presents with symptoms usually described in ASIA syndrome (arthralgia, morning stiffness, dry mouth and eyes, POTS, and neurological complaints compatible with small-fiber neuropathy) after getting extent tattoos. ASIA syndrome has not been previously described following exposure to tattoo ink, but sarcoidosis, considered one of the classical examples of ASIA syndrome, has been associated with tattoos [23, 52]. The fact that ink components commonly include aluminum and other metals, and that our model patient had higher levels of autoantibodies against G-protein-coupled receptors, similar to cases of silicone incompatibility syndrome, sicca syndrome, and POTS after exposure to aluminum, other metals, silicone, and vaccines, validates our hypothesis [1, 6–8, 16, 53]. Furthermore, removing the adjuvants had been shown to improve the clinical presentation and the laboratory markers in ASIA syndrome [8], suggesting that tattoo removal with laser technique could be a potential solution for ASIA syndrome following tattoo.

References

1. Shoenfeld, Y. and Agmon-Levin, N. (2011). "ASIA" – autoimmune/inflammatory syndrome induced by adjuvants. *J. Autoimmun.* 36: 4–8.
2. Molina, V. and Shoenfeld, Y. (2005). Infection, vaccines and other environmental triggers of autoimmunity. *Autoimmunity* 38: 235–245.
3. Inbar, R., Weiss, R., Tomljenovic, L. et al. (2017). Behavioral abnormalities in female mice following administration of aluminum adjuvants and the human papillomavirus (HPV) vaccine Gardasil. *Immunol. Res.* 65: 136–149.
4. Nancy, A.-L. and Shoenfeld, Y. (2008). Chronic fatigue syndrome with autoantibodies--the result of an augmented adjuvant effect of hepatitis-B vaccine and silicone implant. *Autoimmun. Rev.* 8: 52–55.
5. Kagan, P., Halpert, G., Amital, H. et al. (2020). Autoimmune/inflammatory syndrome induced by adjuvant associated with a metal implant in the mouth; explantation was followed by recovery. *Isr. Med. Assoc. J.* 9: 516–517.
6. Schiff, A., Jiries, N., Goldsztein, S. et al. (2020). A possible association of orthopedic metal implants and ASIA syndrome. *Rheumatology* 60 (3): e95–e96. https://doi.org/10.1093/rheumatology/keaa481.
7. Watad, A., Sharif, K., and Shoenfeld, Y. (2017). The ASIA syndrome: basic concepts. *Mediterr. J. Rheumatol.* 28: 64–69.
8. Borba, V., Malkova, A., Basantsova, N. et al. (2020). Classical examples of the concept of the ASIA syndrome. *Biomolecules* 10: 1436.
9. Cárdenas-Roldán, J., Rojas-Villarraga, A., and Anaya, J.-M. (2013). How do autoimmune diseases cluster in families? A systematic review and meta-analysis. *BMC Med.* 11: 73.
10. Steiner, S., Becker, S.C., Hartwig, J. et al. (2020). Autoimmunity-related risk variants in PTPN22 and CTLA4 are associated with ME/CFS with infectious onset. *Front. Immunol.* 11: 578.
11. Watad, A., Quaresma, M., Brown, S. et al. (2017). Autoimmune/inflammatory syndrome induced by adjuvants (Shoenfeld's syndrome) - an update. *Lupus* 26: 675–681.
12. David, P., Watad, A., Halpert, G., and Shoenfeld, Y. (2021). Tattoo as a possible trigger for autoimmune syndrome induced by adjuvants. *Glob. J. Med. Res.* 21: 65–70.
13. Borkenhagen, A., Mirastschijski, U., Petrowski, K., and Brähler, E. (2019). Tattoos in Germany: prevalence, demographics, and health orientation. *Bundesgesundheitsblatt Gesundheitsforschung Gesundheitsschutz* 62: 1077–1082.
14. Balasubramanian, I., Burke, J.P., and Condon, E. (2013). Painful, pigmented lymphadenopathy secondary to decorative tattooing. *Am. J. Emerg. Med.* 31: 1001.e1–1001.e2.
15. Bäumler, W. (2020). Chemical hazard of tattoo colorants. *Presse Med.* 49: 104046.
16. Islam, P.S., Chang, C., Selmi, C. et al. (2016). Medical complications of tattoos: a comprehensive review. *Clin. Rev. Allergy Immunol.* 50: 273–286.
17. Lian, I.-B., Wen, I.-R., and Su, C.-C. (2018). Incidence of sicca syndrome is 3.6 fold higher in areas with farm soils high in chromium and nickel. *J. Formos. Med. Assoc.* 117: 685–690.

18. Drenovska, K., Shahid, M., and Vassileva, S. (2020). Nickel and skin: from allergy to autoimmunity. *Endocr. Metab. Immune Disord. Drug Targets* 20: 1032–1040.
19. Al-Mogairen, S.M., Meo, S.A., Al-Arfaj, A.S. et al. (2010). Nickel-induced allergy and contact dermatitis: does it induce autoimmunity and cutaneous sclerosis? An experimental study in Brown Norway rats. *Rheumatol. Int.* 30: 1159–1164.
20. Mariette, X. and Criswell, L.A. (2018). Primary Sjögren's syndrome. *N. Engl. J. Med.* 378: 931–939.
21. Kluger, N. (2018). Tattoo-associated uveitis with or without systemic sarcoidosis: a comparative review of the literature. *J. Eur. Acad. Dermatol. Venereol.* 32: 1852–1861.
22. Izumikawa, K., Motoi, N., Takaya, H. et al. (2011). A case of concurrent sarcoidosis, aortitis syndrome and Crohn's disease. *Intern. Med.* 50: 2915–2917.
23. Torres, L.K. and Faiz, S.A. (2014). Tattoos and sarcoidosis. *N. Engl. J. Med.* 370: e34.
24. Bindoli, S., Dagan, A., Torres-Ruiz, J.J. et al. (2016). Sarcoidosis and autoimmunity: from genetic background to environmental factors. *Isr. Med. Assoc. J.* 18: 197–202.
25. Valeyre, D., Prasse, A., Nunes, H. et al. (2014). Sarcoidosis. *Lancet* 383: 1155–1167.
26. Orellana Rios, J., Verdaguer Díaz, J.I., Agee, J., and Theodore Smith, R. (2018). Tattoo associated retinochoroiditis. *Arch. Soc. Esp. Oftalmol.* 93: 193–197.
27. Klímová, A., Heissigerová, J., Říhová, E. et al. (2017). Tattoo-associated uveitis. *Ces a Slov Oftalmol Cas Ces Oftalmol Spol a Slov Oftalmol Spol* 73: 30–33.
28. Moschos, M.M. and Guex-Crosier, Y. (2004). Retinal vasculitis and cystoid macular edema after body tattooing: a case report. *Klin. Monbl. Augenheilkd.* 221: 424–426.
29. Reddy, A.K., Shildkrot, Y., Newman, S.A., and Thorne, J.E. (2015). T-Lymphocyte predominance and cellular atypia in tattoo-associated uveitis. *JAMA Ophthalmol.* 133: 1356–1357.
30. Sheldon, R.S., Grubb, B.P. 2nd, Olshansky, B. et al. (2015). 2015 heart rhythm society expert consensus statement on the diagnosis and treatment of postural tachycardia syndrome, inappropriate sinus tachycardia, and vasovagal syncope. *Heart Rhythm.* 12: e41–e63.
31. Li, H., Yu, X., Liles, C. et al. (2014). Autoimmune basis for postural tachycardia syndrome. *J. Am. Heart Assoc.* 3: e000755.
32. Gunning, W.T. 3rd, Kvale, H., Kramer, P.M. et al. (2019). Postural orthostatic tachycardia syndrome is associated with elevated G-protein coupled receptor autoantibodies. *J. Am. Heart Assoc.* 8: e013602–e013602.
33. Fedorowski, A., Li, H., Yu, X. et al. (2017). Antiadrenergic autoimmunity in postural tachycardia syndrome. *Europace* 19: 1211–1219.
34. Dubey, D., Hopkins, S., and Vernino, S. (2016). M1 and M2 muscarinic receptor antibodies among patients with postural orthostatic tachycardia syndrome: potential disease biomarker. *J. Clin. Neuromuscul. Dis.* 17: 179S.
35. Iodice, V., Low, D.A., Mathias, C.J. et al. (2015). Small fibre neuropathy and collagen IV reduction in postural tachycardia syndrome and joint hypermobility syndrome. *Auton. Neurosci.* 192: 125.
36. Haensch, C.-A., Tosch, M., Katona, I. et al. (2014). Small-fiber neuropathy with cardiac denervation in postural tachycardia syndrome. *Muscle Nerve* 50: 956–961.
37. Shoenfeld, Y., Ryabkova, V.A., Scheibenbogen, C. et al. (2020). Complex syndromes of chronic pain, fatigue and cognitive impairment linked to autoimmune dysautonomia and small fiber neuropathy. *Clin. Immunol.* 214: 108384.
38. Park, K., Haberberger, R.V., Gordon, T.P., and Jackson, M.W. (2011). Antibodies interfering with the type 3 muscarinic receptor pathway inhibit gastrointestinal motility and cholinergic neurotransmission in Sjögren's syndrome. *Arthritis Rheum.* 63: 1426–1434.
39. Malysheva, O., Pierer, M., Wagner, U. et al. (2008). Association between beta2 adrenergic receptor polymorphisms and rheumatoid arthritis in conjunction with human leukocyte antigen (HLA)-DRB1 shared epitope. *Ann. Rheum. Dis.* 67: 1759–1764.
40. Jazdzewski, K., Bednarczuk, T., Stepnowska, M. et al. (2007). beta-2-Adrenergic receptor gene polymorphism confers susceptibility to Graves disease. *Int. J. Mol. Med.* 19: 181–186.
41. Metcalf, J.V., Bhopal, R.S., Gray, J. et al. (1997). Incidence and prevalence of primary biliary cirrhosis in the city of Newcastle upon Tyne, England. *Int. J. Epidemiol.* 26: 830–836.
42. Cabral-Marques, O., Marques, A., Giil, L.M. et al. (2018). GPCR-specific autoantibody signatures are associated with physiological and pathological immune homeostasis. *Nat. Commun.* 9: 5224.

43. Xu, B.Y., Huang, D., Pirskanen, R., and Lefvert, A.K. (2000). beta-2-adrenergic receptor gene polymorphisms in myasthenia gravis (MG). *Clin. Exp. Immunol.* 119: 156–160.
44. Smith, A.J., Jackson, M.W., Wang, F. et al. (2005). Neutralization of muscarinic receptor autoantibodies by intravenous immunoglobulin in Sjögren syndrome. *Hum. Immunol.* 66: 411–416.
45. Vera-Lastra, O., Rojas-Milán, E., Peralta-Amaro, A.L. et al. (2020). Autoimmune/inflammatory syndrome induced by methylmethacrylate associated to seronegative antiphospholipid syndrome and diffuse large B-cell non-Hodgkin's lymphoma. *Lupus* 29: 1292–1296.
46. Goldman, A. and Wollina, U. (2019). Polymethylmethacrylate-induced nodules of the lips: clinical presentation and management by intralesional neodymium:YAG laser therapy. *Dermatol. Ther.* 32: e12755.
47. Goldman, A., Staub, H., and Wollina, U. (2018). Hypercalcemia due to polymethylmethacrylate injections? (literature review and case reports). *Georgian Med. News* 17–20.
48. Goldman, A. and Wollina, U. (2018). Intralesional neodymium YAG laser to treat complications of polymethylmethacrylate. *Open access Maced J Med Sci* 6: 1636–1641.
49. Ahn, K.J., Zheng, Z., Kwon, T.R. et al. (2017). Pattern analysis of laser-tattoo interactions for picosecond- and nanosecond-domain 1064-nm neodymium-doped yttrium-aluminum-garnet lasers in tissue-mimicking phantom. *Sci. Rep.* 7: 1533.
50. Khunger, N., Molpariya, A., and Khunger, A. (2015). Complications of tattoos and tattoo removal: stop and think before you ink. *J Cutan Aesthet Surg* 8: 30–36.
51. Colaris, M.J.L., de Boer, M., van der Hulst, R.R., and Cohen Tervaert, J.W. (2017). Two hundreds cases of ASIA syndrome following silicone implants: a comparative study of 30 years and a review of current literature. *Immunol. Res.* 65: 120–128.
52. Ostheimer, T.A., Burkholder, B.M., Leung, T.G. et al. (2014). Tattoo-associated uveitis. *Am. J. Ophthalmol.* 158: 637–43.e1.
53. Guimarães, L.E., Baker, B., Perricone, C., and Shoenfeld, Y. (2015). Vaccines, adjuvants and autoimmunity. *Pharmacol. Res.* 100: 190–209.

15 The Sick Building Syndrome as a Part of the Autoimmune (Autoinflammatory) Syndrome Induced by Adjuvant

Asher Pardo[1] and Eitan Israeli[2]

[1]Department of Occupational and Environmental Health, School of Public Health - Tel Aviv University and the Institute for Occupational Safety and Hygiene, Tel Aviv, Israel

[2]Zabludowicz Center for Autoimmune Diseases, Sheba Medical Center, Tel-Hashomer, Israel

Introduction

The association between environmental quality and health was established early in human history and documented in a treatise entitled "Airs, Waters and Places," part of a group of medical treatises known collectively as the Hippocratic Corpus, attributed to Hippocrates and Hippocratic writers (c. 400 BCE) [1]. The majority of people of all ages spend more than 80% of their time indoors at home, at work, or at leisure – due to changes in lifestyle, work and organizational patterns, and technologies that make the outside accessible from indoors [2, 3]. Even a vehicle may be considered an indoor environment, entailing exposure to low levels of fuel vapors and combustion products as well as to outdoor pollution infiltrating the vehicle's internal space. Thus, today's lifestyle increases people's exposures to their indoor environments, which may sometimes possess poor quality and result in an adverse health impact [4]. Sick building syndrome (SBS) is a term coined for a set of several clinically recognizable symptoms and ailments without a clear cause, reported by occupants of a building [5, 6]. The symptoms and discomfort experienced by the occupants often interfere with their normal function and correlate with times of their presence in the building. The phenomenon has occurred predominantly in nonindustrial modern buildings, including offices, schools, health care centers, and residential buildings, where airtight building envelops and air conditioning or forced ventilation are present. The American Society for Heating, Refrigeration and Air Conditioning Engineering (ASHRAE) has defined a sick building as one where at least 20% of occupants report health symptoms and discomfort associated with their staying in the building, and relief upon leaving the building, but where no definitive cause of the problem can be identified [7]. Another definition regards SBS to be present if there is an onset of two or more symptoms of SBS at least twice followed by a rapid resolution after leaving

Autoimmune Disorders: Adjuvants and Other Risk Factors in Pathogenesis, First Edition.
Edited by Abdulla Watad, Nicola Luigi Bragazzi, and Yehuda Shoenfeld.

the building [8, 9]. Methodological problems make it difficult to identify direct causality between elements associated with a building and the reported symptoms, because so many other unrelated factors may also cause such symptoms. However, epidemiological evidence regarding the syndrome has accumulated over recent decades in different types of settings all over the world [10, 11]. Complaints attributed to workers during working hours are reported much more commonly than those reported by the general public. While SBS may be of a subjective nature and its symptoms frequently reversible, the term building-related illness (BRI) is used when a clinically defined illness is clearly associated with a specific agent in a building's indoor environment. In extreme cases where the causes of SBS have not been identified, and remediation has not been effective, the occupants may abandon the building, thereby creating a "building crisis."

Manifestations of SBS

Transient and long-lasting health effects experienced by occupants subjected to SBS have been found to be associated with many of the environmental agents and factors that determine indoor air quality (IAQ) [7, 12–19]. It is worth noting at the outset, however, that there is a significant subjective component in building occupants' feelings, attitudes, and priorities regarding their indoor environments. Irritation of the eyes and the upper respiratory tract, burning sensations and rhinitis, breathing difficulties and respiratory disorders, tightness in the chest, nonspecific CNS symptoms (headaches, dizziness and fatigue, nausea, difficulties in concentrating, etc.), allergies, asthma, and dry and itchy skin rashes have all been reported by occupants and appear to be associated with the complex chemical environment and poor IAQ, although in many cases the relation to specific agents as a direct cause has not been clear. Table 15.1 presents the most prevalent SBS symptoms found in various studies. Urinary 8-hydroxydeoxyguanosine (8-OHdG) has been suggested as a predictor of oxidative stress to be associated with SBS complaints [23]. Spores released from molds growing on damp walls and other surfaces have been associated with the development of respiratory illness including hypersensitivity pneumonitis and increased risk for sarcoidosis. Multiple chemical sensitivity (MCS), also termed idiopathic environmental intolerance (IEI) by the World Health Organization (WHO) [29], although deemed controversial by clinicians, has also been postulated to be a possible result of initial exposure to high concentrations of a chemical culprit followed by an exposure to low concentrations over time in the indoor environment (MCS has been found higher in allergic patients than in nonallergic patients) [30, 31]. Such a clinical syndrome and other building-related illnesses imply that complex environments may trigger impaired health outcomes, including "functional somatic syndromes" as the "Autoimmune (Autoinflammatory) Syndrome Induced by Adjuvants" (ASIA) [32, 33].

Development of SBS: potential hazards and sources

Indoor health hazards are conveniently classified into categories including chemical, physical, biological, ergonomic, psychosocial, and personal, any of which as well as their combinations may comprise a background for the development of SBS [21]. A large volume of research and practice has focused on indoor environmental quality (IEQ) and SBS in the context of office work, examining the physical, structural, and functional features of a building and its facilities as well as the nature of the effects of the office environment on the health of the occupants and their well-being [19, 24, 34]. However, the symptoms and adverse health outcomes associated with SBS have also been evidenced in health care premises and schools and other public and official buildings [27, 28, 35]. A vast number of chemicals affecting air quality, many with multiple sources, has reportedly been detected in indoor air [20, 34, 36–40], and there is evidence that some of these chemicals are associated with SBS symptoms. A categorial list of sources of indoor chemical

Table 15.1 Prevalence percentage of symptoms associated with sick building syndrome.

Nasal	Ocular	Throat	Skin (various areas)	Headache	Fatigue	Location	References
66	53	—	33	19	30	Hospital	[20]
1.7	7.1	5.7	5.6	2.4	8	Offices	[14]
28	25.1	24.3	45.3	—	—	Hospital	[21]
48.7	39–40	15.8	20.3	38.9	32.3	Offices	[17]
27.9	40.4	20	11.3	16.7	—	Offices	[22]
19	29.7	7.2	1.6	1.8	26.3	Offices	[23]
15.7	23.4	—	2.1	—	—	Offices	[24]
56.5	38.7	48.7	25.7	45.1	66.5	General	[25]
13.9	—	—	7.7	—	—	Confined spaces	[13]
25.4 (M)	27.4	28.6	20.5	36.9	20	Offices	[10]
28.4 (F)	37.9	40.1	19.5	50.9	29.5		
34.2 (M)	17.2	19.5	32.4	13.2	27.2	General	[26]
27.9 (F)	33.2	31.8	57.5	27.0	33.7		
26	8	—	13	45.1	—	School	[27]
—	51.3	27.6	26	26	40	Hospital	[28]

M, males; F, females.

pollutants is presented in Environmental Protection Agency (EPA) documents [4]. Construction materials from which the building is made may degrade, giving rise to airborne particulate matter, while off-gassing and volatile organic compounds (VOCs) may be emitted from plaster boards and drywall as well as pressed wood boards and paints. Combustion processes and tobacco smoke are sources of respirable particles and gasses and vapors, including carbon monoxide as well as formaldehyde and benzene, which are known as human carcinogens. The content of the building, including furniture, equipment, and appliances as well as products used or stored inside the building, is another source of particulate matter and volatiles (formaldehyde, VOCs) and semivolatile organics (SVOC) such as phthalate esters, halogenated ethers, and trihalomethanes. These contaminants are released from a variety of indoor sources and household products such as paints, pressed wood and wood preservatives, plastics, carpets and upholstery, glues, ink ingredients and other graphic items, printers and photocopiers, cleansers, disinfectants, air fresheners, aerosol sprays, insecticides, and fibrous insulation materials attached to ventilation and air-conditioning systems [41]. Occupants' activity inside a building is a source of mechanical dispersion of materials, such as cellulose particles from used paper and processed toner particles from printers. Notably, ozone, which may be a cause of oxidative stress, may be emitted from laser printers and photocopiers, especially old ones, as well as from ozone generators installed to remove airborne contaminants and improve indoor environments [41, 42]. Occupants themselves may be a source of VOCs, and suspended solid and liquid particles released from personal use of consumables such as deodorants and odorous perfumes.They may also cause a secondary dispersion of dusts originating outdoors but adhering to shoes and clothing. Infiltration of outdoor air pollution and suspended soil particulate comprise a further source of many chemical pollutants as does the radioactive radon gas that can infiltrate buildings through cracks or gaps in structures and is a known human carcinogen and one of the leading causes of lung cancer. Water supplies may contain volatiles that can be released while the water is in use. In addition to the sources noted above, one should consider other sources of indoor air pollution that are typical to residential buildings but may be present in public buildings as well. These sources pertain to cooking, tobacco smoking, and heating sources such as fireplaces using wood and coal. Carbon monoxide, a by-product of incomplete combustion, is present in such places. According to a past EPA estimation, the indoor concentrations of some pollutants may be two to five times higher than those typical outdoors. Much emphasis has been put on thermal comfort, ventilation, illumination, and acoustics as the physical agents affecting the quality of the indoor environment and the well-being and comfort of buildings' occupants [21, 43, 44]. Changes in temperature, humidity, thermal radiation, air speed, and outdoor fresh air have been associated with occupants' complaints as well as transient health symptoms and have been widely discussed in the scientific literature over recent decades [45, 46]. Electromagnetic fields have also been suggested as a factor contributing to the effects of SBS and assumed, but not confirmed, to be associated with nervous system symptoms such as headache, fatigue, and burning sensations [36, 47]. Among the physical factors, flaws in the heating, ventilation and air conditioning (HVAC) system, inadequate ventilation, and a lack of sufficient fresh air intake or air filtration have been considered as key reasons for the development of an SBS [19, 43, 48, 49]. The frequency of complaints among occupants in mechanically ventilated and air-conditioned offices has been found to be 30–200% higher than among their counterparts in naturally ventilated offices [50]. These factors have been linked to the overall occupants' comfort and "building-related symptoms" rather than relating them directly to specific morbidity. Biological agents have also been addressed as factors affecting IEQ and the health of people exposed at their work as well as in their homes [38, 51]. Although the evidence supporting a clear causality between bioaerosols and the outcomes mentioned above is not strong in the context of SBS, scientists regard indoor bioaerosols as contributing factors to SBS together with the other possible causes, namely chemical contaminants and unpleasant odors, inadequate ventilation, thermal discomfort, and psychological factors. Analyses of bioaerosols have revealed bacteria, fungi, allergens, endotoxins, and mycotoxins, some of them in concentrations exceeding recommended standards in occupational hygiene guidelines. A diversity of fungal spores dispersed from molds growing on damp and wet surfaces has been shown to exist in indoor bioaerosols [7]. Pathogenic species have been detected among these spores including Aspergillus, Penicillium, Alternaria, and Cladosporium species. *Pseudomonas aeruginosa* is an opportunistic human pathogen specie found indoors. Researchers have emphasized the importance of molds and their mycotoxins in the SBS phenomenon [51]. Recently, findings regarding an association between indoor microbiome exposure and SBS have been published [52].

The association between indoor exposure to bacteria and SBS has been attributed to different classes such as gammaproteobacteria, cyanobacteria, and firmicutes. Airborne endotoxins originating from cell walls of dead gram-negative bacteria are suspected as one of the biological agents associated with the health effects of bioaerosols. These microorganisms and other bioaerosols may cause or enhance respiratory infections as well as triggering or exacerbating hypersensitivity disease, allergies, asthma, and skin lesions and rash, especially in adults and children with a weak or compromised immune system [53, 54]. Fungi and bacteria are not alone in the indoor biological environment relevant to SBS. Viruses, parasites, specific insects and rodents, dust mites, pet hair, and dander and pollens are all classified as potential hazardous sources that may directly or as vectors lead to adverse health effects [36]. Flu viruses and the SARS-CoV-2 virus that has generated the COVID-19 pandemic have well demonstrated the powerful potential hazard of biological agents in the indoor environment, and, likewise, other viruses and bacteria may lead to an outburst of infectious and communicable diseases. Contaminated drinking water which can potentially be aerosolized indoors can be a source of legionella pneumophila known to affect the lungs and cause the Legionnaires' disease. Apart from the attempts to demonstrate associations among chemical, physical, and biological exposure factors in the indoor environment and the development of SBS, researchers have suggested that personal factors, anxiety and depression, environmental discomfort, and job strain may be associated with symptoms of SBS and other work-related symptoms [13, 26, 55, 56]. Other risk factors noted in the scientific literature as associated with SBS include job satisfaction, stress and burnout, the layout of the physical space in offices, and interrelations between employers and employees and among employees themselves. Stress and burnout are considered prominent today among the psychosocial agents impacting worker health and are suggested to be important in the etiology of SBS [17, 44]. They are affected by organizational and personal factors such as physical and mental workload and job demands, responsibility, sense of control, autonomy at work, organizational justice and hindrances, and home–work conflict as well as personal resilience, impaired work relations, and bullying. Ergonomics and the interaction between the human mind and body and the physical environment inside the building must also be considered as contributing factors to the overall well-being and satisfaction of the building's occupants on the one hand and the development of SBS on the other [22]. Musculoskeletal disorders (MSDs) are commonly considered to be consequences of poor ergonomics. In principle, the study and practice of ergonomics engages diverse disciplines, including those related to the human body and its anatomy, physiology, and psychology as well as those related to structural and functional features of the building such as its architecture, interior design, workspaces, and microclimate [57]. The ergonomics of the workplace environment also considers the nature of tasks as well as equipment used and organizational elements, thereby overlapping with factors affecting the psychosocial environment and its impact on workers' health [58]. Productivity and absence from work are two outcomes affected by SBS and IAQ in general. These topics are investigated among office employees in recent and ongoing research projects [43, 59]. Age and sex seem to play a role as risk factors for SBS in residential environments, with young people and females being at higher risk [7, 22]. Increased risk in these environments has also been associated with a medical history of allergies and mental illness, smoking indoors, and special housing specifications for the indoor environment [25].

Conventional and green buildings

Comparisons between conventional and green buildings, including conceptual differences and advantages and disadvantages, have been published in the scientific and professional literature [60]. The "green building" concept is aimed at the conservation of energy, water, and natural resources as well as on effective management of waste, so as to maintain environmental sustainability and optimize residents' general health. Green buildings are also intended to reduce environmental impact throughout their life cycle and improve IAQ through use of environmentally friendly natural resources, materials, and processes [34]. New building materials introduced in recent decades have low emission rates of VOC and SVOC and contribute to the improvement of green buildings' IAQ [61]. Nonetheless, dissatisfaction of occupants and building-related symptoms and illnesses in green buildings have continued to emerge and, although less pronounced in frequency and intensity, bear similar characteristics to those prevailing in the indoor environment of conventional buildings [62]. In an attempt to discuss the reasons for this dissatisfaction, it has been suggested that energy-efficient measures, while consistent with the concepts of energy conservation and sustainability, may nevertheless lead to poor IAQ. Increased thermal insulation and air-tightening measures aimed at saving energy, together with lower rates of outdoor air ventilation, are among these measures [63]. As in conventional buildings, emissions arising from the contents of these new buildings and occupants' activities as well as ergonomic, personal, and psychosocial factors may be additional contributors.

Legal requirements and regulations

Despite the significant prevalence of poor IAQ, there is a remarkable worldwide paucity of assigned regulatory standards and provisions covering the different aspects of the issue. Regulatory occupational exposure and ambient atmosphere standards have been promulgated and issued by many nations to protect workers and the public. However, these standards and other related regulations do not relate specifically to IAQ or SBS in their definitions of nonindustrial environments although the content of some regulatory requirements such as those for adequate ventilation could be implemented to maintain adequate IAQ. There are nonregulatory standards regarding IAQ, e.g. ANSI/*ASHRAE* Standards *62.1* and 62.2 used worldwide [64–66], and a set of guidelines for IAQ developed by the WHO and covering selected pollutants and radon [67]. A few countries and states, e.g. China, California, and New Jersey, have issued specific regulations regarding IAQ. Others such as Japan, South Korea, and Taiwan have partial lists of mandatory IAQ standards for chemical and biological pollutants. Guidelines specifying good practice in managing IAQ as well as performance-based codes exist in various countries. To date, European Union legislation lacks specific reference directives on IAQ although some pre-legislative initiatives exist [68], and there are reference guidelines, documents, and protocols produced by different organizations. The EPA in the United States encourages home owners and public building managers to adopt IAQ guidelines particularly during renovation projects and home retrofitting for improved energy efficiency [69]. Regulations governing the enforcement of IAQ in developing countries either do not exist or are very limited.

SBS and Autoimmune (Autoinflammatory) Syndrome Induced by Adjuvants (ASIA)

During the past two decades, different terms have been used to describe a group of medical conditions having similar symptoms. In the 1990s, the term "functional somatic syndromes" was applied to several syndromes, including additionally to SBS, MCS, repetition stress injury, the side effects of silicone breast implants, the Gulf war syndrome (GWS), chronic fatigue syndrome (CFS), the irritable bowel syndrome, and fibromyalgia (FM) [70]. Patients with these functional somatic syndromes have high self-diagnoses, and their symptoms are often refractory to reassurance, explanation, and standard symptomatic treatment. During the past decade, another term has been used to describe these syndromes – "medically unexplained symptoms" [71, 72]. These same syndromes – SBS, CFS, GWS, MCS, and FM – are defined solely on the basis of symptoms rather than by medical signs. The relationship of such symptoms and syndromes to environmental exposure is often debated, as is the distinction among the various syndromes. Shoenfeld et al. [73] suggested that four conditions – siliconosis, macrophagic myofaciitis (MMF), the GWS, and postvaccination phenomena – sharing clinical and pathogenic resemblances, may be included under a common syndrome entitled the "Autoimmune (Autoinflammatory) Syndrome Induced by Adjuvants" (ASIA). The authors further proposed several major and minor criteria that, although requiring further validation, may aid in the diagnosis of this newly defined syndrome (Table 15.2). We propose here that SBS may also be included as a part of the "**Shoenfeld's syndrome**." Comparison of the clinical manifestations, symptoms, and signs of the four conditions described by Shoenfeld et al. with those described for SBS shows that nine out of 11 main symptom entries in Table 15.2 (adapted from [73]) that exist in the four conditions of ASIA also occur in SBS. These symptoms are myalgia, arthralgias, chronic fatigue, neurological cognitive impairment, fever, gastrointestinal and respiratory symptoms, skin manifestations, and appearance of autoantibodies. The only missing denominator in SBS is the diagnosis of defined autoimmune disease. Symptoms of SBS were described in tens of thousands of people worldwide, although in the relevant studies, the proportion of patients suffering from each clinical manifestation is not always reported by definite percentage [74–78]. SBS as a medical condition also fits well with the criteria suggested by Shoenfeld for ASIA (Box 15.1). The first and most relevant major criterion consistent with **Shoenfeld's syndrome** is "Exposure to an external stimuli (infection, vaccine, silicone, and **adjuvant**) prior to clinical manifestations." In SBS, there is always preexposure to external stimuli in the building environment. Most of the environmental compounds implicated in SBS – VOCs, hydrocarbons, organic allergens, molds, mycotoxins, phthalates, etc. – may be regarded as **environmental adjuvants** [51, 79–82]. Environmental factors that comprise an immune **adjuvant** effect have been recognized for several decades. These adjuvants (i.e. silicone, aluminum, pristane, and

Table 15.2 The prevalence of clinical manifestations: MMF, silicone-related disease, GWS, postvaccination events, and SBS.

Symptoms	MMF N = 250	Silicone N = 100	GWS N = 4600	Post vaccines N = 30000	SBS N = 20000
Myalgias/myopathy/muscle weakness	+++	+++	+	+	+
Arthralgias/arthritis	+++	+++	++	+	+
Chronic fatigue/sleep disturbances	+++	+++	+++	+	++
Neurological/cognitive impairments	+	++	++	+	+
Fever	+	NR	NR	+	+
Gastrointestinal	+	NR	+	+	+
Respiratory	NR	NR	+	+	+
Skin		+	+	+	+
Diagnosis of defined autoimmune disease	+ 33% MS	+	NR	+/–	NR
Antibodies	NR	+	+	NR	+
Increased ESR	++	NR	NR	+	NR

MS, multiple sclerosis; NR, not reported.
The prevalence of signs and symptoms was defined as (+) if reported in <30% of subjects, (++) in 30–60%, and (+++) if present in more than >60% of subjects.Source: Adapted from Shoenfeld et al. [73].

Box 15.1 Suggested criteria for the diagnosis of "ASIA".

Major Criteria:

- Exposure to an external stimuli (infection, vaccine, silicone, and adjuvant) prior to clinical manifestations.
- The appearance of "typical" clinical manifestations:
  - myalgia, myositis, or muscle weakness.
  - Arthralgia and/or arthritis.
  - Chronic fatigue, unrefreshing sleep, or sleep disturbances.
  - Neurological manifestations (especially associated with demyelization)
  - Cognitive impairment and memory loss
  - Pyrexia and dry mouth

Minor Critcria:

- The appearance of autoantibodies or antibodies directed at the suspected adjuvant
- Removal of inciting agent induces improvement
- Typical biopsy of involved organs
- Other clinical manifestations (i.e. irritable bowel syndrome)
- Specific HLA (i.e. HLA DRB1 and HLA DQB1)
- Evolvement of an autoimmune disease (i.e. MS and SSc)

Source: Shoenfeld et al. [73]/with permission of Elsevier.

infectious components) have been found to induce autoimmunity by themselves in different animal models and may possibly provoke autoimmune or autoinflammatory diseases (AI/AIFDs) in humans [83–85]. Exposure to these substances has been documented in the four medical conditions included in ASIA, suggesting that the common denominator to these syndromes is a trigger entailing adjuvant activity. The other major criterion suggested by Shoenfeld for ASIA is "The appearance of 'typical' clinical manifestations," among which a large proportion are symptoms typical to SBS, including myalgia, chronic fatigue, sleep disturbances, neurological manifestations, cognitive impairment, and dry mouth. Some of the minor criteria suggested by Shoenfeld for ASIA are also met in SBS patients: "the appearance of antibodies directed at the suspected adjuvant, or in some cases auto-antibodies" [86–89]; Patients with documented exposure to molds in SBS have elevated titers of antibodies (IgA, IgM, and IgG) to neural-specific antigens when compared with healthy controls [86]. In a mouse model, exposure to molds caused a significant increase in total serum IgG(2a) and interferon gamma [88], and the presence of serum IgE specific to fungi was found to be connected with building-related syndrome in individuals working in damp and moldy buildings [89]. The next criterion – "The removal of the inflicting agent induces improvement" – is very typical to SBS [78]. The last minor criterion – "Evolvement of an autoimmune disease" – is not met distinctively, but there is evidence to suggest an increased risk for autoimmunity [78]. In this study, Gray et al. showed that subjects exposed to mixed mold mycotoxins in a water-damaged building exhibited high risk for producing autoantibodies to nuclei, smooth muscle, CNS and PNS myelin (IgG, IgM, and IgA), and neurofilament. Odds ratio for each autoantibody were significant at 95% confidence intervals, showing an increased risk for autoimmunity. The patients reported a greater frequency and intensity of symptoms, particularly neurological and inflammatory symptoms when compared with controls. (Other abnormal immune parameters were detected in the patients: immune activation markers, with elevated levels of CD+CD26+, CD8+HLR-DR+, CD5+CD25+, and CD8+CD38+ phenotypes on peripheral blood, and decreased complement-receptor-bearing T-suppressor, CD8+CD11b+, cells). **Neurogenic switching** has been proposed as a crossover mechanism between immunogenic inflammation and neurogenic inflammation [90].

Neurogenic inflammation occurs when substance P and other neuropeptides released from sensory neurons produce an inflammatory response, whereas immunogenic inflammation results from the binding of antigen to antibody or leukocyte receptors. Neurogenic switching has been proposed to result when a sensory impulse from a site of activation is rerouted via the CNS to a distant location, producing neurogenic inflammation at the second site. Exposure to an allergen or chemical irritant at one site leads to a sensory nerve impulse. For allergens, mast cells degranulation leads to the release of histamine and other mediators, and histamine binds receptors on sensory nerves. Both histamine and substance P can bind effector cells, such as endothelial cells, mucus-secreting cells, and bronchial smooth muscle cells to produce inflammation. For chemical substances, receptors on peripheral nerves are directly triggered, and when the impulse reaches the CNS, it is redirected to another peripheral location, leading to release of substance P and other neuropeptides and producing inflammation at the second site. An alternative hypothesis is that immunogenic switching occurs, with release of cytokines that act on distant cells even in the brain. These two mechanisms may explain how allergens, infectious agents, adjuvants, etc. can exacerbate conditions such as asthma, migraine, arthritis, and other symptoms descried in SBS and in the other ASIA-related syndromes. It can also explain how respiratory or gut irritants lead to symptoms at other sites in these disorders.

Conclusion

Changes have occurred in the indoor environment over the past 30 years as a result of technological progress and with it the introduction of new construction materials, green concepts such as energy conservation and "the green building," and new capital and consumer goods. Economic factors and the characteristics of employment and even the lifestyles of building occupants, especially of young people, have also changed. The possible roles of these changes require further exploration. Hence, the assessment of the occurrence and prevalence of new, additional risk factors is warranted for different indoor environments, be they industrial, commercial, offices, public premises and services, or residential. Shoenfeld et al. [73] suggested that four conditions – siliconosis, MMF, the GWS, and postvaccination phenomena that share clinical and pathogenic resemblances – may be included under a common syndrome entitled the "Autoimmune (Autoinflammatory) Syndrome Induced by Adjuvants" (ASIA). Comparison of the clinical manifestations, symptoms, and signs of the 4 conditions described by Shoenfeld et al. with those described for SBS shows that 9 out of 10 main symptoms are in correlation in all 5 conditions, namely myalgia, arthralgias, chronic fatigue, neurological cognitive impairment, fever, gastrointestinal and respiratory symptoms, skin manifestations, and appearance of autoantibodies. The authors further proposed several major and minor criteria, which, although requiring further validation, may aid in the diagnosis of this newly defined syndrome. We propose here that SBS may also be included as a part of "**Shoenfeld's syndrome**."

References

1. Lee, E. (2019). Environmental health perspectives in the ancient world. Senior honors thesis. Department of Classics, University of North Carolina at Chapel Hill. https://cdr.lib.unc.edu/concern/honors_theses/k0698c819 (last modified 15 May 2019; cited 2 December 2021).
2. Roberts, T. (2016). We spend 90% of our time indoors. Says who?https://www.buildinggreen.com/blog/we-spend-90-our-time-indoors-says-who [cited 2 December 2021].
3. Klepeis, N., Nelson, W.C., Ott, W.R. et al. (2001). The national human activity pattern survey (NAHPS): a resource for assessing exposure to environmental pollutants. *J. Expo. Anal. Environ. Epidemiol.* 11: 231–252.
4. United States Environmental Protection Agency (2021). Indoor air quality. Washington, DC: United States Environmental Protection Agency. http://www.epa.gov/report-environment/indoor-air-quality (Last updated 7 September 2021; cited 2 December 2021).
5. World Health Organization (1982). Indoor air pollutants: exposure and health effects. EURO reports and studies 78. Copenhagen: Regional Office for Europe, pp. 1–42. https://www.aivc.org/sites/default/files/airbase_1609.pdf (cited 2 December 2021).
6. Passarelli, G.R. (2009). Sick building syndrome: an overview to raise awareness. *J. Build. Apprais.* 5 (1): 55–66.
7. Fanger, P.O. (1988). Hidden olfs in sick buildings. *ASHRAE.* 30: 40–43.
8. Nag, P.K. (2019). Sick building syndrome and other building-related illnesses. In: *Office Buildings*, Design Science and Innovation, 53–103. Singapore: Springer.
9. Wai, T.K. and Willem, H.C. (2011). Perceptions and physiological responses to indoor air quality. In: *Encyclopedia of Environmental Health*, 2e (ed. J.O. Nriagu), 78–84. Elsevier Inc.
10. Marmot, A.F., Eley, J., Stafford, M. et al. (2006). Building health: an epidemiological study of "sick building syndrome" in the Whitehall II study. *Occup. Environ. Med.* 63 (4): 283–289.
11. Epstein, Y. (1994). Sick building syndrome. *Harefuah* 147 (7): 607–608. (Hebrew).
12. Sakellaris, I., Saraga, D., Mandin, C. et al. (2021). Association of subjective health symptoms with indoor air quality in European office buildings: The OFFICEAIR project. *Indoor Air* 31: 426–439.
13. Magnavita, N. (2015). Work-related symptoms in indoor environments: a puzzling problem for the occupational physician. *Int. Arch. Occup. Environ. Health* 88 (2): 185–196.
14. Azuma, K., Ikeda, K., Kagi, N. et al. (2015). Prevalence and risk factors associated with nonspecific building-related symptoms in office employees in Japan: relationships between work environment, indoor air quality and occupational stress. *Indoor Air* 25: 499–511.
15. Tsai, D.H., Lin, J.S., and Chan, C.C. (2012). Office workers' sick building syndrome and indoor carbon dioxide concentrations. *J. Occup. Environ. Hyg.* 9: 345–351.
16. Lan, L., Wargocki, P., Wyon, D.P. et al. (2011). Effects of thermal discomfort in an office on perceived air quality, SBS symptoms, physiological responses, and human performance. *Indoor Air* 21 (5): 376–390. https://doi.org/10.1111/j.1600-0668.2011.00714.x.

17. Hedge, A., Erickson, W.A., and Rubin, G. (1996). Predicting sick building syndrome at the individual and aggregate levels. *Environ. Int.* 22: 3–19.
18. Mendell, M., Sieber, W., Dong, M., et al. (1996). Symptom prevalence distributions in U.S. office buildings investigated by NIOSH for indoor environmental quality complaints. *Proceedings of the Seventh International Conference on Indoor Air Quality and Climate*, pp. 877–882, Nagoya, Japan (21–26 July 1996).
19. Burge, S., Hedge, A., Wilson, S. et al. (1987). Sick building syndriome: a study of 4373 office workers. *Annals Occ. Hyg.* 31 (4A): 493–504.
20. Chang, C.J., Yang, H.H., Wang, Y.F. et al. (2015). Prevalence of sick building syndrome-related symptoms among hospital workers in confined and open working spaces. *Aerosol Air Qual. Res.* 15: 2378–2384.
21. Akova, I., Kilic, E., Sumer, H. et al. (2020). Prevalence of sick building syndrome in hospital staff and its relationship with indoor environmental quality. *Int. J. Environ. Health Res.* 31 (8): 1–16.
22. Lee, S., Park, M.H., and Jeong, B.Y. (2018). Gender differences in public office workers' satisfaction, subjective symptoms and musculoskeletal complaints in workplace and office environments. *Int. J. Occup. Saf. Ergon.* 24 (2): 165–170.
23. Lu, C.Y., Ma, Y.C., Lin, J.M. et al. (2007). Oxidative stress associated with indoor air pollution and sick building syndrome-related symptoms among office workers in Taiwan. *Inhal. Toxicol.* 19 (1): 57–65.
24. Lu, C.Y., Tsai, M.C., Muo, C.H. et al. (2018). Personal, psychosocial and environmental factors related to sick building syndrome in official employees of Taiwan. *Int. J. Environ. Res. Public Health* 15 (1): 7–15.
25. Suzuki, N., Nakayama, Y., Nakaoka, H. et al. (2021). Risk factors for the onset of sick building syndrome: a cross-sectional survey of housing and health in Japan. *Int. Build Environ.* 202: 107976.
26. Runeson, R., Wahlstedt, K., Wieslander, G. et al. (2006). Personal and psychosocial factors and symptoms compatible with sick building syndrome in the Swedish workforce. *Indoor Air* 16: 445–453.
27. Sahlberg, B., Smedje, G., and Norback, D. (2002). Sick building syndrome (SBS) among school employees in the county of Uppsala, Sweden. *Proceedings of the 9th International Conference on Indoor Air Quality and Climate*, pp. 494–499, Monterey, California (30 June–5 July 2002).
28. Sayan, H. and Dulger, S. (2021). Evaluation of the relationship between sick building syndrome complaints among hospital employees and indoor environmental quality. *Med. Lav.* 112 (2): 153–161.
29. International Programme on Chemical Safety (UNEP–ILO–WHO) (1996). Conclusions and recommendations of a workshop on multiple chemical sensitivities (MCS). *Regul. Toxicol. Pharmacol.* 24: S188, Article No. 0095–S189.
30. Jeong, I., Kim, I., Park, H.J. et al. (2014). Allergic diseases and multiple chemical sensitivity in Korean adults. *Allergy, Asthma Immunol. Res.* 6 (5): 409–414.
31. Gibson, P.R. and Lindberg, A. (2011). Physicians' perceptions and practices regarding patient reports of multiple chemical sensitivity. *ISRN Nurs.* 838930, 1–838935. https://doi.org/10.5402/2011/838930.
32. Tuuminen, T., Hyvonen, S., Lohi, J.J. et al. (2021). Dysregulation of the autonomous nervous system in patients with advanced sick building syndrome. *J. Otolaryngol. Neurotol. Res.* 4 (1): 97–111.
33. Israeli, E. and Pardo, A. (2011). The sick building syndrome as a part of the autoimmune (auto-inflammatory) syndrome induced by adjuvants. *Mod. Rheumatol.* 21 (3): 235–239.
34. Mannan, M. and Al-Ghamdi, S.G. (2021). Review indoor air quality in buildings: a comprehensive review on the factors influencing air pollution in residential and commercial structure. *Int. J. Environ. Res. Public Health* 18 (6): 3276.
35. Miladinovic, B., Nikolic, M., Stankovic, A. et al. (2019). Assessment of sick building syndrome among employees in the commercial centers in Nis Serbia. *Occup. Environ. Med.* 76 (Suppl 1): A1–A109. https://doi.org/10.1136/OEM-2019-EPI.231.
36. Dovjak, M. and Kukec, A. (2019). Identification of health risk factors and their parameters. In: *Creating Healthy and Sustainable Buildings: An Assessment of Health Risk Factors*, 83–120. Springer https://doi.org/10.1007/978-3-030-19412-3_3.
37. Amodio, M., Dambruoso, P.R., and de Gennaro, G. (2014). Indoor air quality (IAQ) assessment in a multistorey shopping mall by high-spatial-resolution monitoring of volatile organic compounds (VOC). *Environ. Sci. Pollut. Res.* 21: 13186–13195.
38. Bernstein, J.A., Alexis, N., Bacchus, H. et al. (2008). The health effects of nonindustrial indoor air pollution. *J. Allergy Clin. Immunol.* 121: 585–591.
39. Saijo, Y., Kish, R., Sata, F. et al. (2004). Symptoms in relation to chemicals and dampness in newly built dwellings. *Int. Arch. Occup. Environ. Health* 77: 461–470.

40. Leaderer, B., Naeher, L., and Jan, T. (1999). Indoor, outdoor, and regional summer and winter concentrations of PM_{10}, $PM_{2.5}$, $SO_4^{2}-$, H^+, NH_4^+, NO_3-, NH_3, and nitrous acid in homes with and without kerosene space heaters. *Environ. Health Perspect.* 107: 223–231.
41. Weschler, C.J. (2000). Ozone in indoor environments: concentration and chemistry. *Indoor Air* 10: 269–288.
42. Hubbard, H.F., Coleman, B.K., Sarwar, G. et al. (2005). Effects of an ozone-generating air purifier on indoor secondary particles in three residential dwellings. *Indoor Air* 15: 432–444.
43. Al Horr, Y., Arif, M., Katafigiotou, M. et al. (2016). Impact of indoor environmental quality on occupant well-being and comfort: a review of the literature. *Int. J. Sustain. Built Environ.* 5 (1): 1–11.
44. Rashid, M. and Zimring, C. (2008). A review of the empirical literature on the relationships between indoor environment and stress in health care and office settings. Problems and prospects of sharing evidence. *Environ. Behav.* 40 (2): 151–190.
45. Rizzo, G., Beccali, M., and Nucara, A. (2004). Thermal comfort. In: *Encyclopedia of Energy*, vol. 6 (ed. C.J. Cleveland), 55–64. Elsevier Inc.
46. Fanger, P.O. (1970). *Thermal Comfort. Analysis and Applications in Environmental Engineering*, 1–244. Copenhagen, Denmark: Danish Technical Press.
47. World Health Organization (2015). The international EMF project – progress report, p. 19. https://cdn.who.int/media/docs/default-source/radiation-international-emf-project-reports/emf-iac-2015-progress-report.pdf?sfvrsn=e74f20af_2 (cited 5 December 2021).
48. Wargocki, P., Sundell, J., Bishof, W. et al. (2002). Ventilation and health in non-industrial indoor environments: report from a European multidisciplinary scientific consensus meeting (EUROVEN). *Indoor Air* 12 (2): 113–128.
49. Seppanen, O. and Fisk, W.J. (2002). Association of ventilation system type with SBS symptoms in office workers. *Indoor Air* 12 (2): 98–112.
50. United States Environmental Protection Agency, Washington DC (2007). The EPA cost of illness handbook. (last updated 12 April 2007; cited 5 December 2021).
51. Straus, D. (2009). Molds, mycotoxins, and sick building syndrome. *Toxicol. Ind. Health* 25 (9–10): 617–635.
52. Fu, X., Norback, D., Yuan, Q. et al. (2021). Association between indoor microbiome exposure and sick building syndrome (SBS) in junior high schools of Johor Bahru. *Malaysia. Sci. Total Environ.* 753: 141904.
53. Laquatra, J. (2019). Indoor air quality. In: *Indoor Environmental Quality* (ed. M.A. Mujeebu). IntechOpen. https://www.intechopen.com/chapters/63822 (cited 5 December 2021).
54. Sharpe, R.A., Bearman, N., Thornton, C.R. et al. (2015). Indoor fungal diversity and asthma: a meta-analysis and systematic review of risk factors. *J. Allergy Clin. Immunol.* 135 (1): 110–122.
55. Lu, C.Y., Tsai, M.C., Muo, C.H. et al. (2017). Personal, psychosocial and environmental factors related to sick building syndrome in official employees of Taiwan. *Int. J. Environ. Res. Public Health* 15 (1): 7–15.
56. Norbak, D. (2009). An update on sick building syndrome. *Curr. Opin. Allergy Clin. Immunol.* 1: 55–59.
57. Mujeebu, M.A. (2019). Introductory chapter: indoor environmental quality. In: *Indoor Environmental Quality* (ed. M.A. Mujeebu). IntechOpen. https://www.intechopen.com/chapters/65121 [cited 5 December 2021].
58. Edmonds, J. (2016). Overview of human factors engineering. In: *Human Factors in the Chemical and Process Industries* (ed. J. Edmonds), 153–167. Amsterdam, Netherlands: Elsevier Inc.
59. Gupta, R., Howard, A., and Zahiri, S. (2020). Defining the link between indoor environment and workplace productivity in a modern UK office building. *Archit. Sci. Rev.* 63 (3-4): 248–261.
60. Debating Science (2016). Optimizing conventional buildings. Course blog of junior year writing in the College of Natural Sciences at the University of Massachusetts Amherst. https://blogs.umass.edu/natsci397a-eross/optimizing-conventional-buildings [cited 7 December 2021].
61. Suzuki, N., Nakaoka, H., Hanazato, M. et al. (2019). Indoor air quality analysis of newly built houses. *Int. J. Environ. Res. Public Health* 16: 4142.
62. Gawande, S., Tiwari, R.R., Narayanan, P. et al. (2020). Indoor air quality and sick building syndrome: are green buildings better than conventional buildings? *Indian J. Occup. Environ. Med.* 24: 30–32.
63. Persily, A.K. and Emmerich, S.J. (2012). Indoor air quality in sustainable, energy efficient buildings. *HVAC R Res.* 18 (1–2): 4–20.
64. American Society of Heating, Refrigerating and Air-Conditioning Engineers (2022). Standard 62.1-2019: ventilation for acceptable indoor air quality. ASHRAE, Inc.
65. American Society of Heating, Refrigerating and Air-Conditioning Engineers (2022). Standard 62.2-2019: ventilation and acceptable indoor air quality in residential buildings. ASHRAE, Inc.

66. American Society of Heating, Refrigerating and Air-Conditioning Engineers (2021). Standard 55-2020: thermal environmental conditions for human occupancy. ASHRAE, Inc.
67. World Health Organization (2010). WHO guidelines for indoor air quality: selected pollutants. Regional Office for Europe, p. 99. https://www.euro.who.int/__data/assets/pdf_file/0009/128169/e94535.pdf [cited 7 December 2021].
68. Settimo, G., Manigrasso, M., and Avino, P. (2020). Indoor air quality: a focus on the European legislation and state-of-the-art research in Italy. *Atmosphere*. 11: 370–388.
69. United States Environmental Protection Agency Energy savings plus health: indoor air quality guidelines. https://www.epa.gov/indoor-air-quality-iaq/energy-savings-plus-health-indoor-air-quality-guidelines (cited 7 December 2021).
70. Barsky, A.J. and Borus, J.F. (1999). Functional somatic syndromes. *Ann. Intern. Med.* 130: 910–921.
71. Kipen, H.M. and Fiedler, N. (2002). Environmental factors in medically unexplained symptoms and related syndromes: the evidence and the challenge. *Environ. Health Perspect.* 110 (Suppl 4): 597–599.
72. Binder, L.M. and Campbell, K.A. (2004). Medically unexplained symptoms and neuropsychological assessment. *J. Clin. Exp. Neuropsychol.* 26: 369–392.
73. Shoenfeld, Y. and Agmon-Levin, N. (2010). "ASIA" – autoimmune (auto-inflammatory) syndrome induced by adjuvant: a new syndrome to be defined. *J. Autoimmun.* 36 (1): 4–8.
74. Assoulin-Daya, Y., Leong, A., Shoenfeld, Y., and Gershwin, M.E. (2002). Studies of sick building syndrome. IV. Mycotoxicosis. *J. Asthma.* 39: 191–201.
75. Chang, C. and Gershwin, M.E. (2004). Indoor air quality and human health: truth vs mass hysteria. *Clin. Rev. Allergy Immunol.* 27: 219–239.
76. Chang, C.C., Ruhl, R.A., Halpern, G.M., and Gershwin, M.E. (1993). The sick building syndrome. I. Definition and epidemiological considerations. *J. Asthma.* 30: 285–295.
77. Mahmoudi, M. and Gershwin, M.E. (2000). Sick building syndrome. III. *Stachybotrys chartarum. J. Asthma.* 37: 191–198.
78. Tsai, Y.J. and Gershwin, M.E. (2002). The sick building syndrome: what is it when it is? *Compr. Ther.* 28: 140–144.
79. Garabrant, D.H. and Dumas, C. (2000). Epidemiology of organic solvents and connective tissue disease. *Arthritis Res.* 2: 5–15.
80. Molina, V. and Shoenfeld, Y. (2005). Infection, vaccines and other environmental triggers of autoimmunity. *Autoimmunity* 38: 235–245.
81. Kanazawa, A. and Kishi, R. (2009). Potential risk of indoor semivolatile organic compounds indoors to human health. *Nippon Eiseigaku Zasshi.* 64: 672–682.
82. Koren, H.S., Graham, D.E., and Devlin, R.B. (1992). Exposure of humans to a volatile organic mixture. III. Inflammatory response. *Arch. Environ. Health* 47: 39–44.
83. Agmon-Levin, N., Paz, Z., Israeli, E., and Shoenfeld, Y. (2009). Vaccines and autoimmunity. *Nat. Rev. Rheumatol.* 5: 648–652.
84. Bar-Meir, E., Eherenfeld, M., and Shoenfeld, Y. (2003). Silicone gel breast implants and connective tissue disease—a comprehensive review. *Autoimmunity* 36: 193–197.
85. Zandman-Goddard, G., Blank, M., Ehrenfeld, M. et al. (1999). A comparison of autoantibody production in asymptomatic and symptomatic women with silicone breast implants. *J. Rheumatol.* 26: 73–77.
86. Campbell, A.W., Thrasher, J.D., Madison, R.A. et al. (2003). Neural autoantibodies and neurophysiologic abnormalities in patients exposed to molds in water-damaged buildings. *Arch. Environ. Health* 58: 464–474.
87. Cooley, J.D., Wong, W.C., Jumper, C.A. et al. (2000). An animal model for allergic penicilliosis induced by the intranasal instillation of viable *Penicillium chrysogenum* conidia. *Thorax* 55: 489–496.
88. Gray, M.R., Thrasher, J.D., Crago, R. et al. (2003). Mixed mold mycotoxicosis: immunological changes in humans following exposure in water-damaged buildings. *Arch. Environ. Health* 58: 410–420.
89. Lander, F., Meyer, H.W., and Norn, S. (2001). Serum IgE specific to indoor moulds, measured by basophil histamine release, is associated with building-related symptoms in damp buildings. *Inflamm. Res.* 50: 227–231.
90. Meggs, W.J. (1995). Neurogenic switching: a hypothesis for a mechanism for shifting the site of inflammation in allergy and chemical sensitivity. *Environ. Health Perspect.* 103: 54–56.

16 Gulf War Syndrome (GWS) and ASIA Syndrome

Efrosiniia Talalai
[1]Sackler Faculty of Medicine, Tel-Aviv University, Tel-Aviv, Israel
[2]Zabludowicz Center for Autoimmune Diseases, Sheba Medical Center, Tel-Hashomer, Israel

Introduction

From the mid-1990 to early 1991, the United Nations Coalition, involving 34 countries, deployed approximately 700,000 military personnel to the Persian Gulf, aiming to liberate Kuwait from Iraq's invasion, a conflict known as the Gulf War (GW). The combat phase of the operation was rapid, consisting of six weeks of aerial bombing, followed by five days of ground invasion [1]. Upon returning from the war, veterans reported a myriad of clinical symptoms, records of which were published in the United States [2–4], United Kingdome [5], Canada [6], Australia [7], Denmark [8], and France [9]. Higher rates of sets of symptoms were found in GW veterans as compared to their nondeployed counterparts. Some of the described symptoms include chronic pain, fatigue, myalgia, impaired cognition, skin rashes, memory impairment, gastrointestinal problems, and sleep disturbances. Early reports concluded that the collection of enigmatic symptoms described with self-reports lacked a distinct pattern of illness, designating the complaints as "unexplained illnesses" [2, 5].

While a degree of individual variation exists between individuals, a remarkably consistent symptomatic profile emerged from hundreds of published reports of various GW populations. Subsequently, clusters of health-related manifestations became recognized as Gulf War Syndrome (GWS) or the Chronic Multisymptom Illness (CMI), lacking an agreement by the medical establishment case definition [10]. The Centers for Disease Control and Prevention (CDC) criteria [11] require one or more symptoms for at least six months from two of the following categories: (i) fatigue, (ii) mood and cognition (depressive symptoms, difficulty remembering/concentrating, anxiety sleep disturbances, and anomic aphasia), and (iii) musculoskeletal pain (joint pain/stiffness). Another frequently used criteria – the Kansas definition [12] – requires self-report of at least three chronic symptoms from the six domains: (i) fatigue and sleep disturbances, (ii) pain, (iii) cognitive/neurologic/mood, (iv) gastrointestinal, (v) respiratory, and (vi) skin symptoms.

Prevalence of GWS

Prevalence of GWS varies among GW veterans due to divergent study populations, case definitions, and symptomatic assessments [10]. For instance, the Devens Cohort found 44.8% prevalence

Autoimmune Disorders: Adjuvants and Other Risk Factors in Pathogenesis, First Edition.
Edited by Abdulla Watad, Nicola Luigi Bragazzi, and Yehuda Shoenfeld.

according to the Kansas definition and 57.7% based on the CDC definition (military unit) [13]. The Kansas definition tends to be more strict due to exclusion of veterans with concurrent diagnosed conditions, and the CDC's criteria are more inclusive but less specific [10]. GWS prevalence is associated with military base placement and time spent in deployment. A lower GWS rate was recorded among veterans who retreated from the war territory in March as compared to those who departed in June/July (odds ratio (OR) = 2.8 and 10.3, respectively) [12]. Regardless of the time spent in the Persian Gulf, soldiers who were stationed in Kuwait and/or Iraq had the highest GWS prevalence (42%), while marine soldiers serving on naval ships had the lowest prevalence (21%) [12]. Decades after the war, several longitudinal studies show persistence of GWS among GW veterans, without improvement or worsening of the condition when controlling for age-related deteriorations by comparison to nondeployed era personnel [13–15].

Heterogeneity of Clinical Manifestations

Meta-analysis of 21 studies [16], consisting of 129,000 GW veterans and GW-era controls from four countries and all military branches, found a total of 56 clinical symptoms reported by the veterans. The highest reported symptom was lacking energy (combined prevalence (CP) = 47%), followed by gastrointestinal symptoms, such as flatulence/burping (CP = 44.6%), unrefreshing sleep (CP = 42.9%), headaches (CP = 42.6%), and fatigue (CP = 40.8%). Other symptoms with CP of 30–40% include memory problems, sleep disturbances, back pain, forgetfulness, joint pain/stiffness, and difficulty concentrating. For all analyzed symptoms, GW veterans had a significantly higher OR as compared to appropriate controls. The greatest odds for experiencing symptoms were cognitive/neurologic/mood symptoms (detachment feeling: OR = 3.59; irritability: OR = 3.21), musculoskeletal pain (muscle weakness: OR = 3.19), gastrointestinal (diarrhea: OR = 3.24), and dermatological (skin rash: OR = 3.18).

Etiology and pathogenesis of GWS

Environmental triggers associated with GWS

Epidemiological studies on health outcomes for GW veterans have recognized environmental factors unique to the GW as etiological agents associated with the syndrome's development [1, 17–19]. Troops in the Persian GW zone were exposed to a complex mixture of hazards, making the establishment of a causal link between discrete exposures and GWS challenging. Investigations were further complicated by unequal exposure for all troops and lack of systematic documentations throughout the war regarding hazards, with information primarily accumulating by recall questionnaires and modeling. Notably, research rolls out psychiatric disorders as the explanation behind the GWS, with Post-Traumatic Stress Disorder (PTSD) rates in GWS veterans being higher than nondeployed servicemen but substantially lower than veterans served in other wars [1]. The potentially hazardous exposures include pesticides, chemical nerve gas agents, pyridostigmine bromide (PB), oil well fires, depleted uranium, multiple vaccines, fuel vapor, exhaust fumes, and psychological/physiological stress. Particular interest transpired in pesticides, PB, low levels of nerve agents, and multiple vaccinations, with varying degrees of evidence supporting the link and pesticides being most consistently identified as a significant GWS risk [1]. To explore the relationship among distinct exposures, their combinations, and the underpinning of GWS manifestations, a substantial body of research has been carried out on animal models. Although it is challenging to design a representative model and interpret the results, they provide ground for understanding the syndrome's pathogenesis, especially in conjunction with health findings from epidemiological studies.

The link between GWS and pesticides

Substantial concern regarding arthropod-borne infectious diseases existed for the coalition troops, prompting vast distribution of pesticides for personal use as sprays, liquids, creams, and powders to apply to skin, clothing, and bedding and to be dispersed in base facilities [1, 20–22]. Some of the potentially hazardous pesticides used include organophosphates (OPs; diazinon, malathion, chlorpyrifos, and dichlorvos), carbamates (carbaryl, methomyl, and propoxur), pyrethroids (permethrin), and organochlorine (lindane) [20]. OPs and carbamates inhibit acetylcholinesterase (AChE), the primary catalyzer of ACh breakdown, leading to overstimulation of cholinergic receptors in the brain and peripheral nerves. While OPs bind to the esterase irreversibly, generating permanent inhibition, carbamates' effect is transient due to the reversible nature of binding and higher metabolism rate [1]. Adverse reactions to AChEs manifest with excessive exposures but are also observed at lower doses in individuals with sensitivity to the compounds [1]. Pyrethroids and lindane are both categorized as neurotoxins on account of affecting neuronal excitability, by interfering with voltage-gated sodium channels and neurotransmitter gamma aminobutyric acid (GABA), respectively [1]. Multivariate analysis shows that GWS is significantly associated with repeated, daily pesticide exposure from uniform treatment and skin application (odds ratio (OR) 3.72 and 2.89, respectively) [17]. An epidemiological study investigating pesticide impact on cognitive impairment found dichlorvos to be the main predictor for poor attention and psychomotor control, and methomyl and lindane to be the best predictors for mood domain complaints in GWS veterans [23]. Animal model studies support association between pesticides and GWS, particularly in terms of neurocognitive deficits [24, 25]. A model examining the low-level OP agent, diisopropyl fluorophosphate, found symptoms of chronic depression, anxiety, and memory impairments, accompanied by hippocampal neuronal damage in rats [24]. A mice model showed deterioration of synaptic integrity in the C3 hippocampal region and altered neuron differentiation in the dentate gyrus in response to chlorpyrifos alone or in combination with PB and permethrin at acute time postexposure. In this study, all exposure combinations generated pronounced pathological changes, but some differences between them existed, presumably reflecting the symptomatic heterogeneity of GWS veterans, stemming from diversity of war experiences [25]. The Research Advisory Committee (RAC) on GWS concluded that the accumulated data provides a compelling case for a causal association between GWS and pesticides, citing a consistent dose–response relationship between them [1].

The link between GWS and nerve agents

There are no reports by the U.S. forces confirming large-scale exposures to chemical weapons, sarin and cyclosarin, during the GW, but concerns regarding low-dose exposures to these agents have been raised. They could occur from the fumes of ammunition storage demolition that an estimated 100,000 U.S. soldiers were exposed to and alleged chemical attacks on account of veterans reporting hearing chemical alarms in military camps [26]. Sarin and cyclosarin are highly toxic chemical weapons that irreversibly inhibit AChE, causing acute cholinergic toxicity that leads to rapid death; therefore, lack of immediate and acute neurotoxicity may have gone undetected. Little is understood regarding the long-term biological impact of low-level chemical weapon exposures, with GWS expanding the knowledge in this area. Self-reports of exposure to chemical/biological weapons, used as proxy for sarin/cyclosarin, were significantly associated with increased rates of four medical chronic conditions, including high blood pressure, diabetes, arthritis, and chronic bronchitis [27]. Moreover, nerve agent exposure has been associated with MRI-assessed brain structural abnormalities, such as decreased gray and white matter volumes and increased ventricle size [28–31] as well as significant reduction in the volume of hippocampal CA2, CA3, and dentate gyrus areas [29, 32]. Corresponding to functional imaging studies, exposure to chemical warfare agents was associated with poorer neuropsychological performance, assessed by objective cognitive tests [33]. Animal models have shown that short-term neurological effects of low-to-moderate doses of sarin generate neurobehavioral alterations [34–36], spinal cord lesions, and swelling [37, 38] as well as increased expression of genes associated with apoptosis and neurodegeneration [39]. Long-term effects (3–6 months) to repeated (five days), low-dose sarin proxy, diisopropyl fluorophosphate, in mice generated chronic depression, anxiety, and neuronal damage in the hippocampus [40]. Incorporation of physiological stress, reminiscent of the wartime, to diisopropyl fluorophosphate mice model yields a stronger positive correlation with the syndrome's symptomatology, such as exacerbation of neuroinflammation [41, 42]. The RAC report concluded that the association between the GWS and chemical warfare agents exposure cannot be ruled out, but inconsistency in study observations makes the link ambiguous [1].

The link between GWS and pyridostigmine bromide (PB)

In hopes to prevent adversities from potential nerve agent attacks, GW soldiers were required to administer prophylactic doses of PB. The U.S. Department of Defense reported that over 5 million doses were supplied to the Persian Gulf during the war, and an estimated 250,000 soldiers administered at least a few PB pills [43]. Given the reversible nature of AChE inhibition by PB with low permeability through the blood–brain barrier (BBB), little risk was expected from prophylactic treatment, particularly considering the dire consequences of nerve agent exposure [26]. However, subsequent epidemiological studies uncovered an association between PB administration and GWS. Multivariate analysis of GW exposures found significantly increased odds for GWS development based on self-reported PB intake (OR = 3.21) [22], and a positive correlation was established between the number of PB pills taken and the severity of GWS symptoms [44, 45]. Animal studies investigating the role of PB in GWS progression are inconsistent, with some reporting no deteriorative effects of PB without secondary mediating factors [42, 46], and others suggesting PB alone to be sufficient in producing physiological alterations, such as alterations in gastrointestinal function, neuroinflammation [47], and locomotor deficits [48]. Remarkable interest in the potential additive effect of PB and physiological stress arose following an early animal model study that found intense stressors to render the BBB more permeable to PB [49]. However, numerous model studies utilizing different species of animals (rats, mice, and guinea pigs) with stressors of various types observed neither gross anatomical disruption of brain blood vessels nor pronounced reduction in AChE activity in the brain [50–52]. On the other hand, combination of PB, DEET, and permethrin produced a significant decrease in ACh in the midbrain, brainstem, and cerebellum of rats, though still without increasing BBB permeability [53]. Synergistic effects of PB and pesticides are supported by a study in which GWS veterans who reported being exposed to both chemicals performed worse on cognitive impairment tests [23]. Although the RAC report concludes that PB is causally associated with GWS [1], the U.S Institute of Medicine argues that there is insufficient evidence to establish a direct association between the long-term GWS symptoms and PB [43].

The link between GWS and multiple vaccinations

Receipt of various vaccines over a short period of time is a frequent feature of military deployment, but vaccines given to the troops for the GW have been a controversial topic due to their association with GWS. Virtually all GW veterans report receiving at least one vaccine in relation to deployment, more than 70% report receiving more than 5%, and 30% report more than 10 [1]. A dose–response relationship was found between the number of symptoms reported by Australian GWS veterans and the number of vaccines received for GW deployment, based on immunization booklets [7]. The total quantity of reported symptoms was associated with having at least 10 vaccines, and no single vaccine or vaccine clusters appear to be behind the observed effect. The multiple vaccinations hypothesis is further supported by the findings in the Kansas study in which nondeployed GW-era veterans who received multiple vaccines had significantly higher prevalence of GWS as compared to those with no vaccine records (11.5% versus 3.7%) [12]. Contrastingly, a large postal U.K. study found an association between multiple vaccines and GWS only when the analysis relied on the veterans' own recollections of the vaccines received and diminished upon analysis restriction to formal immunization records. Overall, biological warfare vaccines were found to be associated with GWS to a greater extent regardless of the vaccine documentation [54, 55]. The highly reactogenic anthrax vaccine generated a particular interest among etiologic studies, culminating with inconclusive results [54, 56]. A small study found anthrax protective antigen PA63 in the serum of all GWS veterans tested [57]. Moreover, antibodies against squalene, a polyunsaturated terpene hydrocarbon adjuvant ingredient in a number of vaccines, were detected in virtually all (95%) of GWS veterans, in contrast to patients with other autoimmune conditions and healthy controls who had no detectable levels of such antibodies [58], though the importance of these exposure-associated markers remains to be elucidated [59]. Lack of supporting evidence from animal studies regarding vaccine involvement in GWS pathology, such as no impact on sleep quality, brain EEG patterns, and immune system responses [60, 61] in marmosets, prompted the RAC report to conclude that the association cannot be ruled out, but the evidence to be sparse in important ways [1].

Genetic basis of individual variation in susceptibility to GWS

The contributions of human leukocyte antigens (HLA) genes to GWS pathogenesis have been suggested by several studies [62–64]. HLA genes are located in the major histocompatibility complex of chromosome 6 and play an important role in immune recognition. GWS protection was observed when six Class II HLA alleles were present, including DRB1*01:01, DRB1*13:02, DRB1*08:11, DQB1*02:02, DPB1*06:01, and DPB*01:01. HLA genes are highly polymorphic, and the number of copies of the protective alleles can even be zero. The severity of GWS symptoms and the number of the six protective HLA alleles exhibited an inverse relationship, and the overall frequency was significantly lower in GWS veterans, compared to the unaffected veterans. The presence of DRB1*13:02 allele was associated with spared subcortical brain atrophy [62]. Interestingly, the allele DRB1*13:02 has been implicated with protective roles in a range of autoimmune conditions, including systemic sclerosis, rheumatoid arthritis, and systemic lupus erythematosus [65]. Therefore, the considerable extent of GWS clinical manifestation may depend on the number of copies of the six protective alleles of the Class II HLA.

Brain defects and central nervous system alterations in veterans with GWS

Research findings in veterans with GWS include significant alterations in brain structure and function that correspond with neurocognitive symptoms characteristic of the syndrome. An associative memory evaluation revealed memory deficit directly linked to the amount of activation in the left hippocampus [66]. Pronounced (~10%) subcortical brain atrophy was reported in GWS, primarily consisting of brainstem, cerebellum, thalamus, and to a lesser degree basal ganglia, amygdala, and diencephalon [67]. The highest decrease in volume was seen in brainstem, consistent with low brainstem metabolism measured with MR spectroscopy [68]. Reduced brainstem volumes were associated with depression severity, and specifically, the shrinkage in pons correlated with the intensity and frequency of fatigue [69]. Declined cerebral blood flow (CBF) velocity upon orthostatic stress, reminiscent of cerebral hypoperfusion associated with cognitive deterioration with increasing age, has also been proposed to contribute to cognitive impairment [70]. Cognitive fatigue has been linked with alterations in neural networks, specifically, impaired modulation in the motivation and reward circuitry [71]. While in healthy controls, the caudate nucleus of the striatum exhibited little activation when performing easier tasks and a significant increase in activity during a more challenging task, the opposite effect was measured in GWS, with moderate activation during the easier task, and a decrease in the activity with the more complex task. This implies a considerable requirement for cognitive resources for executing even an undemanding assignment in veterans with GWS [71].

Epidemiological evidence of neuroinflammation in veterans with GWS was presented by measurement of transporter protein (TSPO), indicative of astrocytes and microglia activation [72]. This phenomenon was recorded in prefrontal, precuneus, primary motor, and somatosensory cortices and has been suggested to contribute to cognitive and mood dysfunction in GWS veterans. Significant peripheral inflammation was neither observed nor correlated with TSPO levels in veterans with GWS. TSPO is also highly expressed in activated macrophages, which under physiological conditions are substantially restricted to the choroid plexus and meninges, but pathology accompanied by alterations in BBB permeability can provide access to the brain parenchyma by these leukocytes [73]. Therefore, it is possible that the observed elevation in the levels of TPSO may be reflective of infiltrated macrophages along with activated astrocytes and microglia.

Peripheral immune abnormalities associated with GWS

Sustaining GWS long term has been attributed to various immune alterations in peripheral circulation found in veterans with GWS [1]. Studies examining the blood serum of veterans for distinct patterns of blood cell count, biomarkers, and cytokines can delineate between GWS and other groups on study-by-study basis, but no consensus exists on the specific GWS immune signatures. The observed inconsistency in immune measurements may be due to chronological progression of GWS and differences in study methodology. Principally, studies observe aberrant plasma cytokine levels in GWS veterans, but the nature of expression varies. For instance, a number of pro-inflammatory cytokines, including IFN gamma, IL-6, IL-2 levels, TNF α, and chemokine CCL5, CXCL8, and CX3CL1 have been found in GWS veterans serum [74], but significant downregulation of TNF α, CCL5, and CXCL8 has also been reported in GWS veterans [75]. Cytokine profiles found in GWS are indicative of mixed Th1, Th2, and Th17 responses [76, 77] found in patients with autoimmune diseases, such as rheumatoid arthritis [78] and Grave's disease [79]. However, in these conditions, altered cellular responses are secondary to diminished immunological self-tolerance, which has not yet been reported in GWS. Circulating of c-reactive protein (CRP), a nonspecific acute-phase inflammation biomarker, is consistently detected in the circulation of veterans with GWS [80–82] and has been positively associated with pain, neurocognitive/mood, respiratory issues, and fatigue but not with gastrointestinal or skin symptom severity [80]. Furthermore, CRP and IL-6 exhibited a positive correlation in GWS [81], a phenomenon related to disease activity in other autoimmune conditions [82]. Other biomarkers associated with chronic inflammation that have been detected in GWS include leptin and brain-derived neurotrophic factor [83].

Abnormal humoral responses have been detected in veterans with GWS, as evidenced by increased immunoglobulin G (IgG) against smooth and striated muscle and immunoglobulin M (IgM) against myelin basic protein (MBP), detected in blood eight years after the war [84]. Furthermore, several autoantibodies (AABs) against neuron- and glial-specific proteins have been significantly elevated in GWS, including a ninefold increase in calcium-calmodulin kinase II (CAMKII) AAB, sevenfold increase in myelin-associated glycoprotein, and 2.5-fold increase in AABs against neurofilaments [85]. Lupus anticoagulant (LA) AABs characterized in various autoimmune conditions were detected in one-quarter of GWS patients, a rate comparable to that observed in lupus patients [86]. These AABs were detected decades upon returning from the war, implying that persistent continuation of degenerative processes may stem from the autoimmune component in the GWS etiology. However, humoral responses may not resemble those of typical autoimmune diseases, evidenced by normal levels of serum antinuclear antibodies (ANA), an AAB against nuclear envelope proteins used in diagnosis of several autoimmune diseases in veterans with GWS [87].

Gut microbiome alterations in GWS

A preliminary study on gut microbiome analysis found significantly different patterns of commensal bacteria in GWS, particularly in veterans with gastrointestinal symptoms [88]. This group also had elevated TNF receptor I in the serum and reported greater levels of chronic pain, fatigue, and sleep disturbances. A decrease in the abundance of bacteria *Roseburia* in the GWS group was suggested to cause GI inflammation, which coincided with nearly doubled circulating TNF-RI. The decrease in the abundance of *Dialister* in the GWS group parallels the literature that this decline is associated with depression [89] and arthritis [90]. The observed positive association between *Ruminococcus* abundance and GWS is also found in lupus nephritis [91] and irritable bowel syndrome [92]. Although larger studies are needed to confirm these associations, this is the first insight into the relations among GWS symptoms, inflammation, and microbiome.

GWS in relation to other multisymptom conditions

Parallels have been drawn between GWS and other conditions that are primarily defined by symptoms, such as fibromyalgia (FM), chronic fatigue syndrome (CFS), and multiple chemical sensitivity (MCS). These conditions overlap in their description and may thus represent aspects of an undetermined entity or correspond with a common underlying physiological idiosyncrasy. Not all GWS patients fit the case definitions for other multisymptom conditions, but a fraction of GW veterans may be diagnosed with either of these disorders. Neurocognitive dysfunction is the overarching similarity among these multisymptom conditions, though neither of them can adequately describe the syndrome affecting GW veterans.

GWS in relation to chronic fatigue syndrome (CFS)

The prevalence of CFS in the general population ranges from 0.4% to 2.5%, relying on self-reports of debilitating fatigue, postexertional malaise, pain, sleep disturbances, cognitive and neurologic changes (memory/concentration issues), and altered immune and autonomic function [93–95]. CFS rates have been reported higher among GW veterans as compared to the general public, ranging up to 5.1% [1]. A study investigating diagnosis of various medical conditions found a 40-time higher CFS rate among GW veterans, as compared to their nondeployed colleagues (1.6% versus 0.1%) [96].

Symptomatic similarities between CFS and GWS prompted the comparison of the two conditions in studies identifying disease-specific signatures. A metabolomic study examining the serum of veterans with GWS found irregularities in 8 out of 46 biochemical pathways analyzed. Five of the 8 pathways were shared with observed metabolic phenotype of males with CFS, but 4 of these 5 pathways were dysregulated in opposite directions, showing how similar clinical manifestations can have different chemical mechanisms [97].

GWS in relation to fibromyalgia (FM)

The prevalence of FM in the general population is 2–3%, with the majority of diagnosis occurring in women [1]. FM diagnosis is essentially based on the presence of widespread pain as well as fatigue, cognitive dysfunction, and nonrestorative sleep, among others [98]. FM prevalence is similar between GW veterans and the general population [1]. However, in the predominantly male population of the given age, FM prevalence would be anticipated to be twice lower [96]. Pathophysiological resemblance between GWS and FM has been observed in terms of spatial similarities of neuroinflammatory markers elevation throughout the cortical areas [99].

GWS in relation to multiple chemical sensitivity (MCS)

MCS describes a pattern of symptoms triggered by low-level exposure to one or more chemicals, with symptom resolution upon exposure withdrawal. The prevalence of MCS varies considerably in the existing literature and is also reported to be increasing with time, with most studies reporting a diagnosed rate of about 7% [100, 101]. The array of symptoms presented by MCS patients correspond well with the symptoms of the GWS, such as fatigue, headache, cognitive impairment, digestive challenges, sleep abnormalities, and mood disturbances [101–104]. MCS diagnosis was recognized in multiple studies examining GW veterans, including studies published in the United States [102, 103], United Kingdome [104], and Canada [105]. Overall, MCS prevalence in GWS veterans ranges from 1.3% to 5.6% and has been consistently higher among GW veterans as compared to nondeployed veterans of the era [1]. Aside from the symptomatic resemblance, CFS and GWS may be linked via genetic predisposition. An association has been made between GWS and a variant of PON1 gene, encoding for a paraoxonase enzyme, which metabolizes OP pesticides and sarin [106]. PON1 has also been shown to function at a slower rate in women with MCS as compared to the controls in a Canadian cohort study [107]. The ramification of these results is that a particular variant of PON1 may predispose to sensitivity to chemical exposures and subsequently develop an illness characterized by multiple symptoms spanning several body systems.

Classification of GWS as part of the autoimmune/inflammatory syndrome induced by adjuvants (ASIA)

The autoimmune/inflammatory syndrome induced by adjuvants (ASIA), also referred to as Shoenfeld's syndrome, encompasses autoimmune conditions that share clinical and pathogenic

Table 16.1 Prevalence of ASIA syndrome clinical manifestations in veterans with GWS.

ASIA syndrome symptomatic criteria	Studies N	GW veterans (%) (95% CI)	GW-era controls (%) (95% CI)	OR (95%CI)
Myalgia	13	23.0 (14.9 to 33.8)	9.5 (5.0 to 17.3)	2.36 (1.91 to 2.92)
Myositis/muscle weakness	5	14.7 (9.8 to 21.5)	4.6 (2.7 to 7.5)	3.19 (2.73 to 3.74)
Arthralgia and/or arthritis	3	10.8 (5.8 to 19.0)	4.4 (1.9 to 9.9)	2.35 (1.67 to 3.30)
Chronic fatigue	15	40.8 (31.4 to 45.6)	14.4 (9.0 to 22.2)	2.74 (2.11 to 3.57)
Unrefreshing sleep/sleep disturbances	12	42.9 (33.1 to 53.4)	21.8 (13.9 to 32.4)	1.91 (1.59 to 2.30)
Neurological manifestations				
Headaches	18	42.6 (33.9 to 51.7)	23.7 (16.0 to 33.6)	1.78 (1.49 to 2.12)
Dizziness	10	19.5 (15.5 to 24.3)	7.9 (5.6 to 11.0)	2.34 (2.06 to 2.67)
Numbness and tingling	8	18.8 (10.5 to 31.4)	8.0 (3.9 to 15.8)	2.32 (1.96 to 2.74)
Cognitive impairment				
Forgetfulness	6	34.8 (25.7 to 45.1)	13.7 (7.5 to 23.7)	2.52 (1.80 to 3.52)
Memory problems	7	39.6 (30.8 to 49.0)	14.9 (9.3 to 22.9)	2.63 (2.10 to 3.30)
Anxiety	8	10.9 (5.8 to 19.6)	3.4 (1.5 to 7.5)	2.68 (2.10 to 3.43)
Difficulty concentrating	11	33.3 (27.0 to 40.3)	12.8 (9.0 to 17.9)	2.47 (2.06 to 2.96)
Feeling depressed	14	17.1 (12.7 to 22.7)	7.2 (4.1 to 12.4)	2.26 (1.88 to 2.71)
Irritability	14	29.9 (21.3 to 40.3)	9.2 (4.8 to 16.9)	3.21 (2.28 to 4.52)
Pyrexia	6	8.8 (4.5 to 16.3)	3.6 (1.7 to 7.6)	2.30 (1.75 to 3.03)
Dry mouth		NA		

ASIA, Autoimmune/inflammatory Syndrome Induced by Adjuvants; GW, Gulf War OR; odds ratio was significant for all symptoms (i.e. 95% CI for the OR did not include null OR).

resemblances and are induced by adjuvants [108]. The major ASIA criteria include exposure to an external stimuli prior to the onset of clinical manifestations, improvement of health with removal of inciting agent, and minor criteria that include appearance of AABs or antibodies against the presumed adjuvant, involvement of specific HLA genes, coexisting autoimmune disease, and other clinical symptoms. GWS meets several of the ASIA-defined indications, including the first and most pertinent major criteria – exposure to external stimuli as an inciting factor for the development of the condition. Most literature regarding GWS agree that external triggers are behind the etiology of the syndrome, suggesting the specific environmental factor to entail adjuvant activity. Juxtaposition of clinical presentations described in the ASIA major criteria and those reported by GWS veterans in a meta-analysis of 21 epidemiological studies reveals overlap in 8 out of 9 main symptom entries (Table 16.1) [16], namely myalgia, myositis, arthralgia, chronic fatigue, sleep disturbances, neurological manifestations, cognitive impairment, and pyrexia, and the only ASIA symptom not reported by GWS veterans is dry mouth. Additional symptoms reported by the GWS veterans but are not a part of the ASIA major criteria are gastrointestinal and dermatological symptoms. Some of the minor ASIA syndrome criteria are also satisfied in GWS, including the presence of AABs as well as antibodies against squalene and genetic predisposition associated with certain HLA haplotypes.

Conclusion

Veterans of the 1990–1991 GW were a part of a relatively short military operation that was deemed a success by the United Nations Coalition. Unfortunately, following the war, many veterans developed lasting health consequences that lacked understanding, were trivialized, or denied.

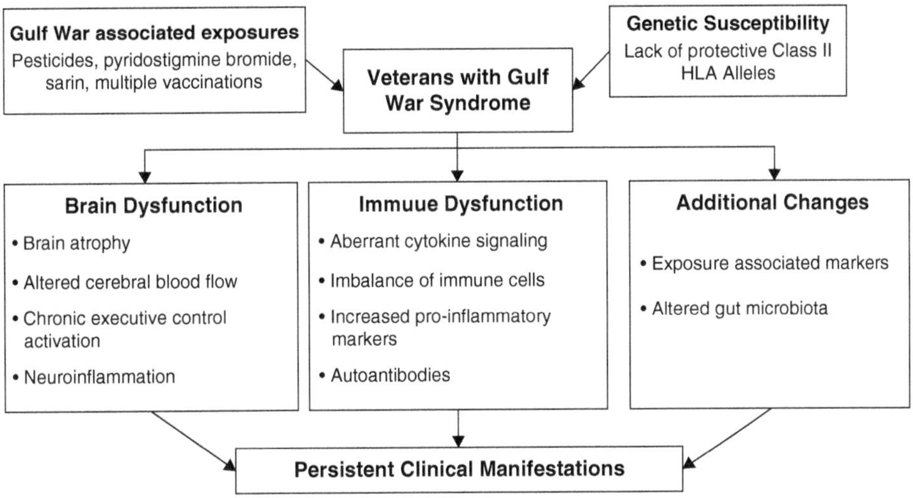

Figure 16.1 Schematic illustration of Gulf War syndrome progression: environmental triggers in genetically predisposed veterans generate a variety of pathophysiological changes, associated with long-term symptoms.

The vast scientific research carried out on the topic since indicates that GWS is a tangible condition developed as a result of neurotoxic environmental exposures encountered by the veterans in the Persian Gulf. GWS is a chronic condition as evidenced by few veterans recovering or having significant improvements with time. One possible unifying explanation behind GWS is the persistent antigen hypothesis based on the findings that the presence of Class II HLA alleles distinguishes healthy GW veterans from those who developed GWS. Lack of protection provided by these alleles hinges on recognition of foreign antigen epitopes and their efficient elimination. This results in chronic, nonspecific inflammation in peripheral circulation as well as CNS that cause fatigue and neurocognitive impairments, among other symptoms. Regardless of the etiology, GWS meets several key ASIA syndrome-defined criteria, including the widely accepted etiology, clinical manifestations, and HLA gene involvement, and is therefore included as part of Shoenfeld's syndrome.

References

1. Binns, J., Barlow, C., Bloom, F. et al. (2008). *Gulf War Illness and the Health of Gulf War Veterans*. Washington, DC: U.S. Government Publishing Office.
2. Gavaghan, H. (1994). NIH panel rejects Persian Gulf syndrome. *Nature* 369 (6475): 8–8.
3. Morbidity and Mortality Weekly Report (MMWR) – CDC. (1995). Unexplained illness among Persian Gulf War veterans in an Air National Guard Unit: preliminary report – August 1990–March 1995.
4. Proctor, S. (1998). Health status of Persian Gulf War veterans: self-reported symptoms, environmental exposures and the effect of stress. *Int. J. Epidemiol.* 27 (6): 1000–1010.
5. Beale, P. (1994). Gulf illness. *BMJ* 308 (6943): 1574–1574.
6. Robinson, A. (1995). Veterans worry that unexplained medical problems a legacy of service during Gulf War. *Can. Med. Assoc. J.* 152 (6): 944–947.
7. Kelsall, H. (2004). Symptoms and medical conditions in Australian veterans of the 1991 Gulf War: relation to immunisations and other Gulf War exposures. *Occup. Environ. Med.* 61 (12): 1006–1013.
8. Ishøy, T. (1999). State of health after deployment in the Persian Gulf. The Danish Gulf War study. *Dan. Med. Bull.* 46 (5): 416–419.
9. Salamon, R., Verret, C., Jutand, M. et al. (2006). Health consequences of the first Persian Gulf War on French troops. *Int. J. Epidemiol.* 35 (2): 479–487.

10. Chronic Multisymptom Illness in Gulf War Veterans (2014). *Case Definitions Reexamined*. National Academies Press.
11. Fukuda, K. (1998). Chronic multisymptom illness affecting air force veterans of the Gulf War. *JAMA* 280 (11): 981.
12. Steele, L. (2000). Prevalence and patterns of Gulf War illness in Kansas veterans: association of symptoms with characteristics of person, place, and time of military service. *Am. J. Epidemiol.* 152 (10): 992–1002.
13. Zundel, C. (2020). Changes in health status in the Ft. Devens Gulf War veterans cohort: 1997–2017. *Neurosci. Insights*. 15: 2633105520952675.
14. Li, B., Mahan, C., Kang, H. et al. (2011). Longitudinal health study of US 1991 Gulf War veterans: changes in health status at 10-year follow-up. *Am. J. Epidemiol.* 174 (7): 761–768.
15. Porter, B., Long, K., Rull, R., and Dursa, E. (2020). Prevalence of chronic multisymptom illness/Gulf War illness over time among millennium cohort participants, 2001 to 2016. *J. Occup. Environ. Med.* 62 (1): 4–10.
16. Maule, A., Janulewicz, P., Sullivan, K. et al. (2018). Meta-analysis of self-reported health symptoms in 1990–1991 Gulf War and Gulf War-era veterans. *BMJ Open* 8 (2): e016086.
17. Steele, L., Sastre, A., Gerkovich, M., and Cook, M. (2012). Complex factors in the etiology of Gulf War illness: wartime exposures and risk factors in veteran subgroups. *Environ. Health Perspect.* 120 (1): 112–118.
18. VA.gov | Veterans Affairs (2015). Publichealth.va.gov. [accessed 5 March 2022]. https://www.publichealth.va.gov/exposures/gulfwar/sources/index.asp.
19. Haley, R. and Tuite, J. (2013). Epidemiologic evidence of health effects from long-distance transit of chemical weapons fallout from bombing early in the 1991 Persian Gulf War. *Neuroepidemiology* 40 (3): 178–189.
20. National Academies of Sciences, Engineering, and Medicine; Health and Medicine Division; Board on Population Health and Public Health Practice; Committee on Gulf War and Health (2018). 5. Pesticides. In: *Gulf War and Health: Volume 11: Generational Health Effects of Serving in the Gulf War*. Washington, DC: National Academies Press (US).
21. The Defense Technical Information Center (2000). *Pesticide Use During the Gulf War: A Survey of Gulf War Veterans*. Santa Monica, CA: National Defense Research Institute (NDRI).
22. DOD (U.S. Department of Defense). (2003). Environmental exposure report: pesticides, final report. Washington, DC: Office of the Special Assistant to the Undersecretary of Defense for Gulf War Illnesses, Medical Readiness, and Military Deployments.
23. Sullivan, K., Krengel, M., Bradford, W. et al. (2018). Neuropsychological functioning in military pesticide applicators from the Gulf War: effects on information processing speed, attention and visual memory. *Neurotoxicol. Teratol.* 65: 1–13.
24. Phillips, K. and Deshpande, L. (2016). Repeated low-dose organophosphate DFP exposure leads to the development of depression and cognitive impairment in a rat model of Gulf War illness. *Neurotoxicology* 52: 127–133.
25. Ojo, J., Abdullah, L., Evans, J. et al. (2013). Exposure to an organophosphate pesticide, individually or in combination with other Gulf War agents, impairs synaptic integrity and neuronal differentiation, and is accompanied by subtle microvascular injury in a mouse model of Gulf War agent exposure. *Neuropathology* 34 (2): 109–127.
26. Michalovicz, L., Kelly, K., Sullivan, K., and O'Callaghan, J. (2020). Acetylcholinesterase inhibitor exposures as an initiating factor in the development of Gulf War illness, a chronic neuroimmune disorder in deployed veterans. *Neuropharmacology* 171: 108073.
27. Zundel, C., Krengel, M., Heeren, T. et al. (2019). Rates of chronic medical conditions in 1991 Gulf War veterans compared to the general population. *Int. J. Environ. Res. Public Health* 16 (6): 949.
28. Heaton, K., Palumbo, C., Proctor, S. et al. (2007). Quantitative magnetic resonance brain imaging in US army veterans of the 1991 Gulf War potentially exposed to sarin and cyclosarin. *Neurotoxicology* 28 (4): 761–769.
29. Chao, L., Rothlind, J., Cardenas, V. et al. (2010). Effects of low-level exposure to sarin and cyclosarin during the 1991 Gulf War on brain function and brain structure in US veterans. *Neurotoxicology* 31 (5): 493–501.
30. Chao, L., Reeb, R., Esparza, I., and Abadjian, L. (2016). Associations between the self-reported frequency of hearing chemical alarms in theater and regional brain volume in Gulf War veterans. *Neurotoxicology* 53: 246–256.
31. Chao, L. and Zhang, Y. (2018). Effects of low-level sarin and cyclosarin exposure on hippocampal microstructure in Gulf War veterans. *Neurotoxicol. Teratol.* 68: 36–46.

32. Chao, L., Kriger, S., Buckley, S. et al. (2014). Effects of low-level sarin and cyclosarin exposure on hippocampal subfields in Gulf War veterans. *Neurotoxicology* 44: 263–269.
33. White, R., Proctor, S., Heeren, T. et al. (2001). Neuropsychological function in Gulf War veterans: relationships to self-reported toxicant exposures. *Am. J. Ind. Med.* 40 (1): 42–54.
34. Hulet, S., McDonough, J., and Shih, T. (2002). The dose–response effects of repeated subacute sarin exposure on guinea pigs. *Pharmacol. Biochem. Behav.* 72 (4): 835–845.
35. Kassa, J., Krejčová, G., and Vachek, J. (2002). The impairment of spatial memory following low-level sarin inhalation exposure and antidotal treatment in rats. *Acta Medica (Hradec Kralove, Czech Republic)*. 45 (4): 149–153.
36. Shih, T., Hulet, S., and McDonough, J. (2006). The effects of repeated low-dose sarin exposure. *Toxicol. Appl. Pharmacol.* 215 (2): 119–134.
37. Husain, K., Pant, S., Raza, S.C. et al. (1995). A comparative study of delayed neurotoxicity in hens following repeated administration of organophosphorus compounds. *Indian J. Physiol. Pharmacol.* 39: 47–50.
38. Husain, K., Vijayaraghavan, R., Pant, S.C. et al. (1993). Delayed neurotoxic effect of sarin in mice after repeated inhalation exposure. *J. Appl. Toxicol.* 13: 143–145.
39. Defense Technical Information Center (2014). *Low-Level Inhalation Exposure to Chemical Nerve Agent Vapor Induces Expression of Neuronal Apoptosis and Regeneration Genes*. Washington, DC: Edgewood Chemical Biological Center.
40. Naughton, S., Hernandez, C., Beck, W. et al. (2018). Repeated exposures to diisopropylfluorophosphate result in structural disruptions of myelinated axons and persistent impairments of axonal transport in the brains of rats. *Toxicology* 406–407: 92–103.
41. O'Callaghan, J., Kelly, K., Locker, A. et al. (2015). Corticosterone primes the neuroinflammatory response to DFP in mice: potential animal model of Gulf War illness. *J. Neurochem.* 133 (5): 708–721.
42. Locker, A., Michalovicz, L., Kelly, K. et al. (2017). Corticosterone primes the neuroinflammatory response to Gulf War illness-relevant organophosphates independently of acetylcholinesterase inhibition. *J. Neurochem.* 142 (3): 444–455.
43. Fulco, C., Liverman, C., and Sox, H. (2000). *Gulf War and Health*, vol. 1. Washington, DC: National Academies Press.
44. Lucas, K., Rowe, P., and Armenian, H. (2007). Latency and exposure-health associations in Gulf War veterans with early fatigue onsets: a case-control study. *Ann. Epidemiol.* 17 (10): 799–806.
45. Golomb, B. (2008). Acetylcholinesterase inhibitors and Gulf War illnesses. *Proc. Natl. Acad. Sci.* 105 (11): 4295–4300.
46. Abou-Donia, M. (1996). Neurotoxicity resulting from coexposure to pyridostigmine bromide, deet, and permethrin: implications of Gulf War chemical exposures. *J. Toxicol. Environ. Health* 48 (1): 35–56.
47. Hernandez, S., Fried, D., Grubišić, V. et al. (2019). Gastrointestinal neuroimmune disruption in a mouse model of Gulf War illness. *FASEB J.* 33 (5): 6168–6184.
48. Abou-Donia, M. (2004). Co-exposure to pyridostigmine bromide, DEET, and/or permethrin causes sensorimotor deficit and alterations in brain acetylcholinesterase activity. *Pharmacol. Biochem. Behav.* 77 (2): 253–262.
49. Friedman, A., Kaufer, D., Shemer, J. et al. (1996). Pyridostigmine brain penetration under stress enhances neuronal excitability and induces early immediate transcriptional response. *Nat. Med.* 2 (12): 1382–1385.
50. Grauer, E., Alkalai, D., Kapon, J. et al. (2000). Stress does not enable pyridostigmine to inhibit brain cholinesterase after parenteral administration. *Toxicol. Appl. Pharmacol.* 164: 301–304.
51. Lallement, G., Foquin, A., Baubichon, D. et al. (1998). Heat stress, even extreme, does not induce penetration of pyridostigmine into the brain of guinea pigs. *Neurotoxicology* 19: 759–766.
52. Shaikh, J. and Pope, C. (2003). Combined forced running stress and subclinical paraoxon exposure have little effect on pyridostigmine-induced acute toxicity in rats. *Toxicology* 190 (3): 221–230.
53. Abdel-Rahman, A., Abou-Donia, S., El-Masry, E. et al. (2004). Stress and combined exposure to low doses of pyridostigmine bromide, DEET, and permethrin produce neurochemical and neuropathological alterations in cerebral cortex, hippocampus, and cerebellum. *J. Toxic. Environ. Health A* 67 (2): 163–192.
54. Unwin, C., Blatchley, N., Coker, W. et al. (1999). Health of UK servicemen who served in Persian Gulf War. *Lancet* 353 (9148): 169–178.
55. Hotopf, M. (2000). Role of vaccinations as risk factors for ill health in veterans of the Gulf war: cross sectional study. *BMJ* 320 (7246): 1363–1367.

56. Gray, G. (2002). Self-reported symptoms and medical conditions among 11,868 Gulf War-era veterans: the Seabee Health Study. *Am. J. Epidemiol.* 155 (11): 1033–1044.
57. Tsilibary, E., Souto, E., Kratzke, M. et al. (2019). Anthrax and Gulf War illness (GWI): evidence for the presence of harmful anthrax antigen PA63 in the serum of veterans with GWI. *J. Neurol. Neuromedicine* 4 (6): 1–9.
58. Asa, P., Cao, Y., and Garry, R. (2000). Antibodies to squalene in Gulf War syndrome. *Exp. Mol. Pathol.* 68 (1): 55–64.
59. Lippi, G., Targher, G., and Franchini, M. (2010). Vaccination, squalene and anti-squalene antibodies: facts or fiction? *Eur. J. Intern. Med.* 21 (2): 70–73.
60. Williams, K., Mann, T., Chamberlain, S. et al. (2006). Multiple vaccine and pyridostigmine interactions: effects on EEG and sleep in the common marmoset. *Pharmacol. Biochem. Behav.* 84 (2): 282–293.
61. Griffiths, G., Hornby, R., Jagger, C. et al. (2006). Development of methods to measure humoral immune responses against selected antigens in the common marmoset (Callithrix jacchus) and the effect of pyridostigmine bromide administration. *Int. Immunopharmacol.* 6 (12): 1755–1764.
62. James, L., Engdahl, B., Leuthold, A., and Georgopoulos, A. (2016). Brain correlates of human leukocyte antigen (HLA) protection in Gulf War illness (GWI). *EBioMedicine*. 13: 72–79.
63. Christova, P., James, L., Carpenter, A. et al. (2020). Human leukocyte antigen (HLA) alleles prevent metabolically-induced inflammation and cerebrocortical thinning in Gulf War illness. *J. Neurol. Neuromedicine* 5 (3): 16–27.
64. James, L., Christova, P., Engdahl, B. et al. (2017). Human leukocyte antigen (HLA) and Gulf War illness (GWI): HLA-DRB1*13:02 spares subcortical atrophy in Gulf War veterans. *EBioMedicine*. 26: 126–131.
65. Furukawa, H., Oka, S., Tsuchiya, N. et al. (2016). The role of common protective alleles HLA-DRB1*13 among systemic autoimmune diseases. *Genes Immun.* 18 (1): 1–7.
66. Odegard, T., Cooper, C., Farris, E. et al. (2013). Memory impairment exhibited by veterans with Gulf War illness. *Neurocase* 19 (4): 316–327.
67. Christova, P., James, L., Engdahl, B. et al. (2017). Subcortical brain atrophy in Gulf War illness. *Exp. Brain Res.* 235 (9): 2777–2786.
68. Haley, R., Marshall, W., McDonald, G. et al. (2000). Brain abnormalities in Gulf War Syndrome: evaluation with 1H MR spectroscopy. *Radiology* 215 (3): 807–817.
69. Zhang, Y., Avery, T., Vakhtin, A. et al. (2020). Brainstem atrophy in Gulf War illness. *Neurotoxicology* 78: 71–79.
70. Falvo, M., Lindheimer, J., and Serrador, J. (2018). Dynamic cerebral autoregulation is impaired in veterans with Gulf War illness: a case-control study. *PLoS One* 13 (10): e0205393.
71. Wylie, G., Genova, H., Dobryakova, E. et al. (2019). Fatigue in Gulf War illness is associated with tonically high activation in the executive control network. *NeuroImage Clin.* 21: 101641.
72. Alshelh, Z., Albrecht, D., Bergan, C. et al. (2020). In-vivo imaging of neuroinflammation in veterans with Gulf War illness. *Brain Behav. Immun.* 87: 498–507.
73. Lopes Pinheiro, M., Kooij, G., Mizee, M. et al. (2016). Immune cell trafficking across the barriers of the central nervous system in multiple sclerosis and stroke. *Biochim. Biophys. Acta (BBA) - Mol. Basis Dis.* 1862 (3): 461–471.
74. Nkiliza, A., Joshi, U., Evans, J. et al. (2021). Adaptive immune responses associated with the central nervous system pathology of Gulf War illness. *Neurosci. Insights*. 16: 263310552110184.
75. Khaiboullina, S., DeMeirleir, K., Rawat, S. et al. (2015). Cytokine expression provides clues to the pathophysiology of Gulf War illness and myalgic encephalomyelitis. *Cytokine* 72 (1): 1–8.
76. Skowera, A., Hotopf, M., Sawicka, E. et al. (2004). Cellular immune activation in Gulf War veterans. *J. Clin. Immunol.* 24 (1): 66–73.
77. 9. Parkitny, L., Middleton, S., Baker, K., and Younger, J. (2015). Evidence for abnormal cytokine expression in Gulf War illness: a preliminary analysis of daily immune monitoring data. *BMC Immunol.* 16 (1): 1–10.
78. Kidd, P. (2003). Th1/Th2 balance: the hypothesis, its limitations, and implications for health and disease. *Altern. Med. Rev.* 8 (3): 223–246.
79. Rydzewska, M., Jaromin, M., Pasierowska, I. et al. (2018). Role of the T and B lymphocytes in pathogenesis of autoimmune thyroid diseases. *Thyroid. Res.* 11 (1): 1–11.
80. James, L., Engdahl, B., Johnson, R., and Georgopoulos, A. (2019). Gulf War illness and inflammation: association of symptom severity with C-reactive protein. *J. Neurol. Neuromedicine*. 4 (2): 15–19.

81. Butterick, T., Trembley, J., Hocum Stone, L. et al. (2019). Gulf War Illness-associated increases in blood levels of interleukin 6 and C-reactive protein: biomarker evidence of inflammation. *BMC Res. Notes.* 12 (1): 1–5.
82. Pradhan, V., Umare, V., Nadkarni, A. et al. (2017). Do high sensitivity C-reactive protein and serum interleukin-6 levels correlate with disease activity in systemic lupus erythematosus patients? *J. Postgrad. Med.* 63 (2): 92.
83. Johnson, G., Slater, B., Leis, L. et al. (2016). Blood biomarkers of chronic inflammation in Gulf War illness. *PLoS One* 11 (6): e0157855.
84. Vojdani, A. and Thrasher, J. (2004). Cellular and humoral immune abnormalities in Gulf War veterans. *Environ. Health Perspect.* 112 (8): 840–846.
85. Abou-Donia, M., Lapadula, E., Krengel, M. et al. (2020). Using plasma autoantibodies of central nervous system proteins to distinguish veterans with Gulf War illness from healthy and symptomatic controls. *Brain Sci.* 10 (9): 610.
86. James, L., Johnson, R., Lewis, S. et al. (2021). Lupus anticoagulant in Gulf War illness and autoimmune disorders: a common pathway toward autoimmunity. *J. Immunol. Sci.* 5 (1): 14–18.
87. Skowera, A., Stewart, E., Davis, E. et al. (2002). Antinuclear autoantibodies (ANA) in Gulf War-related illness and chronic fatigue syndrome (CFS) patients. *Clin. Exp. Immunol.* 129 (2): 354–358.
88. Janulewicz, P., Seth, R., Carlson, J. et al. (2019). The gut-microbiome in Gulf War veterans: a preliminary report. *Int. J. Environ. Res. Public Health* 16 (19): 3751.
89. Valles-Colomer, M., Falony, G., Darzi, Y. et al. (2019). The neuroactive potential of the human gut microbiota in quality of life and depression. *Nat. Microbiol.* 4 (4): 623–632.
90. Picchianti-Diamanti, A., Rosado, M., and D'Amelio, R. (2018). Infectious agents and inflammation: the role of microbiota in autoimmune arthritis. *Front. Microbiol.* 8: 2696.
91. Azzouz, D., Omarbekova, A., Heguy, A. et al. (2019). Lupus nephritis is linked to disease-activity associated expansions and immunity to a gut commensal. *Ann. Rheum. Dis.* 78 (7): 947–956.
92. Rinninella, E., Raoul, P., Cintoni, M. et al. (2019). What is the healthy gut microbiota composition? A changing ecosystem across age, environment, diet, and diseases. *Microorganisms.* 7 (1): 14.
93. Carruthers, B., Jain, A., De Meirleir, K. et al. (2003). Myalgic encephalomyelitis/chronic fatigue syndrome. *J. Chronic Fatigue Syndr.* 11 (1): 7–115.
94. Reeves, W., Jones, J., Maloney, E. et al. (2007). Prevalence of chronic fatigue syndrome in metropolitan, urban, and rural Georgia. *Popul. Health Metrics* 5 (1).
95. Reyes, M., Nisenbaum, R., Hoaglin, D. et al. (2003). Prevalence and incidence of chronic fatigue syndrome in Wichita, Kansas. *Arch. Intern. Med.* 163 (13): 1530.
96. Eisen, S. (2005). Gulf War veterans' health: medical evaluation of a U.S. Cohort. *Ann. Intern. Med.* 142 (11): 881.
97. Naviaux, R., Naviaux, J., Li, K. et al. (2019). Metabolic features of Gulf War illness. *PLoS One* 14 (7): e0219531.
98. Wolfe, F., Clauw, D., Fitzcharles, M. et al. (2010). The American college of rheumatology preliminary diagnostic criteria for fibromyalgia and measurement of symptom severity. *Arthritis Care Res.* 62 (5): 600–610.
99. Albrecht, D., Forsberg, A., Sandström, A. et al. (2019). Brain glial activation in fibromyalgia – a multi-site positron emission tomography investigation. *Brain Behav. Immun.* 75: 72–83.
100. Meggs, W. (1999). Gulf War syndrome, chronic fatigue syndrome, and the multiple chemical sensitivity syndrome: stirring the cauldron of confusion. *Arch. Environ. Health* 54 (5): 309–311.
101. Kutsogiannis, D. and Davidoff, A. (2001). A multiple center study of multiple chemical sensitivity syndrome. *Arch. Environ. Health* 56 (3): 196–207.
102. Kipen, H., Hallman, W., Kang, H. et al. (1999). Prevalence of chronic fatigue and chemical sensitivities in Gulf registry veterans. *Arch. of Environ. Health* 54 (5): 313–318.
103. Proctor, S., Heaton, K., White, R., and Wolfe, J. (2001). Chemical sensitivity and chronic fatigue in Gulf War veterans: a brief report. *J. Occup. Environ. Med.* 43 (3): 259–264.
104. Reid, S. (2001). Multiple chemical sensitivity and chronic fatigue syndrome in British Gulf War veterans. *Am. J. Epidemiol.* 153 (6): 604–609.
105. Goss Gilroy Inc. (1998). Health Study of Canadian Forces Personnel Involved in the 1991 Conflict in the Persian Gulf: Volume 1: Ottawa Canada.

106. Haley, R., Billecke, S., and La Du, B. (1999). Association of low PON1 Type Q (Type A) arylesterase activity with neurologic symptom complexes in Gulf War veterans. *Toxicol. Appl. Pharmacol.* 157 (3): 227–233.
107. McKeown-Eyssen, G. (2004). Case-control study of genotypes in multiple chemical sensitivity: CYP2D6, NAT1, NAT2, PON1, PON2, and MTHFR. *Int. J. Epidemiol.* 33 (5): 971–978.
108. Watad, A., Sharif, K., and Shoenfeld, Y. (2017). The ASIA syndrome: basic concepts. *Mediterr. J. Rheumatol.* 28 (2): 64–69.

17 Vaccinations in Patients with Autoimmune Diseases

Isa Seida and Naim Mahroum
International School of Medicine, Istanbul Medipol University, Istanbul, Turkey

Risk of infection in patients with AIRD

Infections continue to be a significant cause of morbidity and mortality in AIRD patients, which is due to congregation of both the infectious disease itself and the immunosuppressive treatment.

In relation to influenza, retrospective studies showcased an increased rate of influenza in the elderly (≥65 years) with rheumatic diseases [1, 2]. In one of the studies [2], the odds ratio was 1.56 (95% confidence interval (CI): 1.23–2.02) for hospital admissions relating to either pneumonia or influenza and 2.67 (95% CI: 2.26–3.16) for death. In another study [1], the rate of admission to hospital in AIRD patients was 4.5–7% for those who were unvaccinated compared to 0.8% in healthy unvaccinated controls.

Streptococcus pneumoniae is one of the most common causes of pulmonary infections in AIRD patients [3]. In an analysis of the risk of invasive pneumococcal diseases in patients hospitalized with certain immune-mediated disorders, Wotton and Goldacre [4] found a significantly increased risk for multiple immune-mediated diseases including rheumatoid arthritis (RA), systemic sclerosis (SSc), Sjögren's syndrome (SjS), and systemic lupus erythematosus (SLE).

A study evaluating infection in SLE established the respiratory and urinary tracts alongside skin and soft tissue to be the most frequent sites of infection [5]. Respiratory tract infections were predominantly in hospitalized patients, while urinary and skin infections were more commonplace in outpatients, as shown in numerous studies [6–12]. The causative organisms resemble those of the general population, with *Streptococcus pneumoniae* being the most common agent associated with respiratory tract infections. Another cause of infections in SLE is *Staphylococcus aureus*, which predominantly causes skin and soft tissue infections [13]. In terms of UTIs, the most common causative agent remains *Escherichia coli*. The latter, together with *S. aureus* and *Salmonella*, has been linked to causing bacteremia in SLE patients [9, 14, 15]. Furthermore, the rates of tuberculosis are relatively higher in SLE patients when compared to the general population. A prospective study in Spain observed that the incidence of tuberculosis in SLE patients is sevenfold higher than that of the general population [16].

Similarly, RA patients are thought to have an increased risk of contracting tuberculosis. A study that estimated the relative risk of getting infected with TB in patients receiving nonbiological disease-modifying drugs (DMARDs) found the risk to rise from 2.0 to 10.9 after patients receive DMARDs [17]. An increase in risk from 4.0 to 90.1 following treatment with TNF-alpha was

Autoimmune Disorders: Adjuvants and Other Risk Factors in Pathogenesis, First Edition.
Edited by Abdulla Watad, Nicola Luigi Bragazzi, and Yehuda Shoenfeld.

observed in another study [18]. In Canada, the rate of TB in patient with RA was 45.8/100,000 compared to the base rate of 4.2/100,000 in the general population [19]. An examination of an U.S. cohort found the incidence rate of TB in RA patients as 21.33/100,000 compared to the rate of 9.48/100,000 in controls without RA [20].

Corticosteroid therapy has been linked to increased risk of tuberculosis. A retrospective case control study in the United Kingdom observed from 497 new cases of tuberculosis and 1966 age- and sex-matched controls that the adjusted odds ratio (aOR) for tuberculosis was 2.8 (95% CI 1.0, 7.9) for prednisone equivalent doses less than 15 mg/day and 7.7 (95% CI 2.8, 21.4) for doses larger than 15 mg/day [21]. Another study by Wolfe concluded an increasing risk for tuberculosis ranging from 1.5- to 8.7-fold in patients receiving corticosteroid therapy [22].

Herpes zoster is another infectious agent of importance in patients with AIRD. Smitten et al. evaluated the risk of herpes zoster in RA patients in the United States and United Kingdom [23]. The study recognized RA as a risk factor for herpes zoster infection with an HR of 1.65 and 1.91 when compared to healthy controls, respectively. Investigations of the rates of herpes zoster in SLE found them to be increased by 5- up to 16-fold relative to healthy controls [24–26].

Safety and efficacy of vaccinations in patients with AIRD

Influenza vaccines

As per the updated European Alliance of Associations for Rheumatology (EULAR) recommendations, routine seasonal influenza vaccination is not included in the National Immunization Program (NIP) [27]. However, it is now strongly suggested to deliberate annual vaccination in patients receiving DMARD or glucocorticoids treatment. This recommendation is further empowered by the fact that AIRD patients are at a higher risk of contracting influenza [28].

In a study that evaluated 1668 patients who received vaccination for nonadjuvanted influenza A/California/7/2009(H1N1) virus-like flu strain, Saad et al. concluded that all the analyzed parameters were significantly lower in AIRD in relation to healthy controls [29]. However, about half of the patients received corticosteroid and/or immunosuppressive therapy. The study also focused on nonadjuvanted vaccine preparations in order to rule out the possibility of "adjuvant disease," a phenomenon that was initially described by Schoenfeld et al. in 2011 as it follows exposure to adjuvanted vaccines or other adjuvant-involving substances [30].

Vaccine efficacy in AIRD patients undergoing immunosuppressive treatment is highly variable [31]. Influenza vaccine immunogenicity is thought to be reduced in patients receiving methotrexate [32, 33], rituximab [34–38], and abatacept [32, 37].

Aside from the typical concerns of fever, irritability, headache, pain, and swelling in the injection site, another significant concern is severe anaphylactic reaction to the administration of vaccination. Although such anaphylactic reactions are rare, the rapid onset and potential lethality of the complication require vaccine administrators to have plans for anaphylaxis management in place [39].

Influenza vaccine in SLE

Studies have showcased that inactivated influenza vaccination in SLE patients resulted in lower rates of hospitalization due to infection as well as a decrease in complications seen in SLE patients [40, 41]. The same works have also shown that in patients receiving the trivalent vaccine, no immunization associated flares were detected. Further research emphasized that patients run a greater risk of exacerbations from infection than worsening of SLE disease [42].

However, some studies demonstrated that SLE patients showcase lower immunization rates in comparison to healthy controls [43]; this is especially prominent in patients receiving immunosuppressive treatment [44]. In fact, proper immune response to vaccination relies on both humoral and cell-mediated immunities being effective, but these responses may be compromised in SLE [45]. This potential lowering of immunization rates in SLE dates back to 1978 in two different studies. Williams et al. reported that among 19 vaccinated SLE patients, 47% displayed seroconversion, compared to the 94% found in healthy controls [46]. Similarly, Ristow et al. found that only 48% of SLE patients showcased an increase in titers, compared to the 62% increase in controls [47]. Holvast et al. displayed 56 SLE patients who had lower seroconversions than healthy controls: 43% of patients compared to 94% of controls for A (H1N1), 39% of patients against 88% of controls for A(H3N2), and 41% of patients compared to 71% of the controls for B/Hong Kong [48]. In another research, a similar (or modestly reduced) reaction to the influenza vaccine was described in SLE patients in comparison to healthy controls [44, 49–51]. Booster vaccination four weeks following initial dosage failed to increase seroprotection in SLE. However, despite the lower efficacy of influenza vaccination in SLE, it is still protective [52].

In addition, the potential for exacerbations in SLE has created concerns regarding influenza vaccination in SLE patients [45, 53]. Several cases of SLE flares following influenza immunization have been reported [54]. This is supplemented by the fact that influenza vaccination is thought to cause a 10–15% transient increase in autoantibodies even in the absence of flares [54–57]. The possibility of exacerbation in vaccinating SLE patients was described as early as 1978 by Hess and Hahn who reported 2 SLE patients among 109 individuals immunized with A/NewJersey/76 vaccine [58]. The patients developed renal failure. One patient displayed an active urine sediment, while the other possessed a diffuse proliferative nephritis. Furthermore, an analysis by Del Porto et al. reported that among 14 SLE patients who received the nonadjuvanted TIV (A/New Caledonia/20/99[H1N1], A/Moscow/10/99 [H3N2], B/HongKong/330/2001), 2 of them showed SLE exacerbations [59].

Influenza vaccine in RA

The American College of Rheumatology (ACR) recommends that all patients receive yearly influenza vaccination due to its associations with reducing risk of hospitalizations for septicemia, bacteremia, and/or viremia [38, 60]. Yet, vaccination rates in RA remain low in comparison to the general populations, which is possibly due to the concerns regarding vaccine efficacy and safety in patients receiving immunosuppressive therapies [61]. In fact, data regarding whether DMARDs impair vaccine response in RA remains mixed and subject to debate [62]. A study examining RA patients treated with subcutaneous abatacept with adjunct DMARDs, who received the 2011–2012 trivalent seasonal vaccine, found that 81% of the patients reached protective antibody titer levels 28 days following the administration of the vaccination [61]. Certain studies showed appropriate response in patients receiving DMARDs including TNF-alpha blockers and an increase in titers following split-virion-inactivated influenza vaccine [62]. Moreover, a study examining the trivalent influenza vaccine found out higher titer rates in patients receiving methotrexate only compared to TNF-alpha blockers with or without methotrexate, which suggested that TNF-alpha blockers could potentially lower immunogenicity of the influenza vaccination [63]. Overall, it seems that TNF-alpha blockers have the potential in affecting the efficacy of response to influenza vaccinations in RA patients [62, 63].

Additionally, in certain treatments, timing plays a role in the ability of the vaccine to initiate an appropriate immune response. For example, patients treated with rituximab six to ten months prior to vaccination showed an increase in GMT and $CD19^+$ B-cell numbers [38], while patients who were treated with rituximab four to eight weeks prior to vaccination showed virtually no increase in GMT or $CD19^+$. Another study examining patients receiving methotrexate showed that those who stopped methotrexate two weeks prior to vaccination demonstrated greater response rates than those who did not stop methotrexate treatment [64].

In conclusion, medical literature suggests that the immune response to influenza vaccination in RA patients varies greatly and may or may not be affected by the variety of treatment options available; therefore, vaccine efficacy should be considered and determined on a case-by-case basis.

Influenza vaccine in dermatopolymyositis

The interrelationship between inflammatory myopathies and vaccination has been explored by multiple studies. A prospective study examining the nonadjuvanted, nonlive H1N1/2009 vaccine showcased no association with short-term (21 days) harmful effects in 37 dermatomyositis and 21 polymyositis patients with a mean age of 43.1 years [65]. Additionally, dermatopolymyositis patients receiving any of the variety maintenance drugs still displayed adequate immunogenicity and stable clinical parameters.

A prospective study conducted by Guissa et al. [66] evaluated the safety and efficacy of H1N1 vaccination in juvenile dermatomyositis patients. The study observed 30 patients with a mean age of 15.5 years and concluded that seroconversion was most prominently affected in chronic disease. Another study observing juvenile autoimmune rheumatic disease (ARD) (including juvenile dermatomyositis) found seroprotection to be lower in ARD patients and that glucocorticoid utilization was major factor in lowering antibody levels [67].

Influenza vaccine in fibromyalgia

The overlap among Golf ware syndrome, ASIA, and fibromyalgia suggests a potential role for vaccinations in the pathogenesis of the disorders [68]. For instance, the serum antibody titers of 19 fibromyalgia and 38 control patients who received the split-virion influenza were analyzed [69]. The sera of the patients were tested by hemagglutination (HI) against A/California (H1N1), A/Perth (H3N2), and B/Brisbane. The humoral response was determined to be either a fourfold or greater increase in titer or an increase from a nonprotective baseline level of 1/40. No adverse reactions and no changes in the fibromyalgia status of the patients were observed. The study concluded that influenza vaccination seemed to be both safe and effective in fibromyalgia syndrome patients.

Pneumococcal vaccine in AIRD patients

Infection is the major cause of mortality in AIRD patients with hospital admission due to infections for RA patients being doubled [70, 71]. The immunogenicity of the pneumococcal vaccines largely depends on whether vaccination covers the most common serotypes [72, 73]. The variations in serotypes are largely a reflection of the geography, concomitant diseases, age, vaccine, and antibiotic usage [72].

In a systematic review and meta-analysis aimed to check the immunogenicity, safety, and profile of the side effects related to anti-pneumococcal vaccination in patients with SLE, Adawi and friends concluded that immunization is recommended in all age groups of patients, with the priority given to patients who planned to initiate immunosuppressive treatment [74]. The authors based their conclusion on the risk of pneumococcal infection in this group of patients alongside tolerable side effects and safety profile of the vaccines. Furthermore, Elkayam et al. [75] analyzed antibody response in 42 patients with RA, 20 SLE patients, and 20 controls, following the administration of a single dose of the 23-valent pneumococcal vaccine. The vaccine showed no change in the disease status in neither SLE nor RA. Side effects were minor and limited to diffuse musculoskeletal pain in one patient with RA and pleuritic pain in one SLE patient. Immunogenicity was normal in all patients.

In a prospective, multicenter, double-blind, and randomized placebo control trail, Izumi and colleagues evaluated RA patients vaccinated with PPV-23 [76]. The study found no significant changes in the levels of pneumonia between patients treated with glucocorticoids, methotrexate, or even biological agents. In a meta-analysis that included 232 patients vaccinated by PPV-23 and 114 patients vaccinated by PCV-7, the response seemed to be decreased in RA patients treated with methotrexate and rituximab but remained efficient in TNF-alpha blockers [77]. Kapetanovic et al. [78] also concluded a decrease in efficacy of the PPV-23 vaccine in patients receiving methotrexate, while the efficacy remained normal in TNF-alpha blocker therapy.

Hepatitis B vaccine

HBV vaccine is a recombinant vaccine constituting viral surface antigens emulsified within aluminum hydroxide which serves as its antigen. The vaccine was initially utilized in the early 1980s and has since been linked to multiple adverse events, including immune ones [79, 80]. The WHO recommends vaccination against hepatitis B universally [81].

Recent EULAR recommendations allow nonlive vaccines such as the Hep B one to be used in AIRD patients including those receiving glucocorticoids or DMARD therapy [27].

HBV vaccine in SLE

Kuruma et al. [82] evaluated 28 female SLE patients who fulfilled the ACR classification criteria for SLE [83]. The inclusion criteria constituted of age and anti-dsDNA antibody positivity during the disease. Among the patients enrolled, only one had a positive test following vaccination, suggesting that the vaccine is not likely to induce this specific antibody. Moreover, none of the SLE patients had IgG or IgM anticardiolipin antibodies at baseline nor did they have the antibodies following vaccination. Overall, it seems that HBV vaccination is safe in SLE, and there is no evidence linking it to flares. Nevertheless, in an animal model, mice were vaccinated against HBV at 8 and 12 weeks of age and followed for kidney function among other parameters [84]. Aggravation of renal disease was reported following HBV vaccination. The results were related to the adjuvants added in the vaccine.

HBV vaccine in RA

A longitudinal open-label study examined 46 RA patients, 33 treated strictly with synthetic DMARDs, 13 who received both synthetic and biological DMARDs, and 9 healthy controls [85]. The patients were vaccinated with recombinant hepatitis B vaccines at weeks 0, 4, and 24. Antibody levels were measured eight weeks after the final dose. Seroprotection was decreased in RA patients versus controls (64% versus 100%), while patients receiving DMADs had 50% seroprotection; finally, patients receiving synthetic DMARDs had 69.97% seroprotection.

Elkayam et al. assessed the safety and antibody response of HBV vaccine in RA patients [86]. The study compared 22 patients who received three doses of the HBV vaccine with patients who did not receive the vaccine. No significant changes in patient clinical profiles following vaccination were detected. Of the 22 patients, 15 patients responded to vaccination (68%). Patients with poor response to vaccination tended to be older and experienced increase daytime pain following vaccination.

Quadrivalent HPV vaccine

Studies regarding the interactions between HPV vaccination and AIRD patients are limited. Reports in SLE patients indicated a higher risk of developing chronic HPV infections in comparison to healthy controls [87]. Moreover, SLE patients were found to more likely develop abnormal cervical smears [88, 89]. Two studies have further explored these associations. One is an open-label prospective, pre-postintervention study that examines 27 SLE patients, with 22 among them being juvenile SLE patients [90]. The study evaluated lab parameters, SLEDAI scores, and medications a year prior to the study. Only 20 patients completed the study, and among them, there was a significant decrease in SLEDAI scores (6.14 to 4.49) at seven months following administration of the vaccine. No changes were detected in anti-dsDNA titers and complement levels (C3 and C4) alongside the erythrocyte sedimentation rate which remained stable. Nine patients (33%) experienced flare-ups, five had arthralgia, four had rashes, two had pleuritis, and one had peripheral neuropathy. Regardless, the study declared HPV vaccination as safe and well tolerated in SLE, and HPV immunization was increased by 94% despite patients being treated with prednisone. The second study examined 50 stable SLE patients and 50 controls receiving the quadrivalent HPV vaccine [91]. At month 12, the seroconversion rates of anti-HPV serotypes 6, 11, 16, and 18 in SLE patients and healthy women were 82%, 89%, 95%, and 76% and 98%, 98%, 98%, and 80%, respectively. At the same period, no significant changes in anti-dsDNA titers were detected, and SLEDAI scores remained normal. At 0–2 months, 2 mild to moderate flares were detected; at 3–5 months, 6 mild to moderate and 2 severe flares were detected; finally, at 7–12 months, 2 severe flares were detected. A direct causality was not clearly established between the flares and the HPV vaccine. Seroconversion was 76% in HPV versus 93% in healthy controls.

Moreover, multiple cases of AIRD flare following HPV vaccine administration have been reported. These reports empowered the fact that in a certain small number of individuals, immunization can trigger autoimmunity [92–94].

Tetanus and diphtheria vaccines

An analysis aimed to evaluate vaccine efficacy by determining the IgG anti-diphtheria-antitoxin and tetanus-antitoxoid-IgG through ELISA-examined 279 SLE patients, 158 myasthenia gravis patients, and 208 healthy controls [95]. The study displayed similar responses and immunogenicity in all three groups. The serum concentration of anti-diphtheria antibodies decreased with age in all groups, while anti-tetanus antibodies dropped only in elderly (>60 years). A finding of interest was that in SLE patients (<40 years), the concentration was significantly lower than healthy controls. The study concluded that vaccine efficacy is similar in MG, SLE, and healthy controls.

In a study that dates back to 1984, 18 female patients with Hashimoto's disease were compared to 10 healthy female controls [96]. All participants received aluminum adjuvanted diphtheria-tetanus vaccine. The study detected no notable differences in the immunogenicity in the Hashimoto's disease and control groups. However, a marked rise in tetanus antibodies was observed in 7/10 of the controls and 9 of the patients with Hashimoto's disease. The controls displayed a negative correlation between antibody levels prior to the administration of the vaccine and increase in antibody levels postvaccination. Contrastingly, in Hashimoto's disease, there was no correlation between preimmunization levels and the increase in antibody levels following vaccination. It is thought that this inability to regulate antibody production in response to antigens that are continuously present is likely to have perilous consequences, and such a defect could be associated with the initiation and perpetuation of the autoimmune response in Hashimoto's disease.

References

1. Hak, E., Nordin, J., Wei, F. et al. (2002). Influence of high-risk medical conditions on the effectiveness of influenza vaccination among elderly members of 3 large managed-care organizations. *Clin. Infect. Dis.* 35 (4): 370–377.
2. Nichol, K.L., Wuorenma, J., and von Sternberg, T. (1998). Benefits of influenza vaccination for low-, intermediate-, and high-risk senior citizens. *Arch. Intern. Med.* 158 (16): 1769–1776.
3. van Assen, S., Elkayam, O., Agmon-Levin, N. et al. (2011). Vaccination in adult patients with auto-immune inflammatory rheumatic diseases: a systematic literature review for the European League Against Rheumatism evidence-based recommendations for vaccination in adult patients with auto-immune inflammatory rheumatic diseases. *Autoimmun. Rev.* 10 (6): 341–352.
4. Wotton, C.J. and Goldacre, M.J. (2012). Risk of invasive pneumococcal disease in people admitted to hospital with selected immune-mediated diseases: record linkage cohort analyses. *J. Epidemiol. Community Health* 66 (12): 1177–1181.
5. Danza, A. and Ruiz-Irastorza, G. (2013). Infection risk in systemic lupus erythematosus patients: susceptibility factors and preventive strategies. *Lupus* 22 (12): 1286–1294.
6. Bosch, X., Guilabert, A., Pallares, L. et al. (2006). Infections in systemic lupus erythematosus: a prospective and controlled study of 110 patients. *Lupus* 15 (9): 584–589.
7. Duffy, K.N., Duffy, C.M., and Gladman, D.D. (1991). Infection and disease activity in systemic lupus erythematosus: a review of hospitalized patients. *J. Rheumatol.* 18 (8): 1180–1184.
8. Gladman, D.D., Hussain, F., Ibanez, D., and Urowitz, M.B. (2002). The nature and outcome of infection in systemic lupus erythematosus. *Lupus* 11 (4): 234–239.
9. Goldblatt, F., Chambers, S., Rahman, A., and Isenberg, D.A. (2009). Serious infections in British patients with systemic lupus erythematosus: hospitalisations and mortality. *Lupus* 18 (8): 682–689.
10. Jeong, S.J., Choi, H., Lee, H.S. et al. (2009). Incidence and risk factors of infection in a single cohort of 110 adults with systemic lupus erythematosus. *Scand. J. Infect. Dis.* 41 (4): 268–274.
11. Pryor, B.D., Bologna, S.G., and Kahl, L.E. (1996). Risk factors for serious infection during treatment with cyclophosphamide and high-dose corticosteroids for systemic lupus erythematosus. *Arthritis Rheum.* 39 (9): 1475–1482.

12. Zonana-Nacach, A., Camargo-Coronel, A., Yanez, P. et al. (2001). Infections in outpatients with systemic lupus erythematosus: a prospective study. *Lupus* 10 (7): 505–510.
13. Galindo, M., Mateo, I., and Pablos, J.L. (2005). Multiple avascular necrosis of bone and polyarticular septic arthritis in patients with systemic lupus erythematosus. *Rheumatol. Int.* 25 (1): 72–76.
14. Abramson, S., Kramer, S.B., Radin, A., and Holzman, R. (1985). Salmonella bacteremia in systemic lupus erythematosus. Eight-year experience at a municipal hospital. *Arthritis Rheum.* 28 (1): 75–79.
15. Marcos, M., Fernandez, C., Soriano, A. et al. (2011). Epidemiology and clinical outcomes of bloodstream infections among lupus patients. *Lupus* 20 (9): 965–971.
16. Erdozain, J.G., Ruiz-Irastorza, G., Egurbide, M.V. et al. (2006). High risk of tuberculosis in systemic lupus erythematosus? *Lupus* 15 (4): 232–235.
17. Yamada, T., Nakajima, A., Inoue, E. et al. (2006). Increased risk of tuberculosis in patients with rheumatoid arthritis in Japan. *Ann. Rheum. Dis.* 65 (12): 1661–1663.
18. Gomez-Reino, J.J., Carmona, L., Valverde, V.R. et al. (2003). Treatment of rheumatoid arthritis with tumor necrosis factor inhibitors may predispose to significant increase in tuberculosis risk: a multicenter active-surveillance report. *Arthritis Rheum.* 48 (8): 2122–2127.
19. Brassard, P., Kezouh, A., and Suissa, S. (2006). Antirheumatic drugs and the risk of tuberculosis. *Clin. Infect. Dis.* 43 (6): 717–722.
20. Smitten, A.L., Choi, H.K., Hochberg, M.C. et al. (2008). The risk of hospitalized infection in patients with rheumatoid arthritis. *J. Rheumatol.* 35 (3): 387–393.
21. Jick, S.S., Lieberman, E.S., Rahman, M.U., and Choi, H.K. (2006). Glucocorticoid use, other associated factors, and the risk of tuberculosis. *Arthritis Rheum.* 55 (1): 19–26.
22. Wolfe, F., Michaud, K., Anderson, J., and Urbansky, K. (2004). Tuberculosis infection in patients with rheumatoid arthritis and the effect of infliximab therapy. *Arthritis Rheum.* 50 (2): 372–379.
23. Smitten, A.L., Choi, H.K., Hochberg, M.C. et al. (2007). The risk of herpes zoster in patients with rheumatoid arthritis in the United States and the United Kingdom. *Arthritis Rheum.* 57 (8): 1431–1438.
24. Kahl, L.E. (1994). Herpes zoster infections in systemic lupus erythematosus: risk factors and outcome. *J. Rheumatol.* 21 (1): 84–86.
25. Kang, T.Y., Lee, H.S., Kim, T.H. et al. (2005). Clinical and genetic risk factors of herpes zoster in patients with systemic lupus erythematosus. *Rheumatol. Int.* 25 (2): 97–102.
26. Manzi, S., Kuller, L.H., Kutzer, J. et al. (1995). Herpes zoster in systemic lupus erythematosus. *J. Rheumatol.* 22 (7): 1254–1258.
27. Jansen, M.H.A., Rondaan, C., Legger, G.E. et al. (2022). EULAR/PRES recommendations for vaccination of paediatric patients with autoimmune inflammatory rheumatic diseases: update 2021. *Ann. Rheum. Dis.* .
28. Blumentals, W.A., Arreglado, A., Napalkov, P., and Toovey, S. (2012). Rheumatoid arthritis and the incidence of influenza and influenza-related complications: a retrospective cohort study. *BMC Musculoskelet. Disord.* 13: 158.
29. Saad, C.G., Borba, E.F., Aikawa, N.E. et al. (2011). Immunogenicity and safety of the 2009 non-adjuvanted influenza A/H1N1 vaccine in a large cohort of autoimmune rheumatic diseases. *Ann. Rheum. Dis.* 70 (6): 1068–1073.
30. Shoenfeld, Y. and Agmon-Levin, N. (2011). 'ASIA' - autoimmune/inflammatory syndrome induced by adjuvants. *J. Autoimmun.* 36 (1): 4–8.
31. Friedman, M.A., Curtis, J.R., and Winthrop, K.L. (2021). Impact of disease-modifying antirheumatic drugs on vaccine immunogenicity in patients with inflammatory rheumatic and musculoskeletal diseases. *Ann. Rheum. Dis.* 80 (10): 1255–1265.
32. Adler, S., Krivine, A., Weix, J. et al. (2012). Protective effect of A/H1N1 vaccination in immune-mediated disease–a prospectively controlled vaccination study. *Rheumatology (Oxford)* 51 (4): 695–700.
33. Park, J.K., Lee, M.A., Lee, E.Y. et al. (2017). Effect of methotrexate discontinuation on efficacy of seasonal influenza vaccination in patients with rheumatoid arthritis: a randomised clinical trial. *Ann. Rheum. Dis.* 76 (9): 1559–1565.
34. Arad, U., Tzadok, S., Amir, S. et al. (2011). The cellular immune response to influenza vaccination is preserved in rheumatoid arthritis patients treated with rituximab. *Vaccine* 29 (8): 1643–1648.
35. Lakota, K., Perdan-Pirkmajer, K., Sodin-Semrl, S. et al. (2019). The immunogenicity of seasonal and pandemic influenza vaccination in autoimmune inflammatory rheumatic patients-a 6-month follow-up prospective study. *Clin. Rheumatol.* 38 (5): 1277–1292.

36. Nazi, I., Kelton, J.G., Larche, M. et al. (2013). The effect of rituximab on vaccine responses in patients with immune thrombocytopenia. *Blood* 122 (11): 1946–1953.
37. Ribeiro, A.C., Laurindo, I.M., Guedes, L.K. et al. (2013). Abatacept and reduced immune response to pandemic 2009 influenza A/H1N1 vaccination in patients with rheumatoid arthritis. *Arthritis Care Res.* 65 (3): 476–480.
38. van Assen, S., Holvast, A., Benne, C.A. et al. (2010). Humoral responses after influenza vaccination are severely reduced in patients with rheumatoid arthritis treated with rituximab. *Arthritis Rheum.* 62 (1): 75–81.
39. McNeil, M.M. (2019). Vaccine-associated anaphylaxis. *Curr. Treat Options Allergy.* 6 (3): 297–308.
40. Chang, C.C., Chang, Y.S., Chen, W.S. et al. (2016). Effects of annual influenza vaccination on morbidity and mortality in patients with Systemic Lupus Erythematosus: a nationwide cohort study. *Sci. Rep.* 6: 37817.
41. Stojanovich, L. (2006). Influenza vaccination of patients with systemic lupus erythematosus (SLE) and rheumatoid arthritis (RA). *Clin. Dev. Immunol.* 13 (2–4): 373–375.
42. Lu, C.C., Wang, Y.C., Lai, J.H. et al. (2011). A/H1N1 influenza vaccination in patients with systemic lupus erythematosus: safety and immunity. *Vaccine* 29 (3): 444–450.
43. Wallin, L., Quintilio, W., Locatelli, F. et al. (2009). Safety and efficiency of influenza vaccination in systemic lupus erythematosus patients. *Acta Reumatol. Port.* 34 (3): 498–502.
44. Holvast, A., Huckriede, A., Wilschut, J. et al. (2006). Safety and efficacy of influenza vaccination in systemic lupus erythematosus patients with quiescent disease. *Ann. Rheum. Dis.* 65 (7): 913–918.
45. Holvast, B., Huckriede, A., Kallenberg, C.G., and Bijl, M. (2007). Influenza vaccination in systemic lupus erythematosus: safe and protective? *Autoimmun. Rev.* 6 (5): 300–305.
46. Williams, G.W., Steinberg, A.D., Reinertsen, J.L. et al. (1978). Influenza immunization in systemic lupus eruthematosus. A double-blind trial. *Ann. Intern. Med.* 88 (6): 729–734.
47. Ristow, S.C., Douglas, R.G. Jr., and Condemi, J.J. (1978). Influenza vaccination of patients with systemic lupus erythematosus. *Ann. Intern. Med.* 88 (6): 786–789.
48. Holvast, A., van Assen, S., de Haan, A. et al. (2009). Effect of a second, booster, influenza vaccination on antibody responses in quiescent systemic lupus erythematosus: an open, prospective, controlled study. *Rheumatology (Oxford)* 48 (10): 1294–1299.
49. de Jong, J.C., Palache, A.M., Beyer, W.E. et al. (2003). Haemagglutination-inhibiting antibody to influenza virus. *Dev. Biol. (Basel)* 115: 63–73.
50. Gross, P.A., Hermogenes, A.W., Sacks, H.S. et al. (1995). The efficacy of influenza vaccine in elderly persons. A meta-analysis and review of the literature. *Ann. Intern. Med.* 123 (7): 518–527.
51. Mercado, U., Acosta, H., and Avendano, L. (2004). Influenza vaccination of patients with systemic lupus erythematosus. *Rev. Investig. Clin.* 56 (1): 16–20.
52. Heijstek, M.W., Ott de Bruin, L.M., Borrow, R. et al. (2011). Vaccination in paediatric patients with autoimmune rheumatic diseases: a systemic literature review for the European League against Rheumatism evidence-based recommendations. *Autoimmun. Rev.* 11 (2): 112–122.
53. Aron-Maor, A. and Shoenfeld, Y. (2001). Vaccination and systemic lupus erythematosus: the bidirectional dilemmas. *Lupus* 10 (3): 237–240.
54. Perdan-Pirkmajer, K., Thallinger, G.G., Snoj, N. et al. (2012). Autoimmune response following influenza vaccination in patients with autoimmune inflammatory rheumatic disease. *Lupus* 21 (2): 175–183.
55. Abu-Shakra, M., Zalmanson, S., Neumann, L. et al. (2000). Influenza virus vaccination of patients with systemic lupus erythematosus: effects on disease activity. *J. Rheumatol.* 27 (7): 1681–1685.
56. Older, S.A., Battafarano, D.F., Enzenauer, R.J., and Krieg, A.M. (1999). Can immunization precipitate connective tissue disease? Report of five cases of systemic lupus erythematosus and review of the literature. *Semin. Arthritis Rheum.* 29 (3): 131–139.
57. Vista, E.S., Crowe, S.R., Thompson, L.F. et al. (2012). Influenza vaccination can induce new-onset anticardiolipins but not beta2-glycoprotein-I antibodies among patients with systemic lupus erythematosus. *Lupus* 21 (2): 168–174.
58. Hess, E.V. and Hahn, V. (1978). Influenza immunization in lupus erythematosus: safe, effective? *Ann. Intern. Med.* 88 (6): 833–834.
59. Del Porto, F., Lagana, B., Biselli, R. et al. (2006). Influenza vaccine administration in patients with systemic lupus erythematosus and rheumatoid arthritis. Safety and immunogenicity. *Vaccine* 24 (16): 3217–3223.

60. Chen, C.M., Chen, H.J., Chen, W.S. et al. (2018). Clinical effectiveness of influenza vaccination in patients with rheumatoid arthritis. *Int. J. Rheum. Dis.* 21 (6): 1246–1253.
61. Alten, R., Bingham, C.O. 3rd, Cohen, S.B. et al. (2016). Antibody response to pneumococcal and influenza vaccination in patients with rheumatoid arthritis receiving abatacept. *BMC Musculoskelet. Disord.* 17: 231.
62. Fomin, I., Caspi, D., Levy, V. et al. (2006). Vaccination against influenza in rheumatoid arthritis: the effect of disease modifying drugs, including TNF alpha blockers. *Ann. Rheum. Dis.* 65 (2): 191–194.
63. Kapetanovic, M.C., Saxne, T., Nilsson, J.A., and Geborek, P. (2007). Influenza vaccination as model for testing immune modulation induced by anti-TNF and methotrexate therapy in rheumatoid arthritis patients. *Rheumatology (Oxford)* 46 (4): 608–611.
64. Mehta, P., Sanchez, E., Moraitis, E. et al. (2021). Influenza vaccination and interruption of methotrexate in adult patients in the COVID-19 era: an ongoing dilemma. *Lancet Rheumatol.* 3 (1): e9–e10.
65. Shinjo, S.K., de Moraes, J.C., Levy-Neto, M. et al. (2012). Pandemic unadjuvanted influenza A (H1N1) vaccine in dermatomyositis and polymyositis: immunogenicity independent of therapy and no harmful effect in disease. *Vaccine* 31 (1): 202–206.
66. Guissa, V.R., Pereira, R.M., Sallum, A.M. et al. (2012). Influenza A H1N1/2009 vaccine in juvenile dermatomyositis: reduced immunogenicity in patients under immunosuppressive therapy. *Clin. Exp. Rheumatol.* 30 (4): 583–588.
67. Aikawa, N.E., Campos, L.M., Silva, C.A. et al. (2012). Glucocorticoid: major factor for reduced immunogenicity of 2009 influenza A (H1N1) vaccine in patients with juvenile autoimmune rheumatic disease. *J. Rheumatol.* 39 (1): 167–173.
68. Watad, A., Quaresma, M., Bragazzi, N.L. et al. (2018). The autoimmune/inflammatory syndrome induced by adjuvants (ASIA)/Shoenfeld's syndrome: descriptive analysis of 300 patients from the international ASIA syndrome registry. *Clin. Rheumatol.* 37 (2): 483–493.
69. Ablin, J.N., Aloush, V., Brill, A. et al. (2015). Influenza vaccination is safe and effective in patients suffering from fibromyalgia syndrome. *Reumatismo.* 67 (2): 57–61.
70. Franklin, J., Lunt, M., Bunn, D. et al. (2007). Risk and predictors of infection leading to hospitalisation in a large primary-care-derived cohort of patients with inflammatory polyarthritis. *Ann. Rheum. Dis.* 66 (3): 308–312.
71. Hernandez-Cruz, B., Cardiel, M.H., Villa, A.R., and Alcocer-Varela, J. (1998). Development, recurrence, and severity of infections in Mexican patients with rheumatoid arthritis. A nested case-control study. *J. Rheumatol.* 25 (10): 1900–1907.
72. Hausdorff, W.P., Bryant, J., Paradiso, P.R., and Siber, G.R. (2000). Which pneumococcal serogroups cause the most invasive disease: implications for conjugate vaccine formulation and use, part I. *Clin. Infect. Dis.* 30 (1): 100–121.
73. O'Brien, K.L., Wolfson, L.J., Watt, J.P. et al. (2009). Burden of disease caused by Streptococcus pneumoniae in children younger than 5 years: global estimates. *Lancet* 374 (9693): 893–902.
74. Adawi, M., Bragazzi, N.L., McGonagle, D. et al. (2019). Immunogenicity, safety and tolerability of anti-pneumococcal vaccination in systemic lupus erythematosus patients: an evidence-informed and PRISMA compliant systematic review and meta-analysis. *Autoimmun. Rev.* 18 (1): 73–92.
75. Elkayam, O., Paran, D., Caspi, D. et al. (2002). Immunogenicity and safety of pneumococcal vaccination in patients with rheumatoid arthritis or systemic lupus erythematosus. *Clin. Infect. Dis.* 34 (2): 147–153.
76. Izumi, Y., Akazawa, M., Akeda, Y. et al. (2017). The 23-valent pneumococcal polysaccharide vaccine in patients with rheumatoid arthritis: a double-blinded, randomized, placebo-controlled trial. *Arthritis Res. Ther.* 19 (1): 15.
77. Hua, C., Barnetche, T., Combe, B., and Morel, J. (2014). Effect of methotrexate, anti-tumor necrosis factor alpha, and rituximab on the immune response to influenza and pneumococcal vaccines in patients with rheumatoid arthritis: a systematic review and meta-analysis. *Arthritis Care Res.* 66 (7): 1016–1026.
78. Kapetanovic, M.C., Saxne, T., Sjoholm, A. et al. (2006). Influence of methotrexate, TNF blockers and prednisolone on antibody responses to pneumococcal polysaccharide vaccine in patients with rheumatoid arthritis. *Rheumatology (Oxford)* 45 (1): 106–111.
79. Mikaeloff, Y., Caridade, G., Suissa, S., and Tardieu, M. (2009). Hepatitis B vaccine and the risk of CNS inflammatory demyelination in childhood. *Neurology* 72 (10): 873–880.
80. Stubgen, J.P. (2010). Neuromuscular disorders associated with Hepatitis B vaccination. *J. Neurol. Sci.* 292 (1–2): 1–4.

81. (2004). Hepatitis B vaccines. *Wkly Epidemiol. Rec.* 79 (28): 255–263.
82. Kuruma, K.A., Borba, E.F., Lopes, M.H. et al. (2007). Safety and efficacy of hepatitis B vaccine in systemic lupus erythematosus. *Lupus* 16 (5): 350–354.
83. Hochberg, M.C. (1997). Updating the American College of Rheumatology revised criteria for the classification of systemic lupus erythematosus. *Arthritis Rheum.* 40 (9): 1725.
84. Agmon-Levin, N., Arango, M.T., Kivity, S. et al. (2014). Immunization with hepatitis B vaccine accelerates SLE-like disease in a murine model. *J. Autoimmun.* 54: 21–32.
85. Intongkam, S., Samakarnthai, P., Pakchotanon, R. et al. (2019). Efficacy and safety of hepatitis B vaccination in rheumatoid arthritis patients receiving disease-modifying antirheumatic drugs and/or biologics therapy. *J. Clin. Rheumatol.* 25 (8): 329–334.
86. Elkayam, O., Yaron, M., and Caspi, D. (2002). Safety and efficacy of vaccination against hepatitis B in patients with rheumatoid arthritis. *Ann. Rheum. Dis.* 61 (7): 623–625.
87. Klumb, E.M., Pinto, A.C., Jesus, G.R. et al. (2010). Are women with lupus at higher risk of HPV infection? *Lupus* 19 (13): 1485–1491.
88. Blumenfeld, Z., Lorber, M., Yoffe, N., and Scharf, Y. (1994). Systemic lupus erythematosus: predisposition for uterine cervical dysplasia. *Lupus* 3 (1): 59–61.
89. Nyberg, G., Eriksson, O., and Westberg, N.G. (1981). Increased incidence of cervical atypia in women with systemic lupus erythematosus treated with chemotherapy. *Arthritis Rheum.* 24 (5): 648–650.
90. Soybilgic, A., Onel, K.B., Utset, T. et al. (2013). Safety and immunogenicity of the quadrivalent HPV vaccine in female Systemic Lupus Erythematosus patients aged 12 to 26 years. *Pediatr Rheumatol. Online J.* 11: 29.
91. Mok, C.C., Ho, L.Y., Fong, L.S., and To, C.H. (2013). Immunogenicity and safety of a quadrivalent human papillomavirus vaccine in patients with systemic lupus erythematosus: a case-control study. *Ann. Rheum. Dis.* 72 (5): 659–664.
92. Gatto, M., Agmon-Levin, N., Soriano, A. et al. (2013). Human papillomavirus vaccine and systemic lupus erythematosus. *Clin. Rheumatol.* 32 (9): 1301–1307.
93. Melo Gomes, S., Glover, M., Malone, M., and Brogan, P. (2013). Vasculitis following HPV immunization. *Rheumatology (Oxford)* 52 (3): 581–582.
94. Soldevilla, H.F., Briones, S.F., and Navarra, S.V. (2012). Systemic lupus erythematosus following HPV immunization or infection? *Lupus* 21 (2): 158–161.
95. Csuka, D., Czirjak, L., Hobor, R. et al. (2013). Effective humoral immunity against diphtheria and tetanus in patients with systemic lupus erythematosus or myasthenia gravis. *Mol. Immunol.* 54 (3–4): 453–456.
96. Fawcett, J., Hutton, C., McLachlan, S.M. et al. (1984). Defective regulation of the immune response to tetanus toxoid in Hashimoto's disease. *Immunology* 52 (3): 525–528.

18 Autoimmune Phenomena in Cancer Patients Treated with Immune Checkpoint Inhibitors

Milena Tocut[1,2], Michael Ehrenfeld[2,3], and Gisele Zandman-Goddard[1,2]

[1]Department of Internal Medicine C, Wolfson Medical Center, Holon, Israel
[2]Sackler Faculty of Medicine, Tel Aviv University, Tel Aviv, Israel
[3]Zabludowicz Center for Autoimmune Diseases, Sheba Medical Center, Tel-Hashomer, Israel

Introduction

One of the multiple roles of the immune system is to maintain the equilibrium between cell proliferation and cell death resulting from a fine-tuned interplay of costimulatory and inhibitory pathways [1].

The inhibitory pathways, or the immune checkpoints, preserve self-tolerance and thus prevent autoimmune reactions. T-cell exhaustion is a main contributor to loss of immune equilibrium, followed by tumors development. Exhausted T-cell traits include loss of production of interleukin 2 (IL-2) and other pro-inflammatory cytokines and reduced T-cell proliferation and cytotoxic effect [2]. In addition, T-cell exhaustion enhances expression of immune checkpoints such as PD-1 and CTLA-4. The relationship between T-cell function and checkpoint inhibitors expression is inverse, regarding physiologic mechanisms [1–3].

Immune checkpoint inhibitors (ICIs) or immune-modulatory antibodies have revolutionized the therapy of several particular types of cancers. Antitumor immunity is enhanced by the agent's checkpoint inhibition target, negative regulators, on T cells and are represented by cytotoxic T lymphocytes-associated antigen 4 (CTLA-4), antiprogrammed death (PD)-1, and PD-ligand (L)-1 [4]. Removal of self-tolerance increases the risk to develop autoimmunity, followed by an immune-driven inflammatory toxicity, resulting in immune-related adverse events (irAEs). IrAEs could be systemic, affecting multiple organs of the body, presenting with a mild to fatal forms of clinical manifestations, which further warrant the discontinuation of ICIs therapy [5, 6].

To date, three target ICIs are part of the immune-modulatory therapy. The CTLA-4, PD-1, and PD-L1 pathways mediate immune response at different levels. CTLA-4 controls the amplitude of immunologic response at early stages of T-cell activation, whereas PD-1 and PD-L1 pathways act at

Autoimmune Disorders: Adjuvants and Other Risk Factors in Pathogenesis, First Edition.
Edited by Abdulla Watad, Nicola Luigi Bragazzi, and Yehuda Shoenfeld.

later stages by limiting T-cell activity in the peripheral tissues. These differences partly explain variations in toxicity profiles among anti-CTLA-4, anti-PD-1, and anti-PD-L1 agents and the higher frequency and severity seen with anti-CTAL-4 agents [7].

Ipilimumab (Yervoy), an anti-CTLA-4 antibody, is a negative regulator of T-cell activation by blocking the B7 binding to CTLA-4 downregulatory receptor. Thus, it leads to its unopposed engagement with the positive costimulatory receptor CD28 and subsequent T-cell activation. The negative signal for T-cell activation is enhanced by the binding of CTLA-4 on native T cells in the lymph nodes to B7 and in the antigen-presenting cell (APC) to CD28. The CTLA-4 antibody leads to a vigorous costimulatory signal to all T cells that will combat the overexpressed checkpoint inhibitors. Ipilimumab is primarily used in melanoma [7, 8].

PD-1 and its ligands, PD-L1 and PD-L2, are among the key factors responsible for the inhibitory T-cell signaling, mediating mechanisms of tolerance as well as providing immune homeostasis [9]. The PD-1 and PD-L1 are transmembrane protein receptors expressed on immune T cells, B cells, and natural killer (NK) cells, which regulated IL-12 and interferon (IFN)-gamma cytokines. These agents disturb downregulatory signaling mediated through direct tumor–T-cell interactions [10]. Nivolumab (Opdivo), pembrolizumab (Keytruda), and cemiplimab (Libtayo) are antiprogrammed death PD-1 receptors. Atezolizumab (Tecentriq), avelumab (Bavencio), and durvalumab (Imfinzi) are anti-PD-L1 receptors that block the additional inhibitory pathways followed by increased T-cell activation [11]. The PD1/L1 agents are used in renal cell carcinoma (RCC), melanoma, Hodgkin lymphoma, and nonmetastatic and metastatic non-small cell lung carcinoma (NSCLC) [10, 11].

irAEs reports after ICIs therapy resemble nonclassic autoimmune diseases such as arthritis, nephritis, sicca syndrome, myositis, and polymyalgia-like syndromes [12]. The expanding use of ICIs and the autoimmune consequences of these therapies are only beginning to be fully understood [13].

Incidence and autoimmune irAEs

Reports of irAEs increase linearly with the expanding administration of ICIs. The incidence of irAEs is influenced by several factors including ICIs drug mechanism, initial dosage, mono versus combined therapy, and the final accumulated dosage [14]. The general characteristics of irAEs after ICIs therapy resulting from large cohort trials indicate that incidence of irAEs is higher in patients receiving therapy with an anti-CTLA-4 antibody agent (dose dependent) than in patients treated with a PD-1/PD-L1 antibody agent (dose independent). In addition, lower incidence rates of irAEs were noted in patients who received monotherapy in comparison to combined therapy with CTLA-4 and PD-1 inhibitors [3]. The overall incidence of irAEs that are autoimmune in nature is only 5% [14].

The most frequent irAEs are represented by colitis (25–30%), dermatitis (15–30%), endocrinopathies (5–15%), and pneumonitis (3–5%). ICIs induction of autoimmune colitis has the same clinical and endoscopic features of inflammatory bowel disease. The treatment is the same and was reported to be as effective [15]. Pneumonitis secondary to ICI therapy was also proven to have autoimmune traits, which were proven by bronchoscopy that revealed a lymphocyte-predominant alveolitis. While other pulmonary involvements had been recognized, pneumonitis remains the most severe and life-threatening clinical manifestation [16].

Autoimmune and musculoskeletal irAEs reported include arthralgia and arthritis. Arthralgia irAEs after nivolumab and ipilimumab mono and combined therapy have an incidence rate of 1–43% [1, 2, 17]. In a melanoma trial with 945 patients, arthralgia had an incidence rate of 6.1% in patients treated with ipilimumab ($n = 315$) and 7.7% in patients treated with nivolumab ($n = 316$). ICIs combination therapy with ipilimumab and nivolumab increased the irAEs incidence rate to 10.5% ($n = 314$) as was reported in other similar trials [18]. In another single-center retrospective study of 98 patients treated with ICI, arthralgia was reported with an incidence of 11% after a median of 63 days [19]. Myalgia and muscle weakness following ICIs therapy were also reported. A study that included 33 patients treated with ICI monotherapy reported a myalgia incidence rate of 2–18% [20]. In contrast, muscle weakness after mono or combined ICI therapy was reported in only 1% of patients in a trial of 245 patients and in 12% of patients in a trial of 33 patients who received nivolumab and peptide vaccine combined therapy [21].

Severe irAEs are reported as high as 27% with anti-CTLA-4 compared with 16% with anti-PD-1 agents and may increase to 55% when both therapies are utilized in combination. Fatal and life-threatening irAEs range between 0.36% and 1.23%. Anti-PD-1 has the lowest fatal irAEs incidence rate, whereas combination therapy with anti-PD-1/PDL-1 and anti-CTLA4 has the greatest reported fatal irAEs incidence rate [22].

Inflammatory arthritis

The two major clinical entities observed are polymyalgia rheumatica (PMR)-like syndromes and inflammatory arthritis (IA). The broad spectrum of rheumatologic irAEs includes arthralgia, monoarthritis, oligoarthritis, polyarthritis, psoriatic arthritis, reactive arthritis, remitting seronegative symmetrical synovitis with pitting edema, tenosynovitis, and enthesitis. An overall of 3–7.5% of the patients with ICIs therapy have presented with clinical manifestation of polyarthritis or arthralgia [14, 19, 23, 24]. The joints reported to be involved most frequently were the shoulders, metacarpophalangeal (MCP) joints, and proximal interphalangeal (PIP) joints (50%), followed by the knees (40%), hips, elbows, ankles, and feet [25].

Synovial fluid analysis reveals in most cases a clear inflammatory reaction with polymorphonuclear leucocytes predominance, although lymphocytes were also described. Inflammatory serum markers were elevated in two-thirds of the cases. Antinuclear antibody (ANA), rheumatoid factor (RF), and anti-cyclic-citrullinated peptide antibody (anti-CCP) could be positive, though in rare cases [26]. IA imaging by ultrasound and magnetic resonance imaging (MRI) demonstrated synovitis with inflammatory Doppler features, tenosynovitis, effusions, bone erosions, and enthesitis [27].

To date, IA as part of irAEs was described in case series and retrospective cohort studies [17, 28, 29]. One study reported 13 patients with different types of cancers including melanoma, RCC, small cell, and non-small cell lung carcinoma, who were treated with nivolumab or ipilimumab. Nine patients were reported with IA involving axial joint with negative RF, anti-CCP, and ANA serologic studies. The synovial fluid analysis had inflammatory traits and was further investigated by ultrasound and MRI which also showed joint erosions. Two patients had symptoms suggestive of reactive arthritis. Two patients expressed symptoms resembling reactive arthritis with conjunctivitis, dactylitis, urethritis, and large joint oligo-arthritis, and one patient had large joint polyarthritis resembling spondyloarthritis. Three months after ICI therapy, six patients developed rheumatoid arthritis (RA)-like manifestations with symmetric synovitis of the small hand articulations and large joint involvement [13].

One other study was a nationwide multicenter cohort that included 117 patients, which described 136 irAEs. Forty five patients had symmetric polyarthritis, and 17 patients had PMR-like symptoms. In this study, seronegative symmetric polyarthritis was the most common irAEs supporting other studies that reported rheumatologic manifestations to be the most common irAEs [30]. One more case control study of 8028 patients who were treated with ICI for melanoma and genitourinary malignancies reported 226 patients with rheumatologic irAEs. De novo IA was reported in 118 patients and was more common after combined ICI therapy [31].

Sicca syndrome/Sjögren's syndrome

Altogether, 13% of patients experiencing sicca syndrome were reported to fulfill classification criteria for primary Sjögren's syndrome induced by ICIs. Dry eyes were noted in a trial with 30 patients after combined ICI therapy with ipilimumab in 3% of the patients. Induced dry mouth that was nivolumab dose related was reported in 3–11% of 168 RCC patients. Most cases are anti-RO and anti-LA sero-negative [32, 33].

In a big data study, among 26 patients who received monotherapy with anti-PD-1 and anti-PD-L1 (77% of patients) for lung cancer, melanoma, and other malignancies, dry mouth was noted in 25% of the patients and dry eyes in 17% of patients. Pathologic ocular and oral diagnostic tests were present in 62% and 86% of the patients, respectively. Dry eyes and mouth were not associated with anti-CTLA-4 therapy in this trial [33]. Two more single case reports after ICI therapy were of Sjögren parotitis that responded to steroid therapy and a case of sensory neuropathy with a salivary gland biopsy that confirmed Sjögren's syndrome secondary to pembrolizumab therapy [34].

Myositis and neurological diseases

Several patients, yet less than 1% treated with anti-PD-1/PD-L1, were diagnosed with myositis/polymyositis reported as potentially life-threatening complications. Symptoms include acute or subacute myalgia (38%) and proximal muscle weakness (50%). Other symptoms include oculomotor and bulbar symptoms as well as dyspnea and concurrent critical myocarditis. Associated myasthenia gravis has been described infrequently (up to 15%) [35, 36]. Cases described with myositis had a markedly elevated creatine phosphokinase (CPK) level, though myositis-associated autoantibodies were usually negative. In rare case reports, ANA, anti-Sm, anti-Scl 70, or anti-Jo1 was reported in irAEs-related myositis [13].

Cases of dermatomyositis (DM) were reported after therapy with anti-CTLA-4 and anti-PD-1/PD-L1 [37–41]. The most common symptom is represented by proximal muscle weakness followed by neck weakness, respiratory weakness, and, in rare cases, myocarditis. On blood laboratory tests, CPK is elevated, and rhabdomyolysis may also occur. DM antibodies such as anti-Jo1 are negative. Electromyography shows myopathic patterns, and muscle biopsy depicts inflammation and necrosis.

A fatal case of autoimmune myositis, with positive serologic PL-12-B (alanyl-tRNA snythetase antibodies) and SRP-B antibodies, 26 days after nivolumab therapy was reported. The patients presented with third-degree atrioventricular block and rhabdomyolysis followed by multiorgan failure and death [39]. A few cases of inflammatory myositis with fasciitis were documented [41, 42]. Another example is of a patient who presented with painful symmetrical edema and thickening of the skin of the lower extremities, followed by plantar fascia fibrosis with symptomatic contractures. The diagnosis was confirmed by skin and muscle biopsy, which revealed an inflammatory lymphocyte infiltrate and eosinophils in the plantar fascia [42]. To date, only one case of necrotizing myositis was documented after ICI combination therapy in a patient with metastatic colorectal cancer [43].

Autoimmune diseases

Vasculitis

ICI-induced vasculitis reported so far includes cases of cutaneous leucocytoclastic vasculitis [44], granulomatosis with polyangiitis [45], eosinophilic granulomatosis with polyangiitis, cryoglobulinemic vasculitis, giant cell vasculitis (GCA), and PMR. Serologic tests for cryoglobulins, ANA, ANCA (antineutrophilic antibody), and RF are rarely positive [22]. A meta-analysis reported that GCA, aortitis without other manifestations, and nervous system vasculitis that manifested with angiitis of the central and peripheral nerves were the most common irAEs seen three months after ICI therapy [46].

GCA and PMR were documented in two case reports after CTLA-4 inhibitors therapy. A patient with metastatic melanoma who was treated with ipilimumab presented with arthralgia, morning stiffness, trismus, and left side facial swelling three months after ICI therapy. Diagnostic confirmation of GCA was made by temporal artery biopsy [47]. Also noted were case reports of single-organ vasculitis following ICI therapy, including retinal vasculitis [48], lymphocytic vasculitis of the uterus [49], and aortitis vasculitis [50].

Systemic lupus erythematosus

Anti-PD-L1-induced systemic lupus erythematosus (SLE) has a prevalence of 0.48%, and until 2017, only five cases were reported, after a median time of 10 weeks following anti-PD-L1 therapy. Four patients had subacute cutaneous lupus, and one patient had chilblain lupus. Two patients had clinical criteria for SLE with high titers of ANA, dsDNA, and anti-SSA/SSB without clinical manifestations of Sjögren's syndrome including dry eyes and mouth [51]. A sole case of lupus nephritis was reported after ipilimumab therapy for metastatic melanoma. The patient presented with a new onset of nephrotic range proteinuria. Following investigation, increased titers of anti-ds DNA antibodies were found. The kidney biopsy was consistent with type I lupus nephritis. The immunofluorescence study of the renal tissue showed extramembranous and mesangial deposits of IgG, IgM, C3, and C1q. Further confirmation was made by electron microscopy revealing the presence of granular, electron-dense extramembranous deposits; all these findings supported the diagnosis of type I lupus nephritis. It was noted that after ipilimumab therapy was discontinued, anti-ds DNA titers diminished dramatically [52].

Sarcoidosis

A broad spectrum of irAEs has been rapidly expanding, with the description of various other systemic manifestations, which include sarcoidosis or sarcoid-like reactions, which are by far the most commonly described for both anti-CTLA-4 and PD-1/PD-L1 therapies [53]. Most reported cases have skin and pulmonary clinical manifestations [54]. Upon tissue biopsy, granulomatous inflammation is observed. Other sarcoid organ involvements after ICI therapy were yet to be reported [55].

Organ-specific irAEs determined by specific ICI

Single-organ irAEs are more frequently encountered than systemic irAEs. A meta-analysis of 81 articles published from 22 clinical trials described ICI-induced irAEs investigating systemic involvement in a total of 1265 patients. The irAEs were described from the most common to the least common as follows: dermatologic, vitiligo and dermatitis (44%); gastrointestinal, diarrhea and colitis similar to Crohn's disease (35%); endocrine, hypothyroidism more than hyperthyroidism (6%); and hepatic, hepatitis (5%). Neurologic, ophthalmologic, hematologic, and autoimmune irAEs were rare [14, 56].

A systematic review that included 251 cases reported that organ-specific irAEs were correlated to the ICI agent used. After ipilimumab therapy (234 patients), gastrointestinal irAEs including colitis, hepatitis, and pancreatitis predominated (39.7%), followed by endocrine irAEs such as hypophysitis, hypothyroidism, thyrotoxicosis, and adrenal insufficiency (29.1%). Neurologic, ophthalmic, hematologic, and autoimmune irAEs were rare. The most common related irAEs to pembrolizumab were cutaneous (30%), while nivolumab most common related irAEs were endocrine and pneumonitis that had an equal incidence rate (42.9%). Pembrolizumab and nivolumab gastrointestinal irAEs were not documented [9].

Management and treatment of autoimmune irAEs

Guidelines for managing irAEs were published by the American Society of Clinical Oncology in 2018. These guidelines, based on over 200 publications, are created on a consensus of a multiorganizational panel of experts in all fields related to the irAEs [57]. The severity of each irAEs was quantified by grades from 1 to 4 (based on the Common Terminology Criteria for Adverse Events, published in 2010). In general, low-grade irAEs (grades 1–2) are mild to moderate, do not require hospitalization, and should be treated symptomatically. Higher-grade irAEs are severe to life threatening and typically require hospital admission to observe patients closely and assure that they are responding to therapy [57, 58].

Corticosteroids are the mainstay for low-severity irAEs, administered at a low dose of 0.5–1mg/kg day, for moderate grade 1–2mg/kg/day, and high-dose steroids 2mg/kg/day for severe and life-threatening grades. After resolution of irAE, tapering of corticosteroids dose is recommended [4, 59, 60].

Nonsteroidal anti-inflammatory drugs, intraarticular steroid injections, and nonbiologic disease modifying antirheumatic drugs (DMARDS) such as methotrexate, leflunomide, hydroxychloroquine, and sulfasalazine may be a suitable treatment in mild grade 1 irAEs without discontinuation of ICI therapy [61–63]. For more severe grades of irAEs (grades 3–4), or when irAEs do not resolve with the use of corticosteroids, biologic therapy may be considered, such as TNF inhibitors, anti-IL6, abatacept, anti-IL1, anti-CD20, anti-IL17, and anti-IL23 and 12, as well as intravenous immunoglobulins (IVIG) and Janus kinase (JAK) inhibitors, which have all been described as having a positive effect on the higher-grade irAEs [64–66]. In general, cancer immunotherapy may be continued while most grade 1 events are managed. For grade 2–4 events, immunotherapy should be withheld and can be reinitiated once the irAEs resolve although permanent discontinuation is sometimes warranted [64].

The discontinuation of ICI therapy is recommended for specific cases such as moderate symptoms (grade 2) that persist for at least six weeks (not applicable for endocrinopathies managed properly with hormone replacement) or moderate to severe (grades 2–4) ocular manifestations failing to improve to mild symptoms (grade 1) with topical immunosuppression or systemic therapy after two weeks of therapy or failure to taper glucocorticoids to a dose of 7.5–10mg/day prednisone within 12weeks [4, 67].

Summary

ICIs therapy targeting CTLA-4 and PD-1/PDL-1 are revolutionary in their impact on cancer survival. A significant number of patients on ICI develop irAEs affecting a wide variety of organs. As the incidence of autoimmune irAEs will probably increase after widespread utilization of ICI therapy, a collaboration of oncology and rheumatology physicians will be mandatory for prompt detection, monitoring, and treatment according to guidelines.

It is not clear whether ICI irAEs are distinct from conventional autoimmune diseases or whether the manifestations of irAEs are associated with therapeutic efficacy.

References

1. Cappelli, L.C., Shah, A.A., and Bingham, C.O. (2017). Immune-related adverse effects of cancer immunotherapy – implications for rheumatology. *Rheum. Dis. Clin. N. Am.* 43: 65–78.
2. Yoest, J.M. (2017). Clinical features, predictive correlates, and pathophysiology of immune-related adverse events in immune checkpoint inhibitor treatments in cancer: a short review. *Immunotargets Ther.* 10: 73–82.
3. Dyck, L. and Mills, K.H.G. (2017). Immune checkpoints and their inhibition in cancer and infectious diseases. *Eur. J. Immunol.* 47: 765–779.
4. Kumar, V., Chaudhary, N., Garg, M. et al. (2017). Current diagnosis and management of immune related adverse events (irAEs) induced by immune checkpoint inhibitor therapy. *Front. Pharmacol.* 8: 8–49.
5. Friedman, C.F., Proverbs-Singh, T.A., and Postow, M.A. (2016). Treatment of the immune-related adverse effects of immune checkpoint inhibitors: a review. *JAMA Oncol.* 1: 1346–1353.
6. Day, D. and Hansen, A.R. (2016). Immune-related adverse events associated with immune checkpoint inhibitors. *BioDrugs* 30: 571–584.
7. June, C.H., Warshauer, J.T., and Bluestone, J.A. (2017). Is autoimmunity the Achilles' heel of cancer immunotherapy? *Nat. Med.* 23: 540–547.
8. Cappelli, L.C. and Bingham, C.O. (2021). Spectrum and impact of checkpoint inhibitor-induced irAEs. *Nat. Rev. Rheumatol.* 17: 69–70.

9. Tocut, M., Brenner, R., and Zandman-Goddard, G. (2018). Autoimmune phenomena and disease in cancer patients treated with immune checkpoint inhibitors. *Autoimmun. Rev.* 17: 610–616.
10. Topalian, S.L., Drake, C.G., and Pardoll, D.M. (2015). Immune checkpoint blockade: a common denominator approach to cancer therapy. *Cancer Cell* 27: 450–461.
11. Chan, K.K. and Bass, A.R. (2020). Autoimmune complications of immune checkpoint inhibitors for cancer. *BMJ* 369: 736.
12. Chan, M.M.K., Kefford, R.F., Carlino, M. et al. (2015). Arthritis and tenosynovitis associated with the anti-PD1 antibody pembrolizumab in metastatic melanoma. *J. Immunother.* 38: 37–39.
13. Cappelli, L.C., Gutierrez, A.K., Baer, A.N. et al. (2017). Inflammatory arthritis and sicca syndrome induced by nivolumab and ipilimumab. *Ann. Rheum. Dis.* 76: 43–50.
14. Jiang, Y., Zhang, N., Pang, H. et al. (2019). Risk and incidence of fatal adverse events associated with immune checkpoint inhibitors: a systematic review and meta-analysis. *Ther. Clin. Risk Manag.* 15: 293–302.
15. Prieux-Klotz, C., Dior, M., Damotte, D. et al. (2017). Immune checkpoint inhibitor-induced colitis: diagnosis and management. *Target. Oncol.* 12: 301–308.
16. Shannon, V.R. (2017). Pneumotoxicity associated with immune checkpoint inhibitor therapies. *Curr. Opin. Pulm. Med.* 23: 305–316.
17. Mooradian, M.J., Nasrallah, M., Gainor, J.F. et al. (2019). Musculoskeletal rheumatic complications of immune checkpoint inhibitor therapy: a single center experience. *Semin. Arthritis Rheum.* 48: 1127–1132.
18. Brahmer, J.R., Drake, C.G., Wollner, I. et al. (2010). Phase I study of single-agent anti-programmed death-1 (MDX-1106) in refractory solid tumors: safety, clinical activity, pharmacodynamics, and immunologic correlates. *J. Clin. Oncol.* 28: 3167–3175.
19. Lee, J., Graham, A., and Sion, A. (2019). Evaluation of arthralgias in adult oncology patients receiving immune checkpoint inhibitors. *J. Oncol. Pharm. Pract.* 25: 1867–1872.
20. Hodi, F.S., Lee, S., McDermott, D.F. et al. (2014). Ipilimumab plus sargramostim vs ipilimumab alone for treatment of metastatic melanoma: a randomized clinical trial. *JAMA* 312: 1744–1753.
21. Robert, C., Schachter, J., Long, G.V. et al. (2015). Pembrolizumab versus ipilimumab in advanced melanoma. *N. Engl. J. Med.* 372: 2521–2532.
22. Cappelli, L.C., Gutierrez, A.K., Bingham, C.O., and Shah, A. (2017). Rheumatic and musculoskeletal immune-related adverse events due to immune checkpoint inhibitors: a systematic review of the literature. *Arthritis Care Res.* 69: 1751–1763.
23. Cappelli, L.C., Thomas, M.A., Bingham, C.O. et al. (2020). Immune checkpoint inhibitor-induced inflammatory arthritis as a model of autoimmune arthritis. *Immunol. Rev.* 294: 106–123.
24. Pundole, X., Abdel-Wahab, N., and Suarez-Almazor, M.E. (2019). Arthritis risk with immune checkpoint inhibitor therapy for cancer. *Curr. Opin. Rheumatol.* 31: 293–299.
25. Calabrese, L.H., Calabrese, C., and Cappelli, L.C. (2018). Rheumatic immune-related adverse events from cancer immunotherapy. *Nat. Rev. Rheumatol.* 14: 569–579.
26. Jamal, S., Hudson, M., Aurore Fifi-Mah, A. et al. (2020). Rheumatic immune-related adverse events from cancer immunotherapy: a review for the practicing rheumatologist. *J. Rheumatol.* 47: 166–175.
27. Albayda, J., Dein, E., Shah, A. et al. (2019). Sonographic findings in inflammatory arthritis secondary to immune checkpoint inhibition: a case series. *ACR Open Rheum.* 1: 303.
28. Buder-Bakhaya, K., Benesova, K., Schulz, C. et al. (2018). Characterization of arthralgia induced by PD-1 antibody treatment in patients with metastasized cutaneous malignancies. *Cancer Immunol. Immunother.* 67: 175–182.
29. Moseley, K.F., Naidoo, J., Bingham, C.O. et al. (2018). Immune-related adverse events with immune checkpoint inhibitors affecting the skeleton: a seminal case series. *J. Immunother. Cancer* 6: 104–112.
30. Robertsa, J., Ennis, D., Hudson, M. et al. (2020). Rheumatic immune-related adverse events associated with cancer immunotherapy: a nationwide multi-center cohort. *Autoimmun. Rev.* 19: 102595.
31. Cunningham-Bussel, A., Wang, J., Prisco, L.C. et al. (2022). Predictors of rheumatic immune-related adverse events and de novo inflammatory arthritis after immune checkpoint inhibitor treatment for cancer. *Arthritis Rheumatol.* 74: 527–540.
32. Perdigoto, A.L., Kluger, H., and Herold, K.C. (2021). Adverse events induced by immune checkpoint inhibitors. *Curr. Opin. Immunol.* 69: 29–38.

33. Ramos-Casals, M., Maria, A., Suárez-Almazor, M.E. et al. (2019). Sicca/Sjögren's syndrome triggered by PD-1/PD-L1 checkpoint inhibitors. Data from the International ImmunoCancer Registry (ICIR). *Clin. Exp. Rheumatol.* 37: 114–122.
34. Ghosn, J., Vicino, A., Michielin, O. et al. (2018). A severe case of neuro-Sjögren's syndrome induced by pembrolizumab. *J. Immunother. Cancer* 6: 110.
35. Liewluck, T., Kao, J.C., and Mauermann, M.L. (2018). PD-1 inhibitor-associated myopathies: emerging immune-mediated myopathies. *J. Immunother.* 41: 208–211.
36. Jia-Hung, C., Kang-Yun, L., Chaur-Jong, H. et al. (2017). Coexisting myasthenia gravis, myositis, and polyneuropathy induced by ipilimumab and nivolumab in a patient with non-small-cell lung cancer. *Medicine (Baltimore)* 96: e9262.
37. Shah, M., Tayar, J.H., Abdel-Wahab, N. et al. (2019). Myositis as an adverse event of immune checkpoint blockade for cancer therapy. *Semin. Arthritis Rheum.* 48: 736–740.
38. Aldrich, J., Pundole, X., Tummala, S. et al. (2021). Inflammatory myositis in cancer patients receiving immune checkpoint inhibitors. *Arthritis Rheumatol.* 73: 866–874.
39. Behling, J., Kaes, J., Münzel, T. et al. (2017). New-onset third-degree atrioventricular block because of autoimmune-induced myositis under treatment with anti-programmed cell death-1 (nivolumab) for metastatic melanoma. *Melanoma Res.* 27: 155–158.
40. Kudo, F., Watanabe, Y., Yuki Iwai, Y. et al. (2018). Advanced lung adenocarcinoma with nivolumab-associated dermatomyositis. *Intern. Med.* 57: 2217–2221.
41. Narváez, J., Juarez-López, P., LLuch, J. et al. (2018). Rheumatic immune-related adverse events in patients on anti-PD-1 inhibitors: fasciitis with myositis syndrome as a new complication of immunotherapy. *Autoimmun. Rev.* 17: 1040–1045.
42. Khoja, L., Maurice, C., Chappell, M. et al. (2016). Eosinophilic fasciitis and acute encephalopathtoxicity from pembrolizumab treatment of a patient with metastatic melanoma. *Cancer Immunol. Res.* 4: 175–178.
43. Tauber, M., Cohen, R., Laly, P. et al. (2019). Severe necrotizing myositis associated with long term anti-neoplastic efficacy following nivolumab plus ipilimumab combination therapy. *Clin. Rheumatol.* 38: 601–602.
44. Tolaymat, O.A., Pinkston, O., Wang, B. et al. (2019). Drug-associated vasculitis occurring after treatment with pembrolizumab. *Rheumatology (Oxford)* 58: 1501–1503.
45. Hung, W., Cusnir, I., Syed Habib, S. et al. (2021). Immune checkpoint inhibitor-induced granulomatosis with polyangiitis. *Rheumatology (Oxford)* 60: e190–e191.
46. Daxini, A., Cronin, K., and Sreih, A.G. (2018). Vasculitis associated with immune checkpoint inhibitors-a systematic review. *Clin. Rheumatol.* 3: 2579–2584.
47. Goldstein, B.L., Gedmintas, L., and Todd, D.J. (2014). Drug-associated polymyalgia rheumatica/giant cell arteritis occurring in two patients after treatment with ipilimumab, an antagonist of CTLA-4. *Arthritis Rheumatol.* 66: 768–769.
48. Manusow, J.S., Khoja, L., Pesin, N. et al. (2014). Retinal vasculitis and ocular vitreous metastasis following complete response to PD-1 inhibition in a patient with metastatic cutaneous melanoma. *J. Immunother. Cancer* 2: 41.
49. Minor, D.R., Bunker, S.R., and Doyle, J. (2013). Lymphocytic vasculitis of the uterus in a patient with melanoma receiving ipilimumab. *J. Clin. Oncol.* 31: e356.
50. Loricera, J., Hernández, J.L., García-Castaño, A. et al. (2018). Subclinical aortitis after starting nivolumab in a patient with metastatic melanoma. A case of drug-associated aortitis? *Clin. Exp. Rheumatol.* 36 (Suppl 111): 171.
51. Michot, J.M., Fusellier, M., Champiat, S. et al. (2019). Drug-induced lupus erythematosus following immunotherapy with anti-programmed death-(ligand) 1. *Ann. Rheum. Dis.* 78: e67.
52. Fadel, F., El Karoui, K., and Knebelmann, B. (2009). Anti-CTLA4 antibody-induced lupus nephritis. *N. Engl. J. Med.* 361: 211–212.
53. Lomax, A.J., McGuire, H.M., McNeil, C. et al. (2017). Immunotherapy-induced sarcoidosis in patients with melanoma treated with PD-1 checkpoint inhibitors: case series and immunophenotypic analysis. *Int. J. Rheum. Dis.* 20: 1277–1285.
54. Reddy, S.B., Possick, J.D., Kluger, H.M. et al. (2017). Sarcoidosis following anti-PD-1 and anti-CTLA-4 therapy for metastatic melanoma. *J. Immunother.* 40: 307–311.
55. Danlos, F.X., Pagès, C., Baroudjian, B. et al. (2016). Nivolumab-induced sarcoid-like granulomatous reaction in a patient with advanced melanoma. *Chest* 149: e133–e136.

56. Bertrand, A., Kostine, M., Barnetche, T. et al. (2015). Immune related adverse events associated with anti-CTLA-4 antibodies: systematic review and meta-analysis. *BMC Med.* 13: 211.
57. Brahmer, J.R., Lacchetti, C., Schneider, B.J. et al. (2018). Management of immune-related adverse events in patients treated with immune checkpoint inhibitor therapy: American Society of Clinical Oncology Clinical Practice Guideline. *J. Clin. Oncol.* 36: 1714–1768.
58. Brahmer, J.R., Abu-Sbeih, H., Ascierto, P.A. et al. (2021). Society for immunotherapy of cancer (SITC) clinical practice guideline on immune checkpoint inhibitor-related adverse events. *J. Immunother. Cancer* 9: e002435.
59. Hompson, J.A. (2018). New NCCN guidelines: recognition and management of immunotherapy-related toxicity. *J. Natl. Compr. Cancer Netw.* 16: 594–596.
60. Kostine, M., Finckh, A., Bingham, C.O. et al. (2021). EULAR points to consider for the diagnosis and management of rheumatic immune-related adverse events due to cancer immunotherapy with checkpoint inhibitors. *Ann. Rheum. Dis.* 80: 36–48.
61. Alfaro-Lara, R., Espinosa-Ortega, H.F., and Arce-Salinas, C.A. (2019). Systematic review and meta-analysis of the efficacy and safety of leflunomide and methotrexate in the treatment of rheumatoid arthritis. *Reumatol. Clín.* 15: 133–139.
62. Rempenault, C., Combe, B., Barnetche, T. et al. (2020). Clinical and structural efficacy of hydroxychloroquine in rheumatoid arthritis: a systematic review. *Arthritis Care Res.* 72: 36–40.
63. Abu Samra, K., Valdes-Navarro, M., Lee, S. et al. (2016). A case of bilateral uveitis and papillitis in a patient treated with pembrolizumab. *Eur. J. Ophthalmol.* 26: e46–e48.
64. Johnson, D.H., Zobniw, C.M., Trinh, V.A. et al. (2018). Infliximab associated with faster symptom resolution compared with corticosteroids alone for the management of immune-related enterocolitis. *J. Immunother. Cancer* 6: 10.
65. Draghi, A., Borch, T.H., Radic, H.D. et al. (2019). Differential effects of corticosteroids and anti-TNF on tumor-specific immune responses: implications for the management of irAEs. *Int. J. Cancer* 145: 1408–1413.
66. Esfahani, K. and Miller, W.H. Jr. (2017). Reversal of autoimmune toxicity and loss of tumor response by interleukin-17 blockade. *N. Engl. J. Med.* 376: 1989–1991.
67. Haanen, J.B.A.G., Carbonnel, F., Robert, C. et al. (2017). Management of toxicities from immunotherapy: ESMO clinical practice guidelines for diagnosis, treatment and follow-up. *Ann. Oncol.* 28: 119–142.

19 Heavy Metals in Autoimmune Diseases: Too Much Noise in Autoimmunity

Kassem Sharif[1,2,3] and Howard Amital[2,3,4]

[1]Department of Gastroenterology, Sheba Medical Centre, Tel-Hashomer, Israel
[2]Zabludowicz Center for Autoimmune Diseases, Sheba Medical Center, Tel-Hashomer, Israel
[3]Sackler Faculty of Medicine, Tel Aviv University, Tel Aviv, Israel
[4]Department of Internal Medicine 'B', Sheba Medical Center, Tel-Hashomer, Israel

Chapter highlights

1. Exposure to heavy metals results in the dysregulation of immune processes putatively inducing or exacerbating autoimmune conditions.
2. Heavy metals result in the production of proinflammatory cytokines by activating innate immune pathways as well as directly influence the activation of the adaptive arm.
3. Heavy metals in the exacerbation of various autoimmune diseases including systemic lupus erythematosus, rheumatoid arthritis, and multiple sclerosis.

Introduction

The human body requires high atomic mass metals for a variety of functions. Enzyme cofactors that implement iron utilize this metal in heme-based proteins as oxygen carriers and reactive oxygen species (ROS) scavengers [1, 2]. Another ROS scavenger, superoxide dismutase, uses manganese to decompose superoxide radicals into molecular oxygen and hydrogen peroxide [3]. Glutathione peroxidase is another ROS scavenger that utilizes selenium in its active site [4]. Calcium is a major component of bones and teeth, is used in muscle contractions, and regulates bone mineralization via the enzyme osteopontin [5–7]. Aluminum has long been used as an adjuvant in vaccines to boost immune response to antigens by providing long-lasting antigen exposure, thus providing better immunogenicity [8]. Concerns linked to the use of alum particles emerged following recognition of their causative role in the so-called macrophagic myofasciitis due to biopersistance. Other metals are used in pigmentation, membrane potential maintenance, gas exchange, acid/base balance, and nucleic acid synthesis [9–12].

Autoimmune Disorders: Adjuvants and Other Risk Factors in Pathogenesis, First Edition.
Edited by Abdulla Watad, Nicola Luigi Bragazzi, and Yehuda Shoenfeld.

Despite the numerous required application of metals in biological systems, pathologies from certain metals may be caused if the element is present in any amount, as in the case with arsenic, cadmium, and lead [13]. Alternatively, metals that are normally present in the body may reach abnormally high concentrations, and subsequently precipitate disease, such as poisoning with iron, chromium, and manganese. Classically, symptoms associated with heavy metal poisonings include gastrointestinal dysfunction, neuropathy, and psychiatric disturbances [14–18]. Metal poisoning from hexavalent chromium is genotoxic and may subsequently lead to certain types of cancer [19]. The concentration of heavy metals in the environment is linked with anthropogenic activities, such as gold mining [20].

In recent years, evidence has emerged that highlights how diseases of the immune system, particularly autoimmune diseases, are instigated and propagated by environmental factors. Examples of such factors include geographic location, which has been linked to increased incidences of multiple sclerosis (MS) and type 1 diabetes mellitus (T1DM) [21, 22]. Stress, diet, and activity levels have also been linked to autoimmune diseases [23–25].

Metals, such as aluminum, chromium, nickel, and palladium, have been commonly applied in medicine to enhance the immune response to pathogenic materials [26–28]. As such, it is important to consider the negative impacts of metals on the immune system. This chapter summarizes findings on the impact of metals on autoimmune disorders.

How metals affect the immune system

Metals can be found throughout nature. Within biological systems, these elements facilitate a wide array of functions, including but not limited to redox reactions, generation and removal of ROS, and stability of nucleic acids [29]. There are several mechanisms by which metals can illicit improper responses: types II and III hypersensitivities, which are regulated by the humoral arm of the immune system, and type IV hypersensitivities, which consist primarily of an aberrant T cell-based response [30].

Some metals are known to directly impact the growth and development of B cells, thereby influencing the negative selection against autoantibody-producing B cells. For instance, mercury has been shown to affect B cell development by increasing the production of B cell activating factor of the TNF family, BAFF, and A-proliferation inducing ligand, APRIL [31]. An increase in these factors has resulted in autoantibody production similar to rheumatoid arthritis, SLE, and Sjorgen's syndrome, respectively [32–34].

In the case of cellular-mediated hypersensitivities, such as contact dermatitis and multiple sclerosis, the issue begins with the improper activation of pattern recognition receptors (PRRs) on antigen-presenting cells (APCs). Their subsequent sensitization of naïve T cells to eventually form memory T cells follows [35]. This process begins with APCs and may occur through several independent mechanisms. Allergic hypersensitivity reactions due to nickel affect millions of people worldwide due to T-lymphocyte-triggered delayed-type hypersensitivity reaction. Nickel was found to directly activate the PRR Toll-like receptor 4 (TLR4), which is a crucial proinflammatory mediator. The activation of the TLR4 receptor initiates the MyD88-dependent IKK2/NF-κB pathway in endothelial cells. This activation triggers rapid expression of various surface adhesion molecules required for leukocyte adhesion, as well as activating stress-activated mitogen-activated protein kinase (MAPK) pathways such as p38. The downstream signaling of activated TLR4 provides an activation signal for NF-κB as well as release of IL-1β, IL8, and TNF-α [36–38]. The association of these pathways with autoimmune phenomena has been reported. Toll-like receptor signaling and the MyD88 pathway are key components of the innate immune system and both have noted involvement in the course of type 1 diabetes [39]. The MyD88 pathway and NF-κB activation have also been discussed in association with antiphospholipid syndrome [40]. MyD88 pathway has also been described to be associated with adult-onset still's disease (AOSD) and systemic lupus erythematosus (SLE) [41, 42], and autoimmune sialadenitis, which is present in autoimmune diseases such as Sjögren's syndrome [43].

The inflammasome, which releases IL1β, can be engaged with chromium [44]. Beryllium can activate the innate immune system through the MyD88-mediated release of alarmins, such as DNA [45]. Once the innate immune system is activated, APCs containing metal migrate to the lymph nodes, and can then activate T cells through the formation of haptens, directly promoting the cross-linking of major histocompatibility complexes (MHC) with T cell receptors (TCR), or by creating neoantigens through MHCs rearrangement [46, 47].

Outside of this pathway, metals have other documented effects on T cells. When exposed to palladium, T cells have been shown to skew their production of the TRAV-2*02 region of the TCR. This increases the activity of specific $CD8^+$ T cells [48, 49]. Heavy metals have been shown to influence various aspects of the immune system. Antimony, found mainly in conductors and batteries, used in electronics causes chromosomal aberration and excessive production of active oxygen species through depletion of glutathione and protein-bound sulfhydryl [50, 51]. Cadmium, which is used for producing batteries, pigments, coatings, and plating, has been shown to increase neutrophil recruitment, and results in macrophage immune dysfunction through inhibition of NF-kB and macrophage polarization to an M2 predominant profile causing a humoral medicated Th2 immune response [52, 53]. Furthermore, cadmium results in adaptive immune system activation with subsequent upregulation of proinflammatory markers (TNF-a, IL-1, IL-8, IL-6) and increased expression of adhesion molecules such as ICAM, VCAM, PECAM-1, as well as prostaglandin and cyclooxygenase-2 [54–58]. Lead has been reported to cause alterations to the epigenome with DNA hypomethylation, and increased oxidative stress-related microRNA expression [59]. Like other heavy metals, lead results in the activation of T and B lymphocytes, and activation of the NF-kB pathways. [59, 60].

Exposure to mercury has been shown to be closely related to the development of autoimmunity. Exposure of murine models to mercury results in immune complex glomerulonephritis, autoantibody synthesis, polyclonal activation of T- and B-lymphocytes which causes an increase in proinflammatory cytokines (IL-1b, IL-17, IFN-y) and lower levels of antiinflammatory cytokine including IL-1RA and IL10 [61–63]. Various other mechanisms have been proposed including increased radical oxygen species production and alteration in mitochondrial function.

Several factors explaining aluminum's effects on the immune system have been described and have been detailed in the context of its use as an adjuvant in vaccinations [64]. Pro-phagocytic effects have been noted, in which macrophages plated with aluminum hydroxide resulted in induction of MHC II-type antigen-specific memory responses, thus displaying macrophages' sensitivity to aluminum hydroxide-based adjuvants [65]. Aluminum hydroxide-based adjuvants have been shown to activate endogenous cellular immune responses mediated by the specific targeting of nucleotide-binding oligomerization domain (NOD)-like receptor protein (NLRP3). This activation promotes secretion of pro-inflammatory factors such as IL-1β and IL-18 by macrophages [66]. Increased secretion and expression of IL-4 and IL-10 have been shown in association with aluminum, with IL-4 subsequently inducing proliferation of splenic B cells [67].

Collectively, metals may interact with the immune system at various points to generate hypersensitivities (Figure 19.1)

Metals and systemic lupus erythematosus

SLE is a chronic and severe autoimmune disease of the connective tissues that has a broad spectrum of clinical manifestations [68]. SLE predominantly affects young women, African Americans, and Hispanics. The five-year survival rate of newly diagnosed SLE patients is over 90% [69]. It has been shown that environmental factors work synergistically with genetic predisposition to induce SLE as well as exacerbate its symptoms [70, 71]. Limited data exist on the relationship of heavy

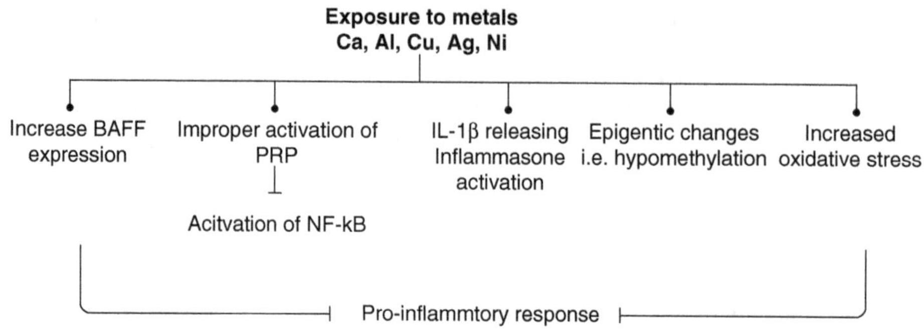

Figure 19.1 The effects of heavy metals on the immune system. *Abbreviations*: Ca, Cadmium; Al, aluminum; Cu, copper; Ag, silver; Ni, nickel; PRR, pattern recognition receptors.

metal exposure to the development of SLE. However, heavy metals have been shown to be associated with disease acceleration in experimental models of SLE.

Nickel and SLE

Data on the link between nickel exposure and SLE induction is sparse. An experimental study involving exposure of SLE-prone mice to nickel showed no exacerbation of disease [72]. Clinically, a case of induced malar rash was documented in a 61-year-old patient with documented SLE, who wore nickel-based eyeglasses. Although the patient's disease was fairly controlled for eight-years, over time she noticed the development of a nonpruritic rash across her nose and cheeks. Upon removal of the nickel-based glasses, her symptoms resolved [73].

Aluminum and SLE

Oral aluminum hydroxide, followed by a simple excision, was reported as a successful treatment for a large subcutaneous calcification in a patient with SLE. Calcinosis cutis is a rare presentation of SLE, and this report may suggest its therapeutic value in the treatment of certain clinical manifestations of SLE. Katz-Agranov et al. note that aluminum-containing vaccinations may be a trigger for postvaccination onset of SLE, although more data is needed to prove an exact causal relationship [74].

Cadmium and SLE

Leffel et al. [75] found that the effects from high doses of cadmium exposure in SLE-prone mice do not manifest in the same manner as those observed in low-dose cadmium exposure. The mice exposed to low doses of cadmium did not have measurable disease; however, mice that were exposed to higher doses of cadmium developed a pattern of measurable results consistent with the induction of SLE. Including increased antic-nuclear antibody production (ANA), deposition of immune complexes, and proteinuria. Additionally, a separate study found increased levels of serum ANA in SLE-prone mice models with oral exposure to cadmium at low concentrations. ANA's pathogenic role has been demonstrated in glomerulonephritis associated with SLE in humans and in mice [76].

Copper and SLE

High concentrations of copper have been measured in patients with SLE, and the level of serum copper has been described as directly related to disease activity and inflammation [77]. A study in 1985 showed that exogenous copper given to rats decreases the formation of lupus erythematosus cells. The rats used in this study were induced with a collagen-like disease, producing SLE-type symptoms, following oral hydralazine administration [78]. In a 2004 double-blind double-placebo study, patients with SLE were administered copper and/or omega-3 fish oils to determine the clinical effect, and the investigators found no significant therapeutic benefits from supplementation with copper [79].

Many patients with SLE are young women of childbearing potential, and avoidance of pregnancy during active disease is vital, as some medications are teratogenic. There are, however, concerns about hormonal disturbances from contraceptives that may exacerbate SLE symptoms or cause flare-ups [80]. A 2005 study conducted by Sánchez-Guerrero et al. compared SLE disease activity in SLE patients who were administered different forms of contraceptives. SLE disease activity was measured in women who used a copper-containing intrauterine device (IUD), women who used a combination of oral contraceptives, and women who took a progestin-only pill. The study found that disease activity remained mild and stable in all groups throughout the trial. The authors did note, however, that severe infections were more frequent in the IUD group [81].

Silver and SLE

There is little data on the linkage of silver to the induction of SLE. Studies conducted in 2003 and 2008 used mice to test whether induction of autoimmunity can be established when administered mercury and silver in the absence of specific susceptible genes. The induction of autoimmunity was assessed by measuring an increase in B-cell activation and antinucleolar autoantibodies. The studies revealed an increase in systemic autoimmunity in mice using these factors, as seen in SLE [82, 83].

Metals and type 1 diabetes mellitus

T1DM is a chronic disorder characterized by insulin deficiency as a result of autoimmune destruction of pancreatic β-cells. The primary cause of T1DM is still largely unknown; however, advances in the field of immunology have contributed to a better understanding of the disease's etiology. It has been shown that genetic susceptibility as well as environmental factors precipitate T1DM. Multiple environmental factors have been shown to induce the disease onset, including viral infections, cow's milk, wheat protein, vitamin D, and other infectious agents. The disease may be found at any age, although diagnosis tends to occur most often between ages 5 and 7, and around the age of puberty. The incidence of T1DM has been increasing worldwide for several decades, which has been thought to occur due to environmental influences [84].

Nickel and T1DM

There has been little documentation on the effects of nickel and T1DM. A 2014 study was conducted on streptozotocin-induced diabetic rats, which showed that silver might be correlated as an antidiabetic agent. Studies revealed reduced blood glucose levels, increased insulin level and expression, increased glucokinase activity, and improved expression of GLUT-2 in rat models [85].

Aluminum and T1DM

A glutamic acid decarboxylase (GAD) vaccine, formulated with aluminum hydroxide (GAD-alum), was tested in a population of T1DM patients ranging in age from 3 to 45. Treatment with GAD in diabetic mice was previously shown to prevent the progression of diabetes when given before the development of hyperglycemia [86].GAD is a major target of the autoimmune response that occurs in T1DM, and the GAD-alum vaccination was tested in patients to preserve insulin production in those who were recently diagnosed. Aluminum was also administered on its own in an additional cohort. Unfortunately, this attempt at antigen-based therapy was not efficacious, and further research is required to better understand the effects of GAD administration [87].

Cadmium and T1DM

Haglund et al. analyzed the Swedish childhood diabetes registry in 1996 as well as the heavy metal content found within groundwater samples in Sweden. Interestingly, in the total study population it was found that, based on the presence of chromium content in the water, chromium was associated with a decreased risk for diabetes [88]. A later study in 2002 analyzed the ultrastructural effects of diabetes and cadmium on the peripheral nervous system. Fifty-two male rats were used as models, and a diabetic condition was induced via intravenous injection of alloxan via the caudal vein. Alloxan is widely used to induce T1DM in animals for experimentation [89]. The sciatic nerve was dissected and analyzed. It was revealed that cadmium toxicity enhances the destructive effect of diabetes on myelinated and unmyelinated fibers of the sciatic nerve, and this situation can cause neuropathy in the peripheral nervous system [90].

A recently published study investigated the association between the accumulation of cadmium exposure below toxic levels and the incidence of diabetes in the general population. The study found no significant relationship of cadmium to diabetes. However, the study population was selected to exclude T1DM patients by selecting participants over the age of 30, in which the prevalence of T1DM is relatively low. In their observations, they were unable to distinguish T1DM patients from type 2 diabetes patients [91].

Copper and T1DM

Copper is an essential trace element and its deficiency can lead to a variety of nutritional and vascular disorders. Al-Saleh et al. [92] measured the maternal-fetal status of various metals and found a significantly higher amount of copper in the umbilical vein of insulin-dependent pregnancies. The fetal-maternal ratio of copper indicated passive placental transport, and the observed altered level of copper is this experiment may have implications for insulin-dependent diabetic pregnancies. Further studies are in progress to determine the possible adverse effects in altered levels of trace elements in pregnant women [92].

Metals and rheumatoid arthritis

Rheumatoid arthritis (RA) is an autoimmune disease that attacks the joints, particularly in the hands and wrists [93]. Although less commonly reported, extra-articular RA, in which patients present with damage to the heart, lungs, and other connective tissues, is documented [94]. While the exact mechanism of RA is unknown, it is understood that a combination of environmental and genetic factors is correlated with disease incidence and prevalence. There is promising evidence that metals play a role in RA. Patients afflicted with RA show an upregulation of metallothionein, a heavy metal scavenger protein. This section summarizes the known studies enumerating the links between specific metals and RA.

Cadmium and RA

As previously mentioned, smoking is a strong environmental risk factor for the development of RA. Smoking increases the levels of citrullinated proteins, which is linked to the upregulation of autoantibodies to these biomolecules, appropriately called antcitrullinated protein antibodies (ACPAs)[95]. Of the many harmful components in cigarette smoke, serum levels of cadmium are greatly elevated in regular smokers [96]. Initially studied in Wistar rats, Ansari et al. showed that cadmium greatly exacerbates the symptoms of rheumatoid arthritis [52].

Joo et al., in a large cross-sectional study of patients from Korea, showed that there is a strong association between serum and urinary levels of cadmium and rheumatoid arthritis (1.30 ± 0.07 versus 1.17 ± 0.01 µg/L, $p < 0.01$) [97]. Interestingly, the study tested for links between rheumatoid arthritis and other metals, including arsenic, manganese, mercury, lead, and zinc but found no significant association.

Nickel and copper in RA

Nickel is currently used in many commonplace items, including jewelry and dental implants. Muris et al. removed nickel-containing dental products in two patients, both of whom reported significantly reduced symptoms related to rheumatoid arthritis, such as pain in the fingers, hands, and joints [98].

Yang et al. demonstrated in a cohort of 122 patients in Taiwan that elevated copper and nickel levels are associated with RA [99].

Aluminum and RA

The immunogenic effects of aluminum are well established, as aluminum-based materials are regularly used as adjuvants for vaccines. Bamonti et al. report that using metal chelation therapy greatly reduced the effects of rheumatoid arthritis on patients, and observed that aluminum was one of the primary metals to be extracted with this treatment [100]. Although interesting, more research should be done to better understand the effects of aluminum in the progression of rheumatoid arthritis.

Metals and multiple sclerosis

MS is a chronic and progressive disease of the central nervous system (CNS) with variable pathologic features. Although the exact cause of MS is unknown, the pathogenesis is thought to be due to an autoimmune reaction against myelin, with the major pathologic mechanisms being inflammation, demyelination, and axon degeneration. Some highly characteristic clinical symptoms and signs of MS include sensory abnormalities in the limbs, vision loss, motor abnormalities, diplopia, gait disturbance, balance problems, sensory abnormalities in the face, Lhermitte sign, vertigo, bladder problems, limb ataxia, acute transverse myelopathy, and pain [101].

Aluminum and MS

Although the exact cause of MS is unknown, toxic heavy metals, such as aluminum, have been thought to be a possible cause of neurodegenerative diseases. Aluminum is commonly found in the environment and is easily ingested by humans. The chronic exposure of aluminum in animals is associated with behavioral, neuropathological, and neurochemical changes. Specifically, aluminum is involved in the production of ROS, which can impair mitochondrial functioning. Research shows that impairments in mitochondrial functioning may play a major role in neurodegenerative disorders [102].

Therefore, Kumar et al. hypothesize that aluminum exposure may be associated with neuropathologies such as MS. Several other neurodegenerative diseases, such as Parkinson's disease, Alzheimer's disease, Friedreich ataxia, and amyotrophic lateral sclerosis, also involve the generation of ROS and mitochondrial dysfunction [103–105].

Fulgenzi et al. aimed to investigate the in vivo impact of heavy metal intoxication on MS progression. The authors assessed the case of a patient diagnosed with MS who has been unsuccessfully treated for years with the currently approved therapies by measuring the patient's toxic heavy metal levels (aluminum, lead, and mercury) in the urine, following treatment with the chelator calcium disodium ethylene diamine tetraacetic acid (EDTA) twice a month [106]. During this treatment regime, the patient experienced improved symptoms, indicating MS remission. The authors hypothesize that these toxic heavy metals, such as aluminum, play a role in the neuroinflammation found in patients with MS. By treating patients with chelator agents, these toxic heavy metals can be converted into complexes that are able to be eliminated in the urine, reducing the overall heavy metal load in the body [106].

Cadmium and MS

Cadmium is mainly ingested by humans during the consumption of vegetables and grains, as well as during the activity of smoking. The harmful effects of cadmium were confirmed several decades ago on industrial workers [107, 108]. Cadmium is able to accumulate in the body, causing organ damage in the brain, kidney, lung, and testis [109]. Usai et al. showed that cadmium can enter neurons via voltage-gated channels [110]. Once inside the neurons, cadmium can impair the functioning of both the peripheral nervous system [111] and CNS [112], resulting in clinical symptoms such as olfactory dysfunction, peripheral neuropathy, neurological disturbances, mental retardation, learning disabilities, motor activity impairment, and behavioral alterations [113]. Cadmium-dependent neurotoxicity has been shown to be related to neurodegenerative diseases including MS [114].

In one study, the researchers demonstrated that cadmium exposure can lead to retrograde axonal transport and neurotoxicity in rat motor neurons [115]. In another study, the cadmium was able to produce ROS, changing membrane fluidity, intracellular calcium levels, lipid peroxidation, and protein carbonylation [116, 117]. Cadmium was also shown to cause neurotoxicity by decreasing GSH levels in both the midbrain and hippocampus, as well as increasing free radicals, mitochondrial membrane dysfunction, and cell apoptosis in brain tissues [118, 119].

There have also been reports showing high levels of cadmium in MS patients [120]. In addition to high levels of cadmium, Aliomrani et al. also showed a relationship between MS patients and glutathione-*s*-transferase levels [120]. The excess cadmium in MS patients is due to environmental exposure from living in industrial areas or from consuming corn, rice, and wheat from industrial areas [121]. Air pollution can also contain cadmium and therefore long-term exposure can potentially have a role in the pathogenesis of MS [122]. In the studies described above, cadmium has been shown to be neurotoxic through the formation of oxidative stress, reduction of antioxidant enzyme activity, and cellular antioxidants.

Copper and MS

Copper is a component of several enzymes found in the brain, regulating neurotransmitter synthesis, iron metabolism, and oxidative defense. In our bodies, copper is able to mediate electron transfer in redox reactions [123]. High concentrations of copper are able to cause oxidative stress by catalyzing the production of hydroxyl radicals and reducing glutathione (GSH), an antioxidant that removes ROS [123].

The role of copper in MS pathology is thought to be due to an excessive amount of copper causing oxidative damage [124–126]. Copper levels in the body can increase via injury to the mitochondrial electron transport system, cytochrome oxidase, and activated glia [127]. However, there have also been findings with conflicting evidence. For example, Sedighi et al. [128] did not show any significant difference between the serum copper levels of MS patients when compared to a control group. Gunther et al. [129] actually showed lower copper concentrations in MS patients, possibly due to gut malabsorption On the other hand, Mana et al. stated that an excessive level of copper could trigger a demyelination attack in the CNS [130].

Riccardis et al. tried to further understand the role of copper in the pathogenesis of MS by comparing the serum and cerebrospinal fluid (CSF) levels of copper in MS patients and a group of control patients. The authors found a significant increase in copper levels in both serum and CSF in the MS group, compared to the control group. To see if this is due to an impairment in copper metabolism, Riccardis et al. measured ceruloplasmin levels and activity in both groups. Their results showed an increase in ceruloplasmin levels and a decrease in the ceruloplasmin activity in the MS group [131].

The researchers were then able to use this data to calculate the total free serum copper levels, showing a significant increase in free serum copper in the MS group. This could possibly lead to the increased level of copper found in the CSF. The decreased ceruloplasmin activity (decreased ability to bind copper) in the MS group could be due to the high oxidative environment found in the serum of MS patients. The alterations in copper levels found in MS patients may play a part in the pathogenesis of MS [131].

It appears that not only an excessive amount of copper but also a deficiency in copper can trigger an attack on myelin in the CNS [130]. Cuprizone, a copper chelator, has been shown to cause both demyelination and remyelination in the CNS of animals. Cuprizone causes demyelination by carrying copper into the CNS and inducing demyelinating lesions due to both oxidative stress and oligodendrocyte toxicity. This can be referred to as experimental autoimmune encephalomyelitis (EAE), the experimental model of MS. More specifically, cuprizone has been shown to demyelinate the corpus callosum, hippocampus, and other white matter regions of the CNS in rodents. In addition, cuprizone causes inhibition of copper-dependent mitochondrial enzymes, cytochrome oxidase, and monoamine oxidase [132, 133]. Overall, this supports the notion that an imbalance of copper homeostasis can induce the formation of ROS and neurodegenerative damage [132, 134–140].

Clioquinol, another copper chelator, has been proven to suppress different neurodegenerative diseases in animal studies [141, 142]. In addition, Choi et al. [143] demonstrated that clioquinol is able to decrease the activation of microglia in the spinal cord of EAE, improving clinical symptoms. These studies show that metal chelator therapy in animal models is able to reverse neuronal degeneration and increase survival in neurodegenerative disorders, such as MS.

Metals and inflammatory bowel disease (IBD)

Inflammatory bowel disease (IBD) includes both ulcerative colitis and Crohn's disease. Ulcerative colitis consists of recurrent episodes of inflammation of the colon starting from the rectum and extending proximally in a continuous fashion. Crohn's disease, on the other hand, is defined by transmural inflammation involving any part of the gastrointestinal system from the mouth to the anus. Both conditions are known to characteristically be caused by sets of interacting genetic and environmental factors.

Aluminum and IBD

Aluminum is a common metal found in the environment and has been found in soil, water, food, and pharmaceutical agents. Multiple hypotheses have been suggested connecting aluminum with the induction and maintenance of Crohn's disease. They include the multiple harmful immune and inflammatory effects of aluminum [144], an aluminum–bacterial interaction [145], and a dietary microparticle association [146, 147], making aluminum a top suspect for the induction and maintenance of Crohn's disease.

Lerner describes the harmful effects of aluminum on the gastrointestinal system and hypothesizes potential mechanisms of aluminum-associated induction and maintenance of Crohn's Disease [144]. Lerner states that urban areas have been shown to have more aluminum contamination, and interestingly, Crohn's disease has been shown to be more prevalent in urban areas as well. In addition, Western lifestyle has been shown to increase aluminum exposure via unique diets and increased exposure to pollution and industrial chemicals [144].

Once absorbed, aluminum is known to have immune-adjuvant activity and the ability to induce granulomatous inflammation, similar to Crohn's disease. Aluminum is absorbed in the gastrointestinal tract via transferrin at sites left vacant by iron [148]. In Crohn's disease, there is low iron intake and stores, and high transferrin levels. This could therefore potentially lead to increased GI aluminum absorption in people with Crohn's disease [149, 150]. Also, individuals with Crohn's disease are known to have a genetically increased intestinal permeability in general [151-156]. In Crohn's disease, there is an increase in DNA damage, and aluminum is also known to induce DNA damage [157–159].

In addition, Perl et al. [145] hypothesize that bacteria, especially mycobacteria, take up aluminum and other trace elements from the gut lumen. This alters their pathogenicity and exacerbates the host's immune response. The aluminum is absorbed through the bacteria's siderophore iron-uptake system and is able to induce a granulomatous inflammatory response, as a result of aluminum's adjuvant properties

Powell et al. hypothesize an association between microparticles and Crohn's disease [147, 160]. Ten microparticles, including highly inert oxides of titanium, aluminum, and silicon, are ingested by individuals with a western diet daily, mainly via food additives. These microparticles are then able to be absorbed by specialized epithelial M cells on the surface of lymphoid tissue, accumulating as a person ages in fixed macrophages at the base of lymphoid follicles. These microparticles are potent adjuvants when ingested with antigenic material. In the intestinal lumen, there are naturally a large amount of potential antigens, proinflammatory biomolecules, and metal cations, modifying these microparticles and thus changing the immune response to these antigens. These modified microparticles generate a $CD8^{+}$ cytotoxic lymphocyte response, as well as the production of the proinflammatory cytokines IL-1 and TNF-alpha [161]. This immune response can be connected to the inflammatory process of Crohn's disease.

Chambrun et al. [162] also aimed to evaluate the effects of environmental aluminum by looking at murine models of colitis. In this study, the authors found that the oral administration of aluminum worsened intestinal inflammation in mice with 2,4,6-trinitrobenzene sulfonic acid and dextran sodium sulfate-induced colitis and chronic colitis in mice that were IL-10 negative. Overall, aluminum was found to increase the duration and intensity of macroscopic and histologic inflammation, colonic myeloperoxidase activity, inflammatory cytokine expression, and decreased the epithelial cell renewal when compared to control mice. Aluminum impaired the intestinal barrier function under basal conditions and induced granuloma formation, as well as stimulated inflammatory cytokine expression by epithelial cells in vitro. These harmful effects of aluminum on intestinal inflammation and repair provide evidence for the possibility of aluminum being an environmental risk factor for IBD [162].

Cadmium, other heavy metals, and IBD

The chronic ingestion of heavy metals from the environment, such as cadmium and copper, can cause pathologies after intestinal absorption and accumulation in specific organs. Breton et al. [163] conducted a study to compare the accumulation and retention of cadmium and lead, as well as their effect on metal balance in primary organs, by looking at the gastrointestinal tract of mice. Different doses of cadmium chloride salts were put in the drinking water of mice for varying lengths of time. Results showed poor accumulation of cadmium in the intestines; however, there were significant changes in the transport, oxidative, and inflammatory status of the small and large intestines due to the ingestion of cadmium. This was measured by changes in the gene expression of certain intestinal markers. The ingestion of cadmium also showed genotoxic effects throughout the gastrointestinal tract.

In addition, current data on cytokines and prostaglandins have been shown to be contradictory, showing either immunosuppressive or proinflammatory activities. In this study by Breton et al., cadmium was not shown to significantly change cytokine expression in the gastrointestinal tract [163].

Overall, based on their results, Breton et al. state that they could not make any conclusions regarding the effect of cadmium on the susceptibility to colitis or its exact role in IBD. The authors call for more studies to evaluate the impact of heavy metals on the microbiota in the gastrointestinal system. This is because the microbiota of the GI tract plays a crucial homeostatic role in the regulatory processes of the host to ingest toxins from the environment [163].

Fazeli et al. [164] evaluate the impact of cadmium on the gastrointestinal tract (GIT) microflora. They found that exposure to cadmium is able to have harmful effects on GIT microflora. Specifically, Fazeli et al. looked at the effect of experimental exposure to cadmium in drinking water on the GIT microflora of mice. Five experimental groups received 23–50 mg/kg cadmium in drinking water and a control group received only water for a total of 45 days. Bacterial counts were then performed on the GIT of the mice. They observed a sharp decrease in all of the microbial species in the intestines of the mice. A smaller effect was seen in the large intestine and rectum relative to the small intestine. Gram-negative bacteria were less sensitive to the cadmium than gram-positive bacteria. In conclusion, cadmium was shown to have a deleterious effect on GIT microflora [164].

Zhai et al. [165]. Also looked at the exposure to heavy metals such as cadmium, lead, copper, and aluminum, and their ability to induce adverse health effects. The authors demonstrated that sub-chronic exposure to cadmium, lead, copper, and aluminum can all induce metal-specific and time-dependent changes in GIT microflora of mice. These alterations in GIT microflora can potentially play a role in inflammatory bowel disease and provide a basis for future studies.

Metals and systemic sclerosis

Systemic sclerosis (SSc) is a systemic inflammatory disorder involving the skin and internal organs characterized by deposition of extracellular matrix resulting in fibrosis and destruction of internal organs. Growing evidence points toward the paramount role of environmental factors in the modulation of epigenetic determinants resulting in disease onset and progression [166]. Several chemical agents have been implicated including for instance crystalline silica among other solvents. Recently, the role of heavy metals piqued the scientific community's interest and various reports aimed to assess the risk of disease development in exposed patients.

The relationship between heavy metals and systemic sclerosis is not broadly studied [167]. However, in a case-control study by Marie et al [168], exposure to heavy metals was shown to confer an increased risk of SSc. In female patients with SSc, higher median levels of antimony ($p = 0.001$), cadmium ($p = 0.0003$), lead ($p = 0.02$), palladium ($p < 0.0001$), and zinc ($p = 0.0003$) were noted. Antimony is a chemical element released from infrared detectors, diodes, lead batteries, and during the manufacture of electronics [169]. Upon exposure, antimony has been shown to alter the epigenome resulting in chromosomal aberration, excess production of active oxygen species, and thus DNA damage [169, 170]. Other metals including Cadmium have been associated with cardiovascular disease, peripheral artery diseases, and diabetes [171, 172]. The mechanism linking exposure to Cadmium with the development of SSc remains unknown; however, it is postulated that cadmium results in the activation of T- and B-lymphocytes, up regulation of cytokines and cell adhesion molecules, and increase of endothelial permeability, moreover, cadmium has been shown to induce vascular dysfunction secondary to oxidative damage [173, 174]. Similarly, evidence from animal model studies has suggested that lead results in T and B lymphocyte activation including cytokine synthesis, upregulation of endothelial nitric oxide synthase, and binding with sulfhydryl bends resulting in organ toxicity from free radicals [168]. Exposure to mercury has been shown to result in an increased prevalence of detectable antinuclear antibodies (OR 8.6 95 CI 4.1–18) and antinucleolar antibodies (OR 30.6 95% CI 7.1–131.9). Experimental models have shown that mercury results in immune complex-mediated glomerulonephritis and autoantibody synthesis (84–85), increased production of pro-inflammatory cytokines (IL-1b, TNF-a, and IFN-y), and decreased levels of antiinflammatory cytokines including IL10, IL1Ra [61, 175].

The production of autoantigens is known to play a vital part as a potential initiator of the autoimmune process. It has been shown that unique protein fragmentation occurs in the presence of heavy metals and can be induced in intact cells exposed to high concentration of those heavy metals, thus pointing toward a pathogenic role in SSc development [176].

Looking at the association between heavy metals and SSc, Forte et al. [177] aimed to quantify the levels of various heavy metals in SSc patients and compare their levels to control. Aluminum was significantly depleted in blood and increased in the urine of SSc patients as compared to controls; moreover, lead was found at higher levels in blood and significantly decreased in SSc. In addition, higher mercury levels were detected in urine of SSc subjects which was associated with higher severity of the disease [177].

Taken together, growing scientific evidence points toward the potential role of heavy metals in disease etiopathogenesis by influencing alteration and modifications of epigenetic determinants. Pathogenic mechanisms pertinent to SSc development remain to be elucidated.

Metals and thyroid disease

Thyroid hormone plays a vital role in the regulation of metabolism, growth, and development of the human body. Thus disruption, by hypersecretion or hyposecretion of thyroid hormone is determinantal and causes detrimental effects on the body's internal balance [178].

Jain assessed the association between selenium, zinc, and copper levels with thyroid function by analyzing the National Health and nutrition examination survey. For males, zinc levels were associated with decreased levels of T4 levels, whereas serum copper was associated with increased levels of T4. Similarly, serum copper was associated with increased levels of T3 and T4 in females [178].

Mercury impairs many physiological processes and thus threatens human health. On the thyroid gland, mercury has been shown to inhibit the biosynthesis of thioredoxin reductase and other selenoenzymes by depletion of selenium [179]. The selective binding of mercury to the thyroid results in disruption in thyroid stimulating hormone production, and inhibition of deiodination [180]. Afrira et al. [181] demonstrated that close to 58% of small-scale miners had mercury levels exceeding the occupational exposure threshold, with significantly decreased levels of T3 ($p < 0.0001$) and T4 ($p < 0.0001$). Mercury levels were significantly negatively correlated with thyroid hormone levels ($p < 0.0001$).

Similarly, Chen et al. showed a negative association between thyroid hormone (T4, T3, and FT3) levels and mercury exposures, it is postulated that mercury results in toxicity by accumulating in the thyroid gland and reducing the uptake of sodium at the sodium/iodine symporter [182]. The thyroid gland has an intrinsic greater affinity for mercury accumulation, and low levels of mercury can result in thyroid inflammation, hypothyroidism, and thyroid depression by replacing iodine at its binding site [181, 183, 184]. Generally, the majority of T3 produced in the body results from deiodination process of T4. Methyl mercury has been shown to cause a coupling defect in the synthesis of iodothyronines, moreover the accumulation of mercury in the liver results in the inhibition of 5′-thyroxine deiodinase type II which is involved in the conversion of T4 to T3[185, 186].

The relationship between manganese and thyroid homeostasis is not well understood, manganese plays a vital role in antioxidation through the manganese superoxide dismutase. It has been postulated that manganese influences the thyroid axis by both the direct dysregulation at the level of thyroid gland or the indirect alteration in dopaminergic control of the thyroid gland and its hormones. It is established that dopamine plays a role in the modulation of TSH secretion. The detrimental effects of manganese on dopaminergic neurons are postulated to result in profound effects on thyroid hormone synthesis [187, 188]. The development of goiter due to manganese was investigated in mice by feeding them excessive amounts of manganese while keeping iodine concentrations at normal. After seven weeks, thyroids from female mice were enlarged, while those from male mice did not become goitrous, on histology thyroid morphology revealed retention of colloid in the lumen [189].

Cadmium has established endocrine-disrupting activities, Chen et al [190] investigated the relationship between thyroid hormones and the levels of cadmium in blood and urine of 4409 adults, and 1109 adolescents. In adults, urinary cadmium was positively associated with T4, T3, FT3, and thyroglobulin (Tg). These results were replicated in another study with an additional finding of elevated blood levels of cadmium being associated with lower levels of TSH, suggesting an overly thyroid disease due to cadmium exposure [191]. Taken together, it is hypothesized that thyroid hormone levels are associated with urinary cadmium burden (urine Cadmium), whereas changes in TSH reflect acute exposure to Cadmium [192]. Luo and Hendryx [193] analyzed 6231 participants aged 20 and older with measurements from 2007 to 2010 of the National Health and Nutrition Examination Survey and demonstrated a positive association between cadmium exposure and thyroglobulin in both sexes, and a positive correlation between cadmium and total T3 among males.

The toxic effect of Cadmium was extensively studied in rat models. Intraperitoneal administration of cadmium resulted in its accumulation in the mitochondria of thyroid follicular epithelial cells and subsequent derangement of the rough endoplasmic reticulum resulting in disruption of active absorption of colloid droplet [194]. Hammouda et al, showed that cadmium accumulates in the thyroid gland and results in the hyposecretion of thyroglobulin [195]. Cadmium has also been shown to influence lymphocytes by upregulating the death receptor "FAS", increase in CD95/Fas complex, and increase the expression of caspase-3 and p-53 [192, 196].

Zinc plays an important role in cellular proliferation and has a role in the catalytic activity of several metalloprotein enzymes. Ertek et al. evaluated the association of zinc levels with thyroid volume in healthy subjects, patients with autoimmune thyroid disease, and patients with nodular goiter. In patients with normal thyroid, zinc levels were significantly associated with free T3 levels ($p < 0.001$). In nodular thyroid group, thyroid volume was negatively correlated with TSH and circulating zinc levels ($p = 0.014$ and $p = 0.045$, respectively). In the autoimmune thyroid disease group – thyroid autoantibodies and zinc were significantly positively correlated [197].

Taken together, heavy metals are shown to influence the function of the thyroid gland through various mechanisms, further investigations are warranted to better delineate the mechanism resulting in thyroid function dysregulation.

Metals and Sjögren disease

Sjögren syndrome (SS) is a chronic disorder characterized by the lymphocytic infiltration of exocrine glands and by B cell hyperreactivity resulting in hypergammaglobulinemia and increased autoantibodies production [198]. Current theories explaining disease etiology are insufficient and the interplay between genetic and environmental factors provides insight into disease etiopathogenetics.

The role of heavy metals in disease etiology is not well elucidated; however, in a report by Lee et al. [199], the association between exposure to heavy metals and SS was investigated and the highest prevalence of SS was located in the area where farm soil contained the highest amounts of chromium. Moreover, the authors note that in their unpublished data, chromium is potent in inducing death of the salivary gland cells compared with other heavy metals. It is imperative that further research is needed to completely elucidate the role of chromium in the pathogenesis of SS.

Metals and autoimmune/inflammatory syndrome induced by adjuvants

Autoimmune/inflammatory syndrome induced by adjuvants is a disease entity that was introduced in 2011 and constitutes a set of closely related immune-mediated disease sharing a common clinical denominator secondary to exposure to adjuvant agents [200]. Adjuvants as previously discussed, describe immunological molecules that function through potentiating antigen-specific immune responses, by prolonging antigen presence in the blood and acting a as delivering vehicle [201]. Adjuvants are known to influence the different arms of the immune system by activating pattern recognition receptors including toll- and NOD-like receptors and C-type lectins [202]. Furthermore, adjuvants are known to activate dendritic cell chemotaxis and antigen presentation to effector cells including B- and T-cells, hence their influence on the adaptive immune system [202]. Adjuvants (including silicone, aluminum, and infectious components) were found to induce autoimmunity in different animal models, hence raising the possibility of provoking autoimmune diseases in humans [203, 204].

Tetramethypendadecane also known as pristine is capable of inducing a lupus-like disease in an SLE animal model, similarly, squalene was shown to induce arthritis in rats and autoantibodies in mice [205, 206]. Intraperitoneal immunization of fish with oil-adjuvanted vaccines resulted in the production of autoantibodies as well as autoimmune phenomenon demonstrated by granulomatous manifestations in the liver and peritoneum, and immune-mediated glomerulonephritis [207]. Additionally, alum-based adjuvant administration in mice resulted in a Sjögren-like disease picture with the development of higher antibody levels, decreased saliva volume, and documented histological inflammatory acinar response [208].

Despite its beneficial effects in the context of vaccine, adjuvants were shown to induce nonspecific constitutional symptoms, including fatigue, mental fog, musculoskeletal cramps, amongst others [200]. More severely, in genetically susceptible individuals, adjuvant administration results in overt immune system activation and thus full-blown autoimmune disease.

Indeed, several conditions were linked to previous exposure to adjuvants including siliconosis, the Gulf war syndrome (GWS), the macrophagic myofasciitis syndrome (MMF), and postvaccination phenomena [200].

Perhaps the most evaluated postvaccination condition is the MMF, which results from the deposition of aluminum which is used in different vaccine preparations and hence results in an immune mediate muscle disease. As a disease entity, it is characterized by local signs at the site of inoculation as well as myalgias, arthralgia, muscle weakness, fatigue, and in rare instances a demyelinating disorder [209, 210]. In various instances, elevation of erythrocyte sedimentation rate, appearance of autoantibodies, and characteristic EMG changes can be documented [211]. Muscle biopsy identifies the presence of large PAS-positive, MHC-1-positive macrophages, and CD 8 T-cells. Such macrophages were shown to contain cytoplasmic crystal material representing aluminum hydroxide. These local lesions were found to result from the high biopersistence of aluminum at the site of inoculation up to several years postvaccination [211].

Similarly, silicone a polymeric molecule commonly used in dental applications, implants, and lubrication, was once thought to be inert [212]. Emerging evidence highlights the role of silicone including particles in the activation of the immune system through various mechanisms including NALP3 inflammasomes, and shifting T cell balance toward a pro-inflammatory profile [213]. In predisposed individuals, silicone breast implants resulted in clinical symptoms including fatigue, weakness, musculoskeletal pain, morning stiffness, dry eye, and mouth [214]. In subjects complaining of silicone breast implants, close to one-third to half of the subjects had Raynaud's phenomenon, some of whom presented with nail fold abnormalities on capillaroscopy [215]. Indeed, in a large database silicone breast implants were associated with an increased risk of diagnosis with autoimmune or rheumatic disease, strongest associated was recorded for Sjögren syndrome, systemic sclerosis, and sarcoidosis [216].

Taken together, while adjuvants are usually well tolerated, ASIA illustrates the role of environmental immune-stimulating agents, in the development of complex autoimmune reactions among individuals bearing a genetic preponderance for autoimmunity [23].

Conclusion

Ample evidence points toward the role of heavy metals in influencing the autoimmune disease process. Evidence from observational studies and animal models highlights the pathogenic role of heavy metals in causing aberrations of cytokine expression and autoantibody production. The interrelation between both factors calls for high clinical suspicion by physicians, as avoiding exposure could result in an improvement in the patient's symptoms. Further research is required to better clarify the specific molecular mechanisms causing the disease processes.

References

1. Thom, C.S., Dickson, C.F., Gell, D.A., and Weiss, M.J. (2013). Hemoglobin variants: biochemical properties and clinical correlates. *Cold Spring Harb. Perspect. Med.* 3 (3): a011858.
2. Vlasova, I.I. (2018). Peroxidase activity of human hemoproteins: keeping the fire under control. *Molecules* 23 (10): 2561.
3. Demicheli, V., Moreno, D.M., and Radi, R. (2018). Human Mn-superoxide dismutase inactivation by peroxynitrite: a paradigm of metal-catalyzed tyrosine nitration in vitro and in vivo. *Metallomics* 10 (5): 679–695.
4. Qazi, I.H., Angel, C., Yang, H. et al. (2018). Selenium, selenoproteins, and female reproduction: a review. *Molecules* 23 (12): 3053.
5. Dorozhkin, S.V. (2017). Calcium orthophosphates (CaPO4): occurrence and properties. *Morphologie* 101 (334): 125–142.

6. Li, M.X. and Hwang, P.M. (2015). Structure and function of cardiac troponin C (TNNC1): Implications for heart failure, cardiomyopathies, and troponin modulating drugs. *Gene* 571 (2): 153–166.
7. Icer, M.A. and Gezmen-Karadag, M. (2018). The multiple functions and mechanisms of osteopontin. *Clin. Biochem.* 59: 17–24.
8. He, P., Zou, Y., and Hu, Z. (2015). Advances in aluminum hydroxide-based adjuvant research and its mechanism. *Hum. Vaccin. Immunother.* 11 (2): 477–488.
9. Solano, F. (2018). On the metal cofactor in the tyrosinase family. *Int. J. Mol. Sci.* 19 (2): 633.
10. Ogawa, H., Shinoda, T., Cornelius, F., and Toyoshima, C. (2009). Crystal structure of the sodium-potassium pump (Na+,K+-ATPase) with bound potassium and ouabain. *Proc. Natl. Acad. Sci. U. S. A.* 106 (33): 13742–13747.
11. Supuran, C.T. (2016). Structure and function of carbonic anhydrases. *Biochem. J.* 473 (14): 2023–2032.
12. Hartwig, A. (2001). Role of magnesium in genomic stability. *Mutat. Res.* 475 (1–2): 113–121.
13. Chowdhury, B.A. and Chandra, R.K. (1987). Biological and health implications of toxic heavy metal and essential trace element interactions. *Prog. Food Nutr. Sci.* 11 (1): 55–113.
14. Miracle, V.A. (2017). Lead poisoning in children and adults. *Dimens. Crit. Care Nurs.* 36 (1): 71–73.
15. Tseng, C.H., Chong, C.K., Tseng, C.P. et al. (2003). Long-term arsenic exposure and ischemic heart disease in arseniasis-hyperendemic villages in Taiwan. *Toxicol. Lett.* 137 (1–2): 15–21.
16. Roth, J.A. (2006). Homeostatic and toxic mechanisms regulating manganese uptake, retention, and elimination. *Biol. Res.* 39 (1): 45–57.
17. Copan, L., Fowles, J., Barreau, T., and McGee, N. (2015). Mercury toxicity and contamination of households from the use of skin creams adulterated with mercurous chloride (Calomel). *Int. J. Environ. Res. Public Health* 12 (9): 10943–10954.
18. Vahabzadeh, M. and Balali-Mood, M. (2016). Occupational metallic mercury poisoning in gilders. *Int. J. Occup. Environ. Med.* 7 (2): 116–122.
19. Chen, Q.Y., DesMarais, T., and Costa, M. (2019). Metals and mechanisms of carcinogenesis. *Annu. Rev. Pharmacol. Toxicol.* 59: 537–554.
20. Fashola, M.O., Ngole-Jeme, V.M., and Babalola, O.O. (2016). Heavy metal pollution from gold mines: environmental effects and bacterial strategies for resistance. *Int. J. Environ. Res. Public Health* 13 (11): 1047.
21. Dahlquist, G. (1998). The aetiology of type 1 diabetes: an epidemiological perspective. *Acta Paediatr. Suppl.* 425: 5–10.
22. Noseworthy, J.H., Lucchinetti, C., Rodriguez, M., and Weinshenker, B.G. (2000). Multiple sclerosis. *N. Engl. J. Med.* 343 (13): 938–952.
23. Segal, Y., Dahan, S., Sharif, K. et al. (2018). The value of autoimmune syndrome induced by adjuvant (ASIA) - shedding light on orphan diseases in autoimmunity. *Autoimmun. Rev.* 17 (5): 440–448.
24. Watad, A., Bragazzi, N.L., Bacigaluppi, S. et al. (2018). Artificial neural networks can be effectively used to model changes of intracranial pressure (ICP) during spinal surgery using different non invasive ICP surrogate estimators. *J. Neurosurg. Sci.* 67 (3): 288–296.
25. Sharif, K., Watad, A., Bragazzi, N.L. et al. (2017). Coffee and autoimmunity: more than a mere hot beverage! *Autoimmun. Rev.* 16 (7): 712–721.
26. Clements, C.J. and Griffiths, E. (2002). The global impact of vaccines containing aluminium adjuvants. *Vaccine* 20 (Suppl 3): S24–S33.
27. Budinger, L. and Hertl, M. (2000). Immunologic mechanisms in hypersensitivity reactions to metal ions: an overview. *Allergy* 55 (2): 108–115.
28. McKee, A.S. and Fontenot, A.P. (2016). Interplay of innate and adaptive immunity in metal-induced hypersensitivity. *Curr. Opin. Immunol.* 42: 25–30.
29. Maret, W. (2016). The metals in the biological periodic system of the elements: concepts and conjectures. *Int. J. Mol. Sci.* 17 (1).
30. Weltzien, H.U., Martin, S.F., and Nicolas, J.F. (2014). T cell responses to contact allergens. *Exp. Suppl.* 104: 41–49.
31. Zheng, Y., Gallucci, S., Gaughan, J.P. et al. (2005). A role for B cell-activating factor of the TNF family in chemically induced autoimmunity. *J. Immunol.* 175 (9): 6163–6168.
32. Groom, J., Kalled, S.L., Cutler, A.H. et al. (2002). Association of BAFF/BLyS overexpression and altered B cell differentiation with Sjögren's syndrome. *J. Clin. Invest.* 109 (1): 59–68.

33. Zhang, J., Roschke, V., Baker, K.P. et al. (2001). Cutting edge: a role for B lymphocyte stimulator in systemic lupus erythematosus. *J. Immunol.* 166 (1): 6–10.
34. Cheema, G.S., Roschke, V., Hilbert, D.M., and Stohl, W. (2001). Elevated serum B lymphocyte stimulator levels in patients with systemic immune-based rheumatic diseases. *Arthritis Rheum.* 44 (6): 1313–1319.
35. Schmidt, M. and Goebeler, M. (2015). Immunology of metal allergies. *J. Dtsch. Dermatol. Ges.* 13 (7): 653–660.
36. Raghavan, B., Martin, S.F., Esser, P.R. et al. (2012). Metal allergens nickel and cobalt facilitate TLR4 homodimerization independently of MD2. *EMBO Rep.* 13 (12): 1109–1115.
37. Schmidt, M. and Goebeler, M. (2011). Nickel allergies: paying the Toll for innate immunity. *J. Mol. Med. (Berl)* 89 (10): 961–970.
38. Schmidt, M., Raghavan, B., Muller, V. et al. (2010). Crucial role for human Toll-like receptor 4 in the development of contact allergy to nickel. *Nat. Immunol.* 11 (9): 814–819.
39. Zipris, D. (2010). Toll-like receptors and type 1 diabetes. *Adv. Exp. Med. Biol.* 654: 585–610.
40. Raschi, E., Testoni, C., Bosisio, D. et al. (2003). Role of the MyD88 transduction signaling pathway in endothelial activation by antiphospholipid antibodies. *Blood* 101 (9): 3495–3500.
41. Chen, D.Y., Lin, C.C., Chen, Y.M. et al. (2013). Involvement of TLR7 MyD88-dependent signaling pathway in the pathogenesis of adult-onset Still's disease. *Arthritis Res. Ther.* 15 (2): R39.
42. Pacheco, G.V., Novelo Noh, I.B., Velasco Cardenas, R.M. et al. (2016). Expression of TLR-7, MyD88, NF-kB, and INF-alpha in B Lymphocytes of Mayan women with systemic lupus erythematosus in Mexico. *Front. Immunol.* 7: 22.
43. Into, T., Niida, S., and Shibata, K.I. (2018). MyD88 signaling causes autoimmune sialadenitis through formation of high endothelial venules and upregulation of LTbeta receptor-mediated signaling. *Sci. Rep.* 8 (1): 14272.
44. Caicedo, M.S., Desai, R., McAllister, K. et al. (2009). Soluble and particulate Co-Cr-Mo alloy implant metals activate the inflammasome danger signaling pathway in human macrophages: a novel mechanism for implant debris reactivity. *J. Orthop. Res.* 27 (7): 847–854.
45. McKee, A.S., Mack, D.G., Crawford, F., and Fontenot, A.P. (2015). MyD88 dependence of beryllium-induced dendritic cell trafficking and CD4(+) T-cell priming. *Mucosal. Immunol.* 8 (6): 1237–1247.
46. Clayton, G.M., Wang, Y., Crawford, F. et al. (2014). Structural basis of chronic beryllium disease: linking allergic hypersensitivity and autoimmunity. *Cell* 158 (1): 132–142.
47. Gamerdinger, K., Moulon, C., Karp, D.R. et al. (2003). A new type of metal recognition by human T cells: contact residues for peptide-independent bridging of T cell receptor and major histocompatibility complex by nickel. *J. Exp. Med.* 197 (10): 1345–1353.
48. Kawano, M., Nakayama, M., Aoshima, Y. et al. (2014). NKG2D(+) IFN-gamma(+) CD8(+) T cells are responsible for palladium allergy. *PLoS One* 9 (2): e86810.
49. Takeda, Y., Suto, Y., Ito, K. et al. (2017). TRAV7-2*02 Expressing CD8(+) T cells are responsible for palladium allergy. *Int. J. Mol. Sci.* 18 (6): 1162.
50. Asakura, K., Satoh, H., Chiba, M. et al. (2009). Genotoxicity studies of heavy metals: lead, bismuth, indium, silver and antimony. *J. Occup. Health* 51 (6): 498–512.
51. Stohs, S.J. and Bagchi, D. (1995). Oxidative mechanisms in the toxicity of metal ions. *Free Radic. Biol. Med.* 18 (2): 321–336.
52. Ansari, M.M. and Neha, K.H.A. (2015). Effect of cadmium chloride exposure during the induction of collagen induced arthritis. *Chem. Biol. Interact.* 238: 55–65.
53. Cox, J.N., Rahman, M.A., Bao, S. et al. (2016). Cadmium attenuates the macrophage response to LPS through inhibition of the NF-kappaB pathway. *Am. J. Physiol. Lung Cell. Mol. Physiol.* 311 (4): L754–l765.
54. Olszowski, T., Gutowska, I., Baranowska-Bosiacka, I. et al. (2018). Cadmium alters the concentration of fatty acids in THP-1 macrophages. *Biol. Trace Elem. Res.* 182 (1): 29–36.
55. Mohajeri, M., Rezaee, M., and Sahebkar, A. (2017). Cadmium-induced toxicity is rescued by curcumin: a review. *BioFactors (Oxford, England)* 43 (5): 645–661.
56. Ohsawa, M., Takahashi, K., and Otsuka, F. (1988). Induction of anti-nuclear antibodies in mice orally exposed to cadmium at low concentrations. *Clin. Exp. Immunol.* 73 (1): 98–102.
57. Svensson, S., Trobos, M., Hoffman, M. et al. (2015). A novel soft tissue model for biomaterial-associated infection and inflammation - bacteriological, morphological and molecular observations. *Biomaterials* 41: 106–121.

58. Fortier, M., Omara, F., Bernier, J. et al. (2008). Effects of physiological concentrations of heavy metals both individually and in mixtures on the viability and function of peripheral blood human leukocytes in vitro. *J. Toxicol. Environ. Health A* 71 (19): 1327–1337.
59. Heo, Y., Parsons, P.J., and Lawrence, D.A. (1996). Lead differentially modifies cytokine production in vitro and in vivo. *Toxicol. Appl. Pharmacol.* 138 (1): 149–157.
60. Vaziri, N.D. (2008). Mechanisms of lead-induced hypertension and cardiovascular disease. *Am. J. Physiol. Heart Circ. Physiol.* 295 (2): H454–H465.
61. Gardner, R.M., Nyland, J.F., Silva, I.A. et al. (2010). Mercury exposure, serum antinuclear/antinucleolar antibodies, and serum cytokine levels in mining populations in Amazonian Brazil: a cross-sectional study. *Environ. Res.* 110 (4): 345–354.
62. Crowe, W., Allsopp, P.J., Watson, G.E. et al. (2017). Mercury as an environmental stimulus in the development of autoimmunity - A systematic review. *Autoimmun. Rev.* 16 (1): 72–80.
63. Hemdan, N.Y.A., Lehmann, I., Wichmann, G. et al. (2007). Immunomodulation by mercuric chloride in vitro: application of different cell activation pathways. *Clin. Exp. Immunol.* 148 (2): 325–337.
64. Seubert, A., Monaci, E., Pizza, M. et al. (2008). The adjuvants aluminum hydroxide and MF59 induce monocyte and granulocyte chemoattractants and enhance monocyte differentiation toward dendritic cells. *J. Immunol.* 180 (8): 5402–5412.
65. Rimaniol, A.C., Gras, G., Verdier, F. et al. (2004). Aluminum hydroxide adjuvant induces macrophage differentiation towards a specialized antigen-presenting cell type. *Vaccine* 22 (23–24): 3127–3135.
66. Li, H., Nookala, S., and Re, F. (2007). Aluminum hydroxide adjuvants activate caspase-1 and induce IL-1beta and IL-18 release. *J. Immunol.* 178 (8): 5271–5276.
67. Jordan, M.B., Mills, D.M., Kappler, J. et al. (2004). Promotion of B cell immune responses via an alum-induced myeloid cell population. *Science* 304 (5678): 1808–1810.
68. Pons-Estel, G.J., Alarcón, G.S., Scofield, L. et al. (2010). Understanding the epidemiology and progression of systemic lupus erythematosus. *Semin. Arthritis Rheum.* 39 (4): 257–268.
69. Petri, M. (2002). Epidemiology of systemic lupus erythematosus. *Best Pract. Res. Clin. Rheumatol.* 16 (5): 847–858.
70. Parks, C.G., de Santos, S.E.A., Barbhaiya, M., and Costenbader, K.H. (2017). Understanding the role of environmental factors in the development of systemic lupus erythematosus. *Best Pract. Res. Clin. Rheumatol.* 31 (3): 306–320.
71. Sarzi-Puttini, P., Atzeni, F., Iaccarino, L., and Doria, A. (2005). Environment and systemic lupus erythematosus: an overview. *Autoimmunity* 38 (7): 465–472.
72. Pollard, K.M., Pearson, D.L., Hultman, P. et al. (1999). Lupus-prone mice as models to study xenobiotic-induced acceleration of systemic autoimmunity. *Environ. Health Perspect.* 107: 729.
73. Kosboth, M., Chin-Loy, A., Lyons, R. et al. (2007). Malar rash caused by metal allergy in a patient with systemic lupus erythematosus. *Nat. Clin. Pract. Rheumatol.* 3 (4): 240–245.
74. Katz-Agranov N, Zandman-Goddard G. Systemic Lupus Erythematosus Induced by Vaccines 1. *Vaccines Autoimmun.*,13:207-22 (2015).
75. Leffel, E.K., Wolf, C., Poklis, A., and White, K.L. (2003). Drinking water exposure to cadmium, an environmental contaminant, results in the exacerbation of autoimmune disease in the murine model. *Toxicology* 188 (2–3): 233–250.
76. Ohsawa, M., Takahashi, K., and Otsuka, F. (1988). Induction of antinuclear antibodies by in vivo and in vitro treatments with cadmium. *Int. J. Immunopharmacol.* 10: 145.
77. Klack, K., Bonfa, E., and Borba Neto, E.F. (2012). Dieta e aspectos nutricionais no lúpus eritematoso sistêmico. *Rev. Bras. Reumatol.* 52 (3): 395–408.
78. Jendryczko, A., Drożdż, M., and Magner, K. (1985). Antilupus activity of copper (II). *Exp. Pathol.* 28 (3): 187–189.
79. Duffy, E.M., Meenagh, G.K., McMillan, S.A. et al. (2004). The clinical effect of dietary supplementation with omega-3 fish oils and/or copper in systemic lupus erythematosus. *J. Rheumatol.* 31 (8): 1551–1556.
80. Chowdhary, V.R. (2017). Broad concepts in management of systemic lupus erythematosus. *Mayo Clin. Proc.* 92 (5): 744–761.
81. Sánchez-Guerrero, J., Uribe, A.G., Jiménez-Santana, L. et al. (2005). A trial of contraceptive methods in women with systemic lupus erythematosus. *N. Engl. J. Med.* 353 (24): 2539–2549.

82. Abedi-Valugerdi, M. (2009). Mercury and silver induce B cell activation and anti-nucleolar autoantibody production in outbred mouse stocks: are environmental factors more important than the susceptibility genes in connection with autoimmunity? *Clin. Exp. Immunol.* 155 (1): 117–124.
83. Hansson, M. and Abedi-Valugerdi, M. (2003). Xenobiotic metal-induced autoimmunity: mercury and silver differentially induce antinucleolar autoantibody production in susceptible H-2s, H-2q and H-2f mice. *Clin. Exp. Immunol.* 131 (3): 405–414.
84. DiMeglio, L.A., Evans-Molina, C., and Oram, R.A. (2018). Type 1 diabetes. *Lancet* 391 (10138): 2449–2462.
85. Alkaladi, A., Abdelazim, A., and Afifi, M. (2014). Antidiabetic activity of zinc oxide and silver nanoparticles on streptozotocin-induced diabetic rats. *Int. J. Mol. Sci.* 15 (2): 2015–2023.
86. Tian, J., Clere-Salzler, M., Herschenfeld, A. et al. (1996). Modulating autoimmune responses to GAD inhibits disease progression and prolongs islet graft survival in diabetes–prone mice. *Nat. Med.* 2 (12): 1348–1353.
87. Wherrett, D.K., Bundy, B., Becker, D.J. et al. (2011). Antigen-based therapy with glutamic acid decarboxylase (GAD) vaccine in patients with recent-onset type 1 diabetes: a randomised double-blind trial. *Lancet* 378 (9788): 319–327.
88. Haglund, B., Ryckenberg, K., Selinus, O., and Dahlquist, G. (1996). Evidence of a relationship between childhood-onset type I diabetes and low groundwater concentration of zinc. *Diabetes Care* 19 (8): 873–875.
89. Rohilla, A. and Ali, S. (2012). Alloxan induced diabetes: mechanisms and effects. *Int. J. Res. Pharmaceut. Biomed. Sci.* 3 (2): 819–823.
90. Demir, N., Akkoyunlu, G., Agar, A. et al. (2002). Effect of cadmium on sciatic nerve in diabetic rats: an ultrastructural study. *Int. J. Neurosci.* 112 (7): 779–796.
91. Moon, S.S. (2013). Association of lead, mercury and cadmium with diabetes in the Korean population: the Korea National Health and Nutrition Examination Survey (KNHANES) 2009–2010. *Diabet. Med.* 30 (4): e143–e148.
92. Al-Saleh, E., Nandakumaran, M., Al-Shammari, M., and Al-Harouny, A. (2004). Maternal–fetal status of copper, iron, molybdenum, selenium and zinc in patients with gestational diabetes. *J. Matern. Fetal Neonatal Med.* 16 (1): 15–21.
93. Lee, D.M. and Weinblatt, M.E. (2001). Rheumatoid arthritis. *Lancet* 358 (9285): 903–911.
94. Turesson, C., O'Fallon, W.M., Crowson, C.S. et al. (2003). Extra-articular disease manifestations in rheumatoid arthritis: incidence trends and risk factors over 46 years. *Ann. Rheum. Dis.* 62 (8): 722–727.
95. Smolen, J.S., Aletaha, D., and McInnes, I.B. (2016). Rheumatoid arthritis. *Lancet* 388 (10055): 2023–2038.
96. Bernhard, D., Rossmann, A., and Wick, G. (2005). Metals in cigarette smoke. *IUBMB Life* 57 (12): 805–809.
97. Joo, S.H., Lee, J., Hutchinson, D., and Song, Y.W. (2019). Prevalence of rheumatoid arthritis in relation to serum cadmium concentrations: cross-sectional study using Korean National Health and Nutrition Examination Survey (KNHANES) data. *BMJ Open* 9 (1): e023233.
98. Muris, J. and Feilzer, A.J. (2006). Micro analysis of metals in dental restorations as part of a diagnostic approach in metal allergies. *Neuro. Endocrinol. Lett.* 27 (Suppl 1): 49–52.
99. Yang, T.H., Yuan, T.H., Hwang, Y.H. et al. (2016). Increased inflammation in rheumatoid arthritis patients living where farm soils contain high levels of copper. *J. Formos. Med. Assoc.* 115 (11): 991–996.
100. Bamonti, F., Fulgenzi, A., Novembrino, C., and Ferrero, M.E. (2011). Metal chelation therapy in rheumatoid arthritis: a case report. Successful management of rheumatoid arthritis by metal chelation therapy. *Biometals* 24 (6): 1093–1098.
101. Leutmezer, F. (2017). Multiple sclerosis – an overview on epidemiology, pathogenesis and diagnosis. *Hamdan Med. J.* 10 (4): 205.
102. Kumar, V. and Gill, K.D. (2009). Aluminium neurotoxicity: neurobehavioural and oxidative aspects. *Arch. Toxicol.* 83 (11): 965–978.
103. Calabrese, V., Lodi, R., Tonon, C. et al. (2005). Oxidative stress, mitochondrial dysfunction and cellular stress response in Friedreich's ataxia. *J. Neurol. Sci.* 233 (1–2, 162): 145.
104. Leuner, K., Hauptmann, S., Abdel-Kader, R. et al. (2007). Mitochondrial dysfunction: the first domino in brain aging and Alzheimer's disease? *Antioxid. Redox Signal.* 9 (10): 1659–1676.
105. Parker, W.D., Ba, J.P., Filley, C.M., and Kleinschmidt-DeMasters, B.K. (1994). Electron transport chain defects in Alzheimer's disease brain. *Neurology* 44 (6): 1090–1090.

106. Fulgenzi, A., Zanella, S.G., Mariani, M.M. et al. (2012). A case of multiple sclerosis improvement following removal of heavy metal intoxication. *Biometals* 25 (3): 569–576.
107. Friberg, L. (1950). Health hazards in the manufacture of alkaline accumulators with special reference to chronic cadmium poisoning; a clinical and experimental study. *Acta Medica Scand. Suppl.* 240: 1–124.
108. Jaishankar, M., Tseten, T., Anbalagan, N. et al. (2014). Toxicity, mechanism and health effects of some heavy metals. *Interdiscip. Toxicol.* 7 (2): 60–72.
109. Jomova, K. and Valko, M. (2011). Advances in metal-induced oxidative stress and human disease. *Toxicology* 283 (2–3): 65–87.
110. Usai, C., Barberis, A., Moccagatta, L., and Marchetti, C. (2008). Pathways of cadmium influx in mammalian neurons. *J. Neurochem.* 72 (5): 2154–2161.
111. Miura, S., Takahashi, K., Imagawa, T. et al. (2013). Involvement of TRPA1 activation in acute pain induced by cadmium in mice. *Mol. Pain* 9: 1744–8069.
112. Marchetti, C. (2014). Interaction of metal ions with neurotransmitter receptors and potential role in neurodiseases. *Biometals* 27 (6): 1097–1113.
113. Wang, B. and Du, Y. (2013). Cadmium and its neurotoxic effects. *Oxidative Med. Cell. Longev.* 2013: 1–12.
114. Sheykhansari, S., Kozielski, K., Bill, J. et al. (2018). Redox metals homeostasis in multiple sclerosis and amyotrophic lateral sclerosis: a review. *Cell Death Dis.* 9 (3): 348.
115. Arvidson, B. (1985). Retrograde axonal transport of cadmium in the rat hypoglossal nerve. *Neurosci. Lett.* 62 (1): 45–49.
116. Kumar, R., Agarwal, A.K., and Seth, P.K. (1996). Oxidative stress-mediated neurotoxicity of cadmium. *Toxicol. Lett.* 89 (1): 65–69.
117. Sinha, M., Manna, P., and Sil, P.C. (2008). Cadmium-induced neurological disorders: prophylactic role of taurine. *J. Appl. Toxicol.* 28 (8): 974–986.
118. López, E., Arce, C., Oset-Gasque, M.J. et al. (2006). Cadmium induces reactive oxygen species generation and lipid peroxidation in cortical neurons in culture. *Free Radic. Biol. Med.* 40 (6): 940–951.
119. Shukla, G.S., Srivastava, R.S., and Chandra, S.V. (1988). Glutathione status and cadmium neurotoxicity: studies in discrete brain regions of growing rats. *Toxicol. Sci.* 11 (1): 229–235.
120. Aliomrani, M., Sahraian, M.A., Shirkhanloo, H. et al. (2017). Correlation between heavy metal exposure and GSTM1 polymorphism in Iranian multiple sclerosis patients. *Neurol. Sci.* 38 (7): 1271–1278.
121. Moradi, A., Honarjoo, N., Etemadifar, M., and Fallahzade, J. (2016). Bio-accumulation of some heavy metals in blood serum of residents in Isfahan and Shiraz, Iran. *Environ. Monit. Assess.* 188 (5): 1–7.
122. Heydarpour, P., Amini, H., Khoshkish, S. et al. (2014). Potential impact of air pollution on multiple sclerosis in Tehran, Iran. *Neuroepidemiology* 43 (3–4): 233–238.
123. Manto, M. (2014). Abnormal copper homeostasis: mechanisms and roles in neurodegeneration. *Toxics* 2 (2): 327–345.
124. Aspli, K.T., Flaten, T.P., Roos, P.M. et al. (2015). Iron and copper in progressive demyelination – new lessons from Skogholt's disease. *J. Trace Elem. Med. Biol.* 31: 183–187.
125. Johnson, S. (2000). The possible role of gradual accumulation of copper, cadmium, lead and iron and gradual depletion of zinc, magnesium, selenium, vitamins B2, B6, D, and E and essential fatty acids in multiple sclerosis. *Med. Hypotheses* 55 (3): 239–241.
126. van Horssen, J., Witte, M.E., Schreibelt, G., and de Vries, H.E. (2011). Radical changes in multiple sclerosis pathogenesis. *Biochim. Biophys. Acta (BBA) - Mol. Basis Dis.* 1812 (2): 141–150.
127. Melo, T.M., Larsen, C., White, L.R. et al. (2003). Manganese, copper, and zinc in cerebrospinal fluid from patients with multiple sclerosis. *Biol. Trace Elem. Res.* 93 (1–3): 1–8.
128. Sedighi, B., Ebrahimi, H.A., Haghdoost, A.A., and Abotorabi, M. (2013). Comparison of serum levels of copper and zinc among multiple sclerosis patients and control group. *Iran. J. Neurol.* 12 (4): 125–128.
129. Günther, P., Baum, P., Then Bergh, F., and Hermann, W. (2009). Morbus Wilson und Multiple Sklerose. *Nervenarzt* 81 (2): 226–228.
130. Maña, P., Fordham, S.A., Staykova, M.A. et al. (2009). Demyelination caused by the copper chelator cuprizone halts T cell mediated autoimmune neuroinflammation. *J. Neuroimmunol.* 210 (1–2): 13–21.
131. De Riccardis, L., Buccolieri, A., Muci, M. et al. (2018). Copper and ceruloplasmin dyshomeostasis in serum and cerebrospinal fluid of multiple sclerosis subjects. *Biochim. Biophys. Acta Mol. Basis Dis.* 1864 (5 Pt A): 1828–1838.

132. Matsushima, G.K. and Morell, P. (2006). The neurotoxicant, cuprizone, as a model to study demyelination and remyelination in the central nervous system. *Brain Pathol.* 11 (1): 107–116.
133. Venturini, G. (1973). Enzymic activities and sodium, potassium and copper concentrations in mouse brain and liver after cuprizone treatment in vivo. *J. Neurochem.* 21 (5): 1147–1151.
134. Groebe, A., Clarner, T., Baumgartner, W. et al. (2009). Cuprizone treatment induces distinct demyelination, astrocytosis, and microglia cell invasion or proliferation in the mouse cerebellum. *Cerebellum* 8 (3): 163–174.
135. Norkute, A., Hieble, A., Braun, A. et al. (2009). Cuprizone treatment induces demyelination and astrocytosis in the mouse hippocampus. *J. Neurosci. Res.* 87 (6): 1343–1355.
136. Silvestroff, L., Bartucci, S., Soto, E. et al. (2010). Cuprizone-induced demyelination in CNP::GFP transgenic mice. *J. Comp. Neurol.* 518 (12): 2261–2283.
137. Skripuletz, T., Lindner, M., Kotsiari, A. et al. (2008). Cortical demyelination is prominent in the murine cuprizone model and is strain-dependent. *Am. J. Pathol.* 172 (4): 1053–1061.
138. Torkildsen, Ø., Brunborg, L.A., Myhr, K.M., and Bø, L. (2008). The cuprizone model for demyelination. *Acta Neurol. Scand.* 117 (s188): 72–76.
139. Wergeland, S., Torkildsen, Ø., Myhr, K.-M. et al. (2012). The cuprizone model: regional heterogeneity of pathology. *APMIS* 120 (8): 648–657.
140. Zatta, P., Raso, M., Zambenedetti, P. et al. (2005). Copper and zinc dismetabolism in the mouse brain upon chronic cuprizone treatment. *Cell. Mol. Life Sci.* 62 (13): 1502–1513.
141. Kaur, D., Yantiri, F., Rajagopalan, S. et al. (2003). Genetic or pharmacological iron chelation prevents MPTP-induced neurotoxicity in vivo. *Neuron* 37 (6): 899–909.
142. Cherny, R.A., Atwood, C.S., Xilinas, M.E. et al. (2001). Treatment with a copper-zinc chelator markedly and rapidly inhibits β-amyloid accumulation in Alzheimer's disease transgenic mice. *Neuron* 30 (3): 665–676.
143. Choi, B.Y., Jang, B.G., Kim, J.H. et al. (2013). Copper/zinc chelation by clioquinol reduces spinal cord white matter damage and behavioral deficits in a murine MOG-induced multiple sclerosis model. *Neurobiol. Dis.* 54: 382–391.
144. Lerner, A. (2007). Aluminum is a potential environmental factor for Crohn's disease induction: extended hypothesis. *Ann. N. Y. Acad. Sci.* 1107 (1): 329–345.
145. Perl, D.P., Fogarty, U., Harpaz, N., and Sachar, D.B. (2004). Bacterial-metal interactions: the potential role of aluminum and other trace elements in the etiology of Crohn's disease. *Inflamm. Bowel Dis.* 10 (6): 881–883.
146. Lomer, M.C.E., Thompson, R.P.H., and Powell, J.J. (2002). Fine and ultrafine particles of the diet: influence on the mucosal immune response and association with Crohn's disease. *Proc. Nutr. Soc.* 61 (1): 123–130.
147. Powell, J.J., Harvey, R.S., and Thompson, R.P. (1996). Microparticles in Crohn's disease–has the dust settled? *Gut* 39 (2): 340–341.
148. Ward, R.J., Zhang, Y., and Crichton, R.R. (2001). Aluminium toxicity and iron homeostasis. *J. Inorg. Biochem.* 87 (1-2): 9–14.
149. Lomer, M.C.E., Kodjabashia, K., Hutchinson, C. et al. (2004). Intake of dietary iron is low in patients with Crohn's disease: a case–control study. *Br. J. Nutr.* 91 (1): 141–148.
150. Revel-Vilk, S., Tamary, H., Broide, E. et al. (2000). Serum transferrin receptor in children and adolescents with inflammatory bowel disease. *Eur. J. Pediatr.* 159 (8): 585–589.
151. Authier, F.-J., Sauvat, S., Christov, C. et al. (2006). Al(OH)3-adjuvanted vaccine-induced macrophagic myofasciitis in rats is influenced by the genetic background. *Neuromuscul. Disord.* 16 (5): 347–352.
152. D'Inca, R., Annese, V., Di Leo, V. et al. (2006). Increased intestinal permeability and NOD2 variants in familial and sporadic Crohn's disease. *Aliment. Pharmacol. Ther.* 23 (10): 1455–1461.
153. Fosmire, G.J., Focht, S.J., and McClearn, G.E. (1993). Genetic influences on tissue deposition of aluminum in mice. *Biol. Trace Elem. Res.* 37 (2–3): 115–121.
154. Fries, W., Renda, M.C., Lo Presti, M.A. et al. (2005). Intestinal permeability and genetic determinants in patients, first-degree relatives, and controls in a high-incidence area of Crohn's disease in Southern Italy. *Am. J. Gastroenterol.* 100 (12): 2730–2736.
155. Schreiber, S. (2006). Slipping the barrier: how variants in CARD15 could alter permeability of the intestinal wall and population health. *Gut* 55 (3): 308–309.

156. Van Rensburg, S.J., Potocnik, F.C.V., De Villiers, J.N.P. et al. (2000). Earlier Age of Onset of Alzheimer's Disease in Patients with Both the Transferrin C2 and Apolipoprotein E-e4 Alleles. *Ann. N. Y. Acad. Sci.* 903 (1 VASCULAR FACT): 200–203.
157. Banasik, A., Lankoff, A., Piskulak, A. et al. (2005). Aluminum-induced micronuclei and apoptosis in human peripheral-blood lymphocytes treated during different phases of the cell cycle. *Environ. Toxicol.* 20 (4): 402–406.
158. Hegde, M.L., Anitha, S., Latha, K.S. et al. (2004). First evidence for helical transitions in supercoiled DNA by amyloid β peptide (1-42) and aluminum: a new insight in understanding Alzheimer's disease. *J. Mol. Neurosci.* 22 (1–2): 19–32.
159. Sawa, T. and Ohshima, H. (2006). Nitrative DNA damage in inflammation and its possible role in carcinogenesis. *Nitric Oxide* 14 (2): 91–100.
160. Lomer, M.C.E., Hutchinson, C., Volkert, S. et al. (2004). Dietary sources of inorganic microparticles and their intake in healthy subjects and patients with Crohn's disease. *Br. J. Nutr.* 92 (6): 947–955.
161. Powell, J.J., Ainley, C.C., Harvey, R.S. et al. (1996). Characterisation of inorganic microparticles in pigment cells of human gut associated lymphoid tissue. *Gut* 38 (3): 390–395.
162. Pineton de Chambrun, G., Body-Malapel, M., Frey-Wagner, I. et al. (2013). Aluminum enhances inflammation and decreases mucosal healing in experimental colitis in mice. *Mucosal Immunol.* 7 (3): 589–601.
163. Breton, J., Le Clère, K., Daniel, C. et al. (2013). Chronic ingestion of cadmium and lead alters the bioavailability of essential and heavy metals, gene expression pathways and genotoxicity in mouse intestine. *Arch. Toxicol.* 87 (10): 1787–1795.
164. Fazeli, M., Hassanzadeh, P., and Alaei, S. (2011). Cadmium chloride exhibits a profound toxic effect on bacterial microflora of the mice gastrointestinal tract. *Hum. Exp. Toxicol.* 30 (2): 152–159.
165. Zhai, Q., Li, T., Yu, L. et al. (2017). Effects of subchronic oral toxic metal exposure on the intestinal microbiota of mice. *Sci. Bull.* 62 (12): 831–840.
166. Gianchecchi, E. and Fierabracci, A. (2015). Gene/environment interactions in the pathogenesis of autoimmunity: new insights on the role of Toll-like receptors. *Autoimmun. Rev.* 14 (11): 971–983.
167. Marie, I. (2019). Systemic sclerosis and exposure to heavy metals. *Autoimmun. Rev.* 18 (1): 62–72.
168. Marie, I., Gehanno, J.F., Bubenheim, M. et al. (2017). Systemic sclerosis and exposure to heavy metals: a case control study of 100 patients and 300 controls. *Autoimmun. Rev.* 16 (3): 223–230.
169. Sundar, S. and Chakravarty, J. (2010). Antimony toxicity. *Int. J. Environ. Res. Public Health* 7 (12): 4267–4277.
170. Marie, I., Gehanno, J.F., Bubenheim, M. et al. (2014). Prospective study to evaluate the association between systemic sclerosis and occupational exposure and review of the literature. *Autoimmun. Rev.* 13 (2): 151–156.
171. Fagerberg, B., Bergstrom, G., Boren, J., and Barregard, L. (2012). Cadmium exposure is accompanied by increased prevalence and future growth of atherosclerotic plaques in 64-year-old women. *J. Intern. Med.* 272 (6): 601–610.
172. Menke, A., Guallar, E., and Cowie, C.C. (2016). Metals in urine and diabetes in US. Adults. *Diabetes* 65 (1): 164–171.
173. Hess, E.V. (2002). Environmental chemicals and autoimmune disease: cause and effect. *Toxicology* 181–182: 65–70.
174. Knoflach, M., Messner, B., Shen, Y.H. et al. (2011). Non-toxic cadmium concentrations induce vascular inflammation and promote atherosclerosis. *Circ J* 75 (10): 2491–2495.
175. Hanley, G.A., Schiffenbauer, J., and Sobel, E.S. (1998). Resistance to HgCl2-induced autoimmunity in haplotype-heterozygous mice is an intrinsic property of B cells. *J. Immunol.* 161 (4): 1778–1785.
176. Casciola-Rosen, L., Wigley, F., and Rosen, A. (1997). Scleroderma autoantigens are uniquely fragmented by metal-catalyzed oxidation reactions: implications for pathogenesis. *J. Exp. Med.* 185 (1): 71–79.
177. Forte, G., Fadda, C., Bocca, B. et al. (2019). Association between exposure to heavy metals and systemic sclerosis: the levels of Al, Cd, Hg, and Pb in blood and urine of patients. *Biol. Trace Elem. Res.* 190 (1): 1–10.
178. Jain, R.B. (2014). Thyroid function and serum copper, selenium, and zinc in general U.S. population. *Biol. Trace Elem. Res.* 159 (1–3): 87–98.
179. Ralston, N.V. and Raymond, L.J. (2010). Dietary selenium's protective effects against methylmercury toxicity. *Toxicology* 278 (1): 112–123.
180. Jonklaas, J., Davidson, B., Bhagat, S., and Soldin, S.J. (2008). Triiodothyronine levels in athyreotic individuals during levothyroxine therapy. *JAMA* 299 (7): 769–777.

181. Afrifa, J., Ogbordjor, W.D., and Duku-Takyi, R. (2018). Variation in thyroid hormone levels is associated with elevated blood mercury levels among artisanal small-scale miners in Ghana. *PLoS One* 13 (8): e0203335.
182. Nishida, M., Yamamoto, T., Yoshimura, Y., and Kawada, J. (1986). Subacute toxicity of methylmercuric chloride and mercuric chloride on mouse thyroid. *J. Pharmacobiodyn* 9 (4): 331–338.
183. Rice, K.M., Walker, E.M. Jr., Wu, M. et al. (2014). Environmental mercury and its toxic effects. *J. Prev. Med. Public Health* 47 (2): 74–83.
184. McGregor, A.J. and Mason, H.J. (1991). Occupational mercury vapour exposure and testicular, pituitary and thyroid endocrine function. *Hum. Exp. Toxicol.* 10 (3): 199–203.
185. Wadaan, M.A.M. (2009). Effects of mercury exposure on blood chemistry and liver histopathology of male rats. *J. Pharmacol. Toxicol.* 4: 126–131.
186. Kawada, J., Nishida, M., Yoshimura, Y., and Mitani, K. (1980). Effects of organic and inorganic mercurials on thyroidal functions. *J. Pharmacobiodyn* 3 (3): 149–159.
187. Soldin, O.P. and Aschner, M. (2007). Effects of manganese on thyroid hormone homeostasis: potential links. *Neurotoxicology* 28 (5): 951–956.
188. Oikawa, S., Hirosawa, I., Tada-Oikawa, S. et al. (2006). Mechanism for manganese enhancement of dopamine-induced oxidative DNA damage and neuronal cell death. *Free Radic. Biol. Med.* 41 (5): 748–756.
189. Kawada, J., Nishida, M., Yoshimura, Y., and Yamashita, K. (1985). Manganese ion as a goitrogen in the female mouse. *Endocrinol. Jpn* 32 (5): 635–643.
190. Chen, A., Kim, S.S., Chung, E., and Dietrich, K.N. (2013). Thyroid hormones in relation to lead, mercury, and cadmium exposure in the National Health and Nutrition Examination Survey, 2007-2008. *Environ. Health Perspect.* 121 (2): 181–186.
191. Yorita Christensen, K.L. (2013). Metals in blood and urine, and thyroid function among adults in the United States 2007-2008. *Int. J. Hyg. Environ. Health* 216 (6): 624–632.
192. Buha, A., Matovic, V., Antonijevic, B. et al. (2018). Overview of cadmium thyroid disrupting effects and mechanisms. *Int. J. Mol. Sci.* 19 (5): 1501.
193. Luo, J. and Hendryx, M. (2014). Relationship between blood cadmium, lead, and serum thyroid measures in US adults - the National Health and Nutrition Examination Survey (NHANES) 2007-2010. *Int. J. Environ. Health Res.* 24 (2): 125–136.
194. Yoshizuka, M., Mori, N., Hamasaki, K. et al. (1991). Cadmium toxicity in the thyroid gland of pregnant rats. *Exp. Mol. Pathol.* 55 (1): 97–104.
195. Hammouda, F., Messaoudi, I., El Hani, J. et al. (2008). Reversal of cadmium-induced thyroid dysfunction by selenium, zinc, or their combination in rat. *Biol. Trace Elem. Res.* 126 (1–3): 194–203.
196. Al-Assaf, A.H., Alqahtani, A.M., Alshatwi, A.A. et al. (2013). Mechanism of cadmium induced apoptosis in human peripheral blood lymphocytes: the role of p53, Fas and Caspase-3. *Environ. Toxicol. Pharmacol.* 36 (3): 1033–1039.
197. Ertek, S., Cicero, A.F., Caglar, O., and Erdogan, G. (2010). Relationship between serum zinc levels, thyroid hormones and thyroid volume following successful iodine supplementation. *Hormones (Athens, Greece)* 9 (3): 263–268.
198. Mavragani, C.P. and Moutsopoulos, H.M. (2014). Sjögren syndrome. *CMAJ* 186 (15): E579–E586.
199. Lee, C.P., Hsu, P.Y., and Su, C.C. (2019). Increased prevalence of Sjögren's syndrome in where soils contain high levels of chromium. *Sci. Total Environ.* 657: 1121–1126.
200. Shoenfeld, Y. and Agmon-Levin, N. (2011). 'ASIA' – Autoimmune/inflammatory syndrome induced by adjuvants. *J. Autoimmun.* 36 (1): 4–8.
201. Di Pasquale, A., Preiss, S., Tavares Da Silva, F., and Garçon, N. (2015). Vaccine adjuvants: from 1920 to 2015 and Beyond. *Vaccines (Basel)* 3 (2): 320–343.
202. Israeli, E., Agmon-Levin, N., Blank, M., and Shoenfeld, Y. (2009). Adjuvants and autoimmunity. *Lupus* 18 (13): 1217–1225.
203. Bar-Meir, E., Eherenfeld, M., and Shoenfeld, Y. (2003). Silicone gel breast implants and connective tissue disease–a comprehensive review. *Autoimmunity* 36 (4): 193–197.
204. Zandman-Goddard, G., Blank, M., Ehrenfeld, M. et al. (1999). A comparison of autoantibody production in asymptomatic and symptomatic women with silicone breast implants. *J. Rheumatol.* 26 (1): 73–77.
205. Reeves, W.H., Lee, P.Y., Weinstein, J.S. et al. (2009). Induction of autoimmunity by pristane and other naturally occurring hydrocarbons. *Trends Immunol.* 30 (9): 455–464.

206. Satoh, M. and Reeves, W.H. (1994). Induction of lupus-associated autoantibodies in BALB/c mice by intraperitoneal injection of pristane. *J. Exp. Med.* 180 (6): 2341–2346.
207. Koppang, E.O., Bjerkas, I., Haugarvoll, E. et al. (2008). Vaccination-induced systemic autoimmunity in farmed Atlantic salmon. *J. Immunol.* 181 (7): 4807–4814.
208. Bagavant, H., Nandula, S.R., Kaplonek, P. et al. (2014). Alum, an aluminum-based adjuvant, induces Sjögren's syndrome-like disorder in mice. *Clin. Exp. Rheumatol.* 32 (2): 251–255.
209. Gherardi, R.K., Coquet, M., Cherin, P. et al. (2001). Macrophagic myofasciitis lesions assess long-term persistence of vaccine-derived aluminium hydroxide in muscle. *Brain J. Neurol.* 124 (Pt 9): 1821–1831.
210. Exley, C., Swarbrick, L., Gherardi, R.K., and Authier, F.J. (2009). A role for the body burden of aluminium in vaccine-associated macrophagic myofasciitis and chronic fatigue syndrome. *Med. Hypotheses* 72 (2): 135–139.
211. Israeli, E., Agmon-Levin, N., Blank, M., and Shoenfeld, Y. (2011). Macrophagic myofaciitis a vaccine (alum) autoimmune-related disease. *Clin. Rev. Allergy Immunol.* 41 (2): 163–168.
212. Price, C.T., Koval, K.J., and Langford, J.R. (2013). Silicon: a review of its potential role in the prevention and treatment of postmenopausal osteoporosis. *Int. J. Endocrinol.* 2013: 316783.
213. Vojdani, A., Campbell, A., and Brautbar, N. (1992). Immune functional impairment in patients with clinical abnormalities and silicone breast implants. *Toxicol. Ind. Health* 8 (6): 415–429.
214. Cohen Tervaert, J.W., Colaris, M.J., and van der Hulst, R.R. (2017). Silicone breast implants and autoimmune rheumatic diseases: myth or reality. *Curr. Opin. Rheumatol.* 29 (4): 348–354.
215. Spiera, R.F., Gibofsky, A., and Spiera, H. (1994). Silicone gel filled breast implants and connective tissue disease: an overview. *J. Rheumatol.* 21 (2): 239–245.
216. Watad, A., Rosenberg, V., Tiosano, S. et al. (2018). Silicone breast implants and the risk of autoimmune/rheumatic disorders: a real-world analysis. *Int. J. Epidemiol.* 47 (6): 1846–1854.

20 The Role of Bisphenol A in ASIA Syndrome

Zora Lazurova
4th Department of Internal Medicine, Pavol Jozef Šafárik University, Kosice, Slovakia

Introduction

There is evidence of a growing prevalence of autoimmune diseases in the past few decades. This can be explained by the development of industrialization, which is leading to a rising exposure of the population to various environmental factors, including bisphenol A (BPA), as well as a mixture of other environmental estrogens and xenobiotics [1, 2]. BPA, a common endocrine disruptor, was first identified to affect the endocrine and primarily the reproductive system. However, further studies revealed its multisystemic effects. BPA plays a role in the etiopathogenesis of several cardiovascular, metabolic, neurological, psychiatric, and oncological disorders, and last but not least, it alters the normal function of the immune system, leading to the development of allergies and autoimmunity [3–7].

The autoimmune/inflammatory syndrome induced by adjuvants (ASIA syndrome), also known as Shoenfeld's syndrome, represents a group of several immune-mediated conditions that are associated with exposure to substances with adjuvant activity, such as silicones, present in various types of implants, i.e. breast implants, or adjuvants used in vaccines, which may lead to postvaccination phenomenon. The manifestation of ASIA syndrome is very heterogeneous; the severity may vary from very mild to severe, and the clinical symptoms may vary from nonspecific, like fatigue, malaise, and myalgia, up to fully presented autoimmune disease [8, 9].

BPA itself has been proven to dysregulate the immune system, exerting the features of an adjuvant. Various pathophysiological mechanisms contributing to the development of systemic, as well as organ-specific, autoimmune diseases have been identified.

Bisphenol A

BPA is an organic, lipophilic, and thermostable substance widely used as a compound in the production of plastics to improve their quality. Due to its molecular structural similarity to endogenous estrogens, BPA is able to bind to estrogen receptors (ERs). Therefore, BPA belongs to the group called environmental estrogens and endocrine disruptors [1].

Autoimmune Disorders: Adjuvants and Other Risk Factors in Pathogenesis, First Edition.
Edited by Abdulla Watad, Nicola Luigi Bragazzi, and Yehuda Shoenfeld.

BPA was first synthetized in 1891 by Russian chemist Alexander Dianin. Initially, it was used as a growth-stimulation substance for poultry and cattle. Later on, when the estrogenic effects were identified, BPA was used for supplementation of estrogens in women. Since the 1950s, it has been used in the production of plastics as a polymerization agent, because of the ability of BPA to improve the quality of plastics, mostly increasing their resistance and thermostability [10].

Since then, the exposure of the population to this xenoestrogen has been rapidly increasing. Recently, it has been found in the urine of more than 93% of U.S. citizens. According to other studies, BPA was confirmed in the serum or urine of 91–99% of the population [11, 12]. The main sources of exposure for humans are plastic bottles, food packages, cans, pipes, clothes, cosmetics, and other plastic subjects of daily use [1, 3].

BPA enters the human body mostly in peroral way by water and food. The absorption from gastrointestinal tract is quite high, but due to the first-pass effect in the liver, BPA is rapidly conjugated into nontoxic metabolites. By the oral route, BPA has low systemic bioavailability, approximately 1–10% and the halftime is a few hours. Despite its high hepatic inactivation after peroral exposure, the total amount of ingested BPA can be occasionally very large; therefore, it represents a significant source of BPA for humans [11]. For example, the study of Carwile et al. found more than 100% increase in urinary BPA levels in individuals after eating a soup from the BPA-lined can [13]. Moreover, due to the lipophilic character of the molecule, percutaneous absorption also represents a significant source. Small dust particles carrying BPA molecules can be inhaled and resorbed from the respiratory system too, though this is the minor source of total exposure.

The molecular structure and configuration of BPA mimic endogenous estrogens; therefore, it can bind to estrogen receptors (ERs; ER-alpha and ER-beta), as well as to estrogen-related receptors (ERRs). BPA exerts direct estrogenic effects, as well as it may regulate the expression of genes and regulate the synthesis of various proteins that mediate its nonestrogenic effects. BPA is also able to bind to other receptors (androgen receptors, receptors for thyroid hormones, peroxisome proliferator-activated receptor gamma – PPAR-gamma, aryl-hydrocarbon receptors, etc.) with lower affinity. Only free BPA is active; some fraction binds to transport proteins, mostly albumin, sex hormone-binding globulin (SHBG), etc. [1–3].

BPA cannot be metabolized and degraded in the organism. The only possible way is nonspecific elimination by the liver, which is mediated by glucuronidation. Due to the lipophilic character of the BPA molecule, some amount can be stored in fat tissue, representing a long-term reservoir of this xenoestrogen [1, 3].

BPA has been demonstrated to exhibit estrogenic activity and many experimental and human studies documented its association with endocrine disorders, especially reproductive and metabolic disturbances [4]. Subsequently, a wide spectrum of BPA effects was described and BPA was identified to play a role in the etiopathogenesis of various other endocrine, as well as cardiovascular, neurological, oncological, and autoimmune diseases [1, 5, 6]. Moreover, several studies documented that intrauterine exposure to BPA may also have an impact on the physiological development of animals and humans, predominantly endocrine, nervous, and immune systems, resulting in a predisposition to certain diseases manifesting in later adulthood [1]. The effects of BPA are dependent on the dose, the duration of exposure, and the co-exposure to other environmental estrogens that can work synergically or even potentiate each other. On the other hand, the effects on the organism may vary and may depend on the age, the comorbidities, and the genetic background of the individual.

In the past few decades, the prevalence of autoimmune diseases has an increasing tendency. It could be explained by the development of industrialization, causing a rising exposure of the population to environmental factors, such as BPA, as well as a mixture of other environmental estrogens and xenobiotics [14, 15]. The term "mosaic of autoimmunity" represents the role of novel exogenous factors in the development of autoimmune diseases. Many environmental factors are implicated, such as geo-epidemiological factors, seasons, UV light, vitamin D, physical activity, stress, hygiene, helminths, certain types of smells, diet, spicy food, coffee, smoking, metals, implanted foreign materials, silicone breast implants, stents and stent-grafts, endoprostheses, and last but not least, environmental chemicals like BPA. All these factors may usually not induce autoimmune diseases themselves, but they participate in the development of autoimmune processes in genetically predisposed patients. Studies have proven that BPA itself, as well as certain other endocrine disruptors, definitely represents an important stone in the mosaic of autoimmunity [14–16]. BPA has been found to be associated with many systemic and organ-specific autoimmune diseases.

Exposure to BPA in health care

ASIA syndrome is predominantly associated with adjuvants from medical exposure, such as silicones, aluminum, or other vaccine-associated adjuvant substances. Health care also represents a significant way of exposure to BPA. It is found in various medical devices including implants, ocular lenses, prostheses, catheters, tubes, and certain dental materials. Previously, the silicone breast implants contained BPA polymers, too; therefore, BPA could possibly contribute to silicone-induced ASIA syndrome. The final exposure may vary depending on the type of material, the duration and frequency of exposure, and the total amount of plastic devices [12].

Bioavailability is up to 10% after oral and transdermal intake, while in parenteral routes of exposure (intravenous, intraperitoneal, subcutaneous), almost 100% of BPA is systemically bioavailable. BPA is conjugated in the liver and the clearance of free BPA from the circulation appears to be relatively fast. However, the degrading process can be impaired in critically ill patients with liver and kidney diseases; therefore, these patients can easily reach the toxic levels of BPA [12].

The highest levels of BPA are expected in patients after acute contact with dental materials, after extracorporeal circulation, and during hemodialysis. Majority of patients in the intensive care units are highly exposed, too. Significant BPA exposure in premature newborns requiring intensive care may have potentially harmful effects for further development, though no exact data are available [12].

Many dental sealants and composites contain BPA. Immediately after implantation, high doses of BPA have been identified in saliva, as well as in blood and urine. The release of BPA decreases within a few days, but mild release may persist for a long time, leading to a chronic exposure [17].

The study of Masereijan et al. found changes in immune system function in children after dental treatment. Patients with BPA-containing sealants had increased activity of B cells after six months of follow-up, when compared to subjects with amalgam fillings. Stimulation of B cells may present a trigger of autoimmunity development, though this study did not continue to follow the prevalence of autoimmune diseases in this population [18].

BPA as an adjuvant

An adjuvant is defined as an additional substance that is able to stimulate the immune system. Various chemicals can have an adjuvant potential. The "classical" adjuvants are chemicals, such as aluminum and squalene, used in vaccines to potentiate the immune response against the antigen. Later, more chemical substances, as well as microbial particles, have been recognized, of which the immunostimulation effect is usually inconvenient. Silicone, as a part of the breast implants and some other prosthetic materials, was one of the first identified [8, 9]. Although there have been no data published yet about BPA and its possible role as an adjuvant, BPA is known to be a common component in various materials of daily use, leading to significant exposure of whole population. Previous studies have revealed its potential to affect almost all levels of immune response, from phagocytosis to humoral immunity, and thereby induce autoimmunity and inflammation in predisposed individuals [15, 16]. Therefore, BPA should be considered as a novel adjuvant.

Pathophysiological mechanisms of BPA-induced autoimmunity

BPA has been shown to have very complex effects on the immune system. Various mechanisms of BPA-induced autoimmunity have been identified. BPA itself has a weak estrogenous activity, and it can also affect the secretion and function of other hormones involved in the modulation of immune responses. In addition, BPA has been shown to directly influence various immunological reactions, and finally, its exposure can result in the loss of self-tolerance and subsequently contribute to the development of autoimmunity [3, 15, 16].

The effects of BPA are mostly mediated by ERs – ER-alpha and ER-beta. Less is known about an orphan receptor estrogen-related receptor-gamma (ERR-gamma), but there is growing evidence about its role in BPA action. Most of the immune cells express ERs; therefore, BPA is able to regulate their activity, proliferation, or differentiation, with effects similar to estrogens. Apart from the mechanisms associated to its estrogenic activity, few more different ways of action are already known. Due to BPA's structural similarity to steroid and thyroid hormones, it also exerts some affinity to androgen receptors and receptors for thyroid hormones. Several other receptors, such as aryl hydrocarbon receptors and PPAR-gamma (peroxisome proliferator-activated receptor), have been found to be the targets for BPA molecules as well. Otherwise, there are few nonspecific mechanisms known, such as increased oxidative stress, affection of ion channels, molecular mimicry, and disruption of liver cytochrome activity, that all may participate in the development of autoimmunity, too [19, 20].

BPA may induce the generation of new epitopes by modulation of endogenous molecules, as well as BPA itself may present as a foreign antigen. Furthermore, BPA affects almost all levels of immune responses, from the innate immunity, through the adaptive reactions, the cytokine secretion, and last but not least, the production of antibodies. Therefore, it may also promote or aggravate already preexisting autoimmune processes [15, 16]. Generally, pathophysiological mechanisms of BPA-induced autoimmunity can be divided into direct and indirect types (Table 20.1).

The actual exposure to BPA in adulthood can be potentially harmful, but also prenatal and early postnatal exposure may markedly influence the development of the immune system and set the function of the immune system to be more "pro-autoimmune" in the future. BPA, as well as many other adjuvants, usually leads to the triggering of autoimmune disease mostly in genetically, or other, predisposed individuals. Moreover, the global exposure to a wide spectrum of many other xenoestrogens can also potentiate the effects of BPA and can work synergically in disrupting normal function of immune system [3, 15, 16].

Direct mechanisms of BPA action on autoimmunity

Cellular immunity

Innate cellular immunity

A nonspecific or innate immune system is the most simple, first-line defense with uniform nonspecific responses against infectious and also some noninfectious triggers. It presents with antigen-independent reactions, not leaving any immunological memory. Innate cellular immunity is represented by phagocytes [mostly macrophages), antigen-presenting cells (APCs), which play a role in the process of phagocytosis, as well as in activation of naive T-cells that are bridging the innate and the adaptive immunity responses. Another mechanism of innate defense is the oxidative stress and the reactive oxygen species (ROS) production, which is actually the least specific and the most primitive form of reaction. Furthermore, more recently identified forms of innate immune mechanisms are neutrophil extracellular traps (NETs) and innate lymphoid cells (ILCs). Affection of any of these parts of innate immune system may be implicated in the development of autoimmunity and BPA has been found to impact almost all mentioned mechanisms participating in innate immune reactions [3, 15, 16, 21, 22] (Figure 20.1).

Table 20.1 The pathophysiological mechanisms of BPA action in the development of autoimmunity.

Direct mechanisms	Cellular immunity	Innate immunity	Oxidative stress Phagocytosis Antigen-presenting cells Neutrophil extracellular traps Innate lymphoid cells
		Adaptive immunity	Th-1/Th-2 dominance Th-17 axis
	Humoral immunity		IgE-mediated autoimmunity IgG2 and IgA
Indirect mechanisms	BPA-binding protein		Protein-disulfide isomerase
	Anti-BPA antibodies		Anti-BPA–albumin antibodies Anti-BPA–PDI antibodies
	Gut microbiota		Estrogen-like changes Local/systemic inflammation
	Hormones		Prolactin Thyroid hormones
	Liver function		Elimination of BPA Activity of CYP P450
	Epigenetics		Methylation Histone modification miRNA

A. Phagocytosis

Phagocytosis is the major mechanism of innate immune defense. It represents one of the first-line reactions responsible for the elimination of infectious or noninfectious triggers and is considered to be a bridge to adaptive immunity.

Regulation of the interplay between phagocytic receptors, responsible for the initiation and maintenance of mechanisms of phagocytosis, and so-called pattern recognition receptors (PRRs), such as toll-like receptors (TLRs), which are implicated in distinguishing the self-antigens from "foreign" antigens, is important in the normal function of macrophages. Affection of some of these receptors may lead to either an increase or decrease in phagocytic activity, or to an alteration of the self-recognition mechanisms that are one of the key factors in self-tolerance breakdown [21].

Evidence suggests that BPA affects the process of phagocytosis in various stages, such as chemotaxis and migration of phagocytes, as well as the function of macrophages itself. However, the results of studies are very inconsistent. BPA has been found to stimulate the chemotaxis by activation of the chemokine ligand 1 (CCL1) signaling pathway [16, 22]. On the other hand, another study revealed that BPA exposure has reduced the chemotactic capacity of neutrophils. TLR-mediated actions of phagocytes have been identified to be stimulated by prenatal BPA exposure in a human study. Overactivated TLRs can bind to autoantigens, thereby contributing to the development of autoimmunity. Stimulation of certain TLRs has led to changes in cytokine production, too [23]. The study of Yang et al. found that low doses of BPA enhanced the activity of macrophages, but on the other hand, higher doses induced their apoptosis [24]. Furthermore, it has been identified that BPA has different effects on various subtypes of macrophages (type M1 and M2). BPA, as well as estradiol exposure, promoted the stimulation of M2 migration. These effects have shown to be mediated by either ERα or ERβ, further activating nuclear factor kappa-light-chain-enhancer of activated B cells (NF-κB), c-Jun N-terminal protein kinase (JNK), Activator protein 1 (AP-1),

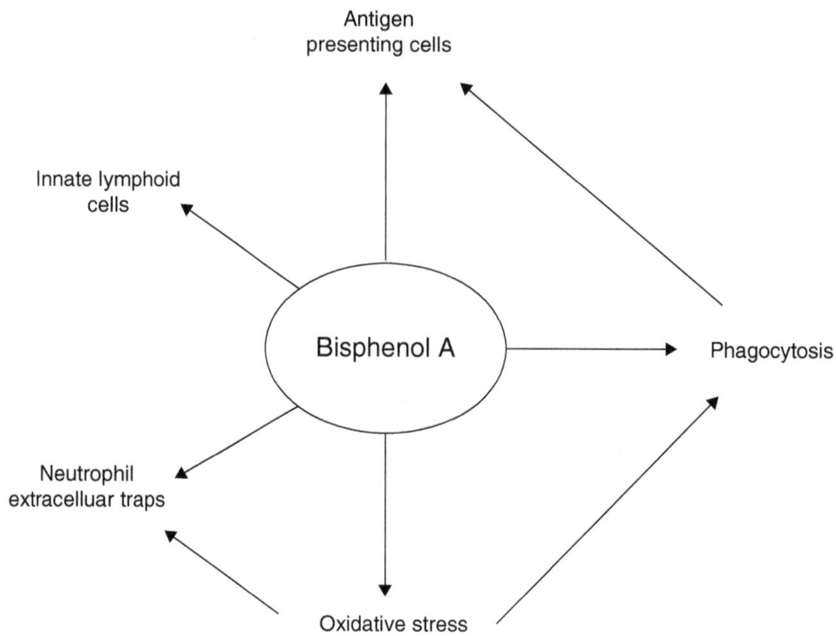

Figure 20.1 The effects of BPA on innate immune responses.

or ERK signaling pathways that are known to be responsible for cell stress reactions, controlling transcription of DNA, cytokine production, and cell survival, generally called the "death" signaling pathways [25]. Another study found that BPA exhibited a synergistic action of ERα and NF-κB transcription factors on NF-kB-associated immune gene expression in macrophages [26]. NF-κB is a proinflammatory mediator, whose deregulated activation is known to be associated with the chronic inflammation and autoimmune diseases and it is a very important factor in maintaining self-tolerance.

Impaired process of phagocytosis can lead to further pathological self-destructive responses of immune system.

B. Antigen-presenting cells (APCs)

Antigen-presenting process is a key mechanism for activation of adaptive immunity, mostly the T-cells. APCs, such as dendritic cells or macrophages, present the antigens on their surface after phagocytosis or receptor-mediated endocytosis. Antigens are usually of foreign origin, but under certain conditions, autoantigens may be presented too, that leads to autoreactivity in predisposed patients [27]. APCs are crucial in maintenance of immune tolerance and in the regulation of immune responses. Chronic activation of dendritic cells by autoantigens generates auto-reactive T and B lymphocytes causing increased production of autoantibodies that finally leads to tissue damage. This mechanism of autoimmunity is common but typically occurs in development of SLE (systemic lupus erythematosus) [27, 28].

It has been demonstrated that BPA can participate in the development of autoimmunity by alteration of antigen-presenting process and also by disruption of elimination of self-activated T-cells, which can play a significant role in etiopathogenesis, as well as in the progression, of autoimmune reactions [15, 16].

Dendritic cells exposed to BPA in combination with tumor necrosis factor-alpha (TNF-alpha) promote CCL1 signaling cascade that induces the Th-2 polarization preferentially. Overactivity of Th-2 lymphocytes and overproduction of their cytokines was previously known to be an "autoimmune profile," but recently, the data about Th1/Th2 dominance in autoimmunity have become more controversial [15, 22, 29]. Most of the published studies are consistent with these data, apart from two studies that describe rather induction of Th-1 activation. First, the study of Cernadas et al. investigated the effect of BPA on the activity of human peripheral blood mononuclear cells and in vitro differentiation of dendritic cells from monocytes. BPA has been shown to increase proliferation of peripheral blood monocytes and upregulate CD1a expression on dendritic cells, a pro-inflammatory biological marker known to trigger Th-1 phenotype polarization of naive CD4 T-cells [30].

Another in vitro study on cell culture found that BPA exposure significantly increased the expression of ERα on monocyte-derived dendritic cells, while ERβ remained unchanged. BPA promoted the expression of HLA-DR via ERα activation, leading to the stimulation of proinflammatory cytokines [3, 31].

The altered activity of APCs may play an important role in autoimmune processes by promotion of T-cell abnormalities with further negative impacts on the cytokine production and affection of T-memory and T-suppressor cells, as well as pathological changes in B-cell function. Therefore, APCs may represent a base for promoting the whole autoimmune cascade.

C. Innate lymphoid cells (ILCs)

ILCs have been recently identified as hematopoietic cells that participate in the regulation of lymphocytes, as well as they represent a substantial source of cytokine production. Furthermore, ILCs are known to be concerned with innate immune responses against infectious or noninfectious triggers, protection of the epithelial barrier, lymphoid organogenesis and inflammation, tissue remodeling, and regulation of homeostasis of tissue stromal cells. ILCs are morphologically similar to T-cells and B-cells; however, they do not express typical lymphoid differential markers. According to their phenotype and the function, three classes of ILCs have been recognized (ILC 1, ILC 2, and ILC 3). There is growing evidence that ILCs play an important role in the development of allergies and autoimmunity, mostly the ILCs type 3 that are proficient in IL-17 production [32]. ILCs have been found to participate in the development of multiple sclerosis, inflammatory bowel diseases, psoriasis, and rheumatic diseases [33].

The study of Malaisé et al. found that prenatal exposure to BPA in mice resulted in a decrease in ILC 3 type in the mucosa of the small intestine, with an increase in IgG response against commensal bacteria in sera [34]. Therefore, alteration of ILCs induced by BPA may represent another possible mechanism by which BPA may potentially contribute to the pathogenesis of autoimmunity; however, more studies are definitely needed to elucidate this hypothesis.

D. Neutrophil extracellular traps (NETs)

NETs are fibrous networks that protrude from the membranes of activated neutrophils. They can be found in a variety of conditions such as infection, malignancy, atherosclerosis, and last but not least, autoimmune diseases, including rheumatoid arthritis, SLE, antineutrophil cytoplasmic antibodies (ANCA)-associated vasculitis, psoriasis, and antiphospholipid syndrome (APS). Under physiological conditions, NETs are formed as antimicrobial reaction, though their production may be induced by environmental factors, such as BPA [35–38].

BPA has been found to increase NET production in a dose-dependent manner. Tong et al. found in their animal in vivo study a significant increase in NET production after exposure to BPA. Moreover, they have also confirmed this association in vitro in human neutrophil cultures, suggesting the stimulating effect of BPA on NETs production in humans too [39]. However, exact mechanisms are still not known, it can be assumed that ROS represents the bridge between BPA exposure and NET formation. However, the direct estrogenic effect on neutrophils cannot be excluded.

Although the NETs represent physiological mechanisms of innate immunity, their inadequate BPA-promoted generation may lead to prolonged extracellular exposure to histone complexes, DNA, and other autoantigens related to NETs. This mechanism can play a role in the development of certain systemic autoimmune diseases in genetically predisposed patients [40].

E. Oxidative stress

ROS play an important role in the development of autoimmunity. Oxidative stress generates damage-associated molecular patterns (DAMPs) or autoantigens that further trigger the innate and adaptive immunity, leading to the dysfunction and cell apoptosis via an inflammatory cascade. Cell damage and apoptosis unveil the self-antigens, promoting the self-tolerance breakdown in predisposed individuals and thus inducing the autodestructing reactions. ROS have been found to be factors in etiopathogenesis of autoimmune diseases generally, but several studies have described their crucial role in the development of systemic scleroderma and vitiligo [41–43].

BPA is known to induce a significant increase in the generation of ROS in a dose-dependent manner. Exposure to even nanomolar doses of BPA causes short, transient bursts of ROS production, while long-term exposure leads to sustained activation of oxidative stress. Free BPA induces ROS production through enzymatic and nonenzymatic mechanisms, generating a variety of free radical species (superoxides, peroxides, hydroxyl radicals, etc.) that exert cytotoxic and DNA-toxic effects [42]. Additionally, BPA also inhibits the expression of antioxidant genes, such as superoxide dismutase, catalase, and reduced form of glutathione (GSH), that further promote the oxidative stress [44].

Increased generation of ROS by neutrophils has been identified after BPA exposure, which was inhibited by the ER-β antagonists, suggesting that BPA's prooxidative effects are explained by its estrogenic activity [45]. In vitro experimental studies have been confirmed by a few human clinical trials. First, the study of Yang et al., who found elevated serum markers of oxidative stress (monodialdehyde and 8-deoxyguanosine) in female postmenopausal patients with increased BPA levels, as well as recently published data of Wang et al., whose study demonstrated that elevated urinary BPA (and bisphenol F) were associated with significantly higher levels of oxidative stress markers in the population of adult men [43, 46].

The production of ROS causes DNA damage, oxidation, and fragmentation of intracellular as well as extracellular proteins and may also be associated with lipid peroxidation, which all lead to alteration of the cellular organelles and result in impairment of normal cellular function. As was already mentioned, exposure to BPA is associated with increased levels of 8-deoxyguanosine, which is a marker of DNA damage induced by DNA toxicity of ROS. Similar markers are oxidized DNA base 8-oxoguanine or 8-hydroxy-2′-deoxyguanosine levels, which have been found to be elevated in certain autoimmune diseases and are considered as markers of oxidative DNA damage in the circulating immune complexes in SLE patients [42, 46, 47].

According to these findings, there is objective evidence that BPA-induced oxidative stress plays a crucial role in initialization of processes leading to the development of autoimmunity. ROS may present a trigger for other mechanisms of innate as well as adaptive immunity.

Adaptive cellular immunity

The adaptive cellular immune responses are mediated by the cytokines, which are mostly produced and regulated by T-lymphocytes. Cytokines are responsible for the maintenance of interplay between cellular innate mechanisms and immunoglobulin secretion. Disruption of the cytokine profile may lead to the dysbalance of immune function, and therefore, trigger the development of autoimmunity [3, 15, 16].

There are generally 5 types of T-cells known: Th-1, Th-2, Th-17 cells, and recently discovered Th1-like Th-17 cells as well as Th-22 cells. All types produce proinflammatory and antiinflammatory cytokines with different predominance [48].

BPA has been found to impact the activity and differentiation of most types of T-lymphocytes, and therefore to affect cytokine production. The scheme of BPA action on various types of T-lymphocytes is presented in Figure 20.2.

A. Th-1 and Th-2 lymphocytes

Recent data indicate that BPA may induce the pathophysiological process of autoimmunity by causing an inappropriate polarization of T-cells and shifting of the cytokine profile from

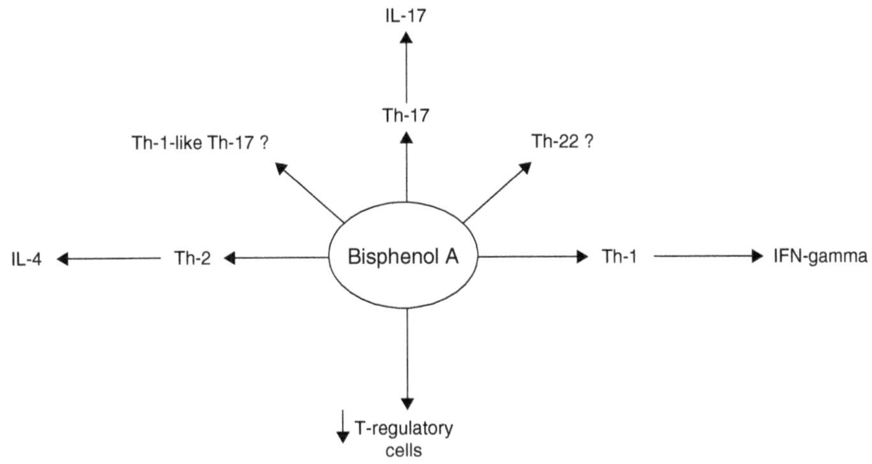

Figure 20.2 BPA effects on T-lymphocytes and cytokine production.

Th-2 dominance into Th-1 dominance [49, 50]. Th-1 cells produce mostly proinflammatory cytokines, such as interferon-gamma (IFN-gamma), while Th-2 lymphocytes generate predominantly antiinflammatory cytokines, especially interleukin-4 (IL-4). It has been found that BPA directly stimulates the production of antigen-specific IFN-gamma in Th-1 cells, but also induces the differentiation and polarization of naive T-cells into Th-1 type [51]. IFN-gamma itself is a significant stimulator of immune responses, but it is able to promote further proinflammatory reactions of innate, adaptive, and humoral immune systems that are associated with autoimmune reactions.

In vivo animal study demonstrated that exposure to BPA in doses equivalent to low human exposure led to the decrease in the number of T-regulatory cells that promoted the loss of self-tolerance and participated in the switch of T-helper lymphocyte dominance [52]. Moreover, Yoshino et al. have found that the prenatal exposure to low doses of BPA may upregulate Th-1 responses later in adulthood [53]. Therefore, the intrauterine development of the immune system may be altered and programmed to increase the risk in autoimmunity development years later during the life.

BPA has been observed to directly affect the secretion of cytokines in all T-lymphocytes. The study of Liu et al. found a significant increase in proinflammatory cytokines – TNF-alpha and IL-6, in contrast with a significant decrease in levels of antiinflammatory regulatory cytokines, such as IL-10 and TGF-beta, after exposure of human monocyte-like cell line to BPA [54].

However, some older studies also revealed the stimulatory effects of BPA on Th-2 lymphocytes, so the data are controversial, and the role of Th1/Th2 polarity in autoimmunity remains unclear and seems to differ in various autoimmune diseases.

B. Th-17 lymphocytes

The alteration of the Th17 axis induced by BPA represents another mechanism in autoimmune reactions. BPA has been shown to activate Th17 cells, leading to the overproduction of proinflammatory cytokine IL-17 that inhibits T-regulatory lymphocyte differentiation and promotes a loss of self-control of immunity [55]. Even prenatal exposure to BPA causes increased proliferation of maternal spleen Th17 lymphocytes and elevated levels of IL-17 were measured in the offspring [56, 57].

However, Th17 pathway overactivation against autoantigens causes type 3 immune complex and complement-mediated hypersensitivity that could play a role in certain autoimmune disorders, such as rheumatoid arthritis; this mechanism has not yet been confirmed in experimental or clinical studies in humans [57].

Humoral immunity

Production of the immunoglobulins against self-antigens is the key factor in the development of autoimmune diseases. Antibody secretion by B-cells and plasmatic cells is mostly regulated by T-helper lymphocytes. It has been found that some endocrine disruptors, including BPA, stimulate proinflammatory cascade of humoral immunity, either directly activating the B-cells or by affection of Th cells and their cytokine secretion [3, 15, 16].

BPA induces the synthesis of IL-4 in T-helper cells, leading to B-lymphocyte class switching into IgE production. What is more, the direct stimulatory effect of BPA on IgE secretion in plasmatic cells has been found [58]. An experimental study demonstrated elevated urinary IgE levels after BPA exposure [59]. Overproduction of IgE is known to be a significant trigger of inflammatory responses and upregulation of the immune system, which may lead to allergic, as well as autoimmune reactions. Previously, it has been thought that elevated levels of IgE probably do not induce the self-destructive reactions and that they are only able to contribute in the already activated autoimmune process. Recently, the special kind, i.e. IgE-mediated autoimmunity, has been identified [60]. While its mechanisms have similar patterns to classical allergy induced by exogenous allergens, this IgE-mediated autoimmunity has been termed "autoallergy" and the target molecules are called "autoallergens." [60]. Autoantibodies in the IgE class may be a possible contributor to the pathogenesis of several autoimmune diseases, such as rheumatoid arthritis, SLE, Grave's disease, multiple sclerosis, and certain dermatological autoimmune disorders like bullous pemphigoid, atopic dermatitis, and psoriasis [60, 61].

Several data suggest that BPA impacts apart from the IgE secretion also other classes of immunoglobulins. In the older study of Yurino et al., BPA exposure was identified to stimulate the activity of B1-cells in vitro [62]. In a murine model of SLE, the group of BPA-treated mice stimulated autoantibody production by B1 cells [63]. An in vivo experimental study found increased IgA and IgG2 production after administration of BPA, which was changed as a consequence of underlying BPA-induced cytokine disturbances. In addition, this study has not investigated subclasses of IgA, but it is known that increased IgA2 subclass shows significant proinflammatory effects. The research in patients with rheumatoid arthritis has found that these patients displayed a shift toward the IgA2 subclass production [64].

BPA appears to stimulate the secretion of immunoglobulins generally, which can increase the levels of autoantibodies in patients with preexisting autoimmune disease.

Indirect mechanisms of BPA action on autoimmunity

BPA may influence the function of the immune system not only by direct effects on immune cells and cytokines, but there are also some other mechanisms known that can indirectly participate in the development of autoimmunity, such as molecular mimicry, hormonal dysbalance, and or affecting the liver function.

BPA-binding protein

Protein disulfide isomerase (PDI) acts as a binding protein for BPA. Physiologically, PDI is one of the major enzymes in the endoplasmic reticulum that catalyzes the formation of disulfide bonds of nascent or misfolded proteins. In addition, later studies demonstrated that it also mediates the effects of various hormones inside the cells, especially estrogens and thyroid hormones, as well as it may act as a reservoir for hormones and regulate their intracellular concentrations [65].

BPA alters the function of the PDI, since it has been found to inhibit isomerase activity of PDI after binding to its molecule; therefore, it may lead to changes in concentrations of some hormones [66]. Moreover, the study of Hiroi et al. demonstrated that binding of BPA to PDI causes the formation of complexes, which present new unknown epitopes potentially promoting antigen–antibody immune reactions [67]. PDI is highly expressed in the central nervous system; therefore, it probably plays a role in autoimmune disorders predominantly affecting brain, such as Parkinson's disease, and multiple sclerosis. [68].

Anti-BPA antibodies

BPA presents as foreign molecule in the organism; therefore, it may act as a new antigen, potentially inducing immune response. Since the structure of BPA may be similar to some endogenous molecules, antibodies against BPA may cross-react with certain self-antigens. Furthermore, as mentioned above, BPA is able to bind to PDI as well as to serum albumin, creating complexes that can represent new epitopes for the immune system, as well [15, 16].

In the study of Vojdani et al., antibodies against the BPA–albumin complexes have been detected in sera of healthy humans [69, 70]. These autoantibodies had the potential to cross-react with some other endogenous structures, such as PDI, myelin basic protein (MBP), and myelin oligodendrocyte protein (MOG). Therefore, it can be assumed that antibodies against BPA itself or complexes of BPA with endogenous proteins may induce autoimmunity, especially in certain neurological autoimmune diseases [69]. Kharazzian et al. found a significant association between antibodies against BPA–albumin complexes and prevalence of alpha-synuclein antibodies that have been previously identified in patients with Parkinson's disease [68].

Since the data are poor, it remains unknown if this effect may be implicated against more endogenous molecules and if BPA may induce a wider spectrum of organ-specific or systemic autoimmune disorders by this mechanism.

Gut microbiota

Gut microbiome plays an important role in the development and regulation of the immune system. It is known that variations in gut bacteria may be important in the pathogenesis of some cardiovascular or metabolic diseases, but there are only limited data about the role of gut microbiome in participation in the development of autoimmunity. The apoptosis of intestinal epithelial cells due to gut dysbiosis that enables the presentation of self-antigens inducing the differentiation of autoreactive Th17 cells and other T helper cells has been documented in several studies [71, 72].

The study of Xu et al. found a shift to "proinflammatory" profile of gut bacteria after BPA exposure in juvenile mice that was also associated with increased risk of diabetes mellitus type 1 in female gender. BPA exposure was related to an increased abundance of *Lachnospiraceae*, *Jeotgalicoccus*, *Ruminococcus*, *Akkermansia*, *Oscillospira*, *Rhodospirillale*, *Anaerofustis*, and *Turicibacter*, and decreased *Sinobacteraceae* and *Koribacteraceae [73]*.

Results of another study also showed significant changes in gut bacteria in mice treated with BPA. They found higher amounts of *Bacteroides*, *Mollicutes*, *Prevotellaceae*, *Erysipelotrichaceae*, *Akkermansia*, *Methanobrevibacter*, and *Sutterella* in individuals exposed to BPA. The same changes in gut microbiome were detected after exposure to ethinylestradiol [74].

BPA, as well as some other environmental estrogens, has been shown to exert estrogenic activity in the gastrointestinal tract that results in changes in gut microbiome, possibly altering the epithelial function and therefore promoting local and systemic inflammation [72–74]. This is the most probable way how can BPA affect gut microbiome and subsequently participate in the development of some autoimmune disorders, such as type 1 diabetes mellitus (T1DM), and especially Crohn's disease or ulcerative colitis.

Hormones

The structure of BPA is similar to estrogens; therefore, most effects of BPA in organisms are mediated by widely expressed ERs, which are also present in the immune cells. Moreover, BPA may mimic some other hormones, such as androgens and thyroid hormones. For example, a molecular mimicry of BPA and thyroid hormones can potentially play a role in the development of thyroid autoimmunity, but no further clinical studies have confirmed this hypothesis [15, 16, 75, 76].

Besides the direct estrogenic activity of BPA, this endocrine disruptor can regulate the secretion of several other hormones, such as prolactin, which is a significant regulator of immune responses. There is evidence that prolactin exerts stimulating effects on immunological responses, i.e. affects antigen-presenting functions, promotes responses to any antigens, including self-antigens, as well as it increases secretion of cytokines and alters B-cell functions [77, 78].

BPA was found to stimulate the production of prolactin, both in vivo as well as in vitro [79]. Estrogens are responsible for the increased release of prolactin. Since BPA has agonistic activity on ERs, it can also stimulate the production of this pituitary hormone. Several human studies observed correlations between urinary or serum BPA levels and prolactin [42, 80]. Moreover, experimental animal studies on mice found that BPA exposure significantly promoted the proliferation of pituitary cells and induced prolactin secretion. Furthermore, BPA concentrations positively correlated with the weight of hypophysis, and higher BPA levels were observed in individuals with prolactinomas [42].

Several studies have reported an association between increased prolactin levels and autoimmune diseases, such as SLE, APS, rheumatoid arthritis, thyroid autoimmunity, T1DM, adrenal insufficiency, and celiac disease [77, 78].

Conclusively, hyperprolactinemia may represent one of the pathophysiological mechanisms of BPA-induced autoimmunity.

Liver function

Impaired hepatic function may indirectly participate in BPA-induced autoimmunity. BPA is largely eliminated from the organism by the liver; therefore, impaired liver functions disrupt the clearance of BPA. Increased levels of this adjuvant secondarily inhibit CYP P450 enzymes, leading to proteomic alteration in immune functions [79, 80]. Higher concentrations of BPA were associated with accelerated production of ROS that promote inflammatory responses. On the other side, it is known that patients with liver diseases have a higher prevalence of autoimmune disorders [42]. The fact that BPA can be one of the possible promoters of immune self-reactive responses in these patients, requires further investigation.

Epigenetics

Epigenetics has been observed to have a crucial role in the development of certain autoimmune diseases. BPA was found to be able to induce DNA hyper- or hypomethylation, as well as histone modification and affection of miRNA synthesis. These changes have the most significant consequences if the exposure to the environmental factor is during the prenatal or early postnatal period [81].

The correlations between increased BPA levels and hypomethylation of the CpG sites of genes responsible for steroidogenesis, immune reactions, and autoimmune thyroid disease have been identified. Whether the BPA-mediated alteration in methylation is related to its estrogenic activity remains unclear. However, a recent study has demonstrated that BPA regulation of methylation was mediated through ERα regulation of DNA methyltransferases (DNMT-1 and 3) expression. Higher urinary BPA levels were found to be associated with hypomethylation of CpG islands on the X-chromosome, attenuating the methylation of genes involved in immune function, transport activity, as well as caspase activity [82].

Additionally, BPA has been found to activate the estrogen-responsible elements, thereby increasing the expression of certain proinflammatory genes, such as NF-Kb. Later, BPA-induced epigenetic changes altering the expression of more genes implicated in the regulation of immune system function, such as Toll-like receptors, have been discovered [83].

Based on these findings, BPA can promote epigenetic changes affecting genes concerned in immune responses, unfortunately not much data on clinical relevance in humans have been published yet.

The role of BPA in autoimmune diseases

Autoimmunity may be targeted against nonspecific, systemic antigens, or epitopes located in just one organ, called organ-specific autoimmune diseases. BPA has been found to play a role in both non-organ-specific and organ-specific autoimmunity; however, clinical data in various autoimmune disorders are quite limited and sometimes even controversial.

BPA and systemic (non-organ-specific) autoimmune diseases

Systemic lupus erythematosus (SLE)

SLE is an autoimmune disease with a very wide spectrum of clinical manifestations. Genetic background plays a key role in pathogenesis, moreover, viral infections, smoking and environment are other major risk factors. Among environmental triggers, the environmental estrogens, such as BPA, are highly discussed [3].

In experimental research, several studies demonstrated that BPA induced a direct structural damage to DNA, which is able to promote anti-dsDNA autoantibodies production [84]. Furthermore, BPA was found to induce the generation of NETs, which represents another important mechanism in the development of SLE. Nevertheless, IgE-mediated autoimmunity has been identified to stimulate antibody production in SLE patients and also increase the disease activity, as described in the chapter Pathophysiological mechanisms of BPA-induced autoimmunity. [85].

One of the most commonly affected organs in patients with SLE are kidneys. A recently published study in an animal model described a possible role of BPA in the exacerbation of preexisting lupus nephritis, though the clinical data on human population are still missing [86].

Antiphospholipid syndrome

APS is an acquired autoimmune-based thrombophilia that can occur as either isolated (primary APS) or coexisting with another systemic autoimmune disease, typically with SLE (secondary APS). There are poor data about BPA and its relation to APS and only one clinical study has been published.

Sugiuiri-Ogasawara et al. studied a group of women with a history of spontaneous abortion and demonstrated a significantly higher prevalence of ANA autoantibodies in patients with high serum BPA levels, although the ANA positivity was not associated with abortions themselves. Moreover, this study did not detect any significant correlations between the levels of antiphospholipid antibodies and serum BPA concentrations [87].

Sjögren's syndrome

Primary Sjögren's syndrome is another systemic autoimmune disease that has been found to be associated with exposure to adjuvants, such as silicones, but BPA seems to be another possible trigger. An in vitro study on dendritic cells from patients suffering from Sjögren's syndrome demonstrated a potentially significant role of BPA in accelerating the disease progression in these patients. After BPA exposure, there were changes in the expression of transcription factors and proinflammatory cytokines that led to further deterioration of this autoimmune disease [31].

BPA and organ-specific autoimmune diseases

BPA and endocrine autoimmunity

Evidence suggests that BPA similarly to other xenoestrogens acts as an endocrine disruptor, affecting various endocrine functions, which was clearly demonstrated in both experimental and large-scale epidemiologic studies [88, 89]. BPA has been shown to have the ability to disrupt thyroid function, the hypothalamic-pituitary axis, as well as ovarian and testicular functions through several mechanisms [90–93]. Although these disrupting mechanisms are relatively well recognized, less is known about the relationship between BPA and endocrine autoimmunity. No data regarding the association of serum or urinary BPA and autoimmune hypophysitis or Addison's disease have been presented to this date. The association with autoimmune thyroid disease, T1DM, and autoimmune ovarian failure has been documented by some authors in a lesser number of studies [3].

Autoimmune thyroid disease and BPA

While the effects of BPA on thyroid hormone action in experimental and in vitro studies seem to be relatively consistent, the association of BPA exposure with thyroid autoimmunity in humans is less recognized. Several studies over the past decade showed that BPA can affect thyroid hormone action through various mechanisms. First, free BPA competitively binds to the thyroid hormone receptor and thereby inhibits the expression of genes regulated by thyroid hormones [94]. Moreover, this xenoestrogen may also interfere with thyroid hormone synthesis, transport, and partially with thyroid hormone metabolism, exerting a potent thyroid-disrupting action [95].

There are limited data on the association of BPA with autoimmune thyroid disease. The study from China did not demonstrate any association between urinary BPA concentration and thyroid autoimmunity; similar results were recently demonstrated in Chinese newborns [96]. Oppositely, Thai NHES reported that serum BPA concentrations were independently associated with thyroid peroxidase (TPO) and thyroglobulin (TG) antibody positivity [97]. Although the results from the studies remain inconsistent, BPA seems to be able to participate in the induction or promotion of thyroid autoimmunity, further resulting in thyroid dysfunction. Indirect proof that BPA may induce thyroid autoimmunity is the observation that dental fillings, which represent a source of human BPA exposure, are associated with anti-TPO and anti-TG positivity. It has been demonstrated that removal of the dental material has led to a decrease in serum levels of both TPOAb and TGAb [98]. Nevertheless, the mechanisms of the relationship between BPA and thyroid autoimmunity require further evaluation.

BPA and premature ovarian failure

Premature autoimmune ovarian failure has been found to be associated with adjuvants. Some cases of POF as a part of ASIA syndrome have been identified after HPV vaccination [99]. There is evidence that BPA exposure is also significantly associated with premature ovarian failure. In various animal models, BPA has been demonstrated to reduce the number of primordial follicles, inhibit the growth of antral follicles, and disrupt steroid hormone synthesis, resulting in fertility reduction [100, 101]. The mechanisms of this ovotoxic effect are still not fully recognized. Whether BPA exposure may stimulate the synthesis of antibodies against various ovarian structures is still unknown and requires further clinical studies.

Diabetes mellitus type 1

While the association of BPA exposure to type 2 diabetes mellitus has been confirmed in several studies, the relationship between BPA and T1DM is suggested by some experimental data. T1DM is a disease resulting from autoimmune destruction of pancreatic beta cells, leading to insulin deficiency and secondarily to the development of T1DM. Animal studies showed that long-term BPA exposure may accelerate spontaneous insulitis and the development of T1DM, especially due to systemic immune alterations [102–104]. The mechanisms of association between BPA exposure and T1DM development are multifactorial and depend on various factors including time of exposure, dose of BPA, sex, age, as well as state of nutrition [102]. In the study of Xu et al., the prenatal BPA exposure had minimal effects on T1DM development in male offspring, whereas it significantly increased the risk of T1DM in female mice [73].

BPA alters the macrophage function in pancreatic beta cells, resulting in an impaired clearance of apoptotic cells, which is a common feature of various autoimmune disorders. Recently, endoplasmic reticulum stress after BPA exposure has also been demonstrated, and it has led to an experimental model of T1DM in rats [105]. Currently, there is only one human study that has not found any association between urinary BPA concentration and T1DM in children [106].

No studies focused on the association of long-term BPA exposure with the presence of autoantibodies specific for autoimmune diabetes mellitus have been published until this time.

BPA and cardiac autoimmunity

BPA is well known to play a role in the etiopathogenesis of certain nonimmunologically mediated cardiovascular diseases, such as arterial hypertension, coronary artery disease, arrhythmias, and hypertrophic cardiomyopathy [6, 107–109]. However, there are some data regarding the association between BPA and cardiac autoimmunity in the current literature.

Myocarditis is a heart disease mostly associated with autoimmune pathogenesis. It can be of infectious and noninfectious origin, although in infectious types, the autoimmune mechanism is also implicated. The infection by Coxackie B3 virus is considered to be the most common cause of myocarditis and can induce the immune reaction against cardiomyocytes. The study of Bruno et al. found a relation between BPA and myocarditis as well as dilated cardiomyopathy in an experimental animal model. Rats exposed to ordinary human-relevant doses of BPA prior to viral infection by Coxackie B3 virus were more prone to develop myocarditis than the control group. Moreover, BPA-exposed rats had more severe disease and they developed dilated cardiomyopathy after myocarditis more commonly [110]. Due to the different distribution of ER-alpha and ER-beta between males and females, BPA tended to have stronger effects on females' myocardium. ER-alpha was found to play a rather protective role, while ER-beta signaling participates in the development of myocarditis [110]. BPA has been previously shown to attenuate the expression of ER-alpha and to upregulate the synthesis of ER-beta in the heart, contributing to its proinflammatory action on the myocardium. Additionally, this study revealed increased prevalence of pericarditis in affected female rats [110, 111]. Evidence suggests that myocarditis may lead to dilated cardiomyopathy due to autoinflammatory damage followed by fibrotic transformation of myocardial tissue. BPA increased the cytokine levels and the intensity of inflammatory process; therefore, rats exposed to BPA had a higher prevalence of post-viral-myocarditis dilated cardiomyopathy [110].

Another study demonstrated that BPA may activate mast cells in the myocardial tissue, which are largely responsible for increased severity of inflammation in females with preexisting myocarditis, leading to more severe heart damage [112].

Previously mentioned studies indicated a possible role of BPA in the pathogenesis and exacerbation of myocarditis, though all the data are obtained from animal research. There are no studies about the association of BPA with autoimmune affection of the heart in humans; therefore, further research is definitely needed.

BPA and gastrointestinal autoimmunity

There is a wide spectrum of autoimmune diseases affecting gastrointestinal, pancreatic, and hepatobiliary tract, but in relation to BPA, the only published data are related to inflammatory bowel disease (IBD). IBD is a group of diseases with two distinct types – Crohn's disease and ulcerative colitis – and other undifferentiated entities. The etiology seems to be multifactorial. Genetic background, environmental factors, and alteration of the gut microbiome may participate in the pathogenesis of IBD. BPA has been shown to exert estrogenic activity in the colon, thereby altering its function. This leads to the development of local inflammation, as well as the induction of changes in gut microbiota that may influence the local and even systemic immune responses [72, 113]. By these mechanisms, BPA probably plays a role in the development of IBD or exacerbation of preexisting colitis.

The experimental animal study of De Luca et al. found an increased clinical, as well as histological activity of colitis in rats exposed to BPA. Also, higher levels of proinflammatory cytokines and changes in concentrations of gut bacterial metabolites have been described, thereby giving a possible explanation to mechanisms of BPA-induced colon inflammation [114].

The study of Javurek et al. demonstrated a significant alteration of gut microbiota after BPA exposure. The changes were almost the same as after ethinylestradiol exposure. Both of them caused sex-dependent changes in gut bacteria colonization. BPA or synthetic estrogen exposure leads to the overgrowth of certain types of bacteria (*i.e. Bacteroides, Mollicutes, Prevotellaceae, Erysipelotrichaceae, Akkermansia, Methanobrevibacter,* and *Sutterella*) that are associated with various diseases, such as IBD, but also with some metabolic disorders and colorectal cancer [74].

Several experimental studies found a relationship between BPA and IBD, but there is a lack of data from human clinical research in this field. The only clinical data available are from an observational National Health and Nutrition Examination Survey (NHANES) study on the U.S. population aged 20–80 years between the years 2005 and 2010 that demonstrated a significant association between exposure to phenols and ulcerative colitis. Furthermore, phenols have been found to be responsible for chronic diarrheal symptoms too. This study observed the presence of functional diarrheal symptoms in more than a quarter of responders who were exposed to phenols, and more than 42% had abnormal markers of inflammation [115]. However, these data reflected the environmental exposure to phenols in general and was not directly focused on BPA.

BPA and neuroautoimmunity

The increasing prevalence of certain autoimmune neurological diseases during the past few decades may be possibly associated with exposure to environmental factors, but the data remain controversial. The most studied association is between BPA and multiple sclerosis.

The study of Rogers et al. found the role of gestational BPA exposure in the development of multiple sclerosis in adulthood in genetically predisposed rats. Furthermore, they have demonstrated a sex-specific response with higher inducibility of this autoimmune disease in male individuals [116]. On the other hand, the results of an older study of Krementsov et al. do not support these data, and the authors do not consider the developmental exposure to BPA as a risk factor for multiple sclerosis [117]. Moreover, both of these studies described no relation between adulthood BPA exposure to higher prevalence of multiple sclerosis [116, 117].

Similarly, as in viral myocarditis, BPA stimulates the inflammation process in Theiler's virus-induced demyelination (TVID), which is considered a mouse model of multiple sclerosis. In infected mice, BPA amplified immune-related gene expression, increased the activity of inflammation, and accelerated the onset of TVID symptoms [118].

Several experimental animal models have demonstrated that BPA may contribute to the development of autoimmune encephalomyelitis and multiple sclerosis, but very few data have been published about such possible effects in humans.

As previously mentioned, BPA has been found to be able to bind to serum albumin and PDI, and these complexes present as new potential epitopes, inducing antibody production. This may lead to cross-reactivity with MBP and myelin oligodendrocyte glycoprotein (MOG), both key molecules in the development of neuroautoimmunity. Kharrazian et al. found a higher prevalence of anti-MBP and anti-MOG autoantibodies in patients with coexisting autoantibodies against BPA–albumin and BPA–PDI complexes [69]. This mechanism may participate in the development of autoimmune demyelination diseases. Whether the autoantibodies to BPA–albumin complexes may also play a role in other autoimmune neurologic disorders remains to be elucidated.

Recently, there has been growing evidence about the possible autoimmune background of Parkinson's disease. The data are not consistent, but alpha-synuclein, being a target for autoimmunity, is highly debated, as well as certain specific changes in innate and adaptive immune reactions in patients with this neurodegenerative disease [119]. Another study of Kharrazian et al. demonstrated that patients with anti-BPA–albumin complex antibodies had higher prevalence of autoantibodies against alpha-synuclein. They also identified a significant positive correlation between the levels of these antibodies [68]. Therefore, BPA may promote the autoimmune processes leading to Parkinson's disease, too.

Conclusion

The ASIA syndrome, also known as Shoenfeld's syndrome, represents a group of several immune-mediated conditions that are associated with exposure to substances with adjuvant activity. There is growing evidence that BPA exerts immunomodulation effects with the potential to induce autoimmunity in already predisposed individuals, thus it should also be considered as an adjuvant. BPA affects the immune system directly, as well as via many indirect mechanisms, leading to potential loss of self-tolerance and development of autoimmune diseases. Several experimental and observational studies have found a relation between BPA and systemic autoimmune diseases, such as SLE and Sjögren's syndrome, as well as organ-specific autoimmunity of thyroid gland, heart, nervous system, large bowel, and diabetes mellitus. Even prenatal exposure to BPA can set the immune system to be more prone to develop autoimmunity later, in adulthood. However, in many cases, the results remain inconsistent or even controversial. Finally, it is thought that BPA participates in the pathogenesis of several autoimmune diseases, but further research is definitely required.

References

1. Jochmanová, I., Lazúrová, Z., Rudnay, M. et al. (2015). Environmental estrogen bisphenol A and autoimmunity. *Lupus* 24 (4–5): 392–399.
2. Rubin, B.S. (2011). Bisphenol A: an endocrine disruptor with widespread exposure and multiple effects. *J. Steroid Biochem. Mol. Biol.* 127 (1–2): 27–34.
3. Gassman, N.R. (2022). Bisphenol A: a multi-modal endocrine disruptor. Issues in Toxicology, Chapter 5, Royal Society of Chemistry, ISBN 978-1-83916-206-0, pp. 106–138.
4. Rochester, J.R. (2013). Bisphenol A and human health: a review of the literature. *Reprod. Toxicol.* 42: 132–155.
5. Lazurova, Z. and Lazurova, I. (2014). The environmental estrogen bisphenol A and its effects on the human organism. *Vnitr. Lek.* 59 (6): 466–471.
6. Gao, X. and Wang, H.S. (2014). Impact of bisphenol a on the cardiovascular system - epidemiological and experimental evidence and molecular mechanisms. *Int. J. Environ. Res. Public Health* 11 (8): 8399–8413.
7. Seachrist, D.D., Bonk, K.W., Ho, S.M. et al. (2016). A review of the carcinogenic potential of bisphenol A. *Reprod. Toxicol.* 59: 167–182.
8. Watad, A., Quaresma, M., Brown, S. et al. (2017). Autoimmune/inflammatory syndrome induced by adjuvants (Shoenfeld's syndrome) - an update. *Lupus* 26 (7): 675–681.
9. Borba, V., Malkova, A., Basantsova, N. et al. (2020). Classical examples of the concept of the ASIA syndrome. *Biomol. Ther.* 10 (10): 1436.
10. Vogel, S.A. (2009). The politics of plastics: the making and unmaking of bisphenol A "safety". *Am. J. Public Health* 99 (S3): S559–S566.
11. Testai E, Hartemann P, Rodriguez-Farré E, et al. (2015). Safety of the use of bisphenol A in medical devices. SCENIHR (Scientific Committee on Emerging and Newly Identified Health Risks). ISSN: 1831-4783, ISBN: 978-92-79-30133-9
12. Choi, J.Y., Lee, J., Huh, D.A. et al. (2022). Urinary bisphenol concentrations and its association with metabolic disorders in the US and Korean populations. *Environ. Pollut.* 15 (295): 118679.
13. Carwile, J.L., Ye, X., Zhou, X. et al. (2011). Canned soup consumption and urinary bisphenol A: a randomized crossover trial. *JAMA* 306: 2218–2220, 20.
14. Wang, L., Wang, F.S., and Gershwin, M.E. (2015). Human autoimmune diseases: a comprehensive update. *J. Intern. Med.* 278 (4): 369–395.
15. Aljadeff, G., Longhi, E., and Shoenfeld, Y. (2018). Bisphenol A: a notorious player in the mosaic of autoimmunity. *Autoimmunity* 51 (8): 370–377.
16. Kharrazian, D. (2014). The potential roles of Bisphenol A (BPA) pathogenesis in autoimmunity. *Autoimmune Dis.* 2014: 743616.

17. Rathee, M., Malik, P., and Singh, J. (2012). Bisphenol A in dental sealants and its estrogen like effect. *Indian J. Endocrinol. Metab.* 16 (3): 339–342.
18. Maserejian, N.N., Shrader, P., Brown, O.A. et al. (2014). Dental sealants and composite restorations and longitudinal changes in immune function markers in children. *Int. J. Paediatr. Dent.* 24 (3): 215–225.
19. MacKay, H. and Abizaid, A. (2018). A plurality of molecular targets: the receptor ecosystem for bisphenol-A (BPA). *Horm. Behav.* 101: 59–67.
20. Rogers, J.A., Metz, L., and Yong, V.W. (2013). Review: Endocrine disrupting chemicals and immune responses: a focus on bisphenol-A and its potential mechanisms. *Mol. Immunol.* 53 (4): 421–430.
21. Huang, F.M., Chang, Y.C., Lee, S.S. et al. (2018). Bisphenol A exhibits cytotoxic or genotoxic potential via oxidative stress-associated mitochondrial apoptotic pathway in murine macrophages. *Food Chem. Toxicol.* 122: 215–224.
22. Guo, H., Liu, T., Uemura, Y. et al. (2010). Bisphenol A in combination with TNF-alpha selectively induces Th2 cell-promoting dendritic cells in vitro with an estrogen-like activity. *Cell. Mol. Immunol.* 7 (3): 227–234.
23. Liao, S.L., Tsai, M.H., Lai, S.H. et al. (2016). Prenatal exposure to bisphenol-A is associated with Toll-like receptor-induced cytokine suppression in neonates. *Pediatr. Res.* 79 (3): 438–444.
24. Yang, M., Qiu, W., Chen, B. et al. (2015). The in vitro immune modulatory effect of bisphenol A on fish macrophages via estrogen receptor α and nuclear factor-κB signaling. *Environ. Sci. Technol.* 49 (3): 1888–1895.
25. Murray, P.J. and Wynn, T.A. (2011). Protective and pathogenic functions of macrophage subsets. *Nat. Rev. Immunol.* 11 (11): 723–737.
26. Huang, F.M., Chang, Y.C., Lee, S.S. et al. (2019). Expression of pro-inflammatory cytokines and mediators induced by bisphenol A via ERK-NFκB and JAK1/2-STAT3 pathways in macrophages. *Environ. Toxicol.* 34 (4): 486–494.
27. Wardowska, A. (2020). The epigenetic face of lupus: Focus on antigen-presenting cells. *Int. Immunopharmacol.* 81: 106262.
28. Biermann, M.H., Veissi, S., Maueröder, C. et al. (2014). The role of dead cell clearance in the etiology and pathogenesis of systemic lupus erythematosus: dendritic cells as potential targets. *Expert. Rev. Clin. Immunol.* 10: 1151–1164.
29. Goto, M., Takano-Ishikawa, Y., Ono, H. et al. (2007). Orally administered bisphenol A disturbed antigen specific immunoresponses in the naïve condition. *Biosci. Biotechnol. Biochem.* 71 (9): 2136–2143.
30. Cernadas, M., Lu, J., Watts, G. et al. (2009). CD1a expression defines an interleukin-12 producing population of human dendritic cells. *Clin. Exp. Immunol.* 155: 523–533.
31. Wang, J., She, C., Li, Z. et al. (2020). In vitro impact of bisphenol A on maturation and function of monocyte-derived dendritic cells in patients with primary Sjögren's syndrome. *Immunopharmacol. Immunotoxicol.* 42 (1): 28–36.
32. Yazdani, R., Sharifi, M., Shirvan, A.S. et al. (2015). Characteristics of innate lymphoid cells (ILCs) and their role in immunological disorders (an update). *Cell. Immunol.* 298 (1–2): 66–76.
33. Xiong, T. and Turner, J.E. (2018). Innate lymphoid cells in autoimmunity and chronic inflammatory diseases. *Semin. Immunopathol.* 40 (4): 393–406.
34. Malaisé, Y., Ménard, S., Cartier, C. et al. (2018). Consequences of bisphenol a perinatal exposure on immune responses and gut barrier function in mice. *Arch. Toxicol.* 92 (1): 347–358.
35. Lee, K.H., Kronbichler, A., Park, D.D. et al. (2017). Neutrophil extracellular traps (NETs) in autoimmune diseases: a comprehensive review. *Autoimmun. Rev.* 16 (11): 1160–1173.
36. Pinegin, B., Vorobjeva, N., and Pinegin, V. (2015). Neutrophil extracellular traps and their role in the development of chronic inflammation and autoimmunity. *Autoimmun. Rev.* 14 (7): 633–640.
37. Berthelot, J.M., Le Goff, B., Neel, A. et al. (2017). NETosis: at the crossroads of rheumatoid arthritis, lupus, and vasculitis. *Joint Bone Spine* 84 (3): 255–262.
38. Meng, H., Yalavarthi, S., Kanthi, Y. et al. (2017). In vivo role of neutrophil extracellular traps in antiphospholipid antibody-mediated venous thrombosis. *Arthritis Rheum.* 69 (3): 655–667.
39. Tong, S., Yang, S., Li, T. et al. (2019). Role of neutrophil extracellular traps in chronic kidney injury by bisphenol-A. *J. Endocrinol.* 241 (2): 125–134.
40. Frangou, E., Chrysanthopoulou, A., Mitsios, A. et al. (2019). REDD1/autophagy pathway promotes thromboinflammation and fibrosis in human systemic lupus erythematosus (SLE) through NETs decorated with tissue factor (TF) and interleukin-17A (IL-17A). *Ann. Rheum. Dis.* 78 (2): 238–248.

41. Doridot, L., Jeljeli, M., Chêne, C. et al. (2019). Implication of oxidative stress in the pathogenesis of systemic sclerosis via inflammation, autoimmunity and fibrosis. *Redox Biol.* 25: 101122.
42. Gassman, N.R. (2017). Induction of oxidative stress by bisphenol A and its pleiotropic effects. *Environ. Mol. Mutagen.* 58 (2): 60–71.
43. Wang, Y., Li, S., and Li, C. (2019). Perspectives of new advances in the pathogenesis of vitiligo: from oxidative stress to autoimmunity. *Med. Sci. Monit.* 25: 1017–1023.
44. Ozaydin, T., Oznurlu, Y., Sur, E. et al. (2018). Effects of bisphenol A on antioxidant system and lipid profile in rats. *Biotech. Histochem.* 93: 231–238.
45. Balistrieri, A., Hobohm, L., Srivastava, T. et al. (2018). Alterations in human neutrophil function by bisphenol A. *Am. J. Phys. Cell Phys.* 315 (5): C636–C642.
46. Yang, Y.J. (2009). Bisphenol A exposure is associated with oxidative stress and inflammation in postmenopausal women. *Environ. Res.* 109 (6): 797–801.
47. Wang, Y.X., Liu, C., Shen, Y. et al. (2019). Urinary levels of bisphenol A, F and S and markers of oxidative stress among healthy adult men: variability and association analysis. *Environ. Int.* 123: 301–309.
48. Miossec, P. and Kolls, J.K. (2012). Targeting IL-17 and TH17 cells in chronic inflammation. *Nat. Rev. Drug Discov.* 11 (10): 763–776.
49. Moudgil, K.D. and Choubey, D. (2011). Cytokines in autoimmunity: role in induction, regulation, and treatment. *J. Interferon Cytokine Res.* 3 (10): 695–703.
50. Yan, H., Takamoto, M., and Sugane, K. (2008). Exposure to bisphenol A prenatally or in adulthood promotes T(H)2 cytokine production associated with reduction of CD4CD25 regulatory T cells. *Environ. Health Perspect.* 116: 514–519.
51. Goto, M., Takano-Ishikawa, Y., Ono, H. et al. (2007). Orally administered bisphenol A disturbed antigen specific immunoresponses in the naive condition. *Biosci. Biotechnol. Biochem.* 71 (9): 2136–2143.
52. Ellis, J.S., Hong, S.H., Zaghouani, H. et al. (2013). Reduced effectiveness of CD4+Foxp3+ regulatory T cells in CD28-deficient NOD.H-2h4 mice leads to increased severity of spontaneous autoimmune thyroiditis. *J. Immunol.* 191 (10): 4940–4949.
53. Yoshino, S., Yamaki, K., Li, X. et al. (2004). Prenatal exposure to bisphenol A up-regulates immune responses, including T helper 1 and T helper 2 responses, in mice. *Immunology* 112 (3): 489–495.
54. Liu, Y., Mei, C., Liu, H. et al. (2014). Modulation of cytokine expression in human macrophages by endocrine-disrupting chemical bisphenol A. *Biochem. Biophys. Res. Commun.* 451: 592–598.
55. Luo, S., Li, Y., Li, Y. et al. (2016). Gestational and lactational exposure to low-dose bisphenol A increases Th17 cells in mice offspring. *Environ. Toxicol. Pharmacol.* 47: 149–158.
56. Wang, G., Li, Y., Li, Y. et al. (2020). Maternal vitamin D supplementation inhibits bisphenol A-induced proliferation of Th17 cells in adult offspring. *Food Chem. Toxicol.* 144: 111604.
57. Kamali, A.N., Noorbakhsh, S.M., Hamedifar, H. et al. (2019). A role for Th1-like Th17 cells in the pathogenesis of inflammatory and autoimmune disorders. *Mol. Immunol.* 105: 107–115.
58. Lee, M.H., Chung, W., Kang, B.Y. et al. (2003). Enhanced interleukin-4 production in CD4+ T-cells and elevated immunoglobulin E levels in antigen-primed mice by Bisphenol A and nonylphenol, endocrine disruptors: involvement of nuclear factor-AT and CA2+. *Immunology* 109 (1): 76–86.
59. Wang, I.J., Chen, C.Y., and Bornehag, C.G. (2016). Bisphenol A exposure may increase the risk of development of atopic disorders in children. *Int. J. Hyg. Environ. Health* 219 (3): 311–316.
60. Maurer, M., Altrichter, S., Schmetzer, O. et al. (2018). Immunoglobulin E-mediated autoimmunity. *Front. Immunol.* 9: 689.
61. Sanjuan, M.A., Sagar, D., and Kolbeck, R. (2016). Role of IgE in autoimmunity. *J. Allergy Clin. Immunol.* 137 (6): 1651–1661.
62. Yurino, H., Ishikawa, S., Sato, T. et al. (2004). Endocrine disruptors (environmental estrogens) enhance autoantibody production by B1 cells. *Toxicol. Sci.* 81 (1): 139–147.
63. Morimoto, S., Nakano, S., Watanabe, T. et al. (2007). Expression of B-cell activating factor of the tumour necrosis factor family (BAFF) in T cells in active systemic lupus erythematosus: the role of BAFF in T cell-dependent B cell pathogenic autoantibody production. *Rheumatology (Oxford)* 46 (7): 1083–1086.
64. Steffen, U., Koeleman, C.A., Sokolova, M.V. et al. (2020). IgA subclasses have different effector functions associated with distinct glycosylation profiles. *Nat. Commun.* 11 (1): 120.
65. Primm, T.P. and Gilbert, H.F. (2001). Hormone binding by protein disulphide isomerase, a high capacity hormone reservoir or the endoplasmic reticulum. *Protein Struct. Folding* 276 (1): 281–286.

66. Hashimoto, S., Shiomoto, K., Okada, K. et al. (2012). The binding site of bisphenol A to protein disulphide isomerase. *J. Biochem.* 151 (1): 35–45.
67. Hiroi, T., Okada, K., Imaoka, S. et al. (2006). Bisphenol A binds to protein disulfide isomerase and inhibits its enzymatic and hormone-binding activities. *Endocrinology* 147 (6): 2773–2780.
68. Kharrazian, D., Herbert, M., and Vojdani, A. (2019). The associations between immunological reactivity to the haptenation of unconjugated bisphenol A to albumin and protein disulfide isomerase with alpha-synuclein antibodies. *Toxics* 7 (2): 26.
69. Kharrazian, D. and Vojdani, A. (2017). Correlation between antibodies to bisphenol A, its target enzyme protein disulfide isomerase and antibodies to neuron-specific antigens. *J. Appl. Toxicol.* 37 (4): 479–484.
70. Vojdani, A., Kharrazian, D., and Mukherjee, P.S. (2015). Elevated levels of antibodies against xenobiotics in a subgroup of healthy subjects. *J. Appl. Toxicol.* 35 (4): 383–397.
71. Molodecky, N. and Kaplan, G. (2010). Environmental risk factors for inflammatory bowel disease. *Gastroenterol. Hepatol.* 6: 339–346.
72. Legaki, E. and Gazouli, M. (2016). Influence of environmental factors in the development of inflammatory bowel disease. *World J. Gastrointest Pharmacol. Ther.* 7: 112.
73. Xu, J., Huang, G., Nagy, T. et al. (2019). Bisphenol A alteration of type 1 diabetes in non-obese diabetic (NOD) female mice is dependent on window of exposure. *Arch. Toxicol.* 93 (4): 1083–1093.
74. Javurek, A., Spollen, W., Johnson, S. et al. (2016). Effects of exposure to bisphenol A and ethinyl estradiol on the gut microbiota of parents and their offspring in a rodent model. *Gut Microbes* 7: 471–485.
75. Moryiama, K., Tagami, T., Akamizu, T. et al. (2002). Thyroid hormone action is disrupted by bisphenol A as an antagonist. *J. Clin. Endocrinol. Metab.* 87 (11): 5185–5190.
76. Davies, J.M. (1997). Molecular mimicry: can epitope mimicry induce autoimmune disease? *Immunol. Cell Biol.* 75 (2): 113–126.
77. Borba, V.V., Zandman-Goddard, G., and Shoenfeld, Y. (2018). Prolactin and autoimmunity. *Front. Immunol.* 9: 73.
78. Borba, V.V., Zandman-Goddard, G., and Shoenfeld, Y. (2019). Prolactin and autoimmunity: the hormone as an inflammatory cytokine. *Best Pract. Res. Clin. Endocrinol. Metab.* 33 (6): 101324.
79. Doherty, D.G. (2016). Immunity, tolerance and autoimmunity in the liver: a comprehensive review. *J. Autoimmun.* 66: 60–75.
80. Namazi, M.R. (2009). Cytochrome-P450 enzymes and autoimmunity: expansion of the relationship and introduction of free radicals as the link. *J. Autoimmune Dis.* 6: 4–6.
81. Xu, J., Huang, G., and Guo, T. (2016). Developmental Bisphenol A exposure modulates immune-related diseases. *Toxics* 4 (4): 23.
82. Kundakovic, M., Gudsnuk, K., Franks, B. et al. (2013). Sex-specific epigenetic disruption and behavioral changes following low-dose in utero bisphenol A exposure. *Proc. Natl. Acad. Sci. U. S. A.* 110 (24): 9956–9961.
83. Khan, D. and Ahmed, S.A. (2015). Epigenetic regulation of non-lymphoid cells by bisphenol A, a model endocrine disrupter: potential implications for immunoregulation. *Front Endocrinol. (Lausanne)* 6: 91.
84. Alhomaidan, H.T., Rasheed, N., Almatrafi, S. et al. (2019). Bisphenol A modified DNA: a possible immunogenic stimulus for anti-DNA autoantibodies in systemic lupus erythematosus. *Autoimmunity* 52 (7-8): 272–280.
85. García-Carrasco, M., Macias-Díaz, S., Mendoza-Pinto, C. et al. (2021). The role of IgE in systemic lupus erythematosus. *Autoimmun. Rev.* 20 (1): 102704.
86. Dong, Y., Zhang, Z., Liu, H. et al. (2020). Exacerbating lupus nephritis following BPA exposure is associated with abnormal autophagy in MRL/lpr mice. *Am. J. Transl. Res.* 12 (2): 649–659.
87. Sugiura-Ogasawara, M., Ozaki, Y., Sonta, S. et al. (2005). Exposure to bisphenol A is associated with recurrent miscarriage. *Hum. Reprod.* 20 (8): 2325–2329.
88. Palioura, E. and Diamanti-Kandarakis, E. (2015). Polycystic ovary syndrome (PCOS) and endocrine disrupting chemicals (EDCs). *Rev. Endocr. Metab. Disord.* 16 (4): 365–371.
89. Bonefeld-Jørgensen, E.C., Long, M., Hofmeister, M.V. et al. (2007). Endocrine-disrupting potential of bisphenol A, bisphenol A dimethacrylate, 4-*n*-nonylphenol, and 4-*n*-octylphenol in vitro: new data and a brief review. *Environ. Health Perspect.* 115 (Suppl 1): 69–76.
90. Kechagias, K.S., Semertzidou, A., Athanasiou, A. et al. (2020). Bisphenol-A and polycystic ovary syndrome: a review of the literature. *Rev. Environ. Health* 35 (4): 323–331. Doi: 10.1515/reveh-2020-0032.

91. Pivonello, C., Muscogiuri, G., Nardone, A. et al. (2020). Bisphenol A: an emerging threat to female fertility. *Reprod. Biol. Endocrinol.* 18 (1): 22.
92. Fernandez, M.O., Bourguignon, N.S., Arocena, P. et al. (2018). Neonatal exposure to bisphenol A alters the hypothalamic-pituitary-thyroid axis in female rats. *Toxicol. Lett.* 285: 81–86.
93. Chianese, R., Viggiano, A., Urbanek, K. et al. (2018). Chronic exposure to low dose of bisphenol A impacts on the first round of spermatogenesis via SIRT1 modulation. *Sci. Rep.* 8 (1): 2961.
94. Zoeller, R.T., Bansal, R., and Parris, C. (2005). Bisphenol-A, an environmental contaminant that acts as a thyroid hormone receptor antagonist in vitro, increases serum thyroxine, and alters RC3/neurogranin expression in the developing rat brain. *Endocrinology* 146 (2): 607–612.
95. Kim, M.J. and Park, Y.J. (2019). Bisphenols and thyroid hormone. *Endocrinol. Metab.* 34: 340–348.
96. Wang, X., Tang, N., Nakayama, S.F. et al. (2020). Maternal urinary bisphenol A concentration and thyroid hormone levels of Chinese mothers and newborns by maternal body mass index. *Environ. Sci. Pollut. Res. Int.* 27 (10): 10939–10949.
97. Chailurkit, L.O., Aekplakorn, W., and Ongphiphadhanakul, B. (2016). The association of serum bisphenol A with thyroid autoimmunity. *Int. J. Environ. Res. Public Health* 13 (11): 1153.
98. Maserejian, N. (2014). Possible association between dental sealants and urinary bisphenol A levels in children warrants additional biomonitoring and safety research. *J. Evid. Based Dent. Pract.* 4 (4): 200–202.
99. Bragazzi, N.L., Hejly, A., Watad, A. et al. (2020). ASIA syndrome and endocrine autoimmune disorders. *Best Pract. Res. Clin. Endocrinol. Metab.* 34 (1): 101412.
100. Vabre, P., Gatimel, N., Moreau, J. et al. (2017). Environmental pollutants, a possible etiology for premature ovarian insufficiency: a narrative review of animal and human data. *Environ. Health* 16 (37): 1–18.
101. Patel, S., Zhou, C., Rattan, S. et al. (2015). Effects of endocrine-disrupting chemicals on the ovary. *Biol. Reprod.* 93 (20): 1–9.
102. Howard, S.G. (2019). Exposure to environmental chemicals and type 1 diabetes: an update. *J. Epidemiol. Community Health* 73 (6): 483–488.
103. Bodin, J., Stene, L.C., and Nygaard, U.C. (2015). Can exposure to environmental chemicals increase the risk of diabetes type 1 development? *Biomed. Res. Int.* 2015: 208947.
104. Bodin, J., Kocbach Bølling, A., Wendt, A. et al. (2015). Exposure to bisphenol A, but not phthalates, increases spontaneous diabetes type 1 development in NOD mice. *Toxicol. Rep.* 2: 99–110.
105. Ahn, C., Kang, H.S., Lee, J.H. et al. (2018). Bisphenol A and octylphenol exacerbate type 1 diabetes mellitus by disrupting calcium homeostasis in mouse pancreas. *Toxicol. Lett.* 295: 162–172.
106. Ince, T., Balcı, A., Yalçın, S.S. et al. (2018). Urinary bisphenol-A levels in children with type 1 diabetes mellitus. *J. Pediatr. Endocrinol. Metab.* 31 (8): 829–836.
107. Yan, S., Song, W., Chen, Y. et al. (2013). Low-dose bisphenol A and estrogen increase ventricular arrhythmias following ischemia-reperfusion in female rat hearts. *Food Chem. Toxicol.* 56: 75–80.
108. Melzer, D., Gates, P., Osborne, N.J. et al. (2012). Urinary bisphenol a concentration and angiography-defined coronary artery stenosis. *PLoS One* 7 (8): e43378.
109. Lazurova, Z. and Tkac, I. (2015). Bisfenol A a jeho vplyv na kardiovaskulárny system. *Intern. Med.* 15 (2): 62–64.
110. Bruno, K.A., Mathews, J.E., Yang, A.L. et al. (2019). BPA alters estrogen receptor expression in the heart after viral infection activating cardiac mast cells and T cells leading to perimyocarditis and fibrosis. *Front. Endocrinol.* 10 (598): 1–16.
111. Koenig, A., Buskiewicz, I., and Huber, S.A. (2017). Age-associated changes in estrogen receptor ratios correlate with increased female susceptibility to coxsackievirus B3-induced myocarditis. *Front. Immunol.* 8: 1585.
112. Stafford, K., Greyner, H., Molina, F. et al. (2014). Bisphenol A (BPA) exacerbates acute myocarditis in female BALB/c by activating mast cells and the inflammasome (HUM1P.302). *J. Immunol.* 192 (Supplement 1): 52.2.
113. Lai, K.P., Chung, Y.T., Li, R. et al. (2016). Bisphenol A alters gut microbiome: comparative metagenomics analysis. *Environ. Pollut.* 218: 923–930.
114. DeLuca, J.A.A., Allred, K.F., Menon, R. et al. (2018). Bisphenol-A alters microbiota metabolites derived from aromatic amino acids and worsens disease activity during colitis. *Exp. Biol. Med.* 243 (10): 864–875.
115. De Silva, P.S., Yang, X., Korzenik, J.R. et al. (2017). Association of urinary phenolic compounds, inflammatory bowel disease and chronic diarrheal symptoms: Evidence from the National Health and Nutrition Examination Survey. *Environ. Pollut.* 229: 621–626.

116. Rogers, J.A., Mishra, M.K., Hahn, J. et al. (2017). Gestational bisphenol-A exposure lowers the threshold for autoimmunity in a model of multiple sclerosis. *Proc. Natl. Acad. Sci. U. S. A.* 114 (19): 4999–5004.
117. Krementsov, D.N., Katchy, A., Laure, K. et al. (2013). Studies in experimental autoimmune encephalomyelitis do not support developmental bisphenol A exposure as an environmental factor in increasing multiple sclerosis risk. *Toxicol. Sci.* 135 (1): 91–102.
118. Brinkmeyer-Langford, C., Rodrigues, A., Kochan, K.J. et al. (2014). Consequences of perinatal bisphenol A exposure in a mouse model of multiple sclerosis. *Autoimmunity* 47 (1): 55–56.
119. Garretti, F., Agalliu, D., Lindestam, A. et al. (2019). Autoimmunity in Pakinson's disease: the role of alpha-synuclein-specific T cells. *Front. Immunol.* 10: 303.

21 Sarcoidosis and Autoimmune Inflammatory Syndrome Induced by Adjuvants: Is There a Connection?

Anna Malkova[1], Yulia Zinchenko[2], Anna Starshinova[3], Igor Kudryavtsev[3,4], Piotr Yablonskiy[1,2], and Yehuda Shoenfeld[5,6]

[1]Laboratory of the Mosaic of Autoimmunity, St. Petersburg State University, Saint Petersburg, Russia
[2]St. Petersburg Research Institute of Phthisiopulmonology, Saint Petersburg, Russia
[3]Almazov National Medical Research Centre, The Research Department, Saint Petersburg, Russia
[4]Department of Immunology, Institution of Experimental Medicine, Petersburg State University, Saint Petersburg, Russia
[5]Reichman university, Herzliya, Israel
[6]Zabludowicz Center for Autoimmune Diseases, Sheba Medical Center, Tel-Hashomer, Israel

Introduction

Sarcoidosis remains a disease with an unknown etiology. According to the existing ideas, based on the data of pathomorphological studies, sarcoidosis is considered a granulomatous disease with an acute, subacute, or chronic course, involving most often (up to 90% of cases) lungs and mediastinal lymph nodes, as well as other organs and tissues, with granuloma formation without caseous necrosis [1]. There are two variants of the acute course of the disease: Lofgren's syndrome with bilateral pulmonary hilar lymphadenopathy, erythema nodosum, fever, polyarthritis, and the Heerfordt-Waldenström syndrome, characterized by parotitis, facial palsy, anterior uveitis, and fever [2].

The problem of finding an etiological factor in studies on sarcoidosis has led to the identification of various infectious agents from bacteria to viral agents and fungi and inorganic factors (silicone, silicates, etc.) [3, 4]. The lack of an etiological factor and understanding of the pathogenesis of the disease leads to the absence of a unified approach to therapy, as well as to the possibility of conducting preclinical studies of the effectiveness of treatment on sarcoidosis models [5].

Autoimmune Disorders: Adjuvants and Other Risk Factors in Pathogenesis, First Edition.
Edited by Abdulla Watad, Nicola Luigi Bragazzi, and Yehuda Shoenfeld.

It is known that a severe progressive course of sarcoidosis can lead to failure of the affected organ, which requires enhanced therapy or even transplantation of healthy tissues [6], which is why it is so important to understand the pathogenesis of the disease to develop patient management.

In recent years, a large number of proponents of the theory of the autoimmune nature of this disease have appeared, which is confirmed by numerous studies [1, 7, 8]. Some authors suggest that prolonged contact of foreign antigens with toll-like receptors of endotheliocytes, macrophages, and dendritic cells leads to activation and epithelioid differentiation of macrophages, which in turn start secreting proinflammatory cytokines (TNF-α, IL-1). Dendritic cells with antigen migrate to the lymph nodes, where they present the antigen to T-lymphocytes. After activation, T-lymphocytes differentiate into $CD4^+$, $CD8^+$, Tx17, Treg, proliferate, and migrate to the focus of inflammation. Accumulation of epithelioid macrophages, T- and B-lymphocytes in the focus of inflammation leads to the formation of epithelioid granulomas without foci of caseous necrosis. Later there is cellular damage by effectors of both humoral (antibodies) and cellular immune response (cytokines of T-lymphocytes). In the chronic form, fibrosis occurs due to Tx17, TNF-α synthesized by macrophages. Perhaps the absence of necrotic masses indicates a constant activation of the immune system by an antigen that cannot be eliminated, which in turn may indicate autoimmune tissue damage [7].

The concept of autoimmune/inflammatory syndrome induced by adjuvants (ASIA), proposed in 2011 by Shoenfeld et al. and the beginning of research on various pathological processes within ASIA, opened new perspectives for understanding sarcoidosis as an autoimmune pathology [9–12].

ASIA signs in sarcoidosis

A certain similarity of ASIA and sarcoidosis as a genetically mediated disease with the development of immunological disorders under the influence of trigger factors raises the question of their connection. This approach allows us to identify autoimmune features in the pathogenesis of this disease, which may bring us closer to understanding it.

Major criteria

Exposure to external factors (infections, vaccines, silicone, adjuvant) before the development of clinical manifestations (prescription from months to several years); removal of the provoking factor causes improvement

Some studies suggest that prolonged contact with inorganic dust, silicates, and print production is associated with the development of sarcoidosis [12–14]. Under laboratory conditions, carbonaceous materials, including the multiwalled carbon nanotubes, have been shown to induce the development of granulomas in lungs with the formation of multinucleated giant cells in mouse models [15–17].

An important role is played by the implantation of various substances, such as silicone, which is widely used in the creation of breast implants, artificial joint shunts for patients with hydrocephalus, catheters, in rhinoplasty and as a part of the dermal fillers. A study by A. Watad, comparing 24,651 patients with silicone implants to 98,604 patients without foreign bodies in the body, showed an increased risk of autoimmune diseases (OR 1.21, 95% CI 1.17–1.26) in female patients with silicone implants, with the strongest associations with sarcoidosis, Sjögren's disease and systemic scleroderma [18, 19]. A case of the development of an acute form of sarcoidosis – Lofgren's syndrome after silicone implantation was described [20, 21], as well as the disease remission after removal of implants, that may suggest a possible link between sarcoidosis and the ASIA syndrome [19, 22]. The role of silicone as a trigger in the development of sarcoidosis may be considered with both local (sarcoid granulomas in the skin at the site of silicone mammoplasty or subcutaneous injection), and, most importantly, systemic manifestations of sarcoidosis with the formation of granulomas in the lung tissue and hilar lymph nodes [23–25]. Cases of the development of pulmonary sarcoidosis with the involvement of the intracranial lymph nodes during the installation of an intragastric silicone balloon are also described; the appearance of radiographic changes in the lung tissue was noted as early as seven days after surgery [26].

When studying the infectious nature of sarcoidosis, the role of viruses, fungi, and bacteria is actively discussed, among which the most attention is paid to *Propionibacterium acnes* and *Mycobacterium tuberculosis* [8]. In numerous studies in patients with sarcoidosis, their genetic material was found in sarcoid granulomas and bronchoalveolar fluid. Activation of peripheral mononuclears in response to mycobacterial antigens has been shown, which may indicate an established immune response against these microorganisms [27, 28]. The effect of mycobacteria on the development of sarcoid granulomas has been shown in animal models (Lewis rats and C57BL/6 mice) [29]. In mouse models, the use of *M. tuberculosis* catalase–peroxidase (mkatg) and *M. tuberculosis* A superoxide dismutase (MSODA) proteins [30, 31], as well as various *P. acnes* proteins [32, 33] showed the development of lung granulomatosis similar in histology to human sarcoid granulomas (recruitment of macrophages and $CD4^{+}$T and $CD45/B220^{+}$ B lymphocytes stimulated by cytokines Th1 and chemokines (TNFα, IFNγ, MCP-1, IL12p40, and IL12p70).

The association of the increase in the incidence of sarcoidosis with the presence of fungi in the dust was noted, in vitro experiments showed the response of peripheral mononuclears when stimulated by antigens of mold fungi found in buildings where office employees worked [34, 35].

One of the main trigger factors in ASIA is the adjuvants contained in vaccines. Postvaccine development of juvenile sarcoidosis has been described in children after BCG administration, most commonly at the site of vaccine administration [36–38]. There have been published clinical cases of the development of sarcoid uveitis, presumably after administration of varicella-zoster virus vaccine (Shingrix) [39], systemic sarcoidosis with sarcoidosis of the tattooed skin [40] and development of retinal vasculitis, similar to changes in sarcoidosis [41] after administration of influenza vaccine, and cutaneous sarcoidosis after Live rubella virus vaccine in a patient with primary immune deficiency [42].

Cases of sarcoid granuloma development in cancer patients deserve special attention. Therefore, there have been described cases of sarcoidosis after administration of a vaccine based on dendritic cells [43] and various peptides of melanoma cells [44].

A case of sarcoid mediastinal lymphadenopathy has been described, presumably after vaccination against COVID-19 [45].

A distinction must be made between the terms "sarcoidosis" and "sarcoid reaction." The latter is characterized by the formation of epithelioid cell granulomas in organs and tissues, in some cases followed by similar clinical symptoms. The main difference between the sarcoid reaction and sarcoidosis is the presence of infectious diseases (i.e. tuberculosis, leishmaniasis, leprosy), tumors (i.e. prostate, breast, lung, colorectal cancer, ovarian, and soft tissue tumors), or other trigger factors. The symptoms of sarcoid reaction are reversed upon removal of the trigger factors. In accordance with this definition, it is possible to assume a link between the sarcoid reaction and the ASIA syndrome. This does not exclude the possibility that in sarcoidosis there is also a trigger factor that just cannot be clearly identified and removed [46, 47].

Therefore, the supposed triggers of sarcoidosis and sarcoid reactions can be biological agents and substances of organic and inorganic origin, whose role in the pathogenesis of sarcoidosis, according to the data analysis, cannot be denied (Table 21.1). At the same time, according to epidemiological studies, the influence of a single provoking factor has not been proven. It is assumed that different factors affect the immune system in different ways, stimulating the immune response leading to the development of sarcoidosis, including the induction of autoimmunity, with genetic factors playing an important role [48–50].

Table 21.1 Suspected organic and inorganic triggers of sarcoidosis development.

Biological triggers	Nonbiological triggers
Bacteria (*M.tuberculosis, Nontuberculous Mycobacterium, P. acnes*)	**Organic compounds** (pine pollen, clay, silicon, etc.)
Fungi	**Metal dust** (aluminum, zirconium, barium, cobalt, copper, titanium, gold, etc.)
Viruses (*human herpes viruses HHV6 and HHV8, retrovirus, cytomegalovirus, Coxsackie virus, rubella virus, adenovirus, etc.*)	**Other inorganic compounds** (talc, photocopy toner powder, fiberglass, etc.)
Vaccines (tuberculosis, flu, cancer)	

Appearance of at least one of the following "typical" clinical manifestations

Clinical manifestations of subacute and chronic sarcoidosis may be either absent or very diverse: associated with lesions of various organs and nonspecific. Up to 50% of patients with pulmonary sarcoidosis report dry cough, dyspnea, and chest pain. Among the nonspecific symptoms, the most common are arthralgia, fatigue (up to 50–70% of patients), chest pain, muscle pain, night sweats, and weight loss. Chronic sarcoidosis is associated with the development of fibrosis (pulmonary and extrapulmonary) and pulmonary arterial hypertension. Adverse prognosis is also associated with the development of lupus pernio, chronic uveitis, hypercalcemia, nephrocalcinosis, cystic bone lesions, and myocardial damage [51, 52].

The development of small fiber neuropathy (SFN) in sarcoidosis deserves special attention. Most often patients complain of burning paresthesias, numbness, and dysfunctions of the cardiovascular, musculoskeletal system, and gastrointestinal tract, which is combined with a decrease in intraepidermal nerve fiber density in the biopsy material [53]. SFN is often found in various autoimmune diseases, which may indicate autoantibody-mediated nerve damage [54].

A more detailed description of the most common clinical manifestations associated with lesions of various organs and a comparison with the clinical manifestations of autoimmune diseases is presented in Table 21.2.

Sarcoidosis often occurs in conjunction with other autoimmune diseases:

- ankylosing spondylitis, granulomatous pulmonary disease, sacroiliitis, and the HLA-B27 genotype typical for spondyloarthritis were detected in patients [55, 56]
- lupus erythematosus [57]
- Sjogren's syndrome [58]
- primary biliary cirrhosis [59]
- Crohn's disease, antiphospholipid syndrome, idiopathic pulmonary fibrosis [60]
- subclinical and clinical hypothyroidism, antithyroid autoantibodies [overall antithyroid peroxidase antibodies (TPOAb)], and in general, thyroid autoimmunity [61]
- Such cases of comorbidity show the possibility of a common pathogenesis of these diseases and confirm the idea of multiautoimmune diseases [62].

Typical biopsy

The main characteristic of sarcoidosis is the formation of noncaseating epithelioid granulomas in various organs, represented by lymphocytes, epithelioid, and giant cells (asteroid and conchoidal bodies). Unlike infectious-mediated granulomas in sarcoidosis, necrotic masses are not

Table 21.2 Clinical manifestations of sarcoidosis typical for autoimmune diseases.

Affected organ	Percentage of occurrence	Clinical manifestations	Clinical manifestations typical for autoimmune diseases
Lymph nodes	95–98%	Lymphadenopathy	
General symptoms	Up to 35%	Fever, unexplained weight loss, fatigue, sleep disturbances	Chronic fatigue, unrelieved sleep, sleep disturbances
			Fever, dry mucous membranes
Eyes	20–50%	Uveitis, retinal vascular changes, lacrimal gland enlargement	Uveitis
Musculoskeletal system	25–39%	Myositis	Myalgia, myositis, muscle weakness
		Muscle weakness	Arthralgia and/or arthritis
		Arthralgia and/or arthritis	
Skin	25%	Papules, nodules, erythema nodosum, lupus pernio, granulomas in the area of tattoos, scars	Rash
Nervous system	10%	Cognitive dysfunction	Neurological manifestations (especially associated with demyelination)
		Small fiber neuropathy (burning paresthesias, numbness, dysfunctions of the cardiovascular, musculoskeletal system, and gastrointestinal tract)	Cognitive disorders, memory impairment, small fiber neuropathy

formed and ACE hyperproduction occurs [7, 63]. The central part of a granuloma is composed of macrophages, modified macrophages, epithelioid cells, and giant cells, with $CD4^+$ T-lymphocytes between them [64]. The peripheral part of a granuloma is predominantly occupied by $CD8^+$ T lymphocytes, fibroblasts, macrophages, and fibrocytes, B lymphocytes are usually very rare in a granuloma [65]. Central fibrinoid may be found [7].

It is important to note the features of lymphocytic infiltration and the general state of the immune system in sarcoidosis, which is similar to some autoimmune diseases [66]. In the presence of autoimmune processes impaired memory and "naïve" B-cells distribution [67, 68], an imbalance of T-helpers and T-follicular helpers toward an increase in the number of T-h17, T-fh17, Th2, a decrease in T-h1, T-regulatory cells [69], imbalance between subpopulations of Tfh cells and regulatory Tfr [70, 71], elevated levels of short-lived, highly differentiated $CD8^+$ T lymphocytes are observed [72].

Thus, in patients with neurosarcoidosis, a high $CD8^+$ T-lymphocytes number was found during immunohistochemical examination of granulomas in autopsies of the meninges and brainstem [73], an increase in the number of mature $CD8^+$ $CD56^+$ T cells, the relative content of which was almost three times higher than the value in the control group [74].

In addition to $CD8^+$ T-lymphocytes, an increase in $CCR4^+$ $CD4^+$ cells number in the peripheral blood was found, as well as an increase in the concentration of the chemokine ligand for this chemokine receptor CCL17 in the blood serum of sarcoidosis patients and locally in the focus of granuloma formation [75]. Excessive Th2 activation in patients with sarcoidosis is also confirmed by the data on an increase in IL-13 mRNA expression, one of the key Th2 cytokines [76]. Moreover, in experiments on laboratory animals [77] and in the analysis of tissue samples obtained from patients [78] overproduction of Th2 cytokines, activation, and differentiation of tissue macrophages toward M2 was shown. M2 macrophages contribute to the development and maintenance of foci of chronic inflammation in tissues, the formation of granulomas, and foci of fibrosis.

There is an assumption about the role of the disturbance of Th1 and Th17 ratio in the formation of granulomas in sarcoidosis [79]. Most researchers have noted increased IL-6, IL-17, IL-22, IFN-γ, and CCL20, synthesized by Th17 in the serum of patients [80] and increased levels of these cytokines, the number of cells involved in their production in the fluid of bronchoalveolar lavage (BAL) and granulomatous tissue [81].

T regulatory cells are immune suppressors and protect from the development of autoimmune diseases. In sarcoidosis, a paradoxical reaction is observed – in the focus of inflammation (in the BAL), a decrease in the number of cells was shown, while in the peripheral blood, on the contrary, an increase. Huang et al. revealed an almost three-fold decrease in the relative number of T-regs in the blood of patients with initially diagnosed sarcoidosis compared with a group of conventionally healthy donors [79]. Furthermore, in many studies, a decrease in the level of the transcription factor T-reg FOXP3 in BAL was noted, which indicates a decrease in cell function [82]. Along with the antiinflammatory cytokines TGF-β and IL-10, an important and relatively poorly studied soluble Treg product is adenosine, which has a pronounced suppressive effect on a wide range of cells of innate and adaptive immunity [83]. When comparing the level of expression of CD39 on regulatory T-cells of peripheral blood, it turned out that the relative content of $CD39^+$ cells is increased both in patients with acute onset and in primary chronic sarcoidosis [84]. Probably, the formation of antiinflammatory adenosine, which is involved in the suppression of hypersensitive immune responses, is one of the key and most common mechanisms of immunosuppression in both acute and chronic sarcoidosis.

In the study of humoral immunity, it was shown that in patients with sarcoidosis, the amount of B-cell-activating factor (BAFF) is significantly higher and, accordingly, Ig-producing B-cells in the lung tissues, while in the blood the level of B-cells in sarcoidosis corresponded to the number in healthy people or was below normal [85]. At the same time, a disbalance of B-cell subtypes was observed. A decrease in the number of memory B-cells, an increase in the number of B-regulatory cells producing IL-10, and hypergammaglobulinemia, correlating with an increase in immunoglobulins in the peripheral blood, were noted in BAL [86]. Hypergammaglobulinemia has been shown in several studies, but no association with disease severity has been found [87].

According to a comprehensive analysis of B- and T-lymphocytes [88, 89], sarcoidosis patients showed an increase in the number of naive B cells, a decrease in memory B cells, and an increase in the number of $CD24^{+++}$ $CD38^{+++}$ and $CD5^+$ $CD27^-$ B cells with regulatory functions, which have been described for many autoimmune diseases. A significantly higher proportion of CXCR5-expressing CD45RA – $CCR7^+$ Th cells was found in patients with sarcoidosis compared with healthy controls, representing an expansion of this subpopulation of memory Th cells in disease.

A comparison of T- and B-lymphocyte subpopulations in sarcoidosis and autoimmune diseases is presented in Table 21.3.

It is important to note that the lymphocyte count can serve as a prognostic factor. Thus, a higher number of CD4 cells and a higher CD4/CD8 ratio was observed in radiologically improved patients and responded better to treatment, while an increasing number of Th17 cells can be predictive for progressive sarcoidosis and may help in the selection of patients with increased risk of lung fibrosis [90]. Low neutrophil count in the BAL fluid was associated with higher chances of spontaneous recovery [91].

Table 21.3 Features of lymphocytic populations in sarcoidosis and autoimmune diseases.

	Sarcoidosis		Autoimmune diseases
	Number in peripheral blood	**Number in BAL**	
CD8 T cells	↑	↑	↑
CD4 T cells	↑	↑	↑
T reg	↑	↓	↓
Suppression of immune responses			
Th17	↑	↑	↑
Cell proliferation activation			
Th 1	↓/↑	↓/↑	↓
Activation of cytotoxic immunity			
Th 2	↑	↑	↑
B cell activation			
Memory B cells	↓	↓	↓
Naïve B cells	↑	↑	↑
Activated B cells	↑	↑	↑

Minor criteria

Appearance of autoantibodies or detection of antibodies against the suspected adjuvant

At the moment, no specific autoantibodies have been identified in sarcoidosis, however, in various studies, autoantibodies to a wide range of antigens have been found in patients, which is very characteristic of ASIA syndrome (Table 21.4). The Shi et al. study showed that patients with sarcoidosis were more likely to have autoantibodies despite no autoimmune disease [98].

According to a comprehensive analysis of antibodies and subpopulations of B-lymphocytes [88] patients with sarcoidosis showed an increase in anti-MCV more than 14U/mL, an increase in

Table 21.4 Detection of various autoantibodies in sarcoidosis patients in various studies.

First author's name, year	Detected AB	Diagnosis
Maddrey WC, 1970 [92]	Antimitochondrial antibodies	Sarcoidosis and chronic liver damage
Fagan EA, 1983 [93]		Sarcoidosis and liver damage
Stanca CM, 2005 [59]		Sarcoidosis and primary biliary cirrhosis
Weinberg I, 2000 [94]	Antinuclear antibodies	Sarcoidosis
	Antibodies to DNA	
Kobak S, 2014 [95, 96]	Antibodies to citrullinated cyclic peptide	
	Rheumatoid factor	
Kinloch AJ, 2018 [97]	Antibodies to vimentin	
A. Malkova, 2021 [88]	Anti-MCV	

"naive" B-cells and a decrease in memory B-cells, and an increase in $CD24^{+++}$ $CD38^{+++}$ B-cells. Based on these data, the research team developed a formula for calculating the *DS* index (1), the use of which suggests the presence of autoimmune inflammation. With an index value of more than seven units (AUC = 0.889) with a sensitivity of 80.56% and a specificity of 93.33%, it is possible to suppose the presence of sarcoidosis (1).

$$DS = (B - naive / B - memory) * (CD38 - B - cells + CD5 - B - cells) * [anti - MCV] / 100D$$

(B-naive/B-memory) – the index of the humoral immune response activity;

(CD38-B-cells + CD5-B-cells) – the total number of regulatory B cells (IL-10 synthesis);

[anti-MCV] – the concentration of anti-MCV, characterizing the presence of autoimmune reactions.

The use of the formula can make it possible to identify patients with the presence of autoimmune inflammation in the pathogenesis of the development of sarcoidosis, which can serve as a recommendation to treat with immunosuppressive therapy and be a prognostic or predictive marker in assessing the course of the disease and therapy efficacy.

Autoantibodies to vimentin and its modifications have been found in various studies in patients with sarcoidosis [88, 97, 99, 100]. There is a hypothesis among researchers about the molecular mimicry of vimentin and mycobacterial proteins [101–103]. Heat shock proteins Mtb-HsP60, Mtb-HsP65, and catalase (mKatG) are considered to participate in cross-reactions with human peptides [28, 104]. However, no publications on the comparison of the structure of vimentin and mycobacterial proteins have been published, which provides new prospects for future research. Serum amyloid A (SSA) is considered to promote TLR2 activation and sustained granulomatous inflammation [31].

Specific HLA (i.e. HLA DRB1, HLA DQB1)

According to recent studies, HLA genotypes are one of the main genetic predisposing factors for autoimmune disease development. Associations with HLA-I class, HLA-II class, and non-HLA genes have been identified, e.g. BTNL2, C4, C6orf10, HSPA1L, LTA, NOTCH4, TAP2, TNF, and VEGF [105].

Of greatest interest is presented in the HLA-DRB1 genotypes, associated with the development of many autoimmune diseases. According to the analysis of the distribution of HLA-DRB1, -DQ1 genotypes in different populations [106] the main predisposing genotypes in the development of sarcoidosis can be identified:

- Lofgren's syndrome HLA-DRB1*01/03, HLA-DQB1*02.01
- Chronic form HLA-DQB1*06.02, HLA-DRB1*07/14/15
- Protective effect HLA-DRB1*01/04

More detailed data on the distribution of genotypes are presented in Table 21.5.

Immunosuppressive therapy

It should be noted that most cases of newly diagnosed sarcoidosis do not require treatment, only dynamic observation is recommended, because in half of the patients, the disease undergoes spontaneous remission within several years [122]. This association is most clearly manifested in sarcoid reactions, one of the features of which is the regression of changes after the removal of the provoking factor.

However, in some patients, the disease may be accompanied by a progressive course with the formation of insufficiency of the affected organ, which requires the appointment of therapy. At the same time, despite the treatment, in a significant number of patients, sarcoidosis will turn into a chronic and progressive form, from 10% to 20% will have consequences, and 6–7% will be fatal [122]. One of the reasons for the complexity of the therapeutic approach is the lack of

Table 21.5 Distribution of HLA-DRB1 genotypes in sarcoidosis patients.

Name of the first author, the year	Patients with sarcoidosis and Lofgren's syndrome	The statistically approved HLA genotypes		Country
		Of predisposition	Protective	
Berlin M, 1997 [107]	Sarcoidosis (n = 122)	DRB1*03, 17	—	Scandinavia
	Lofgren's syndrome (n = 34)	DRB1*17	—	
	Chronic form (n = 57)	DRB1*14, 15	—	
Bogunia-Kubik K, 2001 [108]	Sarcoidosis (n = 53)	DRB1*03	DRB1*11	Poland
Foley, 2001 [109]	Sarcoidosis (n = 345)	DRB1*03	DRB1*01, 04	UK, Poland, Czech Republic
Planck A, 2002 [110]	Lofgren's syndrome (n = 19)	DR B1*17	-	Scandinavia
Rossman MD, 2003 [111]	Sarcoidosis (n = 948)	DRB1*1101, 1501, 1201	DRB1*0401, 0404, 0407, 1503	USA
Sharma SK, 2003 [112]	Sarcoidosis (n = 56)	DRB1*11, 14 (chronic form)	DRB1*07	India
Grunewald, 2010 [113]	Sarcoidosis (n = 724)	DRB1*03, 14, 15	DRB1*01, 03, 07	Scandinavia
Voorter CE, 2005 [114]	Sarcoidosis (n = 149)	DRB1*15:0101 – severe form	—	Netherlands
Papadopoulos KI, 2006 [115]	Sarcoidosis (n = 66)	DRB1*02, 14	—	Germany
Darlington P, 2011 [116]	Patients with sarcoidosis (n = 1000) out of whom had symptoms associated with HS (Heerfordt's syndrome) (n = 83)	DRB1*04 – uveitis	DRB1*04 – system sarcoidosis	Sweden
da Costa CH, 2013 [117]	Sarcoidosis (n = 63)	DRB1*14	DRB1*15, DRB1*16	Brazilia
Ozyilmaz E, 2014 [118]	Pulmonary sarcoidosis (n = 86), Extrapulmonary sarcoidosis (n = 46)	DRB1*15	DRB1*11 - from extra-pulmonary	
Levin AM, 2015 [119]	Sarcoidosis (n = 1277)	DRB1*12, 11	DRB1*03	African Americans
Mortaz E, 2015 [120]	Pulmonary sarcoidosis (n = 51), Extrapulmonary sarcoidosis (n = 39)	DRB1 *7 – pulmonary DRB1 *12 – Extrapulmonary	—	Iran
Yanardag H, 2017 [121]	Sarcoidosis (n = 74)	DRB1*07,14, 15	—	Turkey

unified prognostic markers of the course of the disease, as well as the lack of clarity of the etiological factors and incomplete understanding of the pathogenesis of the disease, which complicates the development of specific treatment methods.

One of the features of sarcoidosis that links it to autoimmune diseases is the response to the therapy commonly used to treat these diseases [123, 124]. No drug for the treatment of sarcoidosis has been approved by the FDA because of the unknown etiology of the disease. This determines the need for additional research on autoimmune pathology in sarcoidosis.

At the moment, the first line of therapy includes glucocorticosteroids (prednisolone, methylprednisolone) [125]. The problem arises in the case of management of patients with intolerance (uncontrolled diabetes mellitus, excessive weight gain, myopathy, osteoporosis), refusal to take this group of drugs, or lack of effect from taking glucocorticosteroids (GCS) (disease progression against the background of an adequate minimum of 10 mg of prednisolone per day for at least three months). Alternatively, immunosuppressive, cytotoxic, and antimalarial agents can be used. The most commonly prescribed second-line drug is methotrexate, and other cytostatics such as leflunomide, azathioprine, and combinations of methotrexate and leflunomide are also possible. Azathioprine affects the synthesis of RNA and DNA thereby suppressing the proliferation of lymphocytes, while exerting a greater effect on cellular immunity than humoral immunity. The exact mechanism by which azathioprine may affect sarcoidosis is unclear [126].

In case of ineffectiveness of the second line of therapy, the next step is to prescribe biological therapy drugs [127]. Targeted TNF therapy was the first biological therapy prescribed to patients with sarcoidosis because TNF-α is secreted by macrophages in patients with active sarcoidosis and plays a key role in the development of sarcoid granuloma. TNF-targeted therapy includes monoclonal antibodies directed against TNF (infliximab, adalimumab, golimumab), a recombinant protein that connects the TNF receptor to the constant end of an IgG1 antibody (etanercept), and a pegylated Fab fragment of a humanized anti-TNF-α monoclonal antibody (certolizumab) [128, 129]. The drugs have different efficacy in different forms of sarcoidosis, but, unfortunately, the data on their use are still insufficient to develop a clear algorithm [130–132].

In the case of contraindications or ineffectiveness, it is possible to use off-label hydroxychloroquine, as well as the use of mycophenolate, cyclophosphamide, or rituximab (these prescriptions are based on experience in the treatment of other immunological lung diseases, with sarcoidosis not fully understood [133, 134].

Sarcoidosis models

Despite the long-term studies on the pathogenesis of sarcoidosis, there are still no reliable models of the disease [135], which would allow to demonstrate the influence of the trigger factor, as well as to determine the etiotropic therapy. In particular, when exposed to various antigens (peptides *M. tuberculosis, P. acne,* carbon nanoparticles) in mouse models, only pulmonary granulomas without fibrosis were obtained. Genetically modified mice developed multiple sites of granulomatosis (lungs, skin, liver, stomach, ganglia), which may indicate the peculiarities of the immune response in healthy mice, allowing more efficient elimination of pathogens. It was also shown that the granulomas obtained in the experiments cannot exist without the continued influence of the adjuvant. The reviewers suggest that sarcoidosis patients are chronically exposed to one or more triggers that promote the development and maintenance of granulomas.

The unambiguous conclusion of all existing reviews and studies devoted to the creation of a model of sarcoidosis is that in the present conditions, it is impossible to achieve this goal, which determines the empiric approach to treatment.

Discussion

According to the analysis, it can be assumed that there are several autoimmune features in the concept of ASIA syndrome in sarcoidosis. The characteristic features confirming this fact include (Figure 21.1):

- connection with the HLA genotype;
- the impact of various trigger factors;

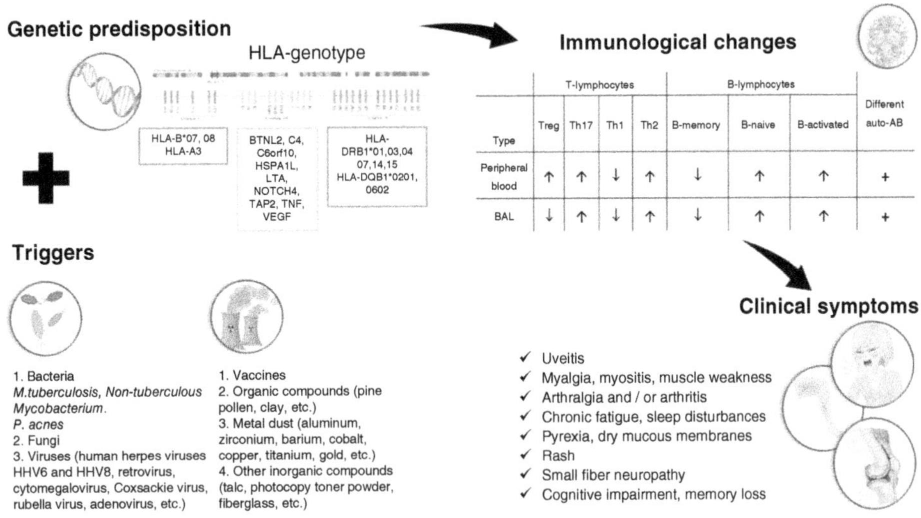

Figure 21.1 ASIA criteria in sarcoidosis.

- improvement of the condition with the elimination of the trigger factor;
- immunological disorders in the form of cytotoxicity of lymphocytes upon stimulation with autoantigens, the presence of autoantibodies, and an imbalance of subpopulations of T- and B-lymphocytes typical for many autoimmune diseases);
- clinical manifestations characteristic of autoimmune pathology;
- histological picture of the disease;
- association with other autoimmune diseases;
- the immunosuppressive therapy efficacy.

However, despite certain associations between sarcoidosis and ASIA, today it is impossible to unambiguously consider all variants of the course of sarcoidosis within the framework of this syndrome. Perhaps, we should talk about different diseases or different "stages" of the course of sarcoidosis, depending on the continuing influence of the trigger factor. The majority of patients with sarcoidosis are prone to self-healing, which can be associated not only with genetic and immunological characteristics but also with an improvement in symptoms due to the possible elimination of trigger factors or cessation of their exposure.

Speaking about the relationship between ASIA and sarcoidosis, it is important to identify a cohort of patients in whom self-healing does not occur, and the course of the disease becomes progressive with the development of fibrosis, organ failure, and generalization of the process. We can assume that in this situation the pathoantigen is not eliminated, and a full-fledged autoimmune disease develops, requiring the appointment of immunosuppressive therapy, which fits into the concept and criteria of ASIA (Figure 21.2).

Analysis of the connection between ASIA and sarcoidosis suggests the need to continue research in the spirit of studying the prognostic and predictive factors that determine the course of the disease and treatment tactics. Questions about the etiological factors, the creation of a model of sarcoidosis, and the justified prescription of immunosuppressive, including biological therapy, remain unanswered, and the relationship between sarcoidosis and ASIA, on the contrary, raises new ones.

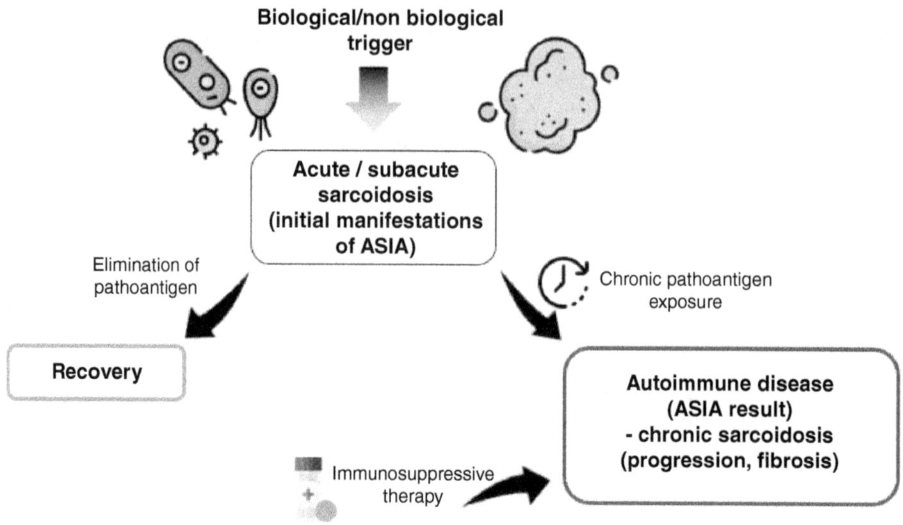

Figure 21.2 Stages of the course of sarcoidosis within the ASIA syndrome.

References

1. Starshinova, A.A., Malkova, A.M., Basantsova, N.Y. et al. (2020). Sarcoidosis as an autoimmune disease. *Front. Immunol.* 10: 2933. https://doi.org/10.3389/FIMMU.2019.02933.
2. Dua, A. and Manadan, A. (2013). Heerfordt's syndrome, or uveoparotid fever. *N. Engl. J. Med.* 369: 458–458. https://doi.org/10.1056/nejmicm1303454.
3. Badar, F., Azfar, S.F., Ahmad, I. et al. (2011). Diagnostic difficulties in differentiating sarcoidosis from tuberculosis, Oman. *Med. J.* 26: 210–211. https://doi.org/10.5001/omj.2011.53.
4. Hunninghake, G.W., Costabel, U., Ando, M. et al. (1999). Statement on sarcoidosis. *Am. J. Respir. Crit. Care Med.* 160: 736–755. https://doi.org/10.1164/ajrccm.160.2.ats4-99.
5. Sellares, J., Strambu, I., Crouser, E.D. et al. (2018). New advances in the development of sarcoidosis models: a synopsis of a symposium sponsored by the Foundation for Sarcoidosis Research. *Sarcoidosis Vasc. Diffuse Lung Dis.* 35: 2–4. https://doi.org/10.36141/svdld.v35i1.7032.
6. Puttgen, K.B. (2014). Diagnosis and management of hemangiomas. *Pediatr. Clin. N. Am.* 61: 383–402. https://doi.org/10.1016/j.pcl.2013.11.010.
7. Broos, C.E., van Nimwegen, M., Hoogsteden, H.C. et al. (2013). Granuloma formation in pulmonary sarcoidosis. *Front. Immunol.* 4: 437. https://doi.org/10.3389/fimmu.2013.00437.
8. Moller, D.R., Rybicki, B.A., Hamzeh, N.Y. et al. (2017). Genetic, immunologic, and environmental basis of sarcoidosis. *Ann. Am. Thorac. Soc.* 14: S429–S436. https://doi.org/10.1513/AnnalsATS.201707-565OT.
9. Zinchenko Yu, Y.P., Basantsova, N., Starshinova, A., and Gilburd, B. (2019). The autoimmune/inflammatory syndrome induced by adjuvants and sarcoidosis. *Med. Alliance* 7: 15–20.
10. Borba, V., Malkova, A., Basantsova, N. et al. (2020). Classical examples of the concept of the ASIA syndrome. *Biomol. Ther.* 10: 1–17. https://doi.org/10.3390/biom10101436.
11. Shoenfeld, Y. and Agmon-Levin, N. (2011). "ASIA" - autoimmune/inflammatory syndrome induced by adjuvants. *J. Autoimmun.* 36: 4–8. https://doi.org/10.1016/j.jaut.2010.07.003.
12. Starshinova, A.A., Malkova, A.M., Zinchenko, Y.S. et al. (2020). Autoimmune component in the etiology of sarcoidosis. *Tuber. Lung Dis.* 98: 54–62. https://doi.org/10.21292/2075-1230-2020-98-5-54-62.
13. Armbruster, C., Dekan, G., and Hovorha, A. (1996). Granulomatous pneumonitis and mediastinal lymphadenopathy due to photocopier toner dust. *Lancet* 348: 690. https://doi.org/10.1016/S0140-6736(05)65119-7.

14. Jordan, H.T., Stellman, S.D., Prezant, D. et al. (2011). Sarcoidosis diagnosed after September 11, 2001, among adults exposed to the World Trade Center disaster. *J. Occup. Environ. Med.* 53: 966–974. https://doi.org/10.1097/JOM.0b013e31822a3596.
15. Ho, C.-C., Chang, H., Tsai, H.-T. et al. (2013). Quantum dot 705, a cadmium-based nanoparticle, induces persistent inflammation and granuloma formation in the mouse lung. *Nanotoxicology* 7: 105–115. https://doi.org/10.3109/17435390.2011.635814.
16. Yanamala, N., Desai, I.C., Miller, W. et al. (2019). Grouping of carbonaceous nanomaterials based on association of patterns of inflammatory markers in BAL fluid with adverse outcomes in lungs. *Nanotoxicology* 13: 1102–1116. https://doi.org/10.1080/17435390.2019.1640911.
17. Huizar, I., Malur, A., Midgette, Y.A. et al. (2011). Novel murine model of chronic granulomatous lung inflammation elicited by carbon nanotubes. *Am. J. Respir. Cell Mol. Biol.* 45: 858–866. https://doi.org/10.1165/rcmb.2010-0401OC.
18. Watad, A., Rosenberg, V., Tiosano, S. et al. (2018). Silicone breast implants and the risk of autoimmune/rheumatic disorders: a real-world analysis. *Int. J. Epidemiol.* 47: 1846–1854. https://doi.org/10.1093/ije/dyy217.
19. Colaris, M.J.L., de Boer, M., van der Hulst, R.R., and Cohen Tervaert, J.W. (2017). Two hundreds cases of ASIA syndrome following silicone implants: a comparative study of 30 years and a review of current literature. *Immunol. Res.* 65: 120–128. https://doi.org/10.1007/s12026-016-8821-y.
20. Barzo, P. and Tamási, L. (1998). Lofgren syndrome after silicone breast prosthesis implantation. *Orv. Hetil.* 139: 23236.
21. Yoshida, T., Tanaka, M., Okamoto, K., and Hirai, S. (1996). Neurosarcoidosis following augmentation mammoplasty with silicone. *Neurol. Res.* 18: 319–320. https://doi.org/10.1080/01616412.1996.11740428.
22. Teuber, S.S., Howell, L.P., Yoshida, S.H., and Gershwin, M.E. (1994). Remission of sarcoidosis following removal of silicone gel breast implants. *Int. Arch. Allergy Immunol.* 105: 404–407. https://doi.org/10.1159/000236791.
23. Chang, K.C., Chan, K.T., Chong, L.Y. et al. (2003). Cutaneous and pulmonary sarcoidosis in a Hong Kong Chinese woman with silicone breast prostheses. *Respirology* 8: 379–382. https://doi.org/10.1046/j.1440--1843.2003.00447.x.
24. Sun, H.H., Sachanandani, N.S., Jordan, B., and Myckatyn, T.M. (2013). Sarcoidosis of the breasts following silicone implant placement. *Plast. Reconstr. Surg.* 131: 939e–940e. https://doi.org/10.1097/PRS.0b013e31828bd964.
25. Colboc, H., Moguelet, P., Bazin, D. et al. (2019). Physicochemical characterization of inorganic deposits associated with granulomas in cutaneous sarcoidosis. *J. Eur. Acad. Dermatol. Venereol.* 33: 198–203. https://doi.org/10.1111/jdv.15167.
26. Stroh, C., Böttger, J., Meyer, F. et al. (2009). Sarcoidosis after adjustable silicone gastric banding – a report of two cases in Germany. *Obes. Facts* 2: 332–334. https://doi.org/10.1159/000235865.
27. Eishi, Y. (2013). Etiologic aspect of sarcoidosis as an allergic endogenous infection caused by *Propionibacterium acnes*. *Biomed. Res. Int.* 2013: 935289. https://doi.org/10.1155/2013/935289.
28. Song, Z., Marzilli, L., Greenlee, B.M. et al. (2005). Mycobacterial catalase-peroxidase is a tissue antigen and target of the adaptive immune response in systemic sarcoidosis. *J. Exp. Med.* 201: 755–767. https://doi.org/10.1084/jem.20040429.
29. Hu, Y., Yibrehu, B., Zabini, D., and Kuebler, W.M. (2017). Animal models of sarcoidosis. *Cell Tissue Res.* 367: 651–661. https://doi.org/10.1007/s00441-016-2526-3.
30. Swaisgood, C.M., Oswald-Richter, K., Moeller, S.D. et al. (2011). Development of a sarcoidosis murine lung granuloma model using *Mycobacterium* superoxide dismutase A peptide. *Am. J. Respir. Cell Mol. Biol.* 44: 166–174. https://doi.org/10.1165/RCMB.2009-0350OC.
31. Chen, E.S., Song, Z., Willett, M.H. et al. (2010). Serum amyloid A regulates granulomatous inflammation in sarcoidosis through toll-like receptor-2. *Am. J. Respir. Crit. Care Med.* 181: 360. https://doi.org/10.1164/RCCM.200905-0696OC.
32. Jiang, D., Huang, X., Geng, J. et al. (2016). Pulmonary fibrosis in a mouse model of sarcoid granulomatosis induced by booster challenge with *Propionibacterium acnes*. *Oncotarget* 7: 33703–33714. https://doi.org/10.18632/ONCOTARGET.9397.
33. Iio, K., Iio, T.U., Okui, Y. et al. (2010). Experimental pulmonary granuloma mimicking sarcoidosis induced by *Propionibacterium acnes* in mice. *Acta Med. Okayama* 64: 75–83. https://doi.org/10.18926/AMO/32852.

34. Terčelj, M., Stopinšek, S., Ihan, A. et al. (2011). In vitro and in vivo reactivity to fungal cell wall agents in sarcoidosis. *Clin. Exp. Immunol.* 166: 87–93. https://doi.org/10.1111/j.1365-2249.2011.04456.x.
35. Terčelj, M., Salobir, B., Harlander, M., and Rylander, R. (2011). Fungal exposure in homes of patients with sarcoidosis – an environmental exposure study. *Environ. Health* 10 (1): 1–6. https://doi.org/10.1186/1476-069X-10-8.
36. Greally, B.M.J.F. and Manning, D. (1989). Sarcoidosis following B.C.G. vaccination in a lymphopaenic boy. *Sarcoidosis* 6: 156–157.
37. Bellet, J.S. and Prose, N.S. (2005). Skin complications of Bacillus Calmette-Guérin immunization. *Curr. Opin. Infect. Dis.* 18: 97–100. https://doi.org/10.1097/01.qco.0000160895.97362.4f.
38. Osborne, G.E.N., Mallon, E., and Mayou, S.C. (2003). Juvenile sarcoidosis after BCG vaccination. *J. Am. Acad. Dermatol.* 48 (5 Suppl): S99–S102. https://doi.org/10.1067/mjd.2003.158.
39. Heydari-Kamjani, M., Vante, I., Uppal, P. et al. (2019). Uveitis sarcoidosis presumably initiated after administration of shingrix vaccine. *Cureus* 11: e4920. https://doi.org/10.7759/CUREUS.4920.
40. Psaltis, N.M., Gardner, R.G., and Denton, W.J. (2014). Systemic sarcoidosis and red dye granulomatous tattoo inflammation after influenza vaccination: a case report and review of literature. *Ocul. Immunol. Inflamm.* 22: 314–321. https://doi.org/10.3109/09273948.2014.891041.
41. Williams, A.A.-B.G.S., Evans, S., and Yeo, D. (2015). Retinal artery vasculitis secondary to administration of influenza vaccine. *BMJ Case Rep.* 2015: bcr2015211971. https://doi.org/10.1136/bcr-2015-211971.
42. Bodemer, C., Sauvage, V., Mahlaoui, N. et al. (2014). Live rubella virus vaccine long-term persistence as an antigenic trigger of cutaneous granulomas in patients with primary immunodeficiency. *Clin. Microbiol. Infect.* 20: O656–O663. https://doi.org/10.1111/1469-0691.12573.
43. Uslu, U. et al. (2017). Sarcoidosis under dendritic cell vaccination immunotherapy in long-term responding patients with metastatic melanoma. *Anticancer Res.* 37: 3243–3248.
44. Bordry, N., Costa-Nunes, C.M., Cagnon, L. et al. (2014). Pulmonary sarcoid-like granulomatosis after multiple vaccinations of a long-term surviving patient with metastatic melanoma, Cancer. *Immunol. Res.* 2: 1148–1153. https://doi.org/10.1158/2326-6066.CIR-14-0143.
45. Bauckneht, M., Aloè, T., Tagliabue, E. et al. (2021). Beyond Covid-19 vaccination-associated pitfalls on [18F]Fluorodeoxyglucose (FDG) PET: a case of a concomitant sarcoidosis. *Eur. J. Nucl. Med. Mol. Imaging* 48: 2661–2662. https://doi.org/10.1007/S00259-021-05360-W.
46. Chopra, A., Nautiyal, A., Kalkanis, A., and Judson, M.A. (2018). Drug-induced sarcoidosis-like reactions. *Chest* 154: 664–677. https://doi.org/10.1016/j.chest.2018.03.056.
47. Tchernev, G., Tana, C., Schiavone, C. et al. (2014). Sarcoidosis vs. sarcoid-like reactions: the two sides of the same coin? *Wien. Med. Wochenschr.* 164: 247–259. https://doi.org/10.1007/s10354-014-0269-x.
48. Semenzato, G. (2005). Access: a case control etiologic study of sarcoidosis. *Sarcoidosis Vasc. Diffuse Lung Dis.* 22: 83–86.
49. Judson, M.A. (2020). Environmental risk factors for sarcoidosis. *Front. Immunol.* 11: 1340. https://doi.org/10.3389/fimmu.2020.01340.
50. Liu, H., Patel, D., Welch, A.M. et al. (2016). Association between occupational exposures and sarcoidosis: an analysis from death certificates in the United States, 1988–1999. *Chest* 150: 289–298. https://doi.org/10.1016/j.chest.2016.01.020.
51. Soto-Gomez, N., Peters, J.I., and Nambiar, A.M. (2016). Diagnosis and management of sarcoidosis. *Am. Fam. Physician* 93: 840–848. www.aafp.org/afp. Accessed September 28, 2021.
52. Polverino, F., Balestro, E., and Spagnolo, P. (2020). Clinical presentations, pathogenesis, and therapy of sarcoidosis: state of the art. *J. Clin. Med.* 9: 2363. https://doi.org/10.3390/jcm9082363.
53. A. Starshinova, Small Fiber Neuropathy in Pulmonary Sarcoidosis and Tuberculosis: Clinical and Histological Correlates, (2020). https://doi.org/10.21203/RS.3.RS-51830/V1.
54. Levine, T.D. (2018). Small fiber neuropathy: disease classification beyond pain and burning. *J. Cent. Nerv. Syst. Dis.* 10: 117957351877170. https://doi.org/10.1177/1179573518771703.
55. Levy, S. and Sandhu, V. (2008). Ankylosing spondylitis and pulmonary sarcoidosis—a case report and discussion of the literature. *J. Rheumatol.* 47: 1733–1734.
56. Stucki, G., Von Felten, A., Speich, R., and Michel, B.A. (1992). Ankylosing spondylitis and sarcoidosis -coincidence or association? Case report and review of the literature. *Clin. Rheumatol.* 11: 436–439. https://doi.org/10.1007/BF02207214.

57. Wesemann, D.R., Costenbader, K.H., and Coblyn, J.S. (2009). Co-existing sarcoidosis, systemic lupus erythematosus and the antiphospholipid antibody syndrome: case reports and discussion from the Brigham and women's hospital lupus center. *Lupus* 18: 202–205. https://doi.org/10.1177/0961203308100483.
58. Santiago, T., Santiago, M., Rovisco, J. et al. (2014). Coexisting primary Sjögren's syndrome and sarcoidosis: coincidence, mutually exclusive conditions or syndrome? *Rheumatol. Int.* 34: 1619–1622. https://doi.org/10.1007/S00296-014-3024-0.
59. Stanca, C.M., Fiel, M.I., Allina, J. et al. (2005). Liver failure in an antimitochondrial antibody-positive patient with sarcoidosis: primary biliary cirrhosis or hepatic sarcoidosis? *Semin. Liver Dis.* 25: 364–370. https://doi.org/10.1055/s-2005-916327.
60. Kobak, S. (2015). Sarcoidosis: a rheumatologist's perspective. *Ther. Adv. Musculoskelet. Dis.* 7: 196–205. https://doi.org/10.1177/1759720X15591310.
61. Fazzi, P., Fallahi, P., and Ferrari, S.M. (2017). Sarcoidosis and thyroid autoimmunity. *Front. Endocrinol. (Lausanne)* 8: 177. https://doi.org/10.3389/fendo.2017.00177.
62. Gokuladhas, S., Schierding, W., Golovina, E. et al. (2021). Unravelling the shared genetic mechanisms underlying 18 autoimmune diseases using a systems approach. *BioRxiv* 12: 693142. https://doi.org/10.1101/2021.03.28.437437.
63. Sakthivel, P. and Bruder, D. (2017). Mechanism of granuloma formation in sarcoidosis. *Curr. Opin. Hematol.* 24: 59–65. https://doi.org/10.1097/MOH.0000000000000301.
64. Oliver, S.J., Kikuchi, T., Krueger, J.G., and Kaplan, G. (2002). Thalidomide induces granuloma differentiation in sarcoid skin lesions associated with disease improvement. *Clin. Immunol.* 102: 225–236. https://doi.org/10.1006/clim.2001.5173.
65. Kita, S., Tsuda, T., Sugisaki, K. et al. (1995). Characterization of distribution of T lymphocyte subsets and activated T lymphocytes infiltrating into sarcoid lesions. *Intern. Med.* 34: 847–855. https://doi.org/10.2169/internalmedicine.34.847.
66. Carvajal Alegria, G., Gazeau, P., Hillion, S. et al. (2017). Could lymphocyte profiling be useful to diagnose systemic autoimmune diseases? *Clin. Rev. Allergy Immunol.* 53: 219–236. https://doi.org/10.1007/S12016-017-8608-5.
67. Nakken, B., Munthe, L.A., Konttinen, Y.T. et al. (2011). B-cells and their targeting in rheumatoid arthritis – current concepts and future perspectives. *Autoimmun. Rev.* 11: 28–34. https://doi.org/10.1016/J.AUTREV.2011.06.010.
68. Hinze, C.H. and Colbert, R.A. (2008). B-cell depletion in Wegener's granulomatosis. *Clin. Rev. Allergy Immunol.* 34: 372–379. https://doi.org/10.1007/S12016-007-8057-7.
69. Knochelmann, H.M., Dwyer, C.J., Bailey, S.R. et al. (2018). When worlds collide: Th17 and Treg cells in cancer and autoimmunity. *Cell. Mol. Immunol.* 15: 458–469. https://doi.org/10.1038/s41423-018-0004-4.
70. Kurata, I., Matsumoto, I., and Sumida, T. (2021). T follicular helper cell subsets: a potential key player in autoimmunity. *Immunol. Med.* 44: 1–9. https://doi.org/10.1080/25785826.2020.1776079.
71. Tangye, S.G., Ma, C.S., Brink, R., and Deenick, E.K. (2013). The good, the bad and the ugly-T FH cells in human health and disease. *Nat. Rev. Immunol.* 13: 412–426. https://doi.org/10.1038/nri3447.
72. Collier, J.L., Weiss, S.A., Pauken, K.E. et al. (2021). Not-so-opposite ends of the spectrum: $CD8^+$ T cell dysfunction across chronic infection, cancer and autoimmunity. *Nat. Immunol.* 22: 809–819. https://doi.org/10.1038/s41590-021-00949-7.
73. D'Errico, S., Bello, S., Cantatore, S. et al. (2011). Immunohistochemical characterisation and TNF-α expression of the granulomatous infiltration of the brainstem in a case of sudden death due to neurosarcoidosis. *Forensic Sci. Int.* 208: e1–e5. https://doi.org/10.1016/j.forsciint.2011.01.021.
74. Katchar, K., Söderström, K., Wahlstrom, J. et al. (2005). Characterisation of natural killer cells and $CD56^+$ T-cells in sarcoidosis patients. *Eur. Respir. J.* 26: 77–85. https://doi.org/10.1183/09031936.05.00030805.
75. Nguyen, Q.P., Deng, T.Z., Witherden, D.A., and Goldrath, A.W. (2019). Origins of $CD4^+$ circulating and tissue-resident memory T-cells. *Immunology* 157: 3–12. https://doi.org/10.1111/imm.13059.
76. Hauber, H.-P., Gholami, D., Meyer, A., and Pforte, A. (2003). Increased interleukin-13 expression in patients with sarcoidosis. *Thorax* 58: 519–524. https://doi.org/10.1136/THORAX.58.6.519.
77. Locke, L.W., Crouser, E.D., White, P. et al. (2019). IL-13–regulated macrophage polarization during granuloma formation in an in vitro human sarcoidosis model. *Am. J. Respir. Cell Mol. Biol.* 60: 84–95. https://doi.org/10.1165/rcmb.2018-0053OC.

78. Shamaei, M., Mortaz, E., Pourabdollah, M. et al. (2018). Evidence for M2 macrophages in granulomas from pulmonary sarcoidosis: a new aspect of macrophage heterogeneity. *Hum. Immunol.* 79: 63–69. https://doi.org/10.1016/j.humimm.2017.10.009.
79. Huang, H., Lu, Z., Jiang, C. et al. (2013). Imbalance between Th17 and regulatory T-cells in sarcoidosis. *Int. J. Mol. Sci.* 14: 21463. https://doi.org/10.3390/IJMS141121463.
80. Ding, J., Dai, J., Cai, H. et al. (2017). Extensively disturbance of regulatory T cells - Th17 cells balance in stage II pulmonary sarcoidosis. *Int. J. Med. Sci.* 14: 1136–1142. https://doi.org/10.7150/ijms.18838.
81. Miedema, J.R., Kaiser, Y., Broos, C.E. et al. (2018). Th17-lineage cells in pulmonary sarcoidosis and Löfgren's syndrome: friend or foe? *J. Autoimmun.* 87: 82–96. https://doi.org/10.1016/j.jaut.2017.12.012.
82. Miyara, M., Amoura, Z., Parizot, C. et al. (2006). The immune paradox of sarcoidosis and regulatory T cells. *J. Exp. Med.* 203: 359–370. https://doi.org/10.1084/jem.20050648.
83. Grant, C.R., Liberal, R., Mieli-Vergani, G. et al. (2015). Regulatory T-cells in autoimmune diseases: challenges, controversies and-yet-unanswered questions. *Autoimmun. Rev.* 14: 105–116. https://doi.org/10.1016/j.autrev.2014.10.012.
84. Kudryavtsev, I.V., Lazareva, N.M., Baranova, O.P. et al. (2019). CD39+ expression by regulatory T cells in pulmonary sarcoidosis and Lofgren's syndrome. *Med. Immunol.* 21: 467–478. https://doi.org/10.15789/1563-0625-2019-3-467-478.
85. Lee, N.S., Barber, L., Akula, S.M. et al. (2011). Disturbed homeostasis and multiple signaling defects in the peripheral blood B-cell compartment of patients with severe chronic sarcoidosis. *Clin. Vaccine Immunol.* 18: 1306–1316. https://doi.org/10.1128/CVI.05118-11.
86. Saussine, A., Tazi, A., Feuillet, S. et al. (2012). Active chronic sarcoidosis is characterized by increased transitional blood B cells, increased IL-10-producing regulatory B cells and high BAFF levels. *PLoS One* 7: e43588. https://doi.org/10.1371/journal.pone.0043588.
87. Belhomme, N., Jouneau, S., Bouzillé, G. et al. (2018). Role of serum immunoglobulins for predicting sarcoidosis outcome: a cohort study. *PLoS One* 13: e0193122. https://doi.org/10.1371/journal.pone.0193122.
88. Malkova, A., Starshinova, A., Zinchenko, Y. et al. (2021). New laboratory criteria of the autoimmune inflammation in pulmonary sarcoidosis and tuberculosis. *Clin. Immunol.* 227: 108724. https://doi.org/10.1016/j.clim.2021.108724.
89. Kudryavtsev, I., Serebriakova, M., Starshinova, A. et al. (2020). Imbalance in B cell and T follicular helper cell subsets in pulmonary sarcoidosis. *Sci. Rep.* 10: 1–10. https://doi.org/10.1038/s41598-020-57741-0.
90. Facco, M., Cabrelle, A., Teramo, A. et al. (2011). Sarcoidosis is a Th1/Th17 multisystem disorder. *Thorax* 66: 144–150. https://doi.org/10.1136/thx.2010.140319.
91. Drent, M., Jacobs, J.A., de Vries, J. et al. (1999). Does the cellular bronchoalveolar lavage fluid profile reflect the severity of sarcoidosis? *Eur. Respir. J.* 13: 1338–1344. https://doi.org/10.1183/09031936.99.13613459.
92. Maddrey, W.C., Johns, C.J., Boitnott, J.K., and Iber, F.L. (1970). Sarcoidosis and chronic hepatic disease: a clinical pathologic study of 20 patients. *Medicine (United States)* 49: 375–395. https://doi.org/10.1097/00005792-197009000-00002.
93. Fagan, E.A., Moore-Gillon, J.C., and Margaret Turner-Warwick, D.M. (1983). Multiorgan granulomas and mitochondrial antibodies. *J. Med.* 308: 572–575.
94. Weinberg, I., Vasiliev, L., and Gotsman, I. (2000). Anti-dsDNA antibodies in sarcoidosis, Semin. *Arthritis Rheum.* 29: 328–331. https://doi.org/10.1016/S0049-0172(00)80019-0.
95. Kobak, S., Yilmaz, H., Sever, F. et al. (2014). Anti-cyclic citrullinated peptide antibodies in patients with sarcoidosis. *J. Vasc. Diffus. Lung Dis.* 31: 206–210.
96. Kobak, S., Yilmaz, H., Sever, F. et al. (2014). The prevalence of antinuclear antibodies in patients with sarcoidosis. *Autoimmune Dis.* 2014: 351852. https://doi.org/10.1155/2014/351852.
97. Kinloch, A.J., Kaiser, Y., Wolfgeher, D. et al. (2018). In situ humoral immunity to vimentin in HLA-DRB1*03+ patients with pulmonary sarcoidosis. *Front. Immunol.* 9: 01516. https://doi.org/10.3389/fimmu.2018.01516.
98. Shi, T.Y., Wen, X.H., Shi, X.H. et al. (2021). Associations between sarcoidosis, autoimmune diseases, and autoantibodies: a single-center retrospective study in China. *Clin. Exp. Med.* 22: 277–283. https://doi.org/10.1007/s10238-021-00737-5.
99. Wahlström, J., Dengjel, J., Persson, B. et al. (2007). Identification of HLA-DR–bound peptides presented by human bronchoalveolar lavage cells in sarcoidosis. *J. Clin. Invest.* 117: 3576. https://doi.org/10.1172/JCI32401.

100. Wahlström, J., Dengjel, J., Winqvist, O. et al. (2009). Autoimmune T cell responses to antigenic peptides presented by bronchoalveolar lavage cell HLA-DR molecules in sarcoidosis. *Clin. Immunol.* 133: 353–363. https://doi.org/10.1016/j.clim.2009.08.008.
101. Ang, S.C. and Moscovic, E.A. (1996). Cross-reactive and species specific *Mycobacterium tuberculosis* antigens in the immunoprofile of Schaumann bodies: a major clue to the etiology of sarcoidosis. *J. Histol. Histopathol.* 11: 125–134.
102. Scadding, J. (1960). *Mycobacterium tuberculosis* in the aetiology of sarcoidosis. *BMJ* 2: 1617–1623.
103. Eberhardt, C., Thillai, M., Parker, R. et al. (2017). Proteomic analysis of Kveim reagent identifies targets of cellular immunity in sarcoidosis. *PLoS One* 12: e01700285. https://doi.org/10.1371/JOURNAL.PONE.0170285.
104. Drake, W.P., Dhason, M.S., Nadaf, M. et al. (2007). Cellular recognition of *Mycobacterium tuberculosis* ESAT-6 and KatG peptides in systemic sarcoidosis. *Infect. Immun.* 75: 527–530. https://doi.org/10.1128/IAI.00732-06.
105. Adrianto, I., Lin, C.P., Hale, J.J. et al. (2012). Genome-wide association study of African and European Americans implicates multiple shared and ethnic specific loci in sarcoidosis susceptibility. *PLoS One* 7: e43907. https://doi.org/10.1371/journal.pone.0043907.
106. Malkova, A., Starshinova, A., Zinchenko, Y. et al. (2020). The opposite effect of human leukocyte antigen genotypes in sarcoidosis and tuberculosis: a narrative review of the literature. *ERJ Open Res.* 6: 00155–02020. https://doi.org/10.1183/23120541.00155-2020.
107. Berlin, M., Fogdell-Hahn, A., Olerup, O. et al. (1997). HLA-DR predicts the prognosis in Scandinavian patients with pulmonary sarcoidosis. *Am. J. Respir. Crit. Care Med.* 156: 1601–1605. https://doi.org/10.1164/ajrccm.156.5.9704069.
108. Bogunia-Kubik, K., Tomeczko, J., Suchnicki, K., and Lange, A. (2001). HLA-DRB1*03, DRB1*11 or DRB1*12 and their respective DRB3 specificities in clinical variants of sarcoidosis. *Tissue Antigens* 57: 87–90. https://doi.org/10.1034/j.1399-0039.2001.057001087.x.
109. Foley, P.J., McGrath, D.S., Puscinska, E. et al. (2001). Human leukocyte antigen-DRB1 position 11 residues are a common protective marker for sarcoidosis. *Am. J. Respir. Cell Mol. Biol.* 25: 272–277. https://doi.org/10.1165/ajrcmb.25.3.4261.
110. Planck, A., Eklund, A., Yamaguchi, E., and Grunewald, J. (2002). Angiotensin-converting enzyme gene polymorphism in relation to HLA-DR in sarcoidosis. *J. Intern. Med.* 251: 217–222. https://doi.org/10.1046/J.1365-2796.2002.00946.X.
111. Rossman, M.D., Thompson, B., Frederick, M. et al. (2003). HLA-DRB1*1101: a significant risk factor for sarcoidosis in blacks and whites. *Am. J. Hum. Genet.* 73: 720. https://doi.org/10.1086/378097.
112. Sharma, S.K., Balamurugan, A., Pandey, R.M. et al. (2003). Human leukocyte antigen-DR alleles influence the clinical course of pulmonary sarcoidosis in Asian Indians. *Am. J. Respir. Cell Mol. Biol.* 29: 225–231. https://doi.org/10.1165/rcmb.2003-0007OC.
113. Grunewald, J., Brynedal, B., Darlington, P. et al. (2010). Different HLA-DRB1 allele distributions in distinct clinical subgroups of sarcoidosis patients. *Respir. Res.* 11: 25. https://doi.org/10.1186/1465-9921-11-25.
114. Voorter, C.E.M., Drent, M., and Van Den Berg-Loonen, E.M. (2005). Severe pulmonary sarcoidosis is strongly associated with the haplotype HLA-DQB1*0602-DRB1*150101. *Hum. Immunol.* 66: 826–835. https://doi.org/10.1016/j.humimm.2005.04.003.
115. Papadopoulos, K.I., Wassmuth, R., Sponsel, T. et al. (2006). Sarcoidosis and autoimmunity: evidence of differential associations with HLA class II markers. *Int. J. Endocrinol. Metab.* 4: 13–18.
116. Darlington, P., Tallstedt, L., Padyukov, L. et al. (2011). HLA-DRB1* alleles and symptoms associated with Heerfordt's syndrome in sarcoidosis. *Eur. Respir. J.* 38: 1151–1157. https://doi.org/10.1183/09031936.00025011.
117. da Costa, C.H., Silva, V.L., Fabricio-Silva, G.M. et al. (2013). A in a cohort of Brazilian patients with sarcoidosis. *Hum. Immunol.* 74: 1326–1332. https://doi.org/10.1016/j.humimm.2013.07.009.
118. Ozyilmaz, E., Goruroglu Ozturk, O., Yunsel, D. et al. (2014). Could HLA-DR B1*11 allele be a clue for predicting extra-pulmonary sarcoidosis? *Sarcoidosis Vasc. Diffuse Lung Dis.* 31: 154–162.
119. Levin, A.A.M., Adrianto, I., Datta, I. et al. (2015). Association of HLA-DRB1 with sarcoidosis susceptibility and progression in African Americans. *Am. J. Respir. Cell Mol. Biol.* 53: 206–216. https://doi.org/10.1165/rcmb.2014-0227OC.

120. Mortaz, E., Sereshki, H.A., Abedini, A. et al. (2015). Association of serum TNF-α, IL-8 and free light chain with HLA-DR B alleles expression in pulmonary and extra-pulmonary sarcoidosis. *J. Inflamm. (Lond).* 12: 21. https://doi.org/10.1186/S12950-015-0066-3.
121. Yanardag, H., Tetikkurt, C., Bilir, M., and Yilmaz, E. (2017). Association of HLA antigens with the clinical course of sarcoidosis and familial disease. *Monaldi Arch. Chest Dis.* 87: 79–84. https://doi.org/10.4081/monaldi.2017.835.
122. Valeyre, D., Prasse, A., Nunes, H. et al. (2014). Sarcoidosis. *Lancet* 383: 1155–1167. https://doi.org/10.1016/S0140-6736(13)60680-7.
123. Korsten, P., Tampe, B., Konig, M.F., and Nikiphorou, E. (2018). Sarcoidosis and autoimmune diseases: differences, similarities and overlaps. *Curr. Opin. Pulm. Med.* 24: 504–512. https://doi.org/10.1097/MCP.0000000000000500.
124. Adler, B.L., Wang, C.J., Bui, T.L. et al. (2019). Anti-tumor necrosis factor agents in sarcoidosis: a systematic review of efficacy and safety, Semin. *Arthritis Rheum.* 48: 1093–1104. https://doi.org/10.1016/j.semarthrit.2018.10.005.
125. Schutt, A.C., Bullington, W.M., and Judson, M.A. (2010). Pharmacotherapy for pulmonary sarcoidosis: a Delphi consensus study. *Respir. Med.* 104: 717–723. https://doi.org/10.1016/j.rmed.2009.12.009.
126. Vorselaars, A.D.M., Wuyts, W.A., Vorselaars, V.M.M. et al. (2013). Methotrexate vs azathioprine in second-line therapy of sarcoidosis. *Chest* 144: 805–812. https://doi.org/10.1378/chest.12-1728.
127. Sweiss, N.J., Welsch, M.J., Curran, J.J., and Ellman, M.H. (2005). Tumor necrosis factor inhibition as a novel treatment for refractory sarcoidosis. *Arthritis Care Res.* 53: 788–791. https://doi.org/10.1002/art.21468.
128. James, W.E. and Baughman, R. (2018). Treatment of sarcoidosis: grading the evidence. *Expert. Rev. Clin. Pharmacol.* 11: 677–687. https://doi.org/10.1080/17512433.2018.1486706.
129. Brito-Zerón, P., Pérez-Alvarez, R., Pallarés, L. et al. (2016). Sarcoidosis: an update on current pharmacotherapy options and future directions. *Expert. Opin. Pharmacother.* 17: 2431–2448. https://doi.org/10.1080/14656566.2016.1258061.
130. Baughman, R.P. and Lower, E.E. (2015). Treatment of Sarcoidosis. *Clin. Rev. Allergy Immunol.* 49: 79–92. https://doi.org/10.1007/s12016-015-8492-9.
131. Hostettler, K.E., Studler, U., Tamm, M., and Brutsche, M.H. (2012). Long-term treatment with infliximab in patients with sarcoidosis. *Respiration* 83: 218–224. https://doi.org/10.1159/000328738.
132. Lahmer, T., Knopf, A., Lanzl, I. et al. (2012). Using TNF-alpha antagonist adalimumab for treatment for multisystem sarcoidosis: a case study. *Rheumatol. Int.* 32: 2367–2370. https://doi.org/10.1007/s00296-011-1968-x.
133. Brill, A.-K., Ott, S.R., and Geiser, T. (2013). Effect and safety of mycophenolate mofetil in chronic pulmonary sarcoidosis: a retrospective study. *Respiration* 86: 376–383. https://doi.org/10.1159/000345596.
134. Hamzeh, N., Voelker, A., Forssén, A. et al. (2014). Efficacy of mycophenolate mofetil in sarcoidosis. *Respir. Med.* 108: 1663–1669. https://doi.org/10.1016/J.RMED.2014.09.013.
135. Besnard, V. and Jeny, F. (2020). Models contribution to the understanding of sarcoidosis pathogenesis: "are there good models of sarcoidosis?". *J. Clin. Med.* 9: 2445. https://doi.org/10.3390/jcm9082445.

22

Sjögren's Syndrome as a Proof of Concept of the Hyperstimulation Syndrome

Vânia Borba[1] and Yehuda Shoenfeld[2,3]
[1]Internal Medicine Departmente, Rehaklik Dussnang AG, Dussnang, Thurgau, Switzerland
[2]Zabludowicz Center for Autoimmune Diseases, Sheba Medical Center, Tel-Hashomer, Israel
[3] Reichman University, Herzelia, Israel

Highlights

- SjS is a multifaceted disease that resembles the ASIA syndrome.
- Pathological hallmark of SjS is focal lymphocyte infiltration in affected glands, accompanied by the production of autoantibodies and inflammatory cytokines, resulting in epithelial damage and disease progression.
- SjS has been described after an adjuvant stimulus (silicone implantation, infections, vaccines, drugs, hormonal dysregulation, etc.) among genetically predisposed individuals, which induces a hyperstimulation of the immune system resulting in the production of autoantibodies, eventually leading to the development of autoimmune diseases and subsequent malignant transformation.
- Patients with pSjS have a 10- to 44-fold greater risk of lymphoma and other cancers when compared to healthy individuals.

Introduction

In 1943, Henrik Sjögren presented for the first time clinical and histologic findings of 19 women who complained of Sicca symptoms. Sjögren's syndrome (SjS) is a progressive systemic autoimmune disease (AID) affecting mainly females in their fourth to fifth decades of life [1]. A genetic predisposition to SjS has been suggested, based on reported increased concordance rates among monozygotic twins and members of the same family [2]. The polymorphic major histocompatibility complex genes are the best documented genetic risk factors for the development of AID. Regarding SjS, DRB1*0301-DQB1*0201-DQA1*0501 haplotypes are the strongest risk factors for the induction of an antibody response and for the development of the disease [3]. Likewise, the

Autoimmune Disorders: Adjuvants and Other Risk Factors in Pathogenesis, First Edition.
Edited by Abdulla Watad, Nicola Luigi Bragazzi, and Yehuda Shoenfeld.

presence of polymorphisms of nonhuman leukocyte antigen genes involved in the interferon (IFN)-1 pathway was also found to be associated with higher susceptibility [4, 5]. The distinctive pathological hallmark of SjS is focal lymphocyte infiltration in affected glands, accompanied by the production of autoantibodies and inflammatory cytokines, leading to epithelial damage and disease progression [6]. Extraglandular complaints have been documented in up to 55% of the patients, and clinical presentation of SjS in younger ages (<35 years) correlates with higher rate of systemic manifestations [7]. Although SjS is considered one of the most common AID, affecting between 1% and 3% of the general population, it is often underestimated or misdiagnosed. It may be present as a primary disease, primary Sjögren's syndrome (pSjS), or in association with other AID such as systemic lupus erythematosus, rheumatoid arthritis, and systemic sclerosis, defining a secondary Sjögren's syndrome (sSjS). Nevertheless, the new *American College of Rheumatology* (ACR)/*European League Against Rheumatism* (EULAR) criteria no longer distinguish between primary and secondary SjS, considering that it may be more accurate to refer to sSjS as "overlapping" with other autoimmune/rheumatic diseases [8, 9]. Anti-Sjögren's syndrome A (anti-SSA/Ro) and B Anti-Sjögren's syndrome A antibodies (anti-SSB/La) autoantibodies are the most specific antinuclear antibodies in primary SjS (pSjS) and are associated with earlier onset, longer disease duration, presence of sicca symptoms, and disease severity [10, 11]. Interestingly, those autoantibodies can be found in sera for up to 20 years before the diagnosis of primary SjS. In this manner, families with multiple cases of AID, autoantibody profiling, along with assessment of genetic risk, enable identification of susceptible individuals in a predisease state [12].

The autoimmune/inflammatory syndrome induced by adjuvants (ASIA) was first introduced in 2011 by Shoenfeld et al. and encompasses a cluster of related immune-mediated diseases, which develop among genetically prone individuals as a result of an adjuvant exposure. In resemblance to ASIA, recent evidence suggests that several agents, such as infections, hormones, vaccines, drugs, or silicone, may act as triggers in determining an abnormal immune response and possibly contributing to the development of SjS [13, 14].

SjS as a classic example of ASIA syndrome

ASIA and SjS divide several common features. Firstly, a shared pathogenic mechanism involving a disruption of the immune system balance, atypical B-cell proliferation, cytokine production, and tissue infiltration. Second, patients with ASIA frequently present clinical features resembling those with SjS [13]. The proposed diagnostic criteria for ASIA include the presence of "typical" clinical manifestations that often comprise fatigue, myalgia and/or muscle weakness, arthralgia and/or arthritis, and dry mouth and/or dry eyes. Certainly, SjS has been described after an adjuvant stimulus among genetically predisposed individuals, which induces a hyperstimulation of the immune system resulting in the production of autoantibodies, eventually leading to the disease development (Figure 22.1) [13]. Unveiling these common pathways will contribute considerably to our understanding and management of both conditions [1].

Hyperstimulation of the immune system in SjS

Inflammation increases tissue damage, leading to functional damage of the affected organs and a chronic inflammatory environment. It has been well recognized that autoreactive B cells and plasma cells contribute to the development of pSjS by cytokine production, antigen presentation, and by producing assorted autoantibodies, including anti-SSA, anti-SSB, and antinuclear antibodies (ANA) [15, 16]. Thus, T helper (Th) cells 1, Th2, Th17, follicular helper T (Tfh) cells, and T/B regulatory cells (Tregs/Bregs), with their characteristic cytokine profiles, have been implicated in the pathogenesis of the disease. Recent studies revealed the pivotal role of Bregs cells

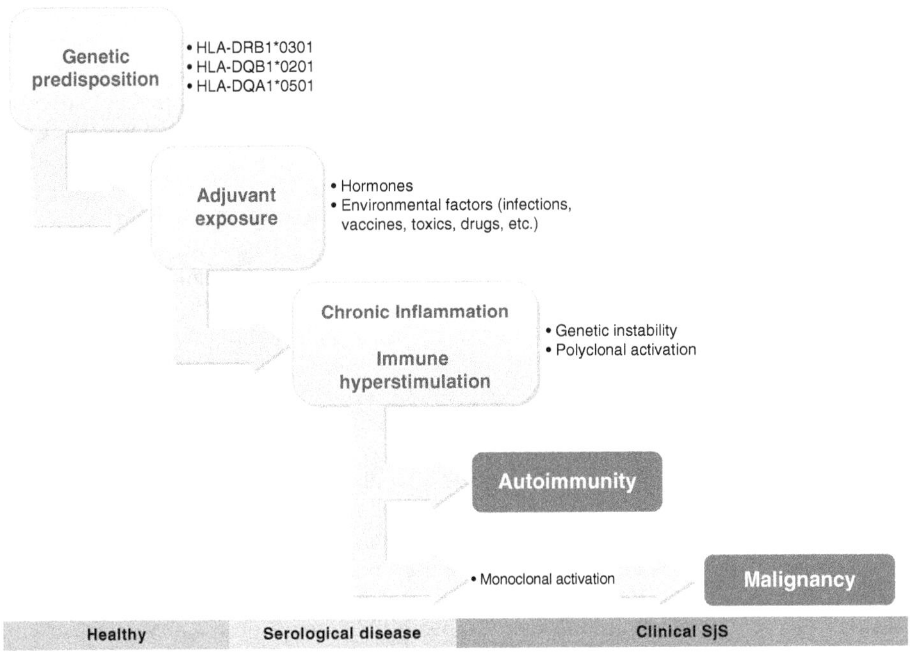

Figure 22.1 Proposed etiopathogenetic mechanisms from genetic susceptibility to the development of autoimmunity and eventual malignant transformation in SjS over time.

in constraining Tfh response in autoimmune pathogenesis [17]. Further, while T cells seem to outweigh in mild lesions, B cells predominate in advanced injuries during disease course. Accordingly, it has been suggested that Th1 and Th17 cells initiate SjS, and as the disease progresses, Th2 and Tfh cells override [14]. In addition, IFN upregulation seems to correlate with severity in clinimetric indexes, such as EULAR Sjögren Syndrome-Disease Activity Index [18]. In addition, the inflammasome activation by the interaction of microbial components, toxins, and mediators of cellular damage with pattern recognition receptors has lately gained some relevance. In pSjS, most studies have focused attention on the NOD-like receptor P3 (NLRP3) inflammasome. When activated, NLRP3 oligomerizes and recruits the adaptor protein, apoptosis-associated speck-like protein, and activates caspase. Hence, NLPR3 and caspase-1 in pSjS salivary glands positively correlate with focal lymphocytic sialadenitis, autoantibodies, and even lymphoma [19, 20]. The lymphomagenesis hypothesis in primary SjS suggests a key role for a continued stimulation of B cells by autoantigens abnormally expressed in the exocrine glands and other organs containing mucosa-associated lymphoid tissue in a multiple-step process where the first event is chronic stimulation at the site of the organs targeted by the autoimmune damage of polyclonal B cells, especially B cells with a rheumatoid factor activity. Moreover, a consequence of polyclonal activation of autoimmune B cells might be the increased frequency of pro-oncogenic factors promoting an abnormal increase of B-cell survival, thus putting the patient at high risk of a malignant transformation [21].

The role of infections

All kinds of infections can be linked with the pathogenesis of SjS [22]. There are three main mechanisms by which infections might trigger AID: antigen mimicry, polyclonal lymphocyte activation, and increased immunogenicity of organ autoantigens secondary to infection-mediated inflammation [23]. Viruses affecting exocrine tissues seem to be able to determine an activation of the innate immune system via Toll-like receptor pathways [24]. A controversial question is whether infections with viruses (such as Epstein–Barr virus (EBV), hepatitis C virus (HCV), human T-cell leukemia virus (HTLV-1), and severe acute respiratory syndrome coronavirus 2 [SARS-CoV-2]) and bacterial agents such as *Helicobacter pylori* (HP) and mycobacteria are candidate causes. Interestingly, some chronic infections have been seen to induce lymphocytic infiltration of the exocrine glands, recurrently indistinguishable from that observed in SjS [25]. Likewise, the identification of virus particles, and the proof of antibodies against pathogens in the sera of SjS patients, has increased the importance of infections in the disease pathogenesis. To support this evidence, Mofors et al. performed a case–control study including 945 SjS patients, in order to identify infections occurring before the diagnosis, during a mean observational time of 16.0 years. It has been concluded that infections increase the risk of developing pSS, most prominently SSA/SSB autoantibody-positive disease, suggesting that microbial triggers of immunity may partake in the pathogenetic process of pSjS [26, 27].

Epstein–Barr virus

Epstein–Barr virus (EBV) is one of the infectious agents proposed as a possible culprit of pSjS. Chronically infecting more than 90% of the world's population, EBV exploits mature B-cell differentiation in germinal center to access the memory B-cell fraction for persistent infection. Despite its ubiquity, infection by EBV is often subclinical, and this invariably reflects the necessity of the virus to preserve its host, balanced with sophisticated host immune mechanisms that maintain viral latency [28]. More than 30 years ago, the relationship between EBV and SjS has already been postulated by Origgi et al. who found that the mean titer of anti-Epstein–Barr nuclear antigen (EBNA) antibodies was significantly higher in SjS patients when compared to controls ($p < 0.001$); moreover, within the SjS population, titers were higher in SSB-positive than in SSB-negative patients ($p < 0.05$) [29]. Hence, Saito et al. found increased EBV-DNA in the salivary gland (SG) of SjS patients, using polymerase chain reaction to detect EBV-DNA in peripheral blood mononuclear cell and tissue biopsies [30]. Interestingly, another research demonstrated that B-cell lines of SjS patients spontaneously produce EBV at a higher frequency and in prominently larger amounts than B-cell lines from patients with rheumatoid arthritis or systemic lupus erythematosus [31]. Furthermore, EBV genome was visualized in autoantibody-producing plasma cells located in the periphery of ectopic lymphoid structures in pSjS, and anti-EBV antibody production was demonstrated within the affected tissue [32]. Indeed, chronic B lymphocyte stimulation in SjS patients was seen to be associated with increased expression of B-cell activating factor, β2 microglobulin, and serum-free light-chain levels [33, 34]. Similar results were recently reported by Sanosyan et al. who observed that β2 microglobulin, kappa lambda light chains, and immunoglobulin G levels were associated with anti-early antigen (EA) antibodies in pSS patients. In addition, β2 microglobulin demonstrated an independent association with anti-EA positivity. The authors conclude that serological evidence of EBV reactivation was more frequently observed and more strongly associated with anti-SSA/B status and B-cell activation markers in pSjS [35]. Kivity et al. have previously reported an association between anti-EA detections and pSjS, which is considered as an indirect evidence of the initiation of lytic replication, and between anti-EA antibodies and the presence of anti-SSA/B autoantibodies [6]. Assorted mechanisms have been considered to justify the effect of EBV on the autoimmune process of SjS, including molecular mimicry among viral EBNA-2 protein, Ro-60 antigen, viral Epstein–Barr virus-encoded small RNAs (EBER)-1/EBER-2 proteins, and La antigen [36, 37]. Besides, genetic susceptibility to $CD8^+$ deficiency and the imbalance between $CD4^+$ and $CD8^+$ T cells (increased of $CD4^+/CD8^+$ ratio) could also promote impaired EBV-specific T-cell response in AID such as SjS [38].

Hepatitis C virus

Hepatitis C virus (HCV) is a global health problem affecting mainly the liver and is often characterized by extrahepatic manifestations mediated by autoimmune reactions, such as arthralgia, vasculitis, and sicca syndrome. Hence, HCV appears to be a trigger for an autoimmune response, as demonstrated by the high percentage of antibodies in the sera of those patients [39, 40]. Aprosin et al. already suggested the involvement of the virus in the etiology of SjS in 1993 [41]. Later on, Koike et al. created transgenic mice with the HCV envelope gene, which interestingly did not induce hepatitis; however, the animals exhibited exocrine inflammation of the salivary and lacrimal glands, confirming that HCV can cause SjS-like pathology [42]. Indeed, HCV patients with Sicca symptomatology and positive autoantibodies could be misdiagnosed as a "primary" SjS [43]. Based on meta-analysis of five cross-sectional and five cohort studies, Wang et al. elucidated a significant positive relationship between HCV infection and development of SjS/Sicca syndrome, with the pooled random effects odds ratio (OR) being 3.31 (95% CI, 1.46–7.48; $p < 0.001$) [44]. Although the role of HCV in causing sialadenitis or SjS is yet to be confirmed, morphological evidence of HCV replication in SG cells has been strongly supported in the literature [45, 46]. Using a large-scale, population-based case–control study in a highly prevalent chronic Hepatitis B Virus (HBV) and HCV infection area, Yeh et al. observed a positive significant association between SjS and chronic HCV infection [47]. Changes in the composition of the saliva suggest that HCV infection can cause Sicca by mechanisms distinct from SjS. Furthermore, a positive correlation was recently observed by Maldonado et al. between HCV RNA-positive epithelial cells and the years of HCV infection. Consistent with the low saliva flow and xerostomia, patients showed changes in several markers of SG acinar and ductal function [48]. Surprisingly, Nagao et al. revealed that the prevalence of SjS in patients with chronic HCV infection was significantly higher than that in patients with chronic HBV infection [49], suggesting that HBV infection protects against AID [50]. This may be explained through an increased risk of extrahepatic manifestations among HCV patients, likely to arise from immunologically triggered mechanisms and virus invasion and replication [51, 52]. In 2017, the ACR has published a new set of criteria for SjS, which concluded that HCV infection is one of the exclusion criteria for primary SjS definition [9, 53].

Other infections

Although virus may exhibit lymphocytic infiltration into exocrine glands, HTLV-1 has been postulated to be another causative agent for SjS [54]. Transgenic mice with HTLV-1 genes showed sialadenitis resembling SjS, but their phenotypic symptoms differed based on the adopted region of the HTLV-1 genes [55]. Lima et al. investigated 272 cases of anti-HTLV-1 antibody-positive patients in Brazil, reporting that 21.7% of them complained about sicca syndrome [56]. Nevertheless, as in Cytomegalovirus (CMV)-infected patients, controverse results have been found among serological studies [6, 29, 57]. For instance, the anti-Ro/SS-A and La/SS-B antibodies detected in the SjS patients showed a negative correlation with viral infections, which could be explained by the inhibitory function of the virus against follicular dendritic cells [55, 58, 59].

Hence, Chen et al. performed a meta-analysis to evaluate the association between HP and SjS, enrolling more than 600 patients. A small but significant higher rate of HP infection among SjS patients in comparison with healthy controls has been noticed [60]. Moreover, serum antibody titers to HP significantly correlated with age, disease duration, disease activity index, and C-reactive protein levels [61, 62]. In a like manner, when compared with healthy subjects and other connective tissue disease patients, cases with SjS have a higher infection rate of HP [63]. Indeed, chronic presence of HP may activate immune system with cytokine production, infiltration of gastric mucosa by neutrophils and macrophages, activation of effector T cells, and antibody production [64].

Along, reports indicate a possible pathogenic and prognostic significance of anti-*Saccharomyces cerevisiae* autoantibodies (ASCA) in SjS, bond already seen among other AID [65]. In a recent study, a nearly 5% prevalence of ASCA was depicted for the first time in an SjS cohort. Impressively, all ASCA positive patients were characterized by anti-SSA/Ro 52/60 and anti-SSB/La positivity, and *S. cerevisiae* mannan displayed high similarity with anti-Ro/60 antibodies [66].

The mechanism of molecular mimicry of self-antigens behind the induction ASCAs may indicate their pathogenic role [67].

Under the light of the recent pandemic, infection with SARS-CoV-2 has been shown to originate excessive pro-inflammatory cytokines formation, although the production of IFN-1 is often blunted. Besides, the prolonged T-cell stimulation, T-cell senescence and exhaustion, and skew toward a Th17 phenotype in patients with Coronavirus disease (COVID-19) pneumonia provided further support on the potential autoimmune capabilities of the virus [68, 69]. Junior et al. exposed a significant increased incidence of pSjS during the COVID-19 pandemic [70]. The first report of pSjS-specific antibodies anti-SSA/Ro in COVID-19-infected patients occurred in two individuals with acute respiratory distress syndrome and no history of AID [53]. Further, the long-term impact of SARS-CoV-2 infection on the host immune system has led to the onset of novel complex chronic clinical manifestations, such as the long-term xerostomia [71]. It has been initially suggested that the xerostomia experienced by COVID-19-infected patients could be due to the neuroinvasive and neurotropic properties of the SARS-CoV-2 [72]. More recently, other studies have confirmed an abundant expression of angiotensin-converting enzyme 2 in squamous epithelial cells of the dorsal tongue, gingiva, buccal tissue, as well as taste bud cells, and submandibular salivary glands, which could justify this symptom [73–75]. Nevertheless, still much is left to discover about the impact of SARS-CoV-2 infection in public health [76].

Ultimately, infectious agents may be still considered essential pathogenic triggers in both induction and perpetuation of immune system dysregulation, which underlies the etiopathogenesis of SjS [77]. Moreover, robust evidence supports a role of infections in the initiation and maintenance of lymphoproliferative damage that affects the long-term prognosis of the disease [78].

Vaccines

Vaccinations represent one of the greatest achievements in the history of medicine, decreasing morbidity and mortality in millions of individuals. Patients with AID, such as SjS, are advised to follow a recommended schedule. Inoculations should preferably be administered during quiescent phases of the diseases due to the possibility to trigger a flare, and for same reason, live attenuated shots should be avoided [79]. Vaccines are able to evoke innate and adaptive immunity through several mechanisms because of their heterogeneous composition: infectious components, adjuvants (aluminum, squalene, etc.), and preservatives [80]. Molecular mimicry may be responsible for the activation of the host's immune response, which, in addition to bacterial and viral antigens, will also target host molecules that share sequence homology or structural similarities with microbial epitopes [81, 82]. Brito-Zerón et al. reported infections as a leading cause of death in SjS, thus stressing the importance to vaccinate the patients for protective immunity [83]. On the other hand, a few case reports have indicated a possible triggering of SjS by different vaccines, such as Influenza and Hepatitis B [84]. Alum, an aluminum-based adjuvant present in many vaccine formulations, was able to induce an SjS-like disease in an experimental *New Zealand Mixed* 2758 strain of mice, associated with ANA positivity, chronic SG dysfunction, and lymphocytic infiltrates within the SG [85]. Because of the increasing evidence about innate immunity as contributor to gland dysfunction in primary SjS, and given the known ability of alum to activate inflammasome pathways, inflammation routes activation triggered by alum may also play a role in induction and progression of SjS [85]. Furthermore, in patients with primary SjS, the A/California/7/2009/H1N1-like virus vaccination leads to a significant increase in the mean levels of anti-SSA/Ro and anti-SSB/La antibodies after 1 year of follow-up [86]. Brauner et al. recently published a study enrolling patients with SjS without immunomodulatory treatment, age- and gender-matched to healthy controls, who were immunized with an H1N1 influenza vaccine and monitored for serological and cellular immune responses. Endosomal toll-like receptor activation of naïve B cells *in vitro* revealed a greater propensity of patient-derived cells to differentiate into plasmablasts and higher production of class-switched IgG [87].

Interestingly, autoantibodies and nonspecific autoimmune and/or rheumatic clinical manifestations may be present long before the development of a clear clinical picture, and adjuvants may represent the "second hit" for the appearance of a full-blown autoimmune rheumatic condition (Figure 22.1) [82, 88].

Silicone and silica

Since the introduction of silicone gel prosthesis in 1962 by *Cronin* and *Gerow*, breast augmentation has become the most performed operation in cosmetic surgery. The external surface of the implants may be smooth or textured and is specifically designed to reduce the risk of leakage of low-molecular-weight silicone [89]. Nonetheless, gel fluid diffusion can be as high as 300 mg/year [90], particularly for older implants. Leaked silicone may cause a histiocytic reaction with foreign-body giant cells, forming granulomas ("siliconomas") even in distant sites of the body [91].

Over the past decades, silicone breast implants (SBI) have been extensively associated with several illnesses, most of them AID [92]. Recent long-term outcome studies on extremely large cohorts suggested higher rates of SjS in patients with SBI. This is consistent with publications dating back in 1984, and with the several case series reported over time [93, 94]. One of the most relevant studies was recently performed by Watad et al., using the computerized databases of *Maccabi Healthcare Services* in Israel, which include up to 20 years of data on 2 million members. The authors analyzed 24,651 SBI recipients and 98,604 matched women without implants. The adjusted OR between women with SBI being diagnosed with any autoimmune/rheumatic disorders was 1.22 (95% CI 1.18–1.26). The strongest association (OR > 1.5, $p < 0.001$) was recorded for SjS, systemic sclerosis, and sarcoidosis (OR of 1.58, 1.63, and 1.98, respectively) [95]. Furthermore, an extensive review of epidemiological studies in the past 10 years by Suh et al. also exhibited evidence affirming an association between SBI and AID. The most commonly recognized diseases were SjS, rheumatoid arthritis, and systemic sclerosis. Explantation of the SBI resulted in alleviation of symptoms in over 50% of patients, strengthening the hypothesis linking SBI to AID [96]. As a matter of fact, women with SBI are more likely to report subsequent diagnosis of SjS. Balk et al. conducted a systematic review regarding breast implants and their association with medical illnesses. An increased statistically significant risk ratio of 2.92 (95% CI 1.01–8.47) in their cumulative evaluation of seven studies investigating SjS in association with SBI was reported [97]. Similar results were found by Coroneos et al. who performed a retrospective cohort study researching the outcomes of 99,993 patients with SBI. Not surprisingly, implants were associated with increased rates of SjS, with a standardized incidence ratio of 8.14 [98].

Silicosis remains an important global health problem, with disease attributed to established and new sources of exposure [99]. Silicon dioxide is the most abundant mineral in earth's crust and appears in amorphous and crystal forms. In many dusty trades, such as mining, sandblasting, and granite cutting, there is an exposure to respiratory particles of crystalline silica [100]. Along the years, assorted reports suggested that silica exposure can precede the onset of SjS, especially in those chronically bared professional groups [100–104]. Interestingly, Ziebelman et al. recently published a case of a patient who simultaneously developed silicosis, scleroderma, and SjS after prolonged exposure to crystalline silica, reinforcing the association of this adjuvant with different AID [105].

Immune checkpoint inhibitors

In recent years, harnessing the power of a patient's immune system to treat cancer has been an increasingly efficacious treatment strategy in oncology [106]. Immune checkpoint inhibitors (ICIs) targeting the cytotoxic T-lymphocyte-associated protein 4 (CTLA-4) and programmed cell death protein 1 (PD-1) pathways have demonstrated not only survival improvements in multiple advanced cancers but also diverse immune-related adverse events [107]. While cancer is considered a "hypoimmune disease," ICI use results in a "hyperimmune" state. The first case of SjS triggered by cancer immunotherapies has been recently published by Cappelli et al. [107], with an increasing number of additional reports since then [108]. Because sicca symptoms are common in the population, with a prevalence reaching up to 30% in persons >65 years of age, their occurrence in a clinical trial may not be attributed to study drug, leading to underreporting [108]. The prevalence of SjS was seen to be 0.3% with anti-PD-1/anti-PD-L1 agents alone, and 2.5% with a combination of anti-PD-1 and anti-CTLA4 agents [109]. Ramos-Casals et al. analyzed the worldwide occurrence of sicca/SjS associated with the use of ICI in patients with cancer, using data from the *International ImmunoCancer Registry*. A total of 26 patients with SjS triggered by ICIs were identified, nevertheless with a very specific profile, different from the idiopathic primary SjS. Authors reported a frequent occurrence in men, higher mean age, predominant immune-negative serological profile, and a notable development of organ-specific autoimmune involvement, despite the poor immunological profile [110]. Indeed, proportions of anti-SSA positivity appear to be much lower than in "classical" pSjS, with a rough mean of 33% of patients with ICI-induced SG dysfunction compared to an approximation of 70% of pSjS patients [111]. Furthermore, by immunohistochemistry, there was a predominant T-lymphocytic infiltrate, with a slight majority of $CD4^+$ over $CD8^+$ T cells and few $CD20^+$ B cells. This pattern is different from characteristic SjS infiltrates where B cells represent 20–62% of all lymphocytes and focus score directly correlating with B-cell ratios [112]. Though the mechanism of sicca syndrome/SjS induced by immunotherapy has not yet been elucidated, the results of these previous studies suggest that an impairment of the PD-1/PD-L1 pathway caused by ICIs triggers the activation of T-lymphocytes, leading to infiltration of the SG epithelium [113, 114].

Autoimmune reactions and the development of novel distinct clinical entities could be regarded as collateral damage, posing new challenges in clinical practice, shedding potentially light on autoimmune pathogenesis as well [115].

Hormonal imbalance

SjS is typified by a strong female predilection, which is also observed among other AID. Growing scientific evidence shows that adult females mount stronger innate and adaptive immunological responses, reflected by a lower risk for serious infections and a better vaccine antibody response [116]. Assorted sex hormones may play a role in the pathogenesis of pSS, mainly dehydroepiandrosterone (DHEA), prolactin (PRL), and estrogen [117–119]. Studies performed using animal models have shown that mice lacking aromatase have destruction of acinar cells of the major SG with age [120], and normal mice that undergo ovariectomy develop apoptosis of the SG epithelial cells [121]. Furthermore, ovariectomy in predisposed mice leads to accelerated onset of a pSjS-like syndrome [122]. Hence, healthy ovariectomized C57BL/6 mice display an exocrinopathy with autoimmune characteristics similar to SjS, including SG focal adenitis, lacrimal glands lesions, Ro/SSA, La/SSB, and α-fodrin autoantibodies [121]. In a recent case–control study, pSjS appearance in women was associated with lower estrogen exposure and lower cumulative menstrual cycling time, when compared to sicca controls. Conversely, an increasing estrogen exposure was negatively associated with development of pSjS [123]. In the case of pSjS, lower cumulative estrogen exposure appears to augment the clinical expression of disease.

Likewise, SjS patients present low levels of androgen hormones, both in the bloodstream and in SG [124]. Hence, the androgens could help maintaining acini structure in healthy SG, while their reduction observed in SjS patients could cause a decrease in integrin expression and a dysregulation of acini architecture [125]. Testosterone may also enhance inflammation, since postmenopausal women with isolated SjS were found to have higher levels of the hormone, which positively correlated with disease activity [126]. In general, androgens drive cell-mediated IFNγ-associated Th1 responses and inhibit antibody production. Probably for this reason, men are less likely to meet the classification criteria for diagnosis of SjS [127, 128].

On the other hand, PRL has a double bioactive function, acting as a hormone and a pro-inflammatory cytokine. It influences the immune system modulation, mainly inhibiting the negative selection of autoreactive B lymphocytes [129, 130]. Furthermore, PRL has an antiapoptotic effect, enhances proliferative response to antigens/mitogens, and enhances the production of immunoglobulins and autoantibodies [131]. Higher levels of PRL were frequently reported among SjS patients when compared to healthy controls [132]. Increased levels of serum PRL are especially evident in patients diagnosed at a young age with active immunological disease, and it correlates to index for internal organ disease. Furthermore, pSjS may be preceded by hyperprolactinemia for many years before diagnosis [133].

Apart from the traditionally considered hormonal and environmental factors, lately, the role of sex chromosomes has drawn much attention. To compensate the gender imbalance, nature has created a defective epigenetic mechanism to silence the second rich in immune-related genes X chromosome. Genes escaping the silencing process transfer the genetic imbalance into the transcriptional and protein level, and therefore contributing to gender differences, as reflected in functions of the innate and adaptive immunity [134].

The crossroad between immune hyperstimulation, SjS, and neoplasms

A complex relationship exists among rheumatic diseases and cancer. This delicate balance among chronic inflammation, hyperstimulation, and malignant cell transformation in neoplasms has been extensively observed but still not well defined. Several studies have shown a high incidence of malignancy associated with SjS, the most common being lymphoma. Together with cryoglobulinemic vasculitis and interstitial lung disease, lymphoma is a systemic complication conferring premature mortality, adding an excess death rate of 9.4 cases per 1000 patient years at risk. Moreover, most rheumatic diseases associated with diffuse large B-cell lymphomas (DLBCLs), in contrast to DLBCLs in the general population, originate from nongerminal center B cells and are possibly a distinct subset within the "DLBCL" category, exhibiting characteristic biological features and clinical behavior [135].

SjS patients display monoclonal immunoglobulins or light chains in their sera from early times on, as well as monoclonal mixed cryoglobulins, suggesting both monoclonal and polyclonal B-cell activation early in the disease course [136]. In the setting of SjS, increased B-cell proliferation driven by the CD40/CD40L interaction may enhance the tendency toward malignancy [137]. Chronic autoantigen stimulation and inflammation represent the major drivers of specific B-cell proliferation and the increase in frequency of their transformation that may promote lymphoma development [138]. This process results in the production of autoantibodies, namely rheumatoid factor, anti-Ro/SSA, and anti-La/SSB. Furthermore, immunoglobulin recombination, somatic mutation, and isotype switching during B-cell development are events that may increase the translocation of oncogenes to immunoglobulin *loci* or tumor suppressor gene inactivation, leading to monoclonal B-cell proliferation [139]. High risk features of lymphoma development include systemic extraepithelial manifestations, low serum levels of complement component C4, and mixed type II cryoglobulinemia [139–141].

Although lymphoma represents the most prevalent malignancy among SjS patients, their higher risk is not exclusive to it. A large meta-analysis was recently performed by Zhong et al., which involved more than 47,607 pSjS patients with the follow-up of more than 452,468 person-year and aimed to investigate the association between pSjS and the risk of malignancy. The results elucidate that pSjS is significantly linked with increased risks of overall malignancy (pooled SIR 2.17, 95% 1.57–3.00), hematological malignancy (pooled SIR 11.55, 95% CI 4.32–30.90), including non-Hodgkin Lymphoma (pooled SIR 13.71, 95% CI 8.83–21.29), Hodgkin lymphoma (pooled SIR 8.84, 95% CI 5.00–15.61), multiple myeloma (pooled SIR 8.27, 95% CI 3.08–22.24), and leukemia (pooled SIR 2.56, 95% CI 1.78–3.69). Nevertheless, an association was also found with solid tumors (pooled SIR 1.39, 95% CI 0.90–2.13), including lung cancer (pooled SIR 1.55, 95% CI 1.29–1.85), thyroid cancer (pooled SIR 2.05, 95% CI 1.20–3.48), nonmelanoma skin cancer (pooled SIR 1.71, 95% CI 1.08–2.72), kidney/urinary tract cancer (pooled SIR 1.36, 95% CI 1.02; 1.81), liver cancer (pooled SIR 1.70, 95% CI 1.13–2.57), and prostate cancer (pooled SIR 1.50, 95% CI 1.02–2.22) [142]. Similar results were obtained by Goulabchand et al. in a nationwide population-based retrospective study from the *French Health Insurance Database*. Higher incidence rates of lymphomas (aHR, 1.97 [95% CI, 1.59–2.43]), Waldenström macroglobulinemia (aHR, 10.8 [6.5–18.0]), leukemia (aHR, 1.61 [1.1–2.4]), and thyroid cancer (aHR, 1.7 [1.1–2.8]) were confirmed among 25,661 hospitalized patients with pSS versus 252,543 matched patients in a median follow-up of 3.96 years [143].

Conclusions

ASIA syndrome encompasses diverse immune-mediated conditions that flourish under the influence of triggering factors among predisposed individuals, which provoke immunological reactions characteristic of AID. Immune system hyperstimulation and chronic inflammatory status induced by an adjuvant stimulus may be implicated not only in SjS disease pathogenesis but also in mechanisms associated with neoplasm development. Interestingly, autoantibodies and nonspecific autoimmune/rheumatic clinical manifestations may be present long before the development of a clear clinical picture, and adjuvants may represent the "second hit" for the appearance of a full-blown autoimmune rheumatic condition. By identifying the major risk factors, it is possible to minimize exposure, which would be expected to lead to decreased disease incidence rates, ameliorate disease severity, and even prevent malignant transformation. This knowledge will allow us in the future to prevent the onset of the disease in susceptible predisposed individuals, adopt personalized preventive and/or therapeutic strategies, and design future studies in order to uncover the blurred lines surrounding these maladies.

Abbreviations

ACR	American College of Rheumatology
AID	Autoimmune diseases
ANA	Antinuclear antibodies
Anti-SSA/Ro	Anti-Sjögren's syndrome A antibodies
Anti-SSB/La)	Anti-Sjögren's syndrome A antibodies
ASCA	Anti-*Saccharomyces cerevisiae* autoantibodies
ASIA	Autoimmune/inflammatory syndrome induced by adjuvants
Bregs	B regulatory cells
CMV	Cytomegalovirus
COVID-19	Coronavirus disease
CTLA-4	Cytotoxic T-lymphocyte-associated protein 4
DHEA	Dehydroepiandrosterone
DLBCL	Diffuse large B-cell lymphoma
EBNA	Epstein–Barr nuclear antigen
EBV	Epstein–Barr virus
EULAR	European League Against Rheumatism
HBV	Hepatitis B virus
HCV	Hepatitis C virus
HP	*Helicobacter pylori*
HTLV-1	Human T-cell leukemia virus
ICI	Immune checkpoint inhibitor
IFN	Interferon

NLRP3	NOD-like receptor P3
OR	Odds ratio
PD-1	Programmed cell death protein 1
PRL	Prolactin
pSjS	Primary Sjögren's syndrome
SARS-CoV-2	Severe acute respiratory syndrome coronavirus 2
SBI	Silicone breast implant
SG	Salivary gland
SjS	Sjögren's syndrome
sSjS	Secondary Sjögren's syndrome
Tfh	Follicular helper T cell
Th	T helper cell
Tregs	T regulatory cell

References

1. Colafrancesco, S., Perricone, C., and Shoenfeld, Y. (2016). Autoimmune/inflammatory syndrome induced by adjuvants and Sjögren's syndrome. *Isr. Med. Assoc. J.* 18 (3–4): 150–153.
2. Bayetto, K. and Logan, R.M. (2010). Sjögren's syndrome: a review of aetiology, pathogenesis, diagnosis and management. *Aust. Dent. J.* 55 (Suppl 1): 39–47.
3. Cruz-Tapias, P., Rojas-Villarraga, A., Maier-Moore, S., and Anaya, J.M. (2012). HLA and Sjögren's syndrome susceptibility. A meta-analysis of worldwide studies. *Autoimmun. Rev.* 11 (4): 281–287.
4. Lessard, C.J., Li, H., Adrianto, I. et al. (2013). Variants at multiple loci implicated in both innate and adaptive immune responses are associated with Sjögren's syndrome. *Nat. Genet.* 45 (11): 1284–1292.
5. Nordmark, G., Kristjansdottir, G., Theander, E. et al. (2009). Additive effects of the major risk alleles of IRF5 and STAT4 in primary Sjögren's syndrome. *Genes Immun.* 10 (1): 68–76.
6. Kivity, S., Arango, M.T., Ehrenfeld, M. et al. (2014). Infection and autoimmunity in Sjögren's syndrome: a clinical study and comprehensive review. *J. Autoimmun.* 51: 17–22.
7. Parisis, D., Chivasso, C., Perret, J. et al. (2020). Current state of knowledge on primary Sjögren's syndrome, an autoimmune exocrinopathy. *J. Clin. Med.* 9 (7): E2299.
8. Wallace, Z.S., Naden, R.P., Chari, S. et al. (2020). The 2019 American college of rheumatology/European league against rheumatism classification criteria for IgG4-related disease. *Ann. Rheum. Dis.* 79 (1): 77–87.
9. Shiboski, C.H., Shiboski, S.C., Seror, R. et al. (2017). 2016 American college of rheumatology/European league against rheumatism classification criteria for primary Sjögren's syndrome: a consensus and data-driven methodology involving three international patient cohorts. *Arthritis Rheumatol.* 69 (1): 35–45.
10. Patel, R. and Shahane, A. (2014). The epidemiology of Sjögren's syndrome. *Clin. Epidemiol.* 6: 247–255.
11. Shen, L. and Suresh, L. (2017). Autoantibodies, detection methods and panels for diagnosis of Sjögren's syndrome. *Clin. Immunol. Orlando. Fla.* 182: 24–29.
12. Theander, E., Jonsson, R., Sjöström, B. et al. (2015). Prediction of Sjögren's syndrome years before diagnosis and identification of patients with early onset and severe disease course by autoantibody profiling. *Arthritis Rheumatol.* 67 (9): 2427–2436.
13. Borba, V., Malkova, A., Basantsova, N. et al. (2020). Classical examples of the concept of the ASIA syndrome. *Biomol. Ther.* 10 (10): E1436.
14. Psianou, K., Panagoulias, I., Papanastasiou, A.D. et al. (2018). Clinical and immunological parameters of Sjögren's syndrome. *Autoimmun. Rev.* 17 (10): 1053–1064.
15. Reed, J.H. (2022). Transforming mutations in the development of pathogenic B cell clones and autoantibodies. *Immunol. Rev.* 307 (1): 101–115.
16. Du, A.X., Gniadecki, R., and Osman, M. (2022). Biomarkers of B cell activation in autoimmune connective tissue diseases: more than markers of disease activity. *Clin. Biochem.* 100: 1–12.
17. Du, W., Han, M., Zhu, X. et al. (2021). The multiple roles of B cells in the pathogenesis of Sjögren's syndrome. *Front. Immunol.* 12: 684999.

18. Bodewes, I.L.A., Al-Ali, S., van Helden-Meeuwsen, C.G. et al. (2018). Systemic interferon type I and type II signatures in primary Sjögren's syndrome reveal differences in biological disease activity. *Rheumatol. Oxf. Engl.* 57 (5): 921–930.
19. Baldini, C., Rossi, C., Ferro, F. et al. (2013). The P2X7 receptor-inflammasome complex has a role in modulating the inflammatory response in primary Sjögren's syndrome. *J. Intern. Med.* 274 (5): 480–489.
20. Baldini, C., Santini, E., Rossi, C. et al. (2017). The P2X7 receptor-NLRP3 inflammasome complex predicts the development of non-Hodgkin's lymphoma in Sjögren's syndrome: a prospective, observational, single-centre study. *J. Intern. Med.* 282 (2): 175–186.
21. Retamozo, S., Brito-Zerón, P., and Ramos-Casals, M. (2019). Prognostic markers of lymphoma development in primary Sjögren syndrome. *Lupus* 28 (8): 923–936.
22. Utomo, S.W. and Putri, J.F. (2020). Infections as risk factor of Sjögren's syndrome. *Open Access Rheumatol. Res. Rev.* 12: 257–266.
23. Bach, J.F. (2005). Infections and autoimmune diseases. *J. Autoimmun.* 25 (Suppl): 74–80.
24. Colafrancesco, S., Perricone, C., Priori, R. et al. (2014). Sjögren's syndrome: another facet of the autoimmune/inflammatory syndrome induced by adjuvants (ASIA). *J. Autoimmun.* 51: 10–16.
25. Ramos-Casals, M., Brito-Zerón, P., and Font, J. (2007). Lessons from diseases mimicking Sjögren's syndrome. *Clin. Rev. Allergy Immunol.* 32 (3): 275–283.
26. Mofors, J., Arkema, E.V., Björk, A. et al. (2019). Infections increase the risk of developing Sjögren's syndrome. *J. Intern. Med.* 285 (6): 670–680.
27. Agmon-Levin, N., Dagan, A., Peri, Y. et al. (2017). The interaction between anti-Ro/SSA and anti-La/SSB autoantibodies and anti-infectious antibodies in a wide spectrum of auto-immune diseases: another angle of the autoimmune mosaic. *Clin. Exp. Rheumatol.* 35 (6): 929–935.
28. Tangye, S.G., Palendira, U., and Edwards, E.S.J. (2017). Human immunity against EBV-lessons from the clinic. *J. Exp. Med.* 214 (2): 269–283.
29. Origgi, L., Hu, C., Bertetti, E. et al. (1988). Antibodies to Epstein-Barr virus and cytomegalovirus in primary Sjögren's syndrome. *Boll. Ist Sieroter. Milan.* 67 (4): 265–274.
30. Saito, I., Servenius, B., Compton, T., and Fox, R.I. (1989). Detection of Epstein-Barr virus DNA by polymerase chain reaction in blood and tissue biopsies from patients with Sjögren's syndrome. *J. Exp. Med.* 169 (6): 2191–2198.
31. Tateishi, M., Saito, I., Yamamoto, K., and Miyasaka, N. (1993). Spontaneous production of Epstein-Barr virus by B lymphoblastoid cell lines obtained from patients with Sjögren's syndrome. Possible involvement of a novel strain of Epstein-Barr virus in disease pathogenesis. *Arthritis Rheum.* 36 (6): 827–835.
32. Croia, C., Astorri, E., Murray-Brown, W. et al. (2014). Implication of Epstein-Barr virus infection in disease-specific autoreactive B cell activation in ectopic lymphoid structures of Sjögren's syndrome. *Arthritis Rheumatol.* 66 (9): 2545–2557.
33. Seo, S., Hong, J.Y., Yoon, S. et al. (2016). Prognostic significance of serum beta-2 microglobulin in patients with diffuse large B-cell lymphoma in the rituximab era. *Oncotarget* 7 (47): 76934–76943.
34. Nocturne, G., Cornec, D., Seror, R., and Mariette, X. (2016). Use of biologics in Sjögren's syndrome. *Rheum. Dis. Clin. N. Am.* 42 (3): 407–417.
35. Sanosyan, A., Daien, C., Nutz, A. et al. (2019). Discrepancy of serological and molecular patterns of circulating Epstein-Barr virus reactivation in primary Sjögren's syndrome. *Front. Immunol.* 10: 1153.
36. Pender, M.P. (2003). Infection of autoreactive B lymphocytes with EBV, causing chronic autoimmune diseases. *Trends Immunol.* 24 (11): 584–588.
37. Whittingham, S., McNeilage, L.J., and Mackay, I.R. (1987). Epstein-Barr virus as an etiological agent in primary Sjögren's syndrome. *Med. Hypotheses* 22 (4): 373–386.
38. Rancan, C., Schirrmann, L., Hüls, C. et al. (2015). Latent membrane protein LMP2A impairs recognition of EBV-infected cells by $CD8^+$ T cells. *PLoS Pathog.* 11 (6): e1004906.
39. Alhazmi, A.A., Almuflihi, A., Aly, M.M. et al. (2021). Hepatitis C-induced Sjögren's syndrome with positive serology: a case report. *Cureus.* 13 (12): e20091.
40. Altomare, A., Corrado, A., Maruotti, N. et al. (2022). HCV and autoimmunity in rheumatic diseases. *Curr. Rheumatol. Rev.* 18 (2): 101–107.
41. Aprosin, Z.G., Serov, V.V., and Lopatkina, T.N. (1993). The hepatitis B virus as a probable etiological factor in Sjögren's disease. *Ter. Arkh.* 65 (4): 73–78.

42. Koike, K., Moriya, K., Ishibashi, K. et al. (1997). Sialadenitis histologically resembling Sjögren syndrome in mice transgenic for hepatitis C virus envelope genes. *Proc. Natl. Acad. Sci. U. S. A.* 94 (1): 233–236.
43. Ramos-Casals, M., García-Carrasco, M., Brito Zerón, M.P. et al. (2002). Viral etiopathogenesis of Sjögren's syndrome: role of the hepatitis C virus. *Autoimmun. Rev.* 1 (4): 238–243.
44. Wang, Y., Dou, H., Liu, G. et al. (2014). Hepatitis C virus infection and the risk of Sjögren or sicca syndrome: a meta-analysis. *Microbiol. Immunol.* 58 (12): 675–687.
45. Arrieta, J.J., Rodríguez-Iñigo, E., Ortiz-Movilla, N. et al. (2001 Jan). In situ detection of hepatitis C virus RNA in salivary glands. *Am. J. Pathol.* 158 (1): 259–264.
46. Toussirot, E., Le Huédé, G., Mougin, C. et al. (2002). Presence of hepatitis C virus RNA in the salivary glands of patients with Sjögren's syndrome and hepatitis C virus infection. *J. Rheumatol.* 29 (11): 2382–2385.
47. Yeh, C.C., Wang, W.C., Wu, C.S. et al. (2016). Association of Sjögrens syndrome in patients with chronic hepatitis virus infection: a population-based analysis. *PLoS One* 11 (8): e0161958.
48. Maldonado, J.O., Beach, M.E., Wang, Y. et al. (2022). HCV infection alters salivary gland histology and saliva composition. *J. Dent. Res.* 101 (5): 534–541.
49. Nagao, Y., Hanada, S., Shishido, S. et al. (2003). Incidence of Sjögren's syndrome in Japanese patients with hepatitis C virus infection. *J. Gastroenterol. Hepatol.* 18 (3): 258–266.
50. Ram, M., Anaya, J.M., Barzilai, O. et al. (2008). The putative protective role of hepatitis B virus (HBV) infection from autoimmune disorders. *Autoimmun. Rev.* 7 (8): 621–625.
51. Agnello, V. and De Rosa, F.G. (2004). Extrahepatic disease manifestations of HCV infection: some current issues. *J. Hepatol.* 40 (2): 341–352.
52. Zignego, A.L., Ferri, C., Pileri, S.A. et al. (2007). Italian association of the study of liver commission on extrahepatic manifestations of HCV infection. Extrahepatic manifestations of hepatitis C virus infection: a general overview and guidelines for a clinical approach. *Dig. Liver Dis.* 39 (1): 2–17.
53. Liu, Z. and Chu, A. (2021). Sjögren's syndrome and viral infections. *Rheumatol. Ther.* 8 (3): 1051–1059.
54. Nakamura, H., Shimizu, T., and Kawakami, A. (2020). Role of viral infections in the pathogenesis of Sjögren's syndrome: different characteristics of Epstein-Barr virus and HTLV-1. *J. Clin. Med.* 9 (5): E1459.
55. Nakamura, H., Tsukamoto, M., Nagasawa, Y. et al. (2022). Does HTLV-1 infection show phenotypes found in Sjögren's syndrome? *Viruses.* 14 (1): 100.
56. Lima, C.M., Santos, S., Dourado, A. et al. (2016). Association of Sicca syndrome with proviral load and proinflammatory cytokines in HTLV-1 infection. *J Immunol Res* 2016: 8402059.
57. Scully, C. (1990). Sjögren's syndrome: no demonstrable association by serology of secondary Sjögren's syndrome with cytomegalovirus. *J. Oral Pathol. Med.* 19 (1): 43–44.
58. Tincani, A., Andreoli, L., Cavazzana, I. et al. (2013). Novel aspects of Sjögren's syndrome in 2012. *BMC Med.* 11: 93.
59. Gugliesi, F., Pasquero, S., Griffante, G. et al. (2021). Human cytomegalovirus and autoimmune diseases: where are we? *Viruses.* 13 (2): 260.
60. Chen, Q., Zhou, X., Tan, W., and Zhang, M. (2018). Association between Helicobacter pylori infection and Sjögren syndrome: a meta-analysis. *Medicine (Baltimore)* 97 (49): e13528.
61. Smyk, D.S., Koutsoumpas, A.L., Mytilinaiou, M.G. et al. (2014). Helicobacter pylori and autoimmune disease: cause or bystander. *World J Gastroenterol: WJG* 20 (3): 613–629.
62. Radić, M. (2014). Role of Helicobacter pylori infection in autoimmune systemic rheumatic diseases. *World J Gastroenterol: WJG* 20 (36): 12839–12846.
63. El Miedany, Y.M., Baddour, M., Ahmed, I., and Fahmy, H. (2005). Sjögren's syndrome: concomitant H. pylori infection and possible correlation with clinical parameters. *Joint Bone Spine.* 72 (2): 135–141.
64. Wang, L., Cao, Z.M., Zhang, L.L. et al. (2022). Helicobacter pylori and autoimmune diseases: involving multiple systems. *Front. Immunol.* 13: 833424.
65. Rinaldi, M., Perricone, R., Blank, M. et al. (2013). Anti-*Saccharomyces cerevisiae* autoantibodies in autoimmune diseases: from bread baking to autoimmunity. *Clin. Rev. Allergy Immunol.* 45 (2): 152–161.
66. Alunno, A., Bistoni, O., Carubbi, F. et al. (2018). Prevalence and significance of anti-*saccharomyces cerevisiae* antibodies in primary Sjögren's syndrome. *Clin. Exp. Rheumatol.* 36 (3): 73–79.
67. Rinaldi, M. (2014). Anti-*saccharomyces cerevisiae* autoantibodies and autoimmune diseases: the sweet and sour of baking yeast. *Isr. Med. Assoc. J.* 16 (10): 616–618.
68. Brito-Zerón, P., Melchor, S., Seror, R. et al. (2021). SARS-CoV-2 infection in patients with primary Sjögren syndrome: characterization and outcomes of 51 patients. *Rheumatol. Oxf. Engl.* 60 (6): 2946–2957.

69. Larionova, R., Byvaltsev, K., Kravtsova, O. et al. (2022). SARS-Cov2 acute and post-active infection in the context of autoimmune and chronic inflammatory diseases. *J. Transl. Autoimmun.* 5: 100154.
70. Martelli Júnior, H., Gueiros, L.A., de Lucena, E.G., and Coletta, R.D. (2021). Increase in the number of Sjögren's syndrome cases in Brazil in the COVID-19 Era. *Oral Dis.* 28 (Suppl 2): 2588–2590.
71. Chowdhury, F., Grigoriadou, S., and Bombardieri, M. (2021). Severity of COVID-19 infection in primary Sjögren's syndrome and the emerging evidence of COVID-19-induced xerostomia. *Clin. Exp. Rheumatol.* 39 (6): 215–222.
72. Dotan, A., Muller, S., Kanduc, D. et al. (2021). The SARS-CoV-2 as an instrumental trigger of autoimmunity. *Autoimmun. Rev.* 20 (4): 102792.
73. Xu, H., Zhong, L., Deng, J. et al. (2020). High expression of ACE2 receptor of 2019-nCoV on the epithelial cells of oral mucosa. *Int. J. Oral. Sci.* 12 (1): 1–5.
74. Sakaguchi, W., Kubota, N., Shimizu, T. et al. (2020). Existence of SARS-CoV-2 entry molecules in the oral cavity. *Int. J. Mol. Sci.* 21 (17): E6000.
75. Szarpak, L., Rafique, Z., Gasecka, A. et al. (2021). A systematic review and meta-analysis of effect of vitamin D levels on the incidence of COVID-19. *Cardiol. J.* 28 (5): 647–654.
76. Halpert, G. and Shoenfeld, Y. (2020). SARS-CoV-2, the autoimmune virus. *Autoimmun. Rev.* 19 (12): 102695.
77. Björk, A., Mofors, J., and Wahren-Herlenius, M. (2020). Environmental factors in the pathogenesis of primary Sjögren's syndrome. *J. Intern. Med.* 287 (5): 475–492.
78. Bartoloni, E., Alunno, A., and Gerli, R. (2019). The dark side of Sjögren's syndrome: the possible pathogenic role of infections. *Curr. Opin. Rheumatol.* 31 (5): 505–511.
79. Furer, V., Rondaan, C., Heijstek, M.W. et al. (2020). 2019 update of EULAR recommendations for vaccination in adult patients with autoimmune inflammatory rheumatic diseases. *Ann. Rheum. Dis.* 79 (1): 39–52.
80. Segal, Y., Dahan, S., Sharif, K. et al. (2018). The value of autoimmune syndrome Induced by adjuvant (ASIA) – shedding light on orphan diseases in autoimmunity. *Autoimmun. Rev.* 17 (5): 440–448.
81. Rizzo, C., Grasso, G., Destro Castaniti, G.M. et al. (2020). Primary Sjögren syndrome: focus on innate immune cells and inflammation. *Vaccine* 8 (2): E272.
82. Soriano, A., Afeltra, A., and Shoenfeld, Y. (2014). Immunization with vaccines and Sjögren's syndrome. *Expert. Rev. Clin. Immunol.* 10 (4): 429–435.
83. Brito-Zerón, P., Kostov, B., Solans, R. et al. (2016). Systemic activity and mortality in primary Sjögren syndrome: predicting survival using the EULAR-SS disease activity index (ESSDAI) in 1045 patients. *Ann. Rheum. Dis.* 75 (2): 348–355.
84. Toussirot, E., Lohse, A., Wendling, D., and Mougin, C. (2000). Sjögren's syndrome occurring after hepatitis B vaccination. *Arthritis Rheum.* 43 (9): 2139–2140.
85. Bagavant, H., Nandula, S., Kaplonek, P. et al. (2013). Alum, an aluminum based adjuvant, induces Sjögren's syndrome-like disorder in mice. *Clin. Exp. Rheumatol.* 32: 251–255.
86. Pasoto, S.G., Ribeiro, A.C., Viana, V.S.T. et al. (2013). Short and long-term effects of pandemic unadjuvanted influenza A(H1N1)pdm09 vaccine on clinical manifestations and autoantibody profile in primary Sjögren's syndrome. *Vaccine* 31 (14): 1793–1798.
87. Brauner, S., Folkersen, L., Kvarnström, M. et al. (2017). H1N1 vaccination in Sjögren's syndrome triggers polyclonal B cell activation and promotes autoantibody production. *Ann. Rheum. Dis.* 76 (10): 1755–1763.
88. Guimarães, L.E., Baker, B., Perricone, C., and Shoenfeld, Y. (2015). Vaccines, adjuvants and autoimmunity. *Pharmacol. Res.* 100: 190–209.
89. Becerra-Gonzales, V.G., Alarcon-Calderon, A., Saint Croix, G., and De La Zerda, D. (2020). Autoimmune/autoinflammatory syndrome induced by adjuvants (ASIA) after a silicone injection. *BMJ Case Rep.* 13 (3): e234832.
90. Yu, L.T., Latorre, G., Marotta, J. et al. (1996). In vitro measurement of silicone bleed from breast implants. *Plast. Reconstr. Surg.* 97 (4): 756–764.
91. Bizjak, M., Selmi, C., Praprotnik, S. et al. (2015). Silicone implants and lymphoma: the role of inflammation. *J. Autoimmun.* 65: 64–73.
92. Watad, A., Bragazzi, N.L., Amital, H., and Shoenfeld, Y. (2019). Hyperstimulation of adaptive immunity as the common pathway for silicone breast implants, autoimmunity, and lymphoma of the breast. *Isr. Med. Assoc. J.* 21 (8): 517–519.

93. Okano, Y., Nishikai, M., and Sato, A. (1984). Scleroderma, primary biliary cirrhosis, and Sjögren's syndrome after cosmetic breast augmentation with silicone injection: a case report of possible human adjuvant disease. *Ann. Rheum. Dis.* 43 (3): 520–522.
94. Akyol, L., Önem, S., Özgen, M., and Sayarlıoğlu, M. (2015). Sjögren's syndrome after silicone breast implantation. *Eur. J. Rheumatol.* 2 (4): 165–166.
95. Watad, A., Rosenberg, V., Tiosano, S. et al. (2018). Silicone breast implants and the risk of autoimmune/rheumatic disorders: a real-world analysis. *Int. J. Epidemiol.* 47 (6): 1846–1854.
96. Suh, L.J., Khan, I., Kelley-Patteson, C. et al. (2022). Breast implant-associated immunological disorders. *J Immunol Res* 2022: 8536149.
97. Balk, E.M., Earley, A., Avendano, E.A., and Raman, G. (2016). Long-term health outcomes in women with silicone gel breast implants: a systematic review. *Ann. Intern. Med.* 164 (3): 164–175.
98. Coroneos, C.J., Selber, J.C., Offodile, A.C. et al. (2019). US FDA breast implant postapproval studies: long-term outcomes in 99,993 patients. *Ann. Surg.* 269 (1): 30–36.
99. Barber, C.M., Fishwick, D., Carder, M., and van Tongeren, M. (2019). Epidemiology of silicosis: reports from the SWORD scheme in the UK from 1996 to 2017. *Occup. Environ. Med.* 76 (1): 17–21.
100. Plavsic, A., Miskovic, R., Bolpacic, J. et al. (2015). Sjögren's syndrome and silicosis – a case report. *Open Access Maced. J. Med. Sci.* 3 (2): 326–330.
101. Astudillo, L., Sailler, L., Ecoiffier, M. et al. (2003). Exposure to silica and primary Sjögren's syndrome in a dental technician. *Rheumatol. Oxf. Engl.* 42 (10): 1268–1269.
102. Orriols, R., Ferrer, J., Tura, J.M. et al. (1997). Sicca syndrome and silicoproteinosis in a dental technician. *Eur. Respir. J.* 10 (3): 731–734.
103. Sanchez-Roman, J., Wichmann, I., Salaberri, J. et al. (1993). Multiple clinical and biological autoimmune manifestations in 50 workers after occupational exposure to silica. *Ann. Rheum. Dis.* 52 (7): 534–538.
104. Puisieux, F., Hachulla, E., Brouillard, M. et al. (1994). Silicosis and primary Gougerot-Sjögren syndrome. *Rev. Med. Interne* 15 (9): 575–579.
105. Ziebelman, A., Raibman-Spector, S., and Gendelman, O. (2022). Three's company: coexistence of silicosis, scleroderma, and Sjögren syndrome in a single patient. *Case Rep. Rheumatol.* 2022: 4487638.
106. Cappelli, L.C., Gutierrez, A.K., Bingham, C.O., and Shah, A.A. (2017). Rheumatic and Musculoskeletal immune-related adverse events due to immune checkpoint inhibitors: a systematic review of the literature. *Arthritis Care Res.* 69 (11): 1751–1763.
107. Cappelli, L.C., Gutierrez, A.K., Baer, A.N. et al. (2017). Inflammatory arthritis and sicca syndrome induced by nivolumab and ipilimumab. *Ann. Rheum. Dis.* 76 (1): 43–50.
108. Warner, B.M., Baer, A.N., Lipson, E.J. et al. (2019). Sicca syndrome associated with immune checkpoint inhibitor therapy. *Oncologist* 24 (9): 1259–1269.
109. Le Burel, S., Champiat, S., Mateus, C. et al. (2017). Prevalence of immune-related systemic adverse events in patients treated with anti-programmed cell death 1/anti-programmed cell death-ligand 1 agents: a single-centre pharmacovigilance database analysis. *Eur. J. Cancer Oxf. Engl.* 1990 (82): 34–44.
110. Ramos-Casals, M., Maria, A., Suárez-Almazor, M.E. et al. (2019). Sicca/Sjögren's syndrome triggered by PD-1/PD-L1 checkpoint inhibitors. Data from the international immunoCancer registry (ICIR). *Clin. Exp. Rheumatol.* 37 (3): 114–122.
111. Pringle, S., Wang, X., Vissink, A. et al. (2020). Checkpoint inhibition-induced sicca: a type II interferonopathy? *Clin. Exp. Rheumatol.* 38 (4): 253–260.
112. Christodoulou, M.I., Kapsogeorgou, E.K., and Moutsopoulos, H.M. (2010). Characteristics of the minor salivary gland infiltrates in Sjögren's syndrome. *J. Autoimmun.* 34 (4): 400–407.
113. Higashi, T., Miyamoto, H., Yoshida, R. et al. (2020). Sjögren's syndrome as an immune-related adverse event of nivolumab treatment for gastric cancer. *Intern. Med.* 59 (20): 2499–2504.
114. Ortiz Brugués, A., Sibaud, V., Herbault-Barrés, B. et al. (2020). Sicca syndrome induced by immune checkpoint inhibitor therapy: optimal management still pending. *Oncologist* 25 (2): e391–e395.
115. Mavragani, C.P. and Moutsopoulos, H.M. (2020). Sicca syndrome following immune checkpoint inhibition. *Clin. Immunol. Orlando. Fla.* 217: 108497.
116. Borba, V.V., Zandman-Goddard, G., and Shoenfeld, Y. (2018). Prolactin and autoimmunity. *Front. Immunol.* 9: 73.

117. Yang, L., Wei, W., He, X. et al. (2018). Influence of hormones on Sjögren's syndrome. *Curr. Pharm. Des.* 24 (35): 4167–4176.
118. Rojas, M., Rodríguez, Y., Ramírez-Santana, C., and Anaya, J.M. (2019). Impact of hyperprolactinemia in a patient with polyautoimmunity. *Clin. Case Rep.* 7 (1): 19–23.
119. Brandt, J.E., Priori, R., Valesini, G., and Fairweather, D. (2015). Sex differences in Sjögren's syndrome: a comprehensive review of immune mechanisms. *Biol. Sex Differ.* 6: 19.
120. Shim, G.J., Warner, M., Kim, H.J. et al. (2004). Aromatase-deficient mice spontaneously develop a lymphoproliferative autoimmune disease resembling Sjögren's syndrome. *Proc. Natl. Acad. Sci. U. S. A.* 101 (34): 12628–12633.
121. Ishimaru, N., Arakaki, R., Watanabe, M. et al. (2003). Development of autoimmune exocrinopathy resembling Sjögren's syndrome in estrogen-deficient mice of healthy background. *Am. J. Pathol.* 163 (4): 1481–1490.
122. Czerwinski, S., Mostafa, S., Rowan, V.S., and Azzarolo, A.M. Time course of cytokine upregulation in the lacrimal gland and presence of autoantibodies in a predisposed mouse model of Sjögren's Syndrome: the influence of sex hormones and genetic background. *Exp. Eye Res.* 128: 15–22. https://pubmed.ncbi.nlm.nih.gov/25218176/.
123. McCoy, S.S., Sampene, E., and Baer, A.N. (2020). Association of Sjögren's syndrome with reduced lifetime sex hormone exposure: a case-control study. *Arthritis Care Res.* 72 (9): 1315–1322.
124. Taiym, S., Haghighat, N., and Al-Hashimi, I. (2004). A comparison of the hormone levels in patients with Sjögren's syndrome and healthy controls. *Oral Surg. Oral Med. Oral Pathol. Oral Radiol. Endod.* 97 (5): 579–583.
125. Porola, P., Laine, M., Virtanen, I. et al. (2010). Androgens and integrins in salivary glands in Sjögren's syndrome. *J. Rheumatol.* 37 (6): 1181–1187.
126. Brennan, M.T., Sankar, V., Leakan, R.A. et al. (2003). Sex steroid hormones in primary Sjögren's syndrome. *J. Rheumatol.* 30 (6): 1267–1271.
127. Girón-González, J.A., Moral, F.J., Elvira, J. et al. (2000). Consistent production of a higher TH1:TH2 cytokine ratio by stimulated T cells in men compared with women. *Eur. J. Endocrinol.* 143 (1): 31–36.
128. Giltay, E.J., Fonk, J.C., von Blomberg, B.M. et al. (2000). In vivo effects of sex steroids on lymphocyte responsiveness and immunoglobulin levels in humans. *J. Clin. Endocrinol. Metab.* 85 (4): 1648–1657.
129. Borba, V.V., Zandman-Goddard, G., and Shoenfeld, Y. (2019). Prolactin and autoimmunity: the hormone as an inflammatory cytokine. *Best Pract. Res. Clin. Endocrinol. Metab.* 33 (6): 101324.
130. Vieira Borba, V. and Shoenfeld, Y. (2019). Prolactin, autoimmunity, and motherhood: when should women avoid breastfeeding? *Clin. Rheumatol.* 38 (5): 1263–1270.
131. Orbach, H. and Shoenfeld, Y. (2007). Hyperprolactinemia and autoimmune diseases. *Autoimmun. Rev.* 6 (8): 537–542.
132. El Miedany, Y.M., Ahmed, I., Moustafa, H., and El Baddini, M. (2004). Hyperprolactinemia in Sjögren's syndrome: a patient subset or a disease manifestation? *Joint Bone Spine.* 71 (3): 203–208.
133. Haga, H.J. and Rygh, T. (1999). The prevalence of hyperprolactinemia in patients with primary Sjögren's syndrome. *J. Rheumatol.* 26 (6): 1291–1295.
134. Chatzis, L.G., Goules, A.V., and Tzioufas, A.G. (2021). Searching for the "X factor" in Sjögren's syndrome female predilection. *Clin. Exp. Rheumatol.* 39 (6): 206–214.
135. Gorodetskiy, V., Probatova, N., Obukhova, T., and Vasilyev, V. (2021). Analysis of prognostic factors in diffuse large B-cell lymphoma associated with rheumatic diseases. *Lupus Sci. Med.* 8 (1): e000561.
136. Brito-Zerón, P., Ramos-Casals, M., Nardi, N. et al. (2005). Circulating monoclonal immunoglobulins in Sjögren syndrome: prevalence and clinical significance in 237 patients. *Medicine (Baltimore)* 84 (2): 90–97.
137. Christodoulou, M.I., Kapsogeorgou, E.K., Moutsopoulos, N.M., and Moutsopoulos, H.M. (2008). Foxp3$^+$ T-regulatory cells in Sjögren's syndrome: correlation with the grade of the autoimmune lesion and certain adverse prognostic factors. *Am. J. Pathol.* 173 (5): 1389–1396.
138. Koff, J.L., Rai, A., and Flowers, C.R. (2018). Characterizing autoimmune disease-associated diffuse large B-cell lymphoma in a SEER-medicare cohort. *Clin. Lymphoma Myeloma Leuk.* 18 (2): e115–e121.
139. Stergiou, I.E., Poulaki, A., and Voulgarelis, M. (2020). Pathogenetic mechanisms implicated in Sjögren's syndrome lymphomagenesis: a review of the literature. *J. Clin. Med.* 9 (12): E3794.

140. Avgoustis, N. and Exarchos, T. (2021). A DSS for predicting lymphoma in primary Sjögren's syndrome patients. *Adv. Exp. Med. Biol.* 1338: 7–11.
141. Theander, E., Manthorpe, R., and Jacobsson, L.T.H. (2004). Mortality and causes of death in primary Sjögren's syndrome: a prospective cohort study. *Arthritis Rheum.* 50 (4): 1262–1269.
142. Zhong, H., Liu, S., Wang, Y. et al. (2022). Primary Sjögren's syndrome is associated with increased risk of malignancies besides lymphoma: a systematic review and meta-analysis. *Autoimmun. Rev.* 21 (5): 103084.
143. Goulabchand, R., Malafaye, N., Jacot, W. et al. (2021). Cancer incidence in primary Sjögren's syndrome: data from the French hospitalization database. *Autoimmun. Rev.* 20 (12): 102987.

23 Gluteal Biopolymer Injections as a Case of ASIA Syndrome

Rojas-Villarraga Adriana[1], María Alejandra Martínez-Ceballos[2], Uribe Rosa[3], and Montealegre Giovanni[4]

[1]Research Institute, Fundación Universitaria de Ciencias de la Salud (FUCS), Bogotá, Colombia
[2]Fundación Oftalmológica Nacional, Bogotá, Colombia and School of Medicine and Health Sciences, Universidad del Rosario, Bogotá, Colombia
[3]Antioquia's Clinic, Itagüí, Colombia
[4]Fundación Universitaria de Ciencias de la Salud (FUCS), Hospital San José, Bogotá, Colombia

Introduction and overview

Recently, there has been an overall 5% increase in surgical and nonsurgical cosmetic procedures. The world leader is the United States with 18.4% (4,310,180 procedures), while other countries, such as Colombia (South America), rank sixth in the world with 2.2% (516,930 procedures) [1–3]. Injectable and resurfacing techniques play an important role in these procedures. Although hyaluronic acid filler is the only Food and Drug Administration (FDA)-approved substance, the use of analog substances from fillers not authorized by the FDA has become popular throughout the world and produces an impact on the health of those they are used on [4–7]. Different terms have been used to describe the disease caused by allogenic substances that are foreign to the body and injected by doctors or unauthorized personnel, e.g. "foreign modeling agent reactions," "allogenic disease," "Iatrogenic allogenosis," "disease by modeling," or "by biopolymers," and "human adjuvant diseases." In general, the materials used are prohibited substances such as industrial oils, silicone, methacrylate, collagen, and paraffin. The use of these substances in the short- or long-term causes diverse manifestations and complications for those who receive them [8–10]. Some authors think that these problems have reached epidemic proportions, especially in Latin America [11–15].

Nowadays, the concept of beauty is related to preestablished social paradigms or socially transformed stereotypes based on the era and culture [16, 17]. In fact, there have been several efforts to define it such as attempting to isolate the various phenotypical (i.e. physical) proportions underlying beauty (i.e. waist-to-hip ratio curvaceousness or the degree of "hourglass shape"). Therefore, many people focus their attention on the fat located on the buttocks in particular, and this influences some individuals to use fillers in that area [18]. According to recent statistics, there were 20,673 buttock augmentation procedures in the United States in 2016 [2]. In Colombia,

Autoimmune Disorders: Adjuvants and Other Risk Factors in Pathogenesis, First Edition.
Edited by Abdulla Watad, Nicola Luigi Bragazzi, and Yehuda Shoenfeld.

information is not complete due to a lack of registration. There are a number of unauthorized and "clandestine" sites with personnel whose training is unknown where these types of procedures are done, and fillers that have not been approved by regulatory agencies are used. This is, therefore, a public health problem because patients put their health and life at risk [19, 20].

In vitro cell effects of biopolymers

The deleterious effects on cell proliferation, cell viability, cytotoxicity effect, inflammatory responses, and expression of inflammatory cytokines in treated cells have been shown through some in vitro studies [21–28]. However, some in vitro studies have shown the absence of those effects, particularly in those that evaluated hyaluronic acid-based dermal filler [27, 29], hyaluronic acid cross-linked with polyethylene glycol [30], or hydroxyapatite spherical particles cross-linked with sodium hyaluronate [31] as well as calcium hydroxylapatite microspheres [32].

At this point, it is important to highlight that biopolymers are recently used in medical areas apart from cosmetic applications, such as cancer imaging identification and oncological therapies [33]. Radu et al. [34] developed in vitro studies using poly 3-hydroxybutyrate-*co*-3-hydroxyvalerate as targeted anticolorectal cancer nanocarrier (bio-nanocarrier) loaded with 5-fluorouracil; the research suggested low cytotoxicity, and it resulted efficiently to kill adenocarcinoma cells. In addition, Taghizadehghalehjoughi et al. [35] developed an in vitro and in vivo animal model with hydrochloride-loaded poly-lactic-*co*-glycolic acid nanoparticles for the treatment of glioblastoma multiforme; the findings were promising due to the results related to significant volume reduction of the extracted tumor. On the other hand, biopolymers are under research in diverse fields of medicine, such as biopolymeric films as delivery vehicles for controlled release of medications to treat chronic skin diseases [36]; natural and synthetic polymer nanocomposites in bone tissue regeneration [37]; 3D-printed biopolymeric encapsulation system for the transplantation of endocrine cells [38]; structured medical hemostatic sponges as a medical devices to stop bleeding and to close the wound [39]; nanodrug carrier for treating rheumatoid arthritis [40]; and biopolymer-based scaffolds for corneal stromal regeneration [41]. These are some examples of potential biopolymers applications; however, through this chapter, we focus on plastic surgery uses.

Clinical consequences of the cosmetic application of biopolymers

The body areas, in cosmetic procedures, where the unknown materials (biopolymers) are most frequently injected are buttocks (8–72%) and breasts (12–16%) [11, 42, 43]. This causes local complications such as ulcers, livedo reticularis, and nodules. The gluteal area is of specific interest because the musculature of this region controls the movements of the hip and supports the back and the iliotibial tract [44, 45]. Therefore, a sitting position will generate more pressure and worsen symptoms. It is also the area that suffers trauma when patients self-medicate with intramuscular medications. What is also well known is that the migration of foreign materials to the lower back is a frequent complication when they are infiltrated subcutaneously. Likewise, when the infiltration is deep, the material migrates to the lower inguinal region, perineum, and lower limbs. It also enters and moves through the endolymphatic tract [8, 42, 43].

The general course of foreign body modeling reaction is quite variable. The spectrum of manifestations fluctuates from mild to severe, depending on the amount of substance infiltrated, the area of application, and the length of exposure as well as other variables (Table 23.1) [46–57]. The initial manifestations usually correspond to a local inflammatory process characterized by pain and continuous or intermittent hyperemia that lasts several months or years after the application of the modeling substance. Subsequently, the migration of the substance to peripheral or distal areas takes place with similar manifestations, progressive local and distant hyperpigmentation, development of a collateral venous network, cutaneous atrophy, and the formation of ulcers. Depending

Table 23.1 Diverse complications by filler type.

Filler type	Clinical complications[a]	In vitro deleterious effects
Calcium hydroxylapatite (caHA)	Infection, pain, swelling, necrosis, arterial embolization, nodule, blindness[b], and blanching[c] [46–49]	• Increases in the secretion of TNF-α, IL-1, IL-8, IL-10, and proMMP-2 and -9 and decreases in the secretion of IL-6 in monocytes culture exposed to caHA[d] [21]
Collagen	Discoloration, blindness[b], maldistribution, infection, skin necrosis, granuloma formation, and foreign body reactions [48, 50]	• Collagen coated with PLLA was phagocyted by one in vitro cell line, and TNF-α was released in cultured cells [22]
Hyaluronic acid	Swelling, infection, nodule, pain, arterial embolization, bleeding, blindness[b], blanching[c], and Tyndall effect[e] [46–49, 51]	• Hyaluronic acid supported the growth of bacterial biofilm in vitro. Multiple needle passes through a biofilm-contaminated surface that resulted in significantly increased contamination of filler material[f] • In a murine in vitro culture system,135-kDa fragments of the hyaluronan induced dendritic cell maturation and initiated alloimmunity acting as an innate immune agonist • In an in vitro analysis, three cellular lines (two keratinocyte cell lines and one human dermal fibroblast) were cultured and exposed to hyaluronic acid cross-linked with 1,4-BDDE or with PEG. PEG-treated cells showed markedly lower cytotoxicity, ROS production, and inflammatory responses than BDDE-treated cells [23–25]
Liquid silicone (oil)[g]	Allergies, blindness[b], inflammatory reactions, migration, granulomatous reactions, rejection, silicone embolism syndrome, ulcers, skin dyschromia, and infections [48, 52, 53]	• Silicone microparticles were phagocyted by one in vitro cell line • Immunoreactivity to medical-grade silicone dermal filler was evaluated in vitro in PBMC. Silicone induced a release of pro-inflammatory cytokines but does not act as a polyclonal activator of CD4+ T cells [22, 26]
Paraffin	Blindness[b], inflammation, infection, embolism, yellowish skin plaques, granulomatous foreign-body reaction (paraffinoma), fistulization, migration, and scarring [48, 54]	
Polyacrylamide hydrogel[h]	Allergic reaction, blindness[b], hypersensitivity reactions, migration, contour abnormalities, abnormal skin sensation, pain, induration, malignant breast tumors, aseptic inflammation, leakage, and hematoma [48, 55, 56]	• Growth of bacterial biofilm in vitro[f] [23]

(Continued)

Table 23.1 (*Continued*)

Filler type	Clinical complications[a]	In vitro deleterious effects
Poly-L-lactic acid (PLLA)	Nodule, granuloma, infection, pain, swelling, bleeding, blindness[b], and paresthesia [46–48, 57]	• Growth of bacterial biofilm in vitro[f] • Cultures exposed to PLLA exhibited a reduction in both cell proliferation and viability compared to control in all time points Histologic analysis showed the presence of multinucleated cells • HAEC were treated with different volume percentages of extract of predegraded PLLA in vitro, and the cell growth curve and morphological changes were examined. The extract of PLLA caused significant growth inhibition and release of NF-κB, VEGF, and VCAM-1 in HAEC with volume percentage dependence [23, 27]
Polymethyl methacrylate[i] (PMMA)	Nodule, localized foreign body reaction, anaphylaxis, blindness[b], infection, and biofilm[j] [47, 48, 51]	• Three in vitro different cell lines could phagocytose polymethylmethacrylate microspheres (<20 μm). • In vitro studies reveal that macrophages rapidly released arachidonic acid and derived inflammatory mediators in response to PMMA particles. However, cells exposed to PMMA are lethally damaged, as reflected by the subsequent leakage of their intracellular LDH [22, 28]

BDDE, Butanediol diglycidyl ether; caHA, Calcium hydroxylapatite; CD4+ T, T lymphocyte (helper); HAEC, Human aortic endothelial cells; IL-1, Interleukin1; IL-10, Interleukin 10; IL-8, Interleukin 8; kDa, Kilodaltons (molecular weight); LDH, Lactate dehydrogenase; NF-κB, Nuclear factor kappa beta; PBMC, Peripheral blood mononuclear cells; PEG, Polyethylene glycol; PLLA, Poly-L-lactic acid; proMMP, Prometalloproteinase; ROS, Reactive oxygen species; TNF-α, Tumor necrosis factor alpha; VCAM-1, Vascular cell adhesion molecule 1; VEGF, Vascular endothelial growth factor.

[a] Most of them from case report, case series, regulatory agencies databases, or medical malpractice litigation databases. Majority of the reports injected in facial area. All of them can produce minor or transient effects such as edema, erythema, mild pain, and ecchymosis.
[b] Facial injection and vascular complications.
[c] Pallor or blanching phase secondary to intraarterial injection.
[d] This was evaluated using nanoporous hydroxyapatite powders synthesized by hard or soft templating but not using other presentations.
[e] Bluish hue that is visible within the skin caused by too superficial placement of dermal filler.
[f] Similar results were shown for polyacrylamide gel and poly-L-lactic acid.
[g] Prohibited by the regulatory agencies due to the evidence of severe side effects.
[h] Mainly reported in breast augmentation with polyacrylamide hydrogel injections.
[i] Microspheres frequently suspended in a water-based carrier gel composed of bovine collagen.
[j] Most frequent with permanent fillers.

on the depth of the infiltration, the substance may be deposited on the fascia, thus affecting the skin with an additional compromise of subcutaneous cellular tissue and the underlying muscles. In Table 23.1, different filler types, the clinical complications, and the in vitro deleterious effects are shown.

ASIA syndrome and gluteal biopolymers

At the systemic level, the patient may develop polyarthralgia, myalgias, and cognitive and sleep disorders. These manifestations have been observed in 60% of the patients who have the autoimmune/inflammatory syndrome induced by adjuvants (ASIA) [58, 59]. Shoenfeld and Agmon-Levin described ASIA syndrome [58, 60] in 2011. The scientific academy has accepted the clinical criteria that Shoenfeld and coworkers recommended for ASIA syndrome [58, 61]. Several of the mechanisms in the pathological pathways of ASIA syndrome include genetic factors [43, 62], innate immune dysregulation, release of inflammatory cytokines, T-cell impairment, altered balance between Th1 and Th2 immune response with an excessive Th1 immune response, specific antigen-driven local immune response through activated Th17 cells, B-cell activation, and epigenetic modifications [63, 64]. Therefore, this disease consists of an antigen-specific response to an adjuvant substance due to its ability to produce widespread activation of various immune cells and inflammatory pathways [58, 65]. As a result, the innate and adaptive immune response is activated, which then increases the local and systemic reaction to antigens by the release of chemokines and cytokines, which, in susceptible individuals, may ultimately lead to the development of autoimmune diseases [63].

A high percentage of patients with foreign body-induced ASIA may develop autoimmune diseases as shown by Cohen Tervaert and Kappel [66] where 50% of patients suffering from silicone implant incompatibility syndrome and associated ASIA syndrome developed a systemic autoimmune disease. Furthermore, Watad et al. [67] found that, compared with women without foreign body modeling agents, the risk of developing an autoimmune disease increased 45%.

Biopolymers have been recognized as adjuvants triggering ASIA syndrome since they are part of the "autoimmune ecology" (i.e. complex interactions between individuals and their environment and the associated mechanisms that lead to a breakdown in immune tolerance and, therefore, to the development of autoimmune diseases) [64, 68].

We performed a comprehensive literature review using PubMed database up to 25 October 2021. Data for this review included ASIA syndrome and specific autoimmune diseases related to biomaterials injected into the gluteal (buttocks) area. The following Medical Subject Heading (MeSH) terms were used: "Rheumatoid arthritis," "Systemic lupus erythematosus," "Arthritis, Rheumatoid," "Dermatomyositis," "Scleroderma," "Antiphospholipid syndrome," "Sjögren's syndrome," "Immunology," and "Autoantibodies," and the key words: "ASIA" and "Autoimmune." Each one was cross-referenced with the following key words: "Adjuvants," "Liquid silicone," "Biopolymer," "Mineral oil," "Bioimplants," "Dermal fills," "Biomaterials," "Plastic surgery," "Paraffin," "Foreign body," "Foreign modeling agent reaction," "NASHA," "Silicone medical grade," "Hyaluronic acid," "Methacrylate," "Methyl methacrylate," "Polyalkylimide," "Collagen," "Rpoly L lactic acid," and "Buttocks," or "Gluteal." Study identification was not restricted by year of publication, language, or country of origin, but it was restricted to humans. The preferred reporting items for systematic reviews and meta-analysis (PRISMA) guidelines were followed in data extraction, analysis, and reporting [69]. The first screening was done by title, and the second by title and abstract when the title did not offer enough information. All the retrieved records were loaded into a database by title, abstract, and PubMed Unique Identifier [PMID number] [Microsoft Excel software® (v. 2013)], after which duplicated records were removed using the PMID. Full-text articles were downloaded into the Mendeley reference manager software (Desktop platform). The articles that were finally included were organized by means of the Microsoft Excel software® (v. 2013). The inclusion criteria were case series or case reports of patients with a diagnosis of ASIA syndrome based on Shoenfeld's criteria [58], or autoimmune diseases diagnosed by internationally validated criteria, and a medical history of infiltration of biopolymers. The exclusion criteria for the first and second screening phases were the following: the title or abstract was not related to ASIA syndrome or autoimmune diseases, the article was related to implant surgery (any material) in breasts or buttocks, it only reported on surgical techniques or complications associated with the procedure, or it did not mention the infiltrated area.

To guarantee the methodological quality of the literature review and avoid the risk of bias in selection of case series and case reports, case report guidelines (CARE) [70] were used, and a high-quality article received a score greater than 10.

Records identified through a database search (PubMed) went up to 11,946. The first screening was done by title (n =96); duplicated records were discarded (n =62); and articles were hand-searched (n =5), resulting in a total of 67 for the first screening (n =63). After the second screening based on the abstract (n =32) and full-text review (n =11), all of them were included: case series and case reports (n =7), prospective cohort (n =2), and cross-sectional (n =2). To recap, the total population of included articles was 352 patients, 95.4% (n =336) had ASIA syndrome; and female gender was the most affected with 90.7% (n =305). The number of patients with ASIA syndrome and/or autoimmune disease in case reports and case [42, 71–76] was 61. Prospective cohort studies [10, 77] reported a sample of 51 patients, 68.6% (n =35) had ASIA syndrome, and 8.5% (n =3) received substances injection in buttocks. Concerning cross-sectional studies [43, 78], they included 240 subjects with ASIA syndrome, and 94% (n =226) of these patients had received biopolymer injections in the gluteal area. Case series and case reports were evaluated with the CARE strategy. All of them had a score greater than 10, which indicated a low risk of bias. The main characteristics of the included studies are shown in Table 23.2.

Authors' experience with patients with biopolymers in the gluteal area and ASIA syndrome

We previously published [3] a case series including first-time consecutive subjects who attended to the plastic surgery department with clinical manifestations of foreign body modeling (i.e. Iatrogenic allogenosis) reaction between May 2016 and December 2016 after the injection of biopolymers or unknown substances in the gluteal region. Those patients were evaluated and followed until 2018 in a search for ASIA syndrome or immunological diseases based on international criteria [ACR/EULAR guidelines for systemic lupus erythematosus (2019), rheumatoid arthritis (2010), and Sjögren's syndrome (2016), respectively].

At baseline, a detailed clinical evaluation and verification of fulfillment of inclusion and exclusion criteria (previous autoimmune disease or neoplastic disease before the exposure to allogenic substances) were done [79]. Follow-up visits every three months with clinical evaluation were done. Clinical evaluation included demographic data, present or previous comorbidities, and familial background (including familial autoimmunity toxic exposure, obstetric outcomes, and other comorbidities). Complete rheumatological examination searching for autoimmune diseases (by a rheumatologist) based on fulfilled standard validated criteria (baseline for exclusion criteria and follow-up) was done. Muscular strength evaluation (MRC) [80], unstimulated whole salivary flow [81], and fatigue based on the functional assessment of chronic illness therapy (FACIT) [82] (those positive were evaluated using the Spanish version of the Fatigue Severity Scale) [83] were measured.

Information regarding biopolymers was collected (date of polymer infiltration, type and volume of the injected substance, area of infiltration, and latency time with foreign body modeling reaction). Diagnostic images were taken, and laboratory tests were done at baseline and repeated annually. Laboratory analysis included acute-phase reactants [C-reactive protein (CRP) and erythrocyte sedimentation rate (ESR)], liver function tests and immunological profile [immunoglobulin levels (IgG-IgM)], Antinuclear Antibodies (ANAs), Antineutrophil Cytoplasmic Antibodies (ANCAs), Rheumatoid Factor (RF), Thyroid Stimulating Hormone (TSH), Free Thyroxine (T4), Antithyroglobulin Antibody Test, and Thyroid Peroxidase Antibody test (TPO).

Table 23.2 Main characteristics of studies including patients with biopolymer gluteal injections and ASIA syndrome development.

Author	Year	*n*	Gluteal area	Diagnostic	Treatment
Pachón S JE	2021	190	190	190 ASIA syndrome	190 Open surgery
López-Mendoza J	2021	11	11	11 ASIA syndrome	4 Ultrasonic-assisted liposuction 4 Open "*en bloc*" excision and primary closure 3 Open "*en bloc*" excision and microsurgical reconstruction 7 Received previous medical treatment
Ali S	2021	1	1	ASIA syndrome induced by liquid silicone	NR
Vera-Lastra O	2020	1	1	ASIA syndrome induced by methyl methacrylate associated with seronegative antiphospholipid syndrome and diffuse large B-cell non-Hodgkin's lymphoma	Cyclophosphamide, doxorubicin, vincristine, prednisone, and rituximab (four cycles)
Alijotas-Reig	2018	45	4/45	45/45 ASIA syndrome 13/45 autoimmune thyroiditis 11/45 panniculitis 8/45 early UCTD 5/45 type 1 diabetes mellitus 3/45 Sjögren's syndrome 3/45 Systemic sclerosis 3/45 seropositive polyarthritis 3/45 leukocytoclastic vasculitis 3/45 Sarcoidosis 2/45 localized scleroderma 2/45 overlap syndrome 2/45 mesenteric panniculitis 2/45 Guillain–Barré 2/45 Crohn's disease 1/45 multiple sclerosis 1/45 ulcerative colitis 1/45 SLE	43/45 Prednisone 33/45 plus chloroquine 19/45 plus NSAIDs 12/45 plus antihistamines 12/45 plus allopurinol 10/45 plus tacrolimus 10/45 surgical procedure
Jara LJ	2017	1	1/1	ASIA syndrome Hemolytic anemia CREST syndrome	Methylprednisolone pulses Danazol Prednisone
Barilaro G	2016	1	1/1	ASIA syndrome	Prednisone
Flores Padilla	2014	1	1/1	ASIA syndrome + RA	Prednisone
Stanford N	2013	36	3/36	20/36 ASIA syndrome	NR
Alijotas-Reig J	2012	15	2/15	ASIA syndrome 2/15 Sjögren's syndrome 2/15 Sicca syndrome 2/15 cutaneous sarcoidosis 2/15 vasculitis 2/15 Morphea/scleroderma 2/15 UCTD	Cyclophosphamide and methotrexate Prednisone Hydroxychloroquine Cetirizine

(*Continued*)

Table 23.2 (*Continued*)

Author	Year	*n*	Gluteal area	Diagnostic	Treatment
Vera-Lastra O	2012	50	36/50	50/50 ASIA syndrome 30/50 autoimmune-rheumatic diseases 20/50 SLE 6/50 Fibromyalgia	Prednisone Methylprednisolone Cyclophosphamide D-penicillamine Colchicine

ASIA, (autoimmune/inflammatory disease induced by adjuvants), CREST syndrome (limited scleroderma); NR, Not reported; NSAID, Nonsteroids anti-inflammatory drugs; RA, Rheumatoid arthritis; SLE, Systemic lupus erythematosus; UCTD, Undifferentiated connective tissue disease.

Of a total of 5014 patients who came during the observation period, 66 had biopolymer gluteal infiltration, only 13 met the inclusion criteria of "first-time clinic visit," while the remaining 53 who came only for follow-up visits were excluded. All of the 13 subjects had received biopolymer injections in the buttocks and were included. Two of them did not complete the two years of follow-up and decided to not provide more information about their clinical history. One patient died during follow-up. In the end, the completed study included 10 ($n = 10$) patients. Aesthetic procedures had been done on all of them in "clandestine clinics" by staff whose training is unknown. Eleven subjects were women, and two were men with gender dysphoria. The mean age was 38.3 years (SD 8.48). Most of the patients were injected with unknown substances. Three received injections of known substances. Two of the three received injections of mineral oil, and one of Biogel. All of them developed local manifestations of foreign body modeling reaction.

The average time between the infiltration of the substance and clinical manifestations of foreign body modeling reaction was 27.8 months (SD 8.48). More than 50% of the patients had familial autoimmunity, and some of them had been exposed to other toxics, and seven patients had had additional aesthetic procedures done. There were no differences in the presentation of the clinical manifestations between those patients who had previous aesthetic procedures and those who did not. During follow-up, three patients developed hypothyroidism, one of whom had elevated antithyroglobulin antibodies. None were positive for other autoantibodies. One patient had elevated IgG/IgM (the other five patients who were evaluated had normal levels). Furthermore, nine patients (out of 12) had an elevated ESR at the last follow-up appointment, while two who had had an elevated ESR at the beginning returned to a normal level. In the case of CRP, 13 had normal levels at the beginning, and the 12 remaining in the study had normal levels at the end. Liver function was elevated in three patients for the first year with normalization during follow-up. Nine patients used oral contraceptive methods. One patient had an alteration in unstimulated whole salivary flow. One woman had 4/5 strength in her lower limbs. The mean FACIT score was 40.6 (SD 9.6). Three patients had significant fatigue (FACIT and high score in the Fatigue Severity Scale). The main patients' characteristics are shown in Table 23.3.

Regarding ASIA diagnosis, 11 patients met Shoenfeld's criteria for ASIA syndrome (see Table 23.4), but three patients were incompletely evaluated for clinical symptoms of ASIA (patients 10, 11, and 13), and four had a very low clinical ASIA score (patients 2, 3, 7, and 12).

Therapeutic approach

The therapeutic approach to this type of pathology is complex because of the diverse anatomical areas in which the modeling material is infiltrated, and the different techniques used. In fact, the approach will differ based on the depth at which the material is placed. Also, in cases where surgery cannot be done or the symptoms are persistent, medical treatment is used [62, 84].

Table 23.3 Clinical characteristics of patients, biopolymer extraction, surgical procedures, and clinical results.

	Age (years)	Gender	Familial AID	Personal AID	Has the material been removed?/ Did the removal induce clinical improvement?	Other cosmetic procedures/ toxic exposure	UWSF	Muscular strength (MRC) Superior/ inferior limbs	FACIT	FSS
1	34	Female	SS[a]	Thyroid disease in pregnancy[b]	No/NA	Mammoplasty augmentation and liposuction/tattoo and hair dyes	N	5/4	25	46
2	44	Female	SS[a]	N	Yes[c]/Yes	Mammoplasty augmentation and liposuction/tattoo and hair dyes	N	5/5	47	9
3	37	Female	N	N	Yes[c]/Yes	N/hair dyes	N	5/5	46	9
4	35	Female	N	Subclinical hypo-thyroidism[b]	Yes[d]/No	Liposuction and lipectomy/tattoo, hair dyes, and muriatic acid	N	5/5	30	59
5	52	Female	Psoriasis[e]	N	No/No	N/tattoo and hair dyes	P	5/5	48	16
6	45	Female	Rheumatoid arthritis[f], hyper-thyroidism[g]	N	Yes[c,d]/Yes	Mammoplasty augmentation and liposuction/tattoo and hair dyes	N	5/5	31	36
7	40	Female	Diabetes type 1[h]	N	No/NA	N/hair dyes and piercing	N	5/5	41	10
8	25	Female	Antiphospholipid syndrome[f], psoriasis[i], and vitiligo[j]	N	Yes[c]/Yes	NA/tattoo	N	5/5	38	37
9	46	Female	Hypothyroidism[f,g]	Hypothyroidism[b]	Yes[c,d]/Yes	Lipectomy/tattoo and hair dyes	N	5/5	50	9

(Continued)

Table 23.3 *(Continued)*

	Age (years)	Gender	Familial AID	Personal AID	Has the material been removed?/ Did the removal induce clinical improvement?	Other cosmetic procedures/ toxic exposure	UWSF	Muscular strength (MRC) Superior/ inferior limbs	FACIT	FSS
10[k]	40	Male	N	N	Yes[l]/No	NA	NA	NA	NA	NA
11[m]	31	Female	NA	NA	No/NA	Mammoplasty augmentation and lipectomy	NA	NA	NA	NA
12	31	Male	N	N	No/NA	Sex reassignment[b], mammoplasty augmentation[b], facial feminization surgery[b], rhinoplasty[b]/ hair dyes	N	5/5	50	9
13[m]	39	Female	NA	NA	No/NA	NA	NA	NA	NA	NA

AID, Autoimmune disease; SS, Sjögren's syndrome; FACIT, Functional Assessment of Chronic Illness Therapy (higher score indicates better quality of life); FSS, Fatigue Severity Scale; MRC, Medical Research Council; N, Negative; NA, Not available; P, Positive; UWSF, Unstimulated whole salivary flow rate (positive if ≤1.5 mm/15 min).

[a] Aunt.
[b] After biopolymer injection.
[c] Butterfly wings technique.
[d] Assisted liposuction (extrainstitutional).
[e] Son.
[f] Mother.
[g] Sister.
[h] Niece.
[i] Cousin.
[j] Uncle.
[k] Death.
[l] Surgical debridement and washout.
[m] Lost follow-up.

Table 23.4 Shoenfeld's criteria for ASIA syndrome.

Patients	Major criteria									Minor criteria			ASIA diagnosis
		"Typical" clinical manifestations											
	Exposure to an external stimuli (infection, vaccine, and silicone) prior to clinical manifestations	Myalgia, myositis, or muscle weakness	Arthralgia and/or arthritis	Chronic fatigue, unrefreshing sleep, or sleep disturbances	Neurological manifestations (especially associated with demyelination)	Cognitive impairment, memory loss	Pyrexia, dry mouth	Removal of inciting agent induces improvement	Typical biopsy of involved organs	The appearance of autoantibodies directed at the suspected adjuvant	Other clinical manifestations (e.g. irritable bowel syndrome)	Evolvement into an autoimmune disease (i.e. MS and SSc)	
1	p	p	p	p	n	p	n	n	na	n		Subclinical hypothyroidism	p
2	p	n	p	n	n	p	n	p	p	n	Iron deficiency anemia, bronchitis	n	p
3	p	n	p	n	n	n	n	p	na	n	Carpal tunnel syndrome	n	p
4	p	p	p	p	n	p	p	n	na	n	Depression, gastroesophageal reflux	Subclinical hypothyroidism	p
5	p	p	p	p	n	p	p	na	na	n	Gastric ulcer, hemorrhoids, facial palsy, blepharospasm, depression, and bradycardia	n	p
6	p	n	n	p	n	n	p	p	na	n	Neurocardiogenic syncope	n	p

(*Continued*)

Table 23.4 *(Continued)*

Patients	Major criteria										Minor criteria		ASIA diagnosis
	"Typical" clinical manifestations												
	Exposure to an external stimuli (infection, vaccine, and silicone) prior to clinical manifestations	Myalgia, myositis, or muscle weakness	Arthralgia and/or arthritis	Chronic fatigue, unrefreshing sleep, or sleep disturbances	Neurological manifestations (especially associated with demyelination)	Cognitive impairment, memory loss	Pyrexia, dry mouth	Removal of inciting agent induces improvement	Typical biopsy of involved organs	The appearance of autoantibodies directed at the suspected adjuvant	Other clinical manifestations (e.g. irritable bowel syndrome)	Evolvement into an autoimmune disease (i.e. MS and SSc)	
7	p	n	n	p	n	n	n	na	na	na	Migraine, gastritis, gastroesophageal reflux disease, and recurrent bacterial vaginosis	n	p
8	p	p	p	p	n	n	n	p	p	n	Gastritis, irritable bowel syndrome, and recurrent urinary tract infection	n	p
9	p	n	p	p	n	p	p	p	p	n	N	Hypothyroidism	p
10[a]	p	p	p	p	na	na	na	n	p	n	N	n	p
11[b]	p	na	na	na	na	na	na	na	na	na	Na	na	na
12	p	n	p	n	n	n	n	na	na	n	N	n	p
13[b]	p	na	na	na	na	na	na	na	na	na	Na	na	na

MS, Multiple sclerosis; n, Negative; na, Not available; p, Positive; SSc, Systemic sclerosis.
Patients recruited in the study for following. The diagnosis of the disease is made with two major criteria or one major plus two minor criteria.
[a] Patient died, during follow-up.
[b] Lost follow-up.
Source: Table taken and adapted from: Shoenfeld and Agmon-Levin [58].

Several surgical techniques have been proposed, which include extensive surgical resection and subsequent reconstruction using local or microsurgical flaps, particularly when the disease affects the mammary and facial areas [85, 86]. There is no standard treatment for gluteal complications from injections of foreign materials [43], and, in addition, the scientific literature is scarce. Gordillo-Hernández et al. [9] retrospectively describe a cohort of 128 patients with human modeling disease, of which 86 cases involved the gluteal region. Although they do not report the exact number of those for whom the material was extracted, they highlighted the use of surgical procedures when medical treatment has failed. They showed that the procedure requires very extensive resections since the substances generally affect the whole anatomical region involved and are widely scattered. Furthermore, the resection causes significant skin-covering defects, which require grafts or flaps of various sizes and generally result in poor and disappointing aesthetic results for patient and surgeons. Martínez Villarreal et al. [11] describe a retrospective case series of 23 patients with foreign modeling agent reaction, 38.5% in buttocks, all of whom had several skin changes such as sclerosis and ulceration as well as systemic complications. Only in the case of 11 patients did they describe a treatment that generally consisted of standard wound technique healing and diverse debridement modalities including surgical debridement with removal of infiltrated areas and reconstructive procedures. They highlighted the fact that surgical removal can be difficult, given that large amounts of injected modeling agent tend to mix with healthy tissue. Other techniques mentioned included conventional liposuction, ultrasound-assisted liposuction, and bloc removal of modeling agents [87].

There is limited and conflicting information regarding the treatment. In some cases, it is necessary to remove the unknown injected substance because of the risk of infection, scarring, severe granulomatous, or inflammatory reaction with significant fibrosis. In addition, there is a lack of information about the criteria for removing the material based on ASIA criteria. This should be considered for upcoming research. That is why our research group proposed a new surgical technique called the "butterfly wings technique." The proposed technique allows a bloc extraction of the exogenous substance with marked improvement in local and systemic symptoms and quality of life. Also, this technique gives good aesthetic results. There was a clinical improvement for all our patients after surgery (five patients of our published case series underwent surgery). The surgical technique (developed by Dr. Montealegre G) is based on the same procedures used for the management of postbariatric patients. This requires the resection of the excess skin after the patient has lost massive weight. Preoperative markings are drawn in the standing position. They consist of sketching a design in the medial area near the intergluteal cleft without exceeding the upper limit of this cleft and without going below the intragluteal fold (Figure 23.1). There are some complications with our technique such as late seroma. However, approximately 80% of the procedure is done by means of a biopolymer bloc removal, the harmony of the gluteal area is maintained, and the surgical wound can be hidden by the underwear.

Other authors have proposed an open meticulous approach safer and keeper technique [78], ultrasonic-assisted liposuction, open *"en bloc"* excision and primary closure, and open *"en bloc"* excision and microsurgical reconstruction with good clinical results [74].

To draw the conclusion regarding surgical procedures, the extraction of biopolymers may be done on asymptomatic patients with a history of immunological disease not justified. Instead, the patient's risk criteria must be considered, mainly taking into account that possibly one of the first steps between the biopolymer injection and later development of ASIA syndrome is the of foreign body modeling reaction (Figure 23.2). Most patients see an improvement in the local and systemic symptoms as well as in their quality of life after the surgical procedure in our experience (Figure 23.3).

Some patients with foreign body modeling reaction have been treated with colchicine for the granulomatous reaction to foreign bodies in response to the injection of exogenous oily substances (mineral, vegetable, or animal) into the dermis or subcutaneous tissue for aesthetic purposes [88, 89]. An improvement has been seen in local manifestations, but a specific immunomodulatory

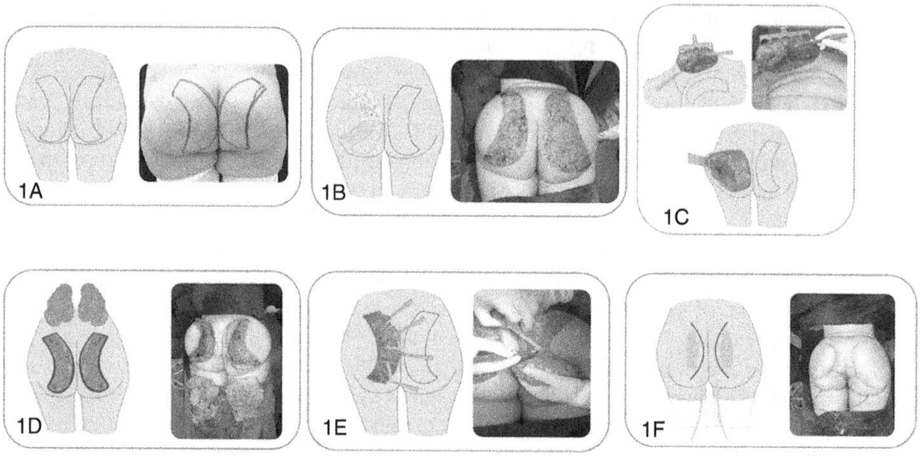

Figure 23.1. Butterfly wings design technique. (a) Preoperative markings are done in the standing position. (b) De-epithelization of the flap. (c) The cellular subcutaneous tissue is dissected to the gluteus major muscle fascia, and subcutaneous tissue elevated to find biopolymers. (d) Bloc resection of biopolymer. (e) Four de-epithelized medial flaps are cut, and each is folded over on itself. Then, they are fixed separately to the muscular fascia. (f) Closed by layers (fat and derma) with polyglactin and a negative pressure system is left and fixed.

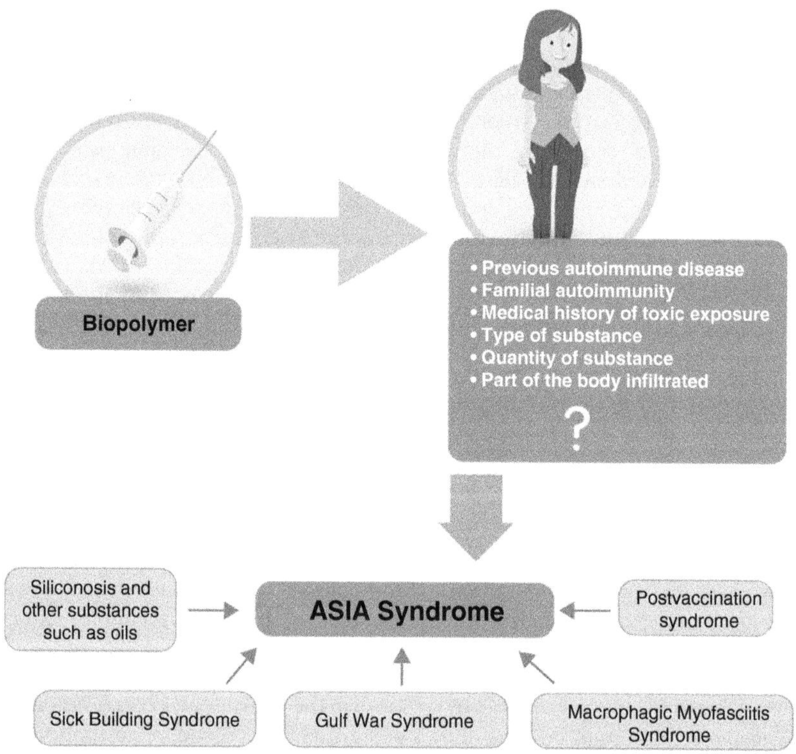

Figure 23.2. Foreign body modeling reaction as a precursor of ASIA syndrome.

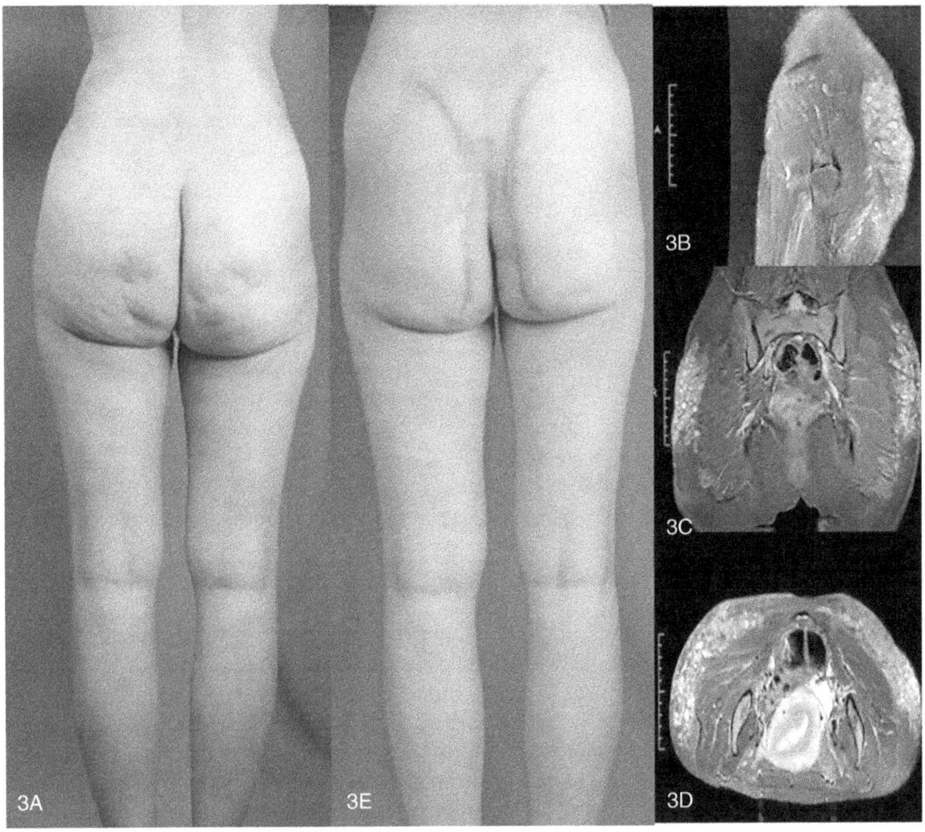

Figure 23.3. Clinical case of a woman with biopolymer injection, magnetic resonance image (MRI) findings, and results after surgery. (a) Presurgical photograph of a 45-year-old woman with a 10-year history. Infiltration of an unknown substance at the level of the buttocks. Changes at the skin level such as hyperpigmentation, nodules, and irregularities are observed. (b) Axial plane of MRI. (c) The sagittal plane of MRI. (d) The coronal plane of MRI. On the three images, a diffuse alteration in the signal intensity of subcutaneous cellular fat tissue on gluteal regions and slight involvement of superficial muscle fibers of the greater gluteus on both sides are observed. (e) Seven months postoperative.

treatment for the manifestations related to foreign body modeling reaction and ASIA cannot yet be established.

Conclusions

Taking the chain-of-events relationship between foreign body modeling reaction and ASIA syndrome, it is our suggestion that this reaction could be considered part of the spectrum of the disease, possibly one of the first steps between the biopolymer injection and later development of ASIA syndrome (Figure 23.2). Gonzalez et al. [90] demonstrated the variable, multiorganic, toxic, immunological, progressive, and fatal outcomes that are triggered following the infiltration

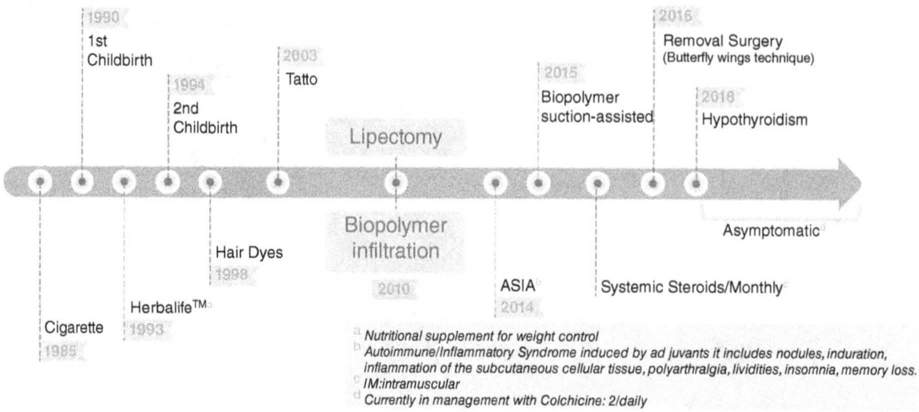

Figure 23.4. Timeline of a patient with some toxic risk factors and biopolymer gluteal injections. Part of the content of the chapter and the tables and figures are published in DOI: 10.1016/j.toxrep.2021.01.011. The publisher license for this copyrighted material was provided by Elsevier and Copyright Clearance Center (License Number 5176511160703).

of some substances by means of an animal model which reproduced pathological effects following infiltration of the substances commonly causing foreign body modeling reaction.

In our previous published case series [3], we found a significant familial autoimmunity background. This, therefore, supports the hypothesis of a predisposed, genetically susceptible host, (i.e. familial autoimmunity or familial autoimmune disease history) who receives two or more different stimuli and then develops an adaptive and innate immune response alteration, which increases the risk of an abnormal clinical response. A total exposure effect on individuals with a genetic predisposition can be hypothesized [68]. An explanatory case from our previous published case series is shown in Figure 23.4. This case shows a possible total exposure effect leading to ASIA syndrome with exposure to toxics such as cigarettes, tattoos, and hair dyes prior to biopolymer infiltration. Therefore, the importance of a comprehensive clinical evaluation is highlighted (familial autoimmunity, preexisting autoimmune phenomena, and previous exposure to toxics), thus balancing the individual risk/benefit of using prosthesis or dermal fillers for aesthetic purposes [42, 43, 64, 72, 73, 91, 92]. Some authors agree that both a preexisting immunologic disease and a genetic predisposition have been found to be important risk factors for the development of ASIA syndrome [61, 93]. In contrast, information associated with exposure to tattoos, cigarette or alcohol consumption, hair dyes, or piercings before or after a filler injection that would explain the development of ASIA was not found through the comprehensive literature review.

Given that all the majority of published patients went to "clandestine" clinics and were treated by personnel whose training was unknown, it is important to consider the need for educational strategies to inform the public of the dangers and damage to one's health involved in going to "clandestine" clinics that provide aesthetic procedures. However, it is necessary to do other types of epidemiological studies focused on public health based on the geoepidemiology of the problem and apply stringent surveillance control.

It is likely that foreign body modeling reaction is a precursor in the spectrum of ASIA syndrome. However, it is necessary to do further well-designed, case–control or prospective cohort studies [94] (including exposed and unexposed subjects and a larger sample size) that would make it possible to analyze why some subjects develop ASIA syndrome and other subjects stay asymptomatic in order to establish predictive models that could help prevent the onset of the disease.

References

1. Aesthetic Society (2019). The aesthetic society's cosmetic surgery National Data Bank: statistics 2019. *Aesthet. Surg. J.* 40: 1–26. https://doi.org/10.1093/ASJ/SJAA144.
2. Heidekrueger, P.I., Juran, S., Ehrl, D. et al. (2017). Global aesthetic surgery statistics: a closer look. *J. Plast. Surg. Hand Surg.* 51: 270–274. https://doi.org/10.1080/2000656X.2016.1248842.
3. Montealegre, G., Uribe, R., Martínez-Ceballos, M.A., and Rojas-Villarraga, A. (2021). ASIA syndrome symptoms induced by gluteal biopolymer injections: case-series and narrative review. *Toxicol. Rep.* 8: 303–314. https://doi.org/10.1016/j.toxrep.2021.01.011.
4. Attenello, N.H. and Maas, C.S. (2015). Injectable fillers: review of material and properties. *Facial Plast. Surg.* 31: 29–34. https://doi.org/10.1055/s-0035-1544924.
5. Reisman, N.R. (2006). Ethics, legal issues, and consent for fillers. *Clin. Plast. Surg.* 33: 505–510. https://doi.org/10.1016/j.cps.2006.08.004.
6. Goldberg, D.J. (2006). Legal ramifications of off-label filler use. *Clin. Plast. Surg.* 33: 597–601. https://doi.org/10.1016/j.cps.2006.08.003.
7. Keizers, P.H.J., Vanhee, C., van den Elzen, E.M.W. et al. (2018). A high crosslinking grade of hyaluronic acid found in a dermal filler causing adverse effects. *J. Pharm. Biomed. Anal.* 159: 173–178. https://doi.org/10.1016/j.jpba.2018.06.066.
8. Coiffman, F. (2008). A new disease: iatrogenic allogenosis. *Cir. Plast. Ibero-Latinoamericana* 34: 1–10.
9. Gordillo-Hernández, J., Alegre-Tamez, E., Torres-Baltazar, I. et al. (2013). Multidisciplinary management of adjuvant human disease by injection of modeling substances. *Cir. Plast. Ibero-Latinoamericana* 39: 269–277. https://doi.org/10.4321/S0376-78922013000300009.
10. Stanford, N. and Montealegre, G. (2013). Iatrogenic allogenosis, findings of a rheumatic disease. *Rev. Colomb. Cir. Plást. y Reconstr.* 19: 28–38.
11. Martínez-Villarreal, A.A., Asz-Sigall, D., Gutiérrez-Mendoza, D. et al. (2017). A case series and a review of the literature on foreign modelling agent reaction: an emerging problem. *Int. Wound J.* 14: 546–554. https://doi.org/10.1111/iwj.12643.
12. Tijerina, J.D., Morrison, S.D., Nolan, I.T. et al. (2019). Celebrity influence affecting public interest in plastic surgery procedures: google trends analysis. *Aesthet. Plast. Surg.* 43: 1669–1680. https://doi.org/10.1007/s00266-019-01466-7.
13. de Almeida, A.T., Banegas, R., Boggio, R. et al. (2017). Diagnosis and treatment of hyaluronic acid adverse events: latin American expert panel consensus recommendations. *Surg. Cosmet. Dermatol.* 9: 204–213. https://doi.org/10.5935/scd1984-8773.20179302.
14. Styperek, A., Bayers, S., Beer, M., and Beer, K. (2013). Nonmedical-grade injections of permanent fillers: medical and medicolegal considerations. *J. Clin. Aesthet. Dermatol.* 6: 22–29.
15. Seok, J., Hong, J.Y., Park, K.Y. et al. (2016). Delayed immunologic complications due to injectable fillers by unlicensed practitioners: our experiences and a review of the literature. *Dermatol. Ther.* 29: 41–44. https://doi.org/10.1111/dth.12298.
16. Ortiz Piedrahíta, V. (2013). Hegemonic, subaltern and/or alternative aesthetic models – a class and gender ethnic-racial approach. *Tabula Rasa* 18: 175–197.
17. Fisher, M.L. and Voracek, M. (2006). The shape of beauty: determinants of female physical attractiveness. *J. Cosmet. Dermatol.* 5: 190–194. https://doi.org/10.1111/j.1473-2165.2006.00249.x.
18. Cornelissen, P.L., Toveé, M.J., and Bateson, M. (2009). Patterns of subcutaneous fat deposition and the relationship between body mass index and waist-to-hip ratio: implications for models of physical attractiveness. *J. Theor. Biol.* 256: 343–350. https://doi.org/10.1016/j.jtbi.2008.09.041.
19. Chayangsu, O., Wanitphakdeedecha, R., Pattanaprichakul, P. et al. (2020). Legal vs. illegal injectable fillers: the adverse effects comparison study. *J. Cosmet. Dermatol.* 19: 1580–1586. https://doi.org/10.1111/jocd.13492.
20. Ortiz-Monasterio, F. and Trigos, I. (1972). Management of patients with complications from injections of foreign materials into the breasts. *Plast. Reconstr. Surg.* 50: 42–47. https://doi.org/10.1097/00006534-197207000-00007.

21. Velard, F., Schlaubitz, S., Fricain, J.C. et al. (2015). In vitro and in vivo evaluation of the inflammatory potential of various nanoporous hydroxyapatite biomaterials. *Nanomedicine* 10: 785–802. https://doi.org/10.2217/nnm.15.12.
22. Morhenn, V.B., Lemperle, G., and Gallo, R.L. (2002). Phagocytosis of different particulate dermal filler substances by human macrophages and skin cells. *Dermatol. Surg.* 28: 484–490. https://doi.org/10.1046/j.1524-4725.2002.01273.x.
23. Saththianathan, M., Johani, K., Taylor, A. et al. (2017). The role of bacterial biofilm in adverse soft-tissue filler reactions: a combined laboratory and clinical study. *Plast. Reconstr. Surg.* 139: 613–621. https://doi.org/10.1097/PRS.0000000000003067.
24. Tesar, B.M., Jiang, D., Liang, J. et al. (2006). The role of hyaluronan degradation products as innate alloimmune agonists. *Am. J. Transplant.* 6: 2622–2635. https://doi.org/10.1111/j.1600-6143.2006.01537.x.
25. Jeong, C.H., Kim, D.H., Yune, J.H. et al. (2021). In vitro toxicity assessment of crosslinking agents used in hyaluronic acid dermal filler. *Toxicol. In Vitro* 70: 105034. https://doi.org/10.1016/j.tiv.2020.105034.
26. Miro-Mur, F., Hindié, M., Kandhaya-Pillai, R. et al. (2009). Medical-grade silicone induces release of proinflammatory cytokines in peripheral blood mononuclear cells without activating T cells. *J. Biomed. Mater. Res. B Appl. Biomater.* 90B: 510–520. https://doi.org/10.1002/jbm.b.31312.
27. Cabral, L.R.B., Teixeira, L.N., Gimenez, R.P. et al. (2020). Effect of hyaluronic acid and poly-l-lactic acid dermal fillers on collagen synthesis: an in vitro and in vivo study. *Clin. Cosmet. Investig. Dermatol.* 13: 701–710. https://doi.org/10.2147/CCID.S266015.
28. Horowitz, S.M., Gautsch, T.L., Frondoza, C.G., and Riley, L. (1991). Macrophage exposure to polymethyl methacrylate leads to mediator release and injury. *J. Orthop. Res.* 9: 406–413. https://doi.org/10.1002/jor.1100090313.
29. Cannella, V., Altomare, R., Leonardi, V. et al. (2020). In vitro biocompatibility evaluation of nine dermal fillers on L929 cell line. *Biomed. Res. Int.* 2020: 8676343. https://doi.org/10.1155/2020/8676343.
30. Marino, F., Cosentino, M., Legnaro, M. et al. (2020). Immune profile of hyaluronic acid hydrogel polyethylene glycol crosslinked: an in vitro evaluation in human polymorphonuclear leukocytes. *Dermatol. Ther.* 33. https://doi.org/10.1111/dth.13388.
31. Liu, Y., Wu, Y., Lin, H. et al. (2018). Study on an injectable biomedical paste using cross-linked sodium hyaluronate as a carrier of hydroxyapatite particles. *Carbohydr. Polym.* 195: 378–386. https://doi.org/10.1016/j.carbpol.2018.04.093.
32. Wollina, U., Wiegand, C., and Hipler, U.C. (2018). Calcium hydroxylapatite microspheres – biocompatibility and clinical effects. *Georgian Med. News* 278: 62–68.
33. Eroglu Mehmet, S., Toksoy Oner, E., Cansever Mutlu, E., and Sennaroglu Bostan, M. (2017). Sugar based biopolymers in nanomedicine; new emerging era for cancer imaging and therapy. *Curr. Top. Med. Chem.* 17: 1507–1520. https://doi.org/10.2174/1568026616666161222101703.
34. Radu, I.C., Hudita, A., Zaharia, C. et al. (2019). Poly(3-hydroxybutyrate-CO-3-hydroxyvalerate) PHBHV biocompatible nanocarriers for 5-FU delivery targeting colorectal cancer. *Drug Deliv.* 26: 318–327. https://doi.org/10.1080/10717544.2019.1582729.
35. Taghizadehghalehjoughi, A., Hacimuftuoglu, A., Cetin, M. et al. (2018). Effect of metformin/irinotecan-loaded poly-lactic-co-glycolic acid nanoparticles on glioblastoma: in vitro and in vivo studies. *Nanomedicine* 13: 1595–1606. https://doi.org/10.2217/nnm-2017-0386.
36. Voss, G.T., Gularte, M.S., de Oliveira, R.L. et al. (2020). Biopolymeric films as delivery vehicles for controlled release of hydrocortisone: promising devices to treat chronic skin diseases. *Mater. Sci. Eng. C* 114. https://doi.org/10.1016/j.msec.2020.111074.
37. Bharadwaz, A. and Jayasuriya, A.C. (2020). Recent trends in the application of widely used natural and synthetic polymer nanocomposites in bone tissue regeneration. *Mater. Sci. Eng. C* 110. https://doi.org/10.1016/j.msec.2020.110698.
38. Farina, M., Chua, C.Y.X., Ballerini, A. et al. (2018). Transcutaneously refillable, 3D-printed biopolymeric encapsulation system for the transplantation of endocrine cells. *Biomaterials* 177: 125–138. https://doi.org/10.1016/j.biomaterials.2018.05.047.
39. Pavliuk, B., Chubka, M., Hroshovyi, T., and Stechyshyn, I. (2020). Characteristics of structured medical hemostatic sponges as a medical devices for stop bleeding and for close the wound. *Pol. Merkur. Lekarski* 48: 422–426.

40. Wang, Z., Zhan, C., Zeng, F., and Wu, S. (2020). A biopolymer-based and inflammation-responsive nanodrug for rheumatoid arthritis treatment: via inhibiting JAK-STAT and JNK signalling pathways. *Nanoscale* 12: 23013–23027. https://doi.org/10.1039/d0nr05551d.
41. Nosrati, H., Ashrafi-Dehkordi, K., Alizadeh, Z. et al. (2020). Biopolymer-based scaffolds for corneal stromal regeneration: a review. *Polim. Med.* 50: 57–64. https://doi.org/10.17219/pim/127653.
42. Alijotas-Reig, J., Esteve-Valverde, E., Gil-Aliberas, N., and Garcia-Gimenez, V. (2018). Autoimmune/inflammatory syndrome induced by adjuvants—ASIA—related to biomaterials: analysis of 45 cases and comprehensive review of the literature. *Immunol. Res.* 66: 120–140. https://doi.org/10.1007/s12026-017-8980-5.
43. Vera-Lastra, O., Medina, G., Cruz-Dominguez, M.D.P. et al. (2012). Human adjuvant disease induced by foreign substances: a new model of ASIA (Shoenfeld's syndrome). *Lupus* 21: 128–135. https://doi.org/10.1177/0961203311429317.
44. Centeno, R.F. and Young, V.L. (2006). Clinical anatomy in aesthetic gluteal body contouring surgery. *Clin. Plast. Surg.* 33: 347–358. https://doi.org/10.1016/j.cps.2006.05.005.
45. Mendieta, C.G. (2006). Classification system for gluteal evaluation. *Clin. Plast. Surg.* 33: 333–346. https://doi.org/10.1016/j.cps.2006.04.006.
46. Rayess, H.M., Svider, P.F., Hanba, C. et al. (2018). A cross-sectional analysis of adverse events and litigation for injectable fillers. *JAMA Facial Plast. Surg.* 20: 207–214. https://doi.org/10.1001/jamafacial.2017.1888.
47. Kim, J.J. and Evans, G.R.D. (2012). Applications of biomaterials in plastic surgery. *Clin. Plast. Surg.* 39: 359–376. https://doi.org/10.1016/j.cps.2012.07.007.
48. Beleznay, K., Carruthers, J.D.A., Humphrey, S., and Jones, D. (2015). Avoiding and treating blindness from fillers: a review of the world literature. *Dermatol. Surg.* 41: 1097–1117. https://doi.org/10.1097/DSS.0000000000000486.
49. Delorenzi, C. (2014). Complications of injectable fillers, part 2: vascular complications. *Aesthet. Surg. J.* 34: 584–600. https://doi.org/10.1177/1090820X14525035.
50. Lucey, P. and Goldberg, D.J. (2014). Complications of collagen fillers. *Facial Plast. Surg.* 30: 615–622. https://doi.org/10.1055/s-0034-1396904.
51. Delorenzi, C. (2013). Complications of injectable fillers, part I. *Aesthet. Surg. J.* 33: 561–575. https://doi.org/10.1177/1090820X13484492.
52. Singh, M., Solomon, I.H., Calderwood, M.S., and Talbot, S.G. (2016). Silicone-induced granuloma after buttock augmentation. *Plast. Reconstr. Surg. Glob. Open* 4: 1–4. https://doi.org/10.1097/GOX.0000000000000618.
53. Bartsich, S. and Wu, J.K. (2010). Silicon emboli syndrome: a sequela of clandestine liquid silicone injections. A case report and review of the literature. *J. Plast. Reconstr. Aesthet. Surg.* 63: e1–e3. https://doi.org/10.1016/j.bjps.2009.04.004.
54. Kontis, T.C. and Rivkin, A. (2009). The history of injectable facial fillers. *Facial Plast. Surg.* 25: 67–72. https://doi.org/10.1055/s-0029-1220645.
55. Lee, S.K., Kim, S.M., Cho, S.H. et al. (2015). Adverse reactions to injectable soft tissue fillers: memorable cases and their clinico-pathological overview. *J. Cosmet. Laser Ther.* 17: 102–108. https://doi.org/10.3109/14764172.2014.968584.
56. Qian, B., Xiong, L., Guo, K. et al. (2020). Comprehensive management of breast augmentation with polyacrylamide hydrogel injection based on 15 years of experience: a report on 325 cases. *Ann. Transl. Med.* 8: 475–475. https://doi.org/10.21037/atm.2020.03.68.
57. Beauvais, D. and Ferneini, E.M. (2020). Complications and litigation associated with injectable facial fillers: a cross-sectional study. *J. Oral Maxillofac. Surg.* 78: 133–140. https://doi.org/10.1016/j.joms.2019.08.003.
58. Shoenfeld, Y. and Agmon-Levin, N. (2011). "ASIA" – autoimmune/inflammatory syndrome induced by adjuvants. *J. Autoimmun.* 36: 4–8. https://doi.org/10.1016/j.jaut.2010.07.003.
59. Vera-Lastra, O., Medina, G., Cruz-Domínguez, M.P. et al. (2018). Autoimmune/inflammatory syndrome induced by mineral oil: a health problem. *Clin. Rheumatol.* 37: 1441–1448. https://doi.org/10.1007/s10067-018-4078-2.
60. Hajdu, S.D., Agmon-Levin, N., and Shoenfeld, Y. (2011). Silicone and autoimmunity. *Eur. J. Clin. Investig.* 41: 203–211. https://doi.org/10.1111/j.1365-2362.2010.02389.x.

61. Cohen Tervaert, J.W. (2020). Autoinflammatory/autoimmunity syndrome induced by adjuvants (ASIA; Shoenfeld's syndrome): a new flame. *Autoimmun. Rev.* 17: 1259–1264. https://doi.org/10.1016/j.autrev.2018.07.003.
62. Alijotas-Reig, J. (2015). Human adjuvant-related syndrome or autoimmune/inflammatory syndrome induced by adjuvants. Where have we come from? Where are we going? A proposal for new diagnostic criteria. *Lupus* 24: 1012–1018. https://doi.org/10.1177/0961203315579092.
63. Perricone, C., Colafrancesco, S., Mazor, R.D. et al. (2013). Autoimmune/inflammatory syndrome induced by adjuvants (ASIA) 2013: unveiling the pathogenic, clinical and diagnostic aspects. *J. Autoimmun.* 47: 1–16. https://doi.org/10.1016/j.jaut.2013.10.004.
64. Anaya, J.M., Ramirez-Santana, C., Alzate, M.A. et al. (2016). The autoimmune ecology. *Front. Immunol.* 7: 00139. https://doi.org/10.3389/fimmu.2016.00139.
65. Segal, Y., Dahan, S., Sharif, K. et al. (2018). The value of autoimmune syndrome induced by adjuvant (ASIA) – shedding light on orphan diseases in autoimmunity. *Autoimmun. Rev.* 17: 440–448. https://doi.org/10.1016/j.autrev.2017.11.037.
66. Cohen Tervaert, J.W. and Kappel, R.M. (2013). Silicone implant incompatibility syndrome (SIIS): a frequent cause of ASIA (Shoenfeld's syndrome). *Immunol. Res.* 56: 293–298. https://doi.org/10.1007/s12026-013-8401-3.
67. Watad, A., Rosenberg, V., Tiosano, S. et al. (2018). Silicone breast implants and the risk of autoimmune/rheumatic disorders: a real-world analysis. *Int. J. Epidemiol.* 47: 1846–1854. https://doi.org/10.1093/ije/dyy217.
68. Anaya, J.M., Restrepo-Jiménez, P., and Ramírez-Santana, C. (2018). The autoimmune ecology: an update. *Curr. Opin. Rheumatol.* 30: 350–360. https://doi.org/10.1097/BOR.0000000000000498.
69. Page, M.J., McKenzie, J.E., Bossuyt, P.M. et al. The PRISMA 2020 statement: an updated guideline for reporting systematic reviews. *BMJ* 2021: 372. https://doi.org/10.1136/bmj.n71.
70. Gagnier, J.J., Kienle, G., Altman, D.G. et al. (2014). The CARE guidelines: consensus-based clinical case report guideline development. *J. Clin. Epidemiol.* 67: 46–51. https://doi.org/10.1016/j.jclinepi.2013.08.003.
71. Flores Padilla, G., Mora Mendoza, B., and Pedraza Montenegro, A. (2014). Síndrome autoinmune/inflamatorio inducido por adyuvante que debuta con manifestaciones pulmonares y articulares. *Reumatol. Clin.* 10: 406–408. https://doi.org/10.1016/j.reuma.2014.01.005.
72. Jara, L.J., García-Collinot, G., Medina, G. et al. (2017). Severe manifestations of autoimmune syndrome induced by adjuvants (Shoenfeld's syndrome). *Immunol. Res.* 65: 8–16. https://doi.org/10.1007/s12026-016-8811-0.
73. Barilaro, G., Spaziani Testa, C., Cacciani, A. et al. (2016). ASIA syndrome, calcinosis cutis and chronic kidney disease following silicone injections. A case-based review. *Immunol. Res.* 64: 1142–1149. https://doi.org/10.1007/s12026-016-8871-1.
74. Lopez-Mendoza, J., Vargas-Flores, E., Mouneu-Ornelas, N., and Altamirano-Arcos, C. (2021). Disease presentation and surgical treatment of patients with foreign-body granulomas and asia syndrome: case series. *Arch. Plast. Surg.* 48: 366–372. https://doi.org/10.5999/aps.2020.02152.
75. Vera-Lastra, O., Rojas-Milán, E., Peralta-Amaro, A.L. et al. (2020). Autoimmune/inflammatory syndrome induced by methylmethacrylate associated to seronegative antiphospholipid syndrome and diffuse large B-cell non-Hodgkin's lymphoma. *Lupus* 29: 1292–1296. https://doi.org/10.1177/0961203320936767.
76. Ali, S., Lakhani, P.M., and Hughes, R. (2021). Autoimmune/inflammatory syndrome induced by buttock augmentation with silicone. *Rheumatol. Adv. Pract.* 5: rkab034. https://doi.org/10.1093/rap/rkab034.
77. Alijotas-Reig, J., Garcia-Gimenez, V., Llurba, E., and Vilardell-Tarrés, M. (2012). Autoimmune/inflammatory syndrome (ASIA) induced by biomaterials injection other than silicone medical grade. *Lupus* 21: 1326–1334. https://doi.org/10.1177/0961203312458838.
78. Jaime Eduardo Pachón, S., Salazar, M.C., Pores, A.M., and Rizo, V.Z. (2021). Clinical and immunological characteristics of patients with biopolymers and autoimmune inflammatory syndrome induced by adjuvants. *Plast. Reconstr. Surg. Glob. Open* 9 (9): e3796. https://doi.org/10.1097/GOX.0000000000003796.
79. Cárdenas-Roldán, J., Rojas-Villarraga, A., and Anaya, J.M. (2013). How do autoimmune diseases cluster in families? A systematic review and meta-analysis. *BMC Med.* 11: 73. https://doi.org/10.1186/1741-7015-11-73.
80. Paternostro-Sluga, T., Grim-Stieger, M., Posch, M. et al. (2008). Reliability and validity of the Medical Research Council (MRC) scale and a modified scale for testing muscle strength in patients with radial palsy. *J. Rehabil. Med.* 40: 665–671. https://doi.org/10.2340/16501977-0235.

81. Navazesh, M. and Kumar, S.K.S. (2008). Measuring salivary flow. *J. Am. Dent. Assoc.* 139: 35S–40S. https://doi.org/10.14219/jada.archive.2008.0353.
82. Hjollund, N.H., Andersen, J.H., and Bech, P. (2007). Assessment of fatigue in chronic disease: a bibliographic study of fatigue measurement scales. *Health Qual. Life Outcomes* 5: 12. https://doi.org/10.1186/1477-7525-5-12.
83. Bernal Vargas, L., Riveros Munévar, F., Vinaccia Alpi, S., and Quiceno Sierra, J.M. (2017). Factorial structure and internal consistency of the Fatigue Severity Scale in Colombian population with chronic diseases. *Enferm. Glob.* 16: 44–49. https://doi.org/10.6018/eglobal.16.2.255821.
84. Novo, R.C., Salgado, C.J., Yim, E. et al. (2016). A staging system for gluteal foreign body reaction to injectables. *J. Plast. Reconstr. Aesthet. Surg.* 69: e174–e179. https://doi.org/10.1016/j.bjps.2016.05.007.
85. Ho, W.-s., Chan, A.C.-w., and Law, B.K.-b. (2001). Management of paraffinoma of the breast: 10 years' experience. *Br. J. Plast. Surg.* 54: 232–234. https://doi.org/10.1054/bjps.2000.3533.
86. Dominguez-Zambrano, A., Haddad-Tame, J.L., Torres-Baltazar, I. et al. (2013). Actual status of adyuvant disease in México and some case examples. *Cir. Plast. Ibero-Latinoamericana* 39: 399–405. https://doi.org/10.4321/S0376-78922013000400010.
87. Rapkiewicz, A.V., Kenerson, K., Hutchins, K.D. et al. (2018). Fatal complications of aesthetic techniques: the gluteal region. *J. Forensic Sci.* 63: 1406–1412. https://doi.org/10.1111/1556-4029.13761.
88. Ramos-e-Silva, M., Pereira, A.L.C., Ramos-e-Silva, S., and Piñeiro-Maceira, J. (2012). Oleoma: rare complication of mesotherapy for cellulite. *Int. J. Dermatol.* 51: 162–167. https://doi.org/10.1111/j.1365--4632.2011.04931.x.
89. Lym, C.I., Nakasato, F.K., Menezes, M.C.S. et al. (2015). Oleoma treated with oral colchicine: report of two cases and review of the literature. *Int. J. Women's Dermatol.* 1: 47–50. https://doi.org/10.1016/j.ijwd.2014.12.004.
90. Gonzalez Castro, L.F., Alviar Rueda, J.D., and Melendez Florez, H.J. (2017). Evaluation of the effects of the application, absorption and deposition of biopolimeros in rodents (iatrogenic allogenosis). *Rev. Colomb. Cir. Plast. y Reconstr.* 23: 46–58.
91. Cukier, J., Beauchamp, R.A., Spindler, J.S. et al. (1993). Association between bovine collagen dermal implants and a dermatomyositis or a polymyositis-like syndrome. *Ann. Intern. Med.* 118: 920–928. https://doi.org/10.7326/0003-4819-118-12-199306150-00002.
92. Alijotas-Reig, J., Fernández-Figueras, M.T., and Puig, L. (2013). Inflammatory, immune-mediated adverse reactions related to soft tissue dermal fillers. *Semin. Arthritis Rheum.* 43: 241–258. https://doi.org/10.1016/j.semarthrit.2013.02.001.
93. Soriano, A., Butnaru, D., and Shoenfeld, Y. (2014). Long-term inflammatory conditions following silicone exposure: the expanding spectrum of the autoimmune/inflammatory syndrome induced by adjuvants (ASIA). *Clin. Exp. Rheumatol.* 32: 151–154.
94. Song, J.W. and Chung, K.C. (2010). Observational studies: cohort and case-control studies. *Plast. Reconstr. Surg.* 126: 2234–2242. https://doi.org/10.1097/PRS.0b013e3181f44abc.

24 The Chemical and Social Landscape of the Modern World and Increased Risk of ASIA

Albert Pinhasov, Elena Shmerkin, and Michael Kirby
Department of Molecular Biology and Adelson School of Medicine,
Ariel University, Ariel, Israel

Introduction

Immunizations or introduction of foreign materials to the body may result in a syndrome known as autoimmune/inflammatory syndrome induced by adjuvants (ASIA [1, 2]), expressed as one of five different autoimmune conditions: undifferentiated connective tissue disease, sarcoidosis, Sjögren's syndrome, silicone implant incompatibility, and immune-related adverse events. Reported cases of ASIA syndrome only number 4500, and it is regarded by most of the medical community as an important but uncommon clinical syndrome [3]. In contrast, autoimmunity is unfortunately a common condition affecting approximately 1 in 15 people, with a higher frequency observed in women (65% of total patient population) [4]. Moreover, current rates of prevalence for autoimmune diseases appear to be increasing, irrespective of changes in diagnostic criteria or clinical assessment tools [5–7]. In addition, there are several inflammation-driven disorders that are increasing in incidence, but are not considered autoimmune disorders, per se (i.e. atopic dermatitis and irritable bowel syndrome, affecting 3% and 15% of the population, respectively [8, 9]), yet are known to be predisposing factors toward development of autoimmune disease [10–14]. Both these conditions, as well as all autoimmune disorders, are known to be epidemiologically associated with urbanization and industrialization [15].

ASIA disorders may become more common health issues than are presently documented, extending beyond the classic five syndromes listed above. Expanded use of adjuvants in vaccines administered against a background of increasing rates of chronic, age-progressive inflammation and increased risk of autoimmunity will likely exacerbate and promote development of autoimmune states. The underlying causes of this background inflammation and autoimmunity are uncertain, but epidemiological evidence points to the incessant exposure to exogenous products of urban and industrial life as well as alterations in the intestinal microbiome and loss of maintenance of stable intestinal permeability [7, 15, 16, reviewed in 17]. Vaccine adjuvants, chemicals specifically selected to enhance immune response in the presence of target antigens, would likely

Autoimmune Disorders: Adjuvants and Other Risk Factors in Pathogenesis, First Edition.
Edited by Abdulla Watad, Nicola Luigi Bragazzi, and Yehuda Shoenfeld.

present additional complications contributing to autoimmunity. Despite this proposition, a recent meta-analysis of association between incidence of autoimmune disease and vaccinations failed to find any increased autoimmunity risk with standard vaccines (e.g. killed or attenuated virus and lipid-adjuvant vaccines), yet the authors acknowledge that genetic or experimental vaccines do not fit their model, and risks from those treatments are as yet unknown [18]. In light of the SARS-Cov-2 pandemic, an array of novel genetic vaccines has been administered *en masse* to the public in many countries, and this population-level interventional approach is likely to become the norm in addressing all future global pandemics. The genetic-based approach allows for a shortened vaccine development time and provides a high degree of disease agent-tailored flexibility. That being said, it is instructive to readdress the potential outcomes of administering genetic vaccines with adjuvants to a population displaying increased rates of chronic inflammatory and autoimmune disorders and assess those risks in their context.

Here, we examine the environmental factors that contribute to the increase in chronic inflammation-associated and autoimmune disorders as well as the potential increased risk of ASIA syndrome. A myriad of diseases are associated with increased intestinal permeability, which may also be the trigger for disease onset. Environmental toxicants have been demonstrated to be the underlying cause of altered gut permeability, driving these inflammation-based changes in allostasis. Additional factors that contribute to autoimmune and chronic inflammation states include adverse early-life events that impose epigenetic changes and heightened hypothalamic–pituitary–adrenal (HPA) axis response leading to substantial increases in intestinal inflammation. Reinforcing these changes, or perhaps preceding them, are alterations in the intestinal microbial ecosystem, a vital component of physiological regulation that can either stabilize against establishment of chronic inflammation states or augment their development. We also review animal models of inflammation that address specific aspects of inflammatory response and can be used to yield clues as to the underlying mechanisms that precipitate autoimmunity and indicate potential means of prevention.

Diseases related to increased intestinal permeability

The influence of exogenous environmental factors in immune activation and chronic inflammatory states has been suspected for at least the past five decades. Epidemiological evidence has accumulated, demonstrating increased rates of autoimmune diseases (multiple sclerosis, rheumatoid arthritis, celiac disease, and asthma) and diseases related to perturbations in metabolism (obesity and diabetes) since the mid-1960s [19–25]. Further, a recorded increase in the incidence rate of IgG and IgE serum antibodies directed against allergens has been noted by immunologists since the 1970s (reviewed in [15]). Recent evidence for increased rates of allergies is demonstrated by changing trends in allergic response. For example, newborns are all IgG-dependent milk protein reactive by age 1 [26], and at least half of the North American, European, and Australian population present with strong IgE-dependent allergen-specific response (reviewed in [15]). These trends in allergic response are somewhat new and have only developed in human populations since the 1960s.

Against this background of increasing autoimmune disease and allergy rates, strong associations with gastrointestinal dysfunction provide mechanistic clues and begin to paint a picture that describes a pandemic industrial and urban phenomenon. Bacterial dysbiosis and loss of epithelial barrier fidelity have been identified as component parts of the pathology of several diseases. These include diseases local to the affected tissue, such as inflammatory bowel [27–29] and celiac [30–32] diseases, as well as diseases affecting organ sites distal to the intestinal tract. Diabetes [33–35], multiple sclerosis [36, 37], nonalcoholic steatohepatitis [38, 39], autoimmune hepatitis [38, 40], hepatic cirrhosis [38, 41, 42], rheumatoid arthritis [43], systemic lupus erythematosus [44], ankylosing spondylitis [45], and obesity [46, 47] also have demonstrated links with increased gut permeability and altered intestinal microbiome. Many of these diseases are intestinal mucosa specific, but some develop among other epithelial barriers. For example, asthma [48, 49], atopic dermatitis [50, 51], allergic rhinitis [52–54], chronic rhinosinusitis [55], and eosinophilic esophagitis [56, 57] are all connected with either the respiratory system or proximal portions of the alimentary tract. Further, at least five different psychiatric and neurological disorders such as autism spectrum disorders [58], Alzheimer's disease [59, 60], Parkinson's disease [59, 61, 62], chronic depression [63–65], and an array of stress-related behavioral disorders [66, 67] have been shown in several studies to have strong links with intestinal dysbiosis and degradation of intestinal epithelial barrier function. Whether these intestinal barrier alterations are causative remains to be proven; however, they are consistent symptom components.

Considering the changing health status of the population with respect to autoimmune, allergic, and chronic inflammatory disorders, the use of vaccines with adjuvants intended to enhance immune response may have unintended negative consequences in this environment. The outcomes may entail development of secondary sequelae or ASIA syndrome, leading to additional complications in patient treatment. Determining the underlying genetic and epigenetic predispositions, psychosocial stressors, and environmental agents that may contribute to chronic inflammation and autoimmunity is therefore of central importance in both understanding disease manifestation and developing a means to counteract or prevent it.

Environmental toxicants and loss of epithelial tight junction fidelity

Regulation of the epithelial barrier is very dynamic by nature, as the system is commonly engaged in mass alteration of tight junction protein expression patterns spatially with respect to the lower alimentary tract proximal–distal axis and both spatially and temporally within the basoapical axis of intestinal villi and crypts. Expression patterns of tight junction proteins change during the process of epithelial cells transitioning from undifferentiated and proliferating states to stable, differentiated cells along the crypt–luminal axis [68]. It is important to mention that these transitions take place on the order of days [69].

Tight junction barriers restrict passage of solutes and bacteria into the paracellular space and are classified into three general groupings (in apicobasal order): tight junction-associated MARVEL proteins (TAMPs), claudins, and cortical thymocyte marker of *Xenopus* (CTX). TAMPs include occludin, MARVELD3, and tricellulin. The precise functions of occludin, an NADH oxidase, are uncertain, but evidence has shown important effects on cellular regulation of energy production and gene expression [70]. Claudins are a broad range of associated structures with four transmembrane domains that regulate both the trans-tight junction voltage and selective paracellular pore diameter. They are classified into two gross categories of claudins, tight and leaky, based on differences in amino acid sequence of the first extracellular loop domain and its selectivity characteristics [71, 72]. The CTX family, despite its name, is highly conserved across all vertebrate species [73] and consists of coxsackie virus and adenovirus receptor (CAR), CXADR like protein (CLMP), and junctional adhesion molecules (JAM-A). JAM-A primarily affects claudin expression, actin–myosin interactions, and, in conjunction with tricellulin, selectivity of paracellular space access.

Noting the dynamically regulated manner governing the expression of tight junction proteins, a variety of agents interact with and affect epithelial barrier maintenance. Some of these factors are endogenous (interleukins [74]; TNFα [75]; glucocorticoids [76]; and protein kinases [77]), some are endemic (bacterial signaling molecules [78, 79]), and some are exogenous (from ingested sources [16]). Among the exogenous sources, a variety of environmental chemicals, some of which are surprisingly common, have been demonstrated to produce potent effects on disruption of the intestinal epithelial barrier. These include detergents, some food additives (emulsifiers and surfactants), microplastics, and nanoparticulates (reviewed in [16]).

Household cleaning agents and laundry and dishwashing detergents have been demonstrated to disrupt tight junction stability in epithelial membranes [15, 80]. Most of the studies conducted focused on pulmonary and dermal epithelium [81, 82]. Modern detergents, mainly based on sodium dodecyl sulfate or sodium dodecylbenzene sulfonate, are very effective cleaners due to additional surfactants and digestive enzymes [81, 83]. Digestive enzymes used in detergents include proteases, lipases, amylases, and cellulases [84]. In lung and skin epithelium, highly diluted concentrations of standard laundry detergents caused reduced expression of claudin 1 in human keratinocyte cultures (detergents 100,000× diluted) and reduced ZO-1 and occludin expression in human bronchial epithelial cell cultures (detergents 25,000× diluted) [81, 82]. These demonstrated effects would also be caused by detergent residues on utensils and in food. Although ingested detergent exposures are likely to be very low, other detergent-like chemicals such as emulsifiers and surfactants are commonly added components of prepared foodstuffs.

The addition of emulsifiers and surfactants in food products is quite recent, only becoming common within the past 50 years. Accumulating evidence implicates these processed food additions as one of several culpable environmental agents contributing to alterations in intestinal barrier permeability and promotion of chronic inflammation states [85–95]. The major emulsifiers used are fatty acid monoglycerides and diglycerides, polysorbate-80 (P80), and carboxymethylcellulose (CMC) at concentrations of up to 2% in prepared foods [91]. Trace levels of these agents can induce chronic inflammation, reduce tight junction protein expression, and drive bacterial translocation to epithelial paracellular space [95]. Their prolific use over the past five decades may at least partially explain the increased incidence of metabolic syndrome and inflammatory bowel disease, as suggested in animal models [93]. Mice fed concentrations of CMC or P80 up to 1% for 12 weeks were pro-obesogenic, developed glucose intolerance, and had chronic, low-level inflammation. When tested with inflammation-prone mouse models lacking either IL-10 or Toll-like receptor five expression, both models developed chronic inflammation, which progressed to colitis.

When we reflect upon the material that defines our modern civilization, it is not steel or aluminum that is the most appropriate choice. The obvious choice for a defining modern material is polymers, specifically plastics. Plastics are a widespread component of everyday life and touch all aspects of our existence. Development of plastics began just prior to the twentieth century but came into common use in the 1950s. Since that time, profound amounts of plastic products have been produced and disposed of with little regard toward recycling strategies, amounting to a one-way destination in landfills and, eventually, the ocean. Plastic polymers break down into smaller particulates through mechanical deformation, as by-products of manufacturing, and through chemical and ultraviolet light degradation. As a consequence, plastics have become a major pollutant [96, 97] and flow through the global food chain [98–101], with even smaller plastic particles becoming airborne contaminants [102]. Termed "microplastic fallout," the airborne contaminants ran the gamut of all common plastics including polypropylene, polystyrene, polyethylene, polyethylene terephthalate, and polyvinyl chloride.

Microplastics are defined as plastic particulates between 5 mm and 1 μm in size [103], with sizes below the minimum defined as nanoplastics. Microplastics equal to or less than 1.5 μm have been demonstrated to readily pass the intestinal epithelial barrier [104]. Exposure of A549 human lung epithelial cells to nanoplastic polystyrene produced a range of proapoptotic effects including increased caspase expression (caspases 3, 8, and 9), cytochrome-c, BAX, and DR5 [105]. Nanopolystyrene produced S-phase cell cycle arrest, increases in inflammatory gene transcription (CCND, CCNE, and Ki67), and increases in markers of inflammation (IL-8, NF-κB, and TNFα). *In silico* modeling of nanoplastic–protein interactions has demonstrated that nanoplastics can bind with and allosterically modify protein structure [106, 107]. Dietary exposure of mice to 5 μm polystyrene for six weeks resulted in marked intestinal dysbiosis, as well as alterations in bacterial primary metabolic pathways, and metabolic disturbances in bile and amino acid metabolism [108]. In addition to environmental plastics sources and despite the obvious dangers, microplastics are intentional components of consumer products (toothpaste, laundry and dishwasher pods, cigarette filters, cosmetics, and hand sanitizers), and nanoparticulates are also being developed as drug delivery vehicles, specifically for their ability to disrupt the intestinal epithelial barrier [109–111].

In addition to exogenous triggers of chronic inflammation, adverse early-life events can epigenetically reprogram for exaggerated stress response and secretion of CRH and cortisol. These increased secretions have long-term negative consequences for normal intestinal function. Furthermore, a population that is sensitive to stress-induced changes in HPA axis function likely exists and represents a particularly vulnerable group.

Early-life stress, vulnerability to psychosocial stress, and role of the HPA axis

Early-life stress, both pre- and postnatal, has a significant impact on the neurological, behavioral, and psychological development of children, with long-term consequences throughout later life [112–114]. There are several theories about the impact of early-life stress on the development of offspring. According to the cumulative stress hypothesis, all adversities throughout life, starting from early childhood, can accumulate and lead to disease development. For example, it was shown that childhood stress has been linked to increased arousal, enhanced processing of negative emotional information, and cognitive deficits, contributing to heightened sensitivity to stress and an increased risk of mental disorders such as major depressive disorder, substance abuse disorders, and posttraumatic stress disorder [115]. Another leading model, the match/mismatch theory, claims that early-life adversity may prepare an organism for later-life exposure to similar ("matching") adversity, resulting in a predicted adaptive response that can help an organism respond to future stresses more effectively. The fact that some individuals who experienced early-childhood stress showed a reduced HPA axis response to acute stress in adulthood supports this theory [116–118].

According to match/mismatch theory as revealed through rodent studies, prenatal stress causes the pregnant dam to produce more glucocorticoids, which pass through the placenta to the fetus, impacting prenatal programming of the HPA axis. Maternal glucocorticoids have been shown to affect fetal hippocampal development, wherein glucocorticoid and mineralocorticoid receptor activation is thought to be required for successful stress adaptation by decreasing the early behavioral stress reaction and increasing stress recovery [112]. Permanent alterations in HPA axis regulation [119, 120] impose changes in enteric glia–mast cell interaction [121] and have been linked to manifestation of irritable bowel syndrome [122]. Early-life stress and poor maternal care also appear to impose epigenetic changes causing sensitization to psychosocial stress and proneness to develop psychiatric disorders [123, 124], which may serve as an origin of inflammation and immune dysregulation in adulthood.

The level of vulnerability to psychosocial stress in females has a notable influence on the development of stress response mechanisms in their offspring. Stress can precipitate states of chronic inflammation [124–126]. Therefore, having a low-threshold response to stress (stress sensitivity) or an exaggerated stress response, whether inborn or postnatally acquired [124, 127], would increase the potential to develop chronic inflammation. However, investigations examining the link between adversity and risk of depression have failed to identify genes associated with inborn sensitivity to stress [128]; thus, an epigenetic mechanism is likely the underlying cause [124]. Nonetheless, a genotypic basis for stress sensitivity may still exist and reside in differences in allele-specific methylation (ASM [129]).

Thus, we have shown that prenatal stress (PRS) has a differential effect on the development of offspring in socially dominant (Dom) and submissive (Sub) mice. In the placentas of Dom dams subjected to PRS, higher levels of glucocorticoid receptor expression and the inactivating enzyme for glucocorticoids, 11β-hydroxysteroid dehydrogenase-2 (11βHSD2), were observed compared with the placentas of control Dom dams [130]. In contrast, the level of the glucocorticoid receptor expression in the placentas of PRS-exposed Sub dams was reduced, without changes in 11βHSD2 content. We propose that PRS causes developmental delays in that PRS-Sub offspring had low birthweights and continue to present with reduced body weight into adulthood compared with their unstressed counterparts.

Due to the strong influence of maternal glucocorticoids and their substantial programming effects (e.g., lastingly altering the expression levels of glucocorticoids and mineralocorticoids, programming hypertension, and influencing hormone levels) on the development of the HPA axis in the fetus, multiple protective mechanisms prevent excessive corticosteroid exposure to the developing fetal brain. Prenatally, placental 11βHSD2 reduces fetal exposure to maternal corticosteroids through rapid inactivation throughout the pregnancy. However, it has been established that repeated prenatal stress, accompanied by an increase in corticosteroids in pregnant dams leads to partial penetration of glucocorticoids through the placental barrier and affects the development of the brain HPA-axis of the fetus [112]. Furthermore, the ability of offspring to adjust to stress-inducing events may be impaired due to the alterations in hippocampal response to glucocorticoids; as a result, stress may trigger the development of behavioral disorders among sensitive individuals [113]. We found that PRS elevated serum corticosterone in Sub offspring and exacerbated anxiety- and depressive-like behavior, while Dom offspring were unaltered by PRS hormonal and behavioral effects. Furthermore, PRS exposure significantly facilitated glucocorticoid receptor recruitment to the hippocampus in Dom mice in response to restraint stress, which could explain their resilience to stressful situations. These findings show that a tendency for adaptive or maladaptive prenatal programming of hippocampal glucocorticoid receptor recruitment is heritable and predicted as a function of social dominance or submissiveness [130]. Stress vulnerability and the nature of the stress response also appear related to an increased risk of obesity that additionally compounds inflammatory load in mouse models [131]. Furthermore, recent studies have revealed links among stress, alteration in intestinal permeability, and dysbiosis of the intestinal microbiome.

Role of the gut-brain axis and intestinal microbiome

The microbiota-gut-brain (MGB) axis is a bidirectional communication system between intestinal microflora and the central nervous system. The intestinal microbiome inhabits a rather large epithelial surface area for interaction, comprising 30% of the total body epithelium (as calculated from [132–134]). The overwhelming majority of intestinal flora falls into two major phyla, Firmicutes and Bacteroides, which represent 99% of the intestinal species [135].

Maintenance of the microbiome for stabilization of normal physiological states has moved to the forefront of medicine and physiology research as a focal point for future intervention strategies geared to treat a wide array of human diseases [135], including mouse model evidence that deficits of intestinal microbiota can induce ultrastructural and metabolic changes in adipose tissues, driving increases in global inflammation [136, 137]. There are strong links between good overall health and intestinal microbiome species diversity, with some genera or species of bacteria denoted as critical for normal human physiology, and others directly connected with disease states. For example, dysbiosis in psoriasis results in a high β-diversity compared with healthy control patients, with psoriatic patients typically presenting with markedly increased abundance of Firmicutes and Actinobacteria and a decreased abundance of Bacteroides [138].

A broader view of MGB axis interactions has evolved to denote specific communication pathways. The gut microbiota communicate with the central nervous system indirectly through chemical messenger mediation from enteroendocrine cells either directed to vagus nerve sensory afferents or via the enteric nervous system communication with the vagus nerve (the vagus nerve actually only contains 20% efferent fibers [139]). Vagal tone imposes a pro–anti-inflammatory effect thought to occur by cholinergic inhibition of cytokine release, as demonstrated *in vitro* with human macrophage cultures (inhibited release of TNFα, IL-1b, IL-6, and IL-18 [140–143]), and also is thought to promote release of an array of bacterial bioactive molecules to the intestinal luminal space (for a listing, see [144]). Further, bacterial products can either augment or inhibit vagal tone, thus acting in either an anti-inflammatory or pro-inflammatory capacity, depending on changes in intestinal epithelial physiology, microbiome species profile, and bacterial metabolism [145–147]. Moreover, intestinal bacteria prompt release of enteroendocrine messengers (e.g., GLP-1, CCK, and PYY) [148] and release an array of their own messengers as lipids [79], polyamines [149], tryptophan metabolites and precursors [150–152], neurotransmitters [135, 148, 151], and a variety of chemical relatives of the above [149].

Bacterial product regulation of tight junction permeability is influenced by a host of chemical messengers but most prominently through the action of short-chain fatty acids (SCFAs). Binding EC_{50}s of SCFAs at target receptors are typically in the μM range or higher, whereas other bacterial products such as long-chain fatty acids, fatty amides, glyceroglycolipids, and sterol lipids produce effects on target receptors at nM to μM ranges [79]. Despite low binding potency, SCFAs are produced by microbiota in copious amounts (ranging from 20 μM to 70 mM, calculated based on [153, 154]), with butyrate, propionate, and acetate being the three main SCFA bacterial products [155, 156]. SCFAs are a mixed bag, which can be summarized in general as promoting increased tight junction fidelity (butyrate) or increased tight junction permeability (acetate and propionate). For example, reduction in butyrate-producing species (e.g., Firmicutes: *Faecalibacterium prausnitzii* and *Roseburia hominis*) is associated with colitis [157]. However, with respect to inflammation, butyrate appears to be primarily anti-inflammatory, whereas acetate and propionate effects vary by cell type and tissue. Therefore, the overall picture of SCFA contributions is complex.

The primary targets of the big three SCFAs are G-protein-coupled receptors (e.g., GPR41, GPR43, GPR81, and GPR109A), and the effects exerted by SCFAs vary from suppressed insulin signaling in adipose tissue to NLRP3 inflammasome activation and increased IL-8 production (reviewed in [79]). Activation of GPRs reduces histone deacetylase activities (primarily by butyrate and propionate) and alters gene expression of cytokine secretion by macrophages and dendritic cells (TNFα, IL-12, and IL-6) [158, 159]. With respect to control of inflammation, butyrate, in particular, has direct effects on stimulating regulatory T-cell (Treg) differentiation through forkhead box P3 (FOXP3), thus mediating the development of inflammatory responses [160, 161]. Butyrate alters the cytokine profile of Th cells, imposing an anti-inflammatory effect [162], and shifts cytokine secretions in dendritic cells and macrophages through a GPR109A-mediated mechanism to reduce secretion of IL-6 and increase IL-10, thus fostering Treg development and inhibiting clonal expansion of pro-inflammatory Th17 cells [163].

The remaining two SCFAs of the big three, acetate and propionate, can also exhibit anti-inflammatory effects. Acetate can also participate in support of normal intestinal permeability through GPR43-mediated mechanisms, regulating inflammation [164] and tight junction fidelity [165]. GPR43 signaling reduces expression of NLRP3, which reduces IL-18 secretion and inflammasome activation [166, 167]. Furthermore, acetate tends to interact more with neutrophils than other immune cells and reduces TNFα production [158, 168]. Propionate and acetate also participate in energy regulatory functions and stimulate epithelial secretion of GLP-1, which is an incretin that regulates gluconeogenesis, glucagon secretion, and insulin response [169]. Regarding serum concentrations of SCFAs, most butyrate is metabolized locally by intestinal epithelial cells, whereas propionate is hepatically eliminated; only acetate attains functional serum concentrations. Therefore, most immunomodulatory effects of SCFAs tend to originate in the intestinal mucosa [169]. SCFA physiological effects described here do not do justice to the full range of their health contributions, which will no doubt be expanded in the near future as the continuing focus of intestinal microbiome research.

Dysbiosis and changes in microbial metabolism impose alterations in the intestinal epithelium and tight junction protein expression, in addition to allowing immune system access to typically restricted chemicals. These changes precipitate inflammatory states, accidental cross-reactivity with foreign antigens, and represent risk factors for autoimmunity. The addition of adjuvants in vaccines on top of these conditions may manifest increased rates of ASIA syndrome. To address the possibility of these consequences, animal models of chronic inflammation are essential tools for understanding the dynamic nature of these processes.

Animal models of chronic inflammation

Biological models are widely used to research inflammation, its functional regulatory mechanisms, and to test anti-inflammatory drugs. Commonly used rodent models of inflammation can be divided into three major types: exogenous administration of endotoxin (e.g., lipopolysaccharide treatment), viable pathogens (e.g., inoculation with *Escherichia coli*), or disruption of the endogenous protective barrier (cecal ligation and puncture model) [170–172]. A fourth class of chronic inflammation model would be inherited vulnerability to stress, as observed in the Sub mouse strain we developed. All of these models have their advantages and disadvantages and address a specific type of question; however, it is still unclear which model is best used in the study of inflammation [170, 172].

Lipopolysaccharide (LPS), the main component of the outer membrane of many Gram-negative bacteria, initiates acute inflammatory responses in mammals and induces a wide range of inflammation symptoms [172, 173]. The lipopolysaccharide treatment model (LPS) is characterized by its ease of use and the rapid development of systemic inflammation accompanied by high levels of inflammatory cytokines TNFα, IL-1, and IL-6 in the blood [172, 174]. It was shown that direct and local LPS injections stimulate microglia by activating the NF-κB signaling pathway and producing neuroinflammation, which leads to an increase in Aβ levels and neuronal cell death resulting in cognitive impairment [175–178]. Thus, the LPS model can be used to study several neurodegenerative disorders such as Alzheimer's and Parkinson's diseases and the role of anti-inflammatory treatment in their prevention [175, 176, 178]. The disadvantage of this model is that it is characterized by early cytokine reactions, which are of shorter duration than seen in humans [170, 172, 174]. Furthermore, potential therapeutic anti-inflammatory agents investigated using the LPS model were ineffective in clinical trials [174, 179]. Overall, the available evidence suggests that LPS can be used to study the pathophysiological processes of systemic inflammation but not sepsis in general [171].

Another type of systemic inflammation paradigm is the peritoneal contamination and infection (PCI) model, based on intraperitoneal injections of stool samples from healthy, nonvegetarian donors to mouse recipients [171]. Donor stool samples contain various aerobic and anaerobic Gram-positive (*Staphylococcus* and *Pseudomonas*) and Gram-negative (*E. coli*) bacteria. Specific steps must be taken in advance to validate this experimental model by verifying the microbiological profile of each stool sample [170]. The advantages of this paradigm are high reproducibility, technical ease, and the rapid development of polymicrobial sepsis [171]. However, the applicability of the PCI model to the research of human systemic inflammation and sepsis is debatable, given that patients rarely have significant bacteremia [170, 171]. Moreover, the success of the model is highly dependent on antibiotic treatment and fluid resuscitation. The clinical course of inflammation in the PCI model is such that it quickly leads to the development of sepsis and death before organ injury occurs. Therefore, mice should be given maintenance antibiotic therapy [170].

The cecal ligation and puncture model (CLP) is used more to study peritonitis and sepsis than systemic inflammation [180, 181]. In this type of model, inflammation develops after the surgical operation. Following a midline laparotomy, the ileocecal valve is ligated, and the cecum is needle-punctured. Perforation of the cecum causes bacterial peritonitis, which is followed by the translocation of mixed enteric bacteria into the blood compartment. Bacteremia causes a systemic inflammatory response, septic shock, and multiorgan dysfunction [170, 182]. This model is considered "the gold standard of sepsis," such as after the CLP procedure, immune, hemodynamic, and metabolic responses in rodents identical to the clinical picture of human sepsis [180–182]. Another benefit of the CLP model is that it may be used to produce acute and chronic inflammation and sepsis of various severity levels [180, 181]. Conversely, it is necessary to standardize the protocol of the CLP procedure since the volume of bowel leakage determines the level of chronic inflammation and further sepsis. In addition, since each laboratory rodent species has its own microbiome characteristics, it is challenging to standardize studies conducted in different laboratories on different rodent species and strains. Moreover, various details of operations that may not be reported in the publications, such as needle size, incision size, and the number of punctures, can significantly impact the amount of pro-inflammatory cytokines released into the peritoneum and blood as well as affect disease progression [170, 171].

Inherited vulnerability to stress in the Sub mouse model can also be used as a model for chronic inflammation. We have found that submissive, stress-sensitive mice have an aging-dependent increase in pro-inflammatory cytokines IL-1β and IL-6 compared with both the background mouse strain (Sabra-M) and their Dom strain counterparts. The outcome of these effects were confirmed by morphological examination, which denoted splenomegaly in Sub males and females recorded postmortem at six months age. Additional confirmation of chronic inflammation in Sub mice is in the form of metabolic alterations, such as lower insulin levels and reduction of an essential factor of anabolic regulation: protein kinase B (Akt) phosphorylation. Furthermore, the reduced Akt-mediated signaling in Sub mice resulted in increased glycogen synthase kinase-3 (GSK3) activation and decreased glycogen levels in the liver, likely due to glycogenesis dysfunction [136]. Moreover, the application of chronic mild stress to Sub mice exacerbates all examined inflammation-associated changes. These data show that innate sensitivity to stress is associated with the development of chronic inflammation. Advantages of this model are the ability to develop inflammation independently, without the addition of endotoxins, bacteria, or surgical interventions, thus providing a high reproducibility and stability from generation to generation. Furthermore, the distinct inherited stress vulnerabilities of Sub mice allow researchers to study the relationship between stress and inflammation under various environmental conditions and developmental windows, including pre- and postnatal stages, aging, and the promotion of various diseases. The disadvantages of this model are the need to generate Dom-Sub mice colonies obtained by selective breeding and the need to confirm their phenotype in each generation in the dominant–submissive relationship test for breeding selection in the next generation.

Thus, different types of chronic inflammation models have their pros and cons. LPS and PCI models are easy to use and quickly develop inflammation with increased levels of pro-inflammatory cytokines [172], but the level of cytokines completely normalizes after 72 hours, and thereafter, inflammation tends to drop to zero [171]. In addition, these models do not fit the clinical picture of the development of chronic inflammation in humans. In the case of multiple injections of bacteria, the PCI model requires clinical monitoring of mice and their treatment with antibiotics. The clinical picture of the development of chronic inflammation and sepsis in humans completely coincides with the CLP model. However, long-term and precise standardization of surgical and postoperative care protocols is required to conduct research using this model. In addition, CLP mice are characterized by a higher mortality rate than LPS and PCI models [171, 181]. The mouse model naturally developing inflammation is the Sub model of innate stress vulnerability, which may present a more accurate depiction of a distinct human demographic, both in its native state and under conditions of psychosocial or chemical stress.

Conclusions

The changing chemical landscape in industrial and postindustrial nations since the latter part of the twentieth century up to today has presented new challenges on a broad population level with respect to inflammatory and autoimmune diseases. The suspected culprits behind these changes in our collective health status are intrinsic elements of modern life and will not likely be replaced or disappear from the environment anytime in the near future. The emerging threat of novel diseases, promulgated by global trade and ease of international travel, presents new challenges to the health care community regarding rapid vaccine development and deployment. The increasing use of mRNA-based vaccines, due to the specificity with which they can be tailored coupled with their shortened development time, will likely become the new normal for future mass immunizations. Use of adjuvants, common components of vaccines, in a population with increasing rates of chronic inflammation and autoimmune disease will likely increase the incidence of ASIA syndromes. The unknown long-term effects of mRNA vaccine use require thorough monitoring and follow-up collection of a wide array of physiological parameters to fully assess their future societal health impact. Animal models of stress sensitivity and chronic inflammation are also indispensable tools in this pursuit toward unraveling the mechanisms behind the population-wide rise in inflammation-based and autoimmune diseases. The Sub mouse strain is of particular utility in that it has demonstrated an innate sensitivity to stress, stress- and toxicant-induced epigenetic alteration of intestinal tight junction expression, and intestinal dysbiosis as a default condition, all suspected components of vulnerability to development of chronic inflammation and autoimmune disease. With regard to ASIA syndrome, use of stress-sensitive mice displaying chronic inflammation treated with adjuvant-laden vaccines as a test model may provide some predictive measures of vaccine-related adverse health outcomes.

References

1. Shoenfeld, Y. and Agmon-Levin, N. (2011). 'ASIA' – autoimmune/inflammatory syndrome induced by adjuvants. *J. Autoimmun.* 36 (1): 4–8.
2. Borba, V., Malkova, A., Basantsova, N. et al. (2020). Classical examples of the concept of the ASIA syndrome. *Biomol. Ther.* 10 (10): 1436.
3. Jara, L.J., Garcia-Collinot, G., Medina, G. et al. (2017). Severe manifestations of autoimmune syndrome induced by adjuvants (Shoenfeld's syndrome). *Immunol. Res.* 65 (1): 8–16.
4. Desai, M.K. and Brinton, R.D. (2019). Autoimmune disease in women: endocrine transition and risk across the lifespan. *Front. Endocrinol. (Lausanne)* 10: 265.
5. Parks, C.G., Miller, F.W., Pollard, K.M. et al. (2014). Expert panel workshop consensus statement on the role of the environment in the development of autoimmune disease. *Int. J. Mol. Sci.* 15 (8): 14269–14297.
6. Lerner, A., Jeremias, P., and Matthias, T. (2015). The world incidence and prevalence of autoimmune diseases is increasing. *Int. J. Celiac. Dis.* 3 (4): 151–155.
7. Lerner, A. and Matthias, T. (2015). Changes in intestinal tight junction permeability associated with industrial food additives explain the rising incidence of autoimmune disease. *Autoimmun. Rev.* 14 (6): 479–489.
8. Canavan, C., West, J., and Card, T. (2014). The epidemiology of irritable bowel syndrome. *Clin. Epidemiol.* 6: 71–80.
9. Avena-Woods, C. (2017). Overview of atopic dermatitis. *Am. J. Manag. Care* 23 (8 Suppl): S115–S123.
10. Ford, A.C., Talley, N.J., Walker, M.M., and Jones, M.P. (2014). Increased prevalence of autoimmune diseases in functional gastrointestinal disorders: case-control study of 23471 primary care patients. *Aliment. Pharmacol. Ther.* 40 (7): 827–834.
11. Wu, L.C., Hwang, C.Y., Chung, P.I. et al. (2014). Autoimmune disease comorbidities in patients with atopic dermatitis: a nationwide case-control study in Taiwan. *Pediatr. Allergy Immunol.* 25 (6): 586–592.
12. Koloski, N., Jones, M., Walker, M.M. et al. (2019). Population based study: atopy and autoimmune diseases are associated with functional dyspepsia and irritable bowel syndrome, independent of psychological distress. *Aliment. Pharmacol. Ther.* 49 (5): 546–555.
13. Oliveira, C. and Torres, T. (2019). More than skin deep: the systemic nature of atopic dermatitis. *Eur. J. Dermatol.* 29 (3): 250–258.
14. Ivert, L.U., Wahlgren, C.F., Lindelof, B. et al. (2021). Association between atopic dermatitis and autoimmune diseases: a population-based case-control study. *Br. J. Dermatol.* 185 (2): 335–342.
15. Akdis, C.A. (2021). Does the epithelial barrier hypothesis explain the increase in allergy, autoimmunity and other chronic conditions? *Nat. Rev. Immunol.* 21 (11): 739–751.

16. Celebi Sozener, Z., Cevhertas, L., Nadeau, K. et al. (2020). Environmental factors in epithelial barrier dysfunction. *J. Allergy Clin. Immunol.* 145 (6): 1517–1528.
17. Pinhasov, A. and Kirby, M. (2022). Linking stress and inflammation - is there a missing piece in the puzzle? *Expert Rev. Clin. Immunol.* **18** (4): 321–323.
18. Petras, M., Lesna, I.K., Danova, J., and Celko, A.M. (2021). Can vaccination trigger autoimmune disorders? A meta-analysis. *Vaccines (Basel)* 9 (8): 821.
19. Bach, J.F. (2002). The effect of infections on susceptibility to autoimmune and allergic diseases. *N. Engl. J. Med.* 347 (12): 911–920.
20. Asher, M.I., Montefort, S., Bjorksten, B. et al. (2006). Worldwide time trends in the prevalence of symptoms of asthma, allergic rhinoconjunctivitis, and eczema in childhood: ISAAC phases one and three repeat multicountry cross-sectional surveys. *Lancet* 368 (9537): 733–743.
21. Eder, W., Ege, M.J., and von Mutius, E. (2006). The asthma epidemic. *N. Engl. J. Med.* 355 (21): 2226–2235.
22. Platts-Mills, T.A. (2015). The allergy epidemics: 1870-2010. *J. Allergy Clin. Immunol.* 136 (1): 3–13.
23. Backman, H., Raisanen, P., Hedman, L. et al. (2017). Increased prevalence of allergic asthma from 1996 to 2006 and further to 2016-results from three population surveys. *Clin. Exp. Allergy* 47 (11): 1426–1435.
24. Grode, L., Bech, B.H., Jensen, T.M. et al. (2018). Prevalence, incidence, and autoimmune comorbidities of celiac disease: a nation-wide, population-based study in Denmark from 1977 to 2016. *Eur. J. Gastroenterol. Hepatol.* 30 (1): 83–91.
25. Pereira, M., Carreira, H., Lunet, N., and Azevedo, A. (2014). Trends in prevalence of diabetes mellitus and mean fasting glucose in Portugal (1987-2009): a systematic review. *Public Health* 128 (3): 214–221.
26. Huang, X., Tsilochristou, O., Perna, S. et al. (2018). Evolution of the IgE and IgG repertoire to a comprehensive array of allergen molecules in the first decade of life. *Allergy* 73 (2): 421–430.
27. Toedter, G., Li, K., Sague, S. et al. (2012). Genes associated with intestinal permeability in ulcerative colitis: changes in expression following infliximab therapy. *Inflamm. Bowel Dis.* 18 (8): 1399–1410.
28. Schoultz, I. and Keita, A.V. (2019). Cellular and molecular therapeutic targets in inflammatory bowel disease-focusing on intestinal barrier function. *Cell* 8 (2).
29. Hou, Q., Huang, J., Ayansola, H. et al. (2020). Intestinal stem cells and immune cell relationships: potential therapeutic targets for inflammatory bowel diseases. *Front. Immunol.* 11: 623691.
30. Fasano, A. (2012). Zonulin, regulation of tight junctions, and autoimmune diseases. *Ann. N. Y. Acad. Sci.* 1258: 25–33.
31. Leffler, D.A., Kelly, C.P., Green, P.H. et al. (2015). Larazotide acetate for persistent symptoms of celiac disease despite a gluten-free diet: a randomized controlled trial. *Gastroenterology* 148 (7): 1311–9 e6.
32. Schumann, M., Siegmund, B., Schulzke, J.D., and Fromm, M. (2017). Celiac disease: role of the epithelial barrier. *Cell. Mol. Gastroenterol. Hepatol.* 3 (2): 150–162.
33. Bosi, E., Molteni, L., Radaelli, M.G. et al. (2006). Increased intestinal permeability precedes clinical onset of type 1 diabetes. *Diabetologia* 49 (12): 2824–2827.
34. Sharma, S. and Tripathi, P. (2019). Gut microbiome and type 2 diabetes: where we are and where to go? *J. Nutr. Biochem.* 63: 101–108.
35. Sorini, C., Cosorich, I., Conte, M.L. et al. (2019). Loss of gut barrier integrity triggers activation of islet-reactive T cells and autoimmune diabetes. *Proc. Natl. Acad. Sci. U. S. A.* 116 (30): 15140–15149.
36. Camara-Lemarroy, C.R., Silva, C., Greenfield, J. et al. (2020). Biomarkers of intestinal barrier function in multiple sclerosis are associated with disease activity. *Mult. Scler.* 26 (11): 1340–1350.
37. Buscarinu, M.C., Fornasiero, A., Romano, S. et al. (2019). The contribution of gut barrier changes to multiple sclerosis pathophysiology. *Front. Immunol.* 10: 1916.
38. Mouries, J., Brescia, P., Silvestri, A. et al. (2019). Microbiota-driven gut vascular barrier disruption is a prerequisite for non-alcoholic steatohepatitis development. *J. Hepatol.* 71 (6): 1216–1228.
39. Fukui, H. (2019). Role of gut dysbiosis in liver diseases: what have we learned so far? *Diseases* 7 (4): 58.
40. Hoffmanova, I., Sánchez, D., Tučková, L. et al. (2018). Celiac disease and liver disorders: from putative pathogenesis to clinical implications. *Nutrients* 10 (7): 892.
41. Ponziani, F.R., Zocco, M.A., Cerrito, L. et al. (2018). Bacterial translocation in patients with liver cirrhosis: physiology, clinical consequences, and practical implications. *Expert Rev. Gastroenterol. Hepatol.* 12 (7): 641–656.
42. Di Ciaula, A., Baj, J., Garruti, G. et al. (2020). Liver steatosis, gut-liver axis, microbiome and environmental factors. a never-ending bidirectional cross-talk. *J. Clin. Med.* 9 (8): 2648.

43. Tajik, N., Frech, M., Schulz, O. et al. (2020). Targeting zonulin and intestinal epithelial barrier function to prevent onset of arthritis. *Nat. Commun.* 11 (1): 1995.
44. Kim, J.W., Kwok, S.K., Choe, J.Y. et al. (2019). Recent advances in our understanding of the link between the intestinal microbiota and systemic lupus erythematosus. *Int. J. Mol. Sci.* 20 (19): 4871.
45. Ciccia, F., Guggino, G., Rizzo, A. et al. (2017). Dysbiosis and zonulin upregulation alter gut epithelial and vascular barriers in patients with ankylosing spondylitis. *Ann. Rheum. Dis.* 76 (6): 1123–1132.
46. Raybould, H.E. (2012). Gut microbiota, epithelial function and derangements in obesity. *J. Physiol.* 590 (3): 441–446.
47. Cox, A.J., West, N.P., and Cripps, A.W. (2015). Obesity, inflammation, and the gut microbiota. *Lancet Diabetes Endocrinol.* 3 (3): 207–215.
48. Xiao, C., Puddicombe, S.M., Field, S. et al. (2011). Defective epithelial barrier function in asthma. *J. Allergy Clin. Immunol.* 128 (3): 549–556. e1-12.
49. Wawrzyniak, P., Wawrzyniak, M., Wanke, K. et al. (2017). Regulation of bronchial epithelial barrier integrity by type 2 cytokines and histone deacetylases in asthmatic patients. *J. Allergy Clin. Immunol.* 139 (1): 93–103.
50. De Benedetto, A., Rafaels, N.M., McGirt, L.Y. et al. (2011). Tight junction defects in patients with atopic dermatitis. *J. Allergy Clin. Immunol.* 127 (3): 773–786. e1-7.
51. Irvine, A.D., McLean, W.H., and Leung, D.Y. (2011). Filaggrin mutations associated with skin and allergic diseases. *N. Engl. J. Med.* 365 (14): 1315–1327.
52. Steelant, B., Wawrzyniak, P., Martens, K. et al. (2019). Blocking histone deacetylase activity as a novel target for epithelial barrier defects in patients with allergic rhinitis. *J. Allergy Clin. Immunol.* 144 (5): 1242–1253 e7.
53. Steelant, B., Seys, S.F., Van Gerven, L. et al. (2018). Histamine and T helper cytokine-driven epithelial barrier dysfunction in allergic rhinitis. *J. Allergy Clin. Immunol.* 141 (3): 951–963 e8.
54. Steelant, B., Farré, R., Wawrzyniak, P. et al. (2016). Impaired barrier function in patients with house dust mite-induced allergic rhinitis is accompanied by decreased occludin and zonula occludens-1 expression. *J. Allergy Clin. Immunol.* 137 (4): 1043–1053 e5.
55. Soyka, M.B., Wawrzyniak, P., Eiwegger, T. et al. (2012). Defective epithelial barrier in chronic rhinosinusitis: the regulation of tight junctions by IFN-gamma and IL-4. *J. Allergy Clin. Immunol.* 130 (5): 1087–1096 e10.
56. Simon, D., Page, B., Vogel, M. et al. (2018). Evidence of an abnormal epithelial barrier in active, untreated and corticosteroid-treated eosinophilic esophagitis. *Allergy* 73 (1): 239–247.
57. Masterson, J.C., Biette, K.A., Hammer, J.A. et al. (2019). Epithelial HIF-1alpha/claudin-1 axis regulates barrier dysfunction in eosinophilic esophagitis. *J. Clin. Invest.* 129 (8): 3224–3235.
58. Fiorentino, M., Sapone, A., Senger, S. et al. (2016). Blood-brain barrier and intestinal epithelial barrier alterations in autism spectrum disorders. *Mol. Autism* 7: 49.
59. Pellegrini, C., Antonioli, L., Colucci, R. et al. (2018). Interplay among gut microbiota, intestinal mucosal barrier and enteric neuro-immune system: a common path to neurodegenerative diseases? *Acta Neuropathol.* 136 (3): 345–361.
60. Kohler, C.A., Maes, M., Slyepchenko, A. et al. (2016). The gut-brain axis, including the microbiome, leaky gut and bacterial translocation: mechanisms and pathophysiological role in Alzheimer's disease. *Curr. Pharm. Des.* 22 (40): 6152–6166.
61. Dutta, S.K., Verma, S., Jain, V. et al. (2019). Parkinson's disease: the emerging role of gut dysbiosis, antibiotics, probiotics, and fecal microbiota transplantation. *J. Neurogastroenterol. Motil.* 25 (3): 363–376.
62. van IJzendoorn, S.C.D. and Derkinderen, P. (2019). The intestinal barrier in Parkinson's disease: current state of knowledge. *J. Parkinsons Dis.* 9 (s2): S323–S329.
63. Rudzki, L. and Maes, M. (2021). From "leaky gut" to impaired glia-neuron communication in depression. *Adv. Exp. Med. Biol.* 1305: 129–155.
64. Maes, M., Kubera, M., Leunis, J.C., and Berk, M. (2012). Increased IgA and IgM responses against gut commensals in chronic depression: further evidence for increased bacterial translocation or leaky gut. *J. Affect. Disord.* 141 (1): 55–62.
65. Ohlsson, L., Gustafsson, A., Lavant, E. et al. (2019). Leaky gut biomarkers in depression and suicidal behavior. *Acta Psychiatr. Scand.* 139 (2): 185–193.

66. Kelly, J.R., Kennedy, P.J., Cryan, J.F. et al. (2015). Breaking down the barriers: the gut microbiome, intestinal permeability and stress-related psychiatric disorders. *Front. Cell. Neurosci.* 9: 392.
67. Madison, A. and Kiecolt-Glaser, J.K. (2019). Stress, depression, diet, and the gut microbiota: human-bacteria interactions at the core of psychoneuroimmunology and nutrition. *Curr. Opin. Behav. Sci.* 28: 105–110.
68. Garcia-Hernandez, V., Quiros, M., and Nusrat, A. (2017). Intestinal epithelial claudins: expression and regulation in homeostasis and inflammation. *Ann. N. Y. Acad. Sci.* 1397 (1): 66–79.
69. Lu, Z., Ding, L., Lu, Q., and Chen, Y.H. (2013). Claudins in intestines: Distribution and functional significance in health and diseases. *Tissue Barriers* 1 (3): e24978.
70. Castro, V., Skowronska, M., Lombardi, J. et al. (2018). Occludin regulates glucose uptake and ATP production in pericytes by influencing AMP-activated protein kinase activity. *J. Cereb. Blood Flow Metab.* 38 (2): 317–332.
71. Mrsny, R.J., Brown, G.T., Gerner-Smidt, K. et al. (2008). A key claudin extracellular loop domain is critical for epithelial barrier integrity. *Am. J. Pathol.* 172 (4): 905–915.
72. Mineta, K., Yamamoto, Y., Yamazaki, Y. et al. (2011). Predicted expansion of the claudin multigene family. *FEBS Lett.* 585 (4): 606–612.
73. Chretien, I., Marcuz, A., Courtet, M. et al. (1998). CTX, a Xenopus thymocyte receptor, defines a molecular family conserved throughout vertebrates. *Eur. J. Immunol.* 28 (12): 4094–4104.
74. Keita, A.V. and Soderholm, J.D. (2010). The intestinal barrier and its regulation by neuroimmune factors. *Neurogastroenterol. Motil.* 22 (7): 718–733.
75. Al-Sadi, R., Guo, S., Ye, D., and Ma, T.Y. (2013). TNF-alpha modulation of intestinal epithelial tight junction barrier is regulated by ERK1/2 activation of Elk-1. *Am. J. Pathol.* 183 (6): 1871–1884.
76. Boivin, M.A., Ye, D., Kennedy, J.C. et al. (2007). Mechanism of glucocorticoid regulation of the intestinal tight junction barrier. *Am. J. Physiol. Gastrointest. Liver Physiol.* 292 (2): G590–G598.
77. Findley, M.K. and Koval, M. (2009). Regulation and roles for claudin-family tight junction proteins. *IUBMB Life* 61 (4): 431–437.
78. Diaz-Garrido, N., Badia, J., and Baldoma, L. (2021). Microbiota-derived extracellular vesicles in interkingdom communication in the gut. *J. Extracell. Vesicles* 10 (13): e12161.
79. Morozumi, S., Ueda, M., Okahashi, N., and Arita, M. (2022). Structures and functions of the gut microbial lipidome. *Biochim. Biophys. Acta Mol. Cell Biol. Lipids* 1867 (3): 159110.
80. Sjo, A., Magnusson, K.E., and Peterson, K.H. (2010). Protein kinase C activation has distinct effects on the localization, phosphorylation and detergent solubility of the claudin protein family in tight and leaky epithelial cells. *J. Membr. Biol.* 236 (2): 181–189.
81. Xian, M., Wawrzyniak, P., Ruckert, B. et al. (2016). Anionic surfactants and commercial detergents decrease tight junction barrier integrity in human keratinocytes. *J. Allergy Clin. Immunol.* 138 (3): 890–893 e9.
82. Wang, M., Tan, G., Eljaszewicz, A. et al. (2019). Laundry detergents and detergent residue after rinsing directly disrupt tight junction barrier integrity in human bronchial epithelial cells. *J. Allergy Clin. Immunol.* 143 (5): 1892–1903.
83. Bajpai, D. and Tyagi, V.K. (2007). Laundry detergents: an overview. *J. Oleo Sci.* 56 (7): 327–340.
84. Leisola, M., Jokela, J., Pastinen, O., and Turunen, O. (2001). Industrial use of enzymes. In: *Medical and Health Sciences*, vol. II (ed. O.O.P. Hanninen and M. Atalay), 130–154. Eolss Publishers.
85. Csaki, K.F. (2011). Synthetic surfactant food additives can cause intestinal barrier dysfunction. *Med. Hypotheses* 76 (5): 676–681.
86. Ilback, N.G., Nyblom, M., Carlfors, J. et al. (2004). Do surface-active lipids in food increase the intestinal permeability to toxic substances and allergenic agents? *Med. Hypotheses* 63 (4): 724–730.
87. Roberts, C.L., Rushworth, S.L., Richman, E., and Rhodes, J.M. (2013). Hypothesis: Increased consumption of emulsifiers as an explanation for the rising incidence of Crohn's disease. *J. Crohns Colitis* 7 (4): 338–341.
88. Traunmuller, F. (2005). Etiology of Crohn's disease: do certain food additives cause intestinal inflammation by molecular mimicry of mycobacterial lipids? *Med. Hypotheses* 65 (5): 859–864.
89. Mine, Y. and Zhang, J.W. (2003). Surfactants enhance the tight-junction permeability of food allergens in human intestinal epithelial Caco-2 cells. *Int. Arch. Allergy Immunol.* 130 (2): 135–142.
90. Bancil, A.S., Sandall, A.M., Rossi, M. et al. (2021). Food additive emulsifiers and their impact on gut microbiome, permeability, and inflammation: mechanistic insights in inflammatory bowel disease. *J. Crohns Colitis* 15 (6): 1068–1079.

91. Cani, P.D. and Everard, A. (2015). Keeping gut lining at bay: impact of emulsifiers. *Trends Endocrinol. Metab.* 26 (6): 273–274.
92. Cani, P.D. (2015). Metabolism: Dietary emulsifiers--sweepers of the gut lining? *Nat. Rev. Endocrinol.* 11 (6): 319–320.
93. Chassaing, B., Koren, O., Goodrich, J.K. et al. (2015). Dietary emulsifiers impact the mouse gut microbiota promoting colitis and metabolic syndrome. *Nature* 519 (7541): 92–96.
94. Aguayo-Patron, S.V. and Calderon de la Barca, A.M. (2017). Old fashioned vs. ultra-processed-based current diets: possible implication in the increased susceptibility to type 1 diabetes and celiac disease in childhood. *Foods* 6 (11): 100.
95. Roberts, C.L., Keita, A.V., Duncan, S.H. et al. (2010). Translocation of Crohn's disease *Escherichia coli* across M-cells: contrasting effects of soluble plant fibres and emulsifiers. *Gut* 59 (10): 1331–1339.
96. Cordier, M. and Uehara, T. (2019). How much innovation is needed to protect the ocean from plastic contamination? *Sci. Total Environ.* 670: 789–799.
97. De-la-Torre, G.E. (2020). Microplastics: an emerging threat to food security and human health. *J. Food Sci. Technol.* 57 (5): 1601–1608.
98. Galloway, T.S. (2015). Micro- and nano-plastics and human health marine anthropogenic litter. In: *Bremerhaven* (ed. M. Bergmann, L. Gutow, and M. Klages). Germany: Springer, Cham.
99. Lehel, J. and Murphy, S. (2021). Microplastics in the food chain: food safety and environmental aspects. *Rev. Environ. Contam. Toxicol.* 259: 1–49.
100. Cverenkarova, K., Valachovicova, M., Mackulak, T. et al. (2021). Microplastics in the food chain. *Life (Basel)* 11: 12, 1349.
101. Kwon, J.H., Kim, J.W., Pham, T.D. et al. (2020). Microplastics in food: a review on analytical methods and challenges. *Int. J. Environ. Res. Public Health* 17 (18): 6710.
102. Allen, S., Allen, D., Phoenix, V.R. et al. (2019). Atmospheric transport and deposition of microplastics in a remote mountain catchment. *Nat. Geosci.* 12: 339–344.
103. Frias, J. and Nash, R. (2019). Microplastics: Finding a consensus on the definition. *Mar. Pollut. Bull.* 138: 145–147.
104. Stock, V., Bohmert, L., Lisicki, E. et al. (2019). Uptake and effects of orally ingested polystyrene microplastic particles in vitro and in vivo. *Arch. Toxicol.* 93 (7): 1817–1833.
105. Xu, M., Halimu, G., Zhang, Q. et al. (2019). Internalization and toxicity: A preliminary study of effects of nanoplastic particles on human lung epithelial cell. *Sci. Total Environ.* 694: 133794.
106. Holloczki, O. and Gehrke, S. (2019). Nanoplastics can change the secondary structure of proteins. *Sci. Rep.* 9 (1): 16013.
107. Holloczki, O. and Gehrke, S. (2020). Can nanoplastics alter cell membranes? *ChemPhysChem* 21 (1): 9–12.
108. Jin, Y., Lu, L., Tu, W. et al. (2019). Impacts of polystyrene microplastic on the gut barrier, microbiota and metabolism of mice. *Sci. Total Environ.* 649: 308–317.
109. Lichtenstein, D., Ebmeyer, J., Meyer, T. et al. (2017). It takes more than a coating to get nanoparticles through the intestinal barrier in vitro. *Eur. J. Pharm. Biopharm.* 118: 21–29.
110. Vita, A.A., Royse, E.A., and Pullen, N.A. (2019). Nanoparticles and danger signals: oral delivery vehicles as potential disruptors of intestinal barrier homeostasis. *J. Leukoc. Biol.* 106 (1): 95–103.
111. Khanna, P., Ong, C., Bay, B.H., and Baeg, G.H. (2015). Nanotoxicity: an interplay of oxidative stress, inflammation and cell death. *Nanomaterials (Basel)* 5 (3): 1163–1180.
112. Smith, K.E. and Pollak, S.D. (2020). Early life stress and development: potential mechanisms for adverse outcomes. *J. Neurodev. Disord.* 12 (1): 34.
113. Gross, M., Romi, H., Miller, A., and Pinhasov, A. (2018). Social dominance predicts hippocampal glucocorticoid receptor recruitment and resilience to prenatal adversity. *Sci. Rep.* 8: 9595.
114. Murlanova, K., Begmatova, D., Weber-Stadlbauer, U. et al. (2022). Double trouble: prenatal immune activation in stress sensitive offspring. *Brain Behav. Immun.* 99: 3–8.
115. van Bodegom, M., Homberg, J.R., and Henckens, M.J.A.G. (2017). Modulation of the hypothalamic-pituitary-adrenal axis by early life stress exposure. *Front. Cell. Neurosci.* 11: 87.
116. Elzinga, B.M., Roelofs, K., Tollenaar, M.S. et al. (2008). Diminished cortisol responses to psychosocial stress associated with lifetime adverse events a study among healthy young subjects. *Psychoneuroendocrinology* 33 (2): 227–237.

117. Bunea, I.M., Szentágotai-Tătar, A., and Miu, A.C. (2017). Early-life adversity and cortisol response to social stress: a meta-analysis. *Transl. Psychiatry* 7 (12): 1–8.
118. Zhang, H., Yao, Z., Lin, L. et al. (2019). Early life stress predicts cortisol response to psychosocial stress in healthy young adults. *Psych J.* 8 (3): 353–362.
119. Ceruso, A., Martinez-Cengotitabengoa, M., Peters-Corbett, A. et al. (2020). Alterations of the HPA axis observed in patients with major depressive disorder and their relation to early life stress: a systematic review. *Neuropsychobiology* 79 (6): 417–427.
120. Hosseini-Kamkar, N., Lowe, C., and Morton, J.B. (2021). The differential calibration of the HPA axis as a function of trauma versus adversity: a systematic review and p-curve meta-analyses. *Neurosci. Biobehav. Rev.* 127: 54–135.
121. McClain, J.L., Mazzotta, E.A., Maradiaga, N. et al. (2020). Histamine-dependent interactions between mast cells, glia, and neurons are altered following early-life adversity in mice and humans. *Am. J. Physiol. Gastrointest. Liver Physiol.* 319 (6): G655–G668.
122. Chang, L., Di Lorenzo, C., Farrugia, G. et al. (2018). Functional bowel disorders: a roadmap to guide the next generation of research. *Gastroenterology* 154 (3): 723–735.
123. Li, M., Fu, X., Xie, W. et al. (2020). Effect of early life stress on the epigenetic profiles in depression. *Front Cell Dev. Biol.* 8: 867.
124. Sur, D., Agranyoni, O., Kirby, M. et al. (2023). Nurture outpaces nature: fostering with an attentive mother alters social dominance in a mouse model of stress sensitivity. *Mol. Psychiatry* **28** (9): 3816–3828.
125. Liu, Y.Z., Wang, Y.X., and Jiang, C.L. (2017). Inflammation: the common pathway of stress-related diseases. *Front. Hum. Neurosci.* 11: 316.
126. Rohleder, N. (2019). Stress and inflammation – the need to address the gap in the transition between acute and chronic stress effects. *Psychoneuroendocrinology* 105: 164–171.
127. Pfeiffer, J.R., Mutesa, L., and Uddin, M. (2018). Traumatic stress epigenetics. *Curr. Behav. Neurosci. Rep.* 5 (1): 81–93.
128. Bahji, A., Forth, E., Hargreaves, T., and Harkness, K. (2021). Genetic markers of the stress generation model: a systematic review. *Psychiatry Res.* 304: 114139.
129. Orjuela, S., Machlab, D., Menigatti, M. et al. (2020). DAMEfinder: a method to detect differential allele-specific methylation. *Epigenetics Chromatin* 13 (1): 25.
130. Gross, M., Romi, H., Gilimovich, Y. et al. (2018). Placental glucocorticoid receptor and 11β-hydroxysteroid dehydrogenase-2 recruitment indicates impact of prenatal adversity upon postnatal development in mice. *Stress* 21 (6): 474–483.
131. Ben-Shachar, M., Daniel, T., Wollman, A. et al. (2023). Inherited stress resiliency prevents the development of metabolic alterations in diet-induced obese mice. *Obesity (Silver Spring)* **31** (8): 2043–2056.
132. Hasleton, P.S. (1972). The internal surface area of the adult human lung. *J. Anat.* 112 (Pt 3): 391–400.
133. Helander, H.F. and Fandriks, L. (2014). Surface area of the digestive tract - revisited. *Scand. J. Gastroenterol.* 49 (6): 681–689.
134. Gallo, R.L. (2017). Human skin is the largest epithlelial surface for interaction with microbes. *J. Invest. Dermatol.* 137 (6): 1213–1214.
135. Cryan, J.F., O'Riordan, K.J., Cowan, C.S.M. et al. (2019). The microbiota-gut-brain axis. *Physiol. Rev.* 99 (4): 1877–2013.
136. Bairachnaya, M., Agranyoni, O., Antoch, M. et al. (2019). Innate sensitivity to stress facilitates inflammation, alters metabolism and shortens lifespan in a mouse model of social hierarchy. *Aging (Albany NY)* 11 (21): 9901–9911.
137. Agranyoni, O., Meninger-Mordechay, S., Uzan, A. et al. (2021). Gut microbiota determines the social behavior of mice and induces metabolic and inflammatory changes in their adipose tissue. *NPJ Biofilms Microbiomes* **7** (1): 28.
138. Shapiro, J., Cohen, N.A., Shalev, V. et al. (2019). Psoriatic patients have a distinct structural and functional fecal microbiota compared with controls. *J. Dermatol.* 46 (7): 595–603.
139. Agostoni, E., Chinnock, J.E., De Daly, M.B. et al. (1957). Functional and histological studies of the vagus nerve and its branches to the heart, lungs and abdominal viscera in the cat. *J. Physiol.* 135 (1): 182–205.
140. Borovikova, L.V., Ivanova, S., Zhang, M. et al. (2000). Vagus nerve stimulation attenuates the systemic inflammatory response to endotoxin. *Nature* 405 (6785): 458–462.

141. Borovikova, L.V., Ivanova, S., Nardi, D. et al. (2000). Role of vagus nerve signaling in CNI-1493-mediated suppression of acute inflammation. *Auton. Neurosci.* 85 (1–3): 141–147.
142. Pavlov, V.A., Wang, H., Czura, C.J. et al. (2003). The cholinergic anti-inflammatory pathway: a missing link in neuroimmunomodulation. *Mol. Med.* 9 (5–8): 125–134.
143. Du, M.H., Luo, H.M., Hu, S. et al. (2013). Electroacupuncture improves gut barrier dysfunction in prolonged hemorrhagic shock rats through vagus anti-inflammatory mechanism. *World J. Gastroenterol.* 19 (36): 5988–5999.
144. Bonaz, B., Sinniger, V., and Pellissier, S. (2017). The vagus nerve in the neuro-immune axis: implications in the pathology of the gastrointestinal tract. *Front. Immunol.* 8: 1452.
145. Bonaz, B., Sinniger, V., and Pellissier, S. (2017). Vagus nerve stimulation: a new promising therapeutic tool in inflammatory bowel disease. *J. Intern. Med.* 282 (1): 46–63.
146. Bernstein, C.N. (2017). The brain-gut axis and stress in inflammatory bowel disease. *Gastroenterol. Clin. N. Am.* 46 (4): 839–846.
147. Bonaz, B. (2018). Is-there a place for vagus nerve stimulation in inflammatory bowel diseases? *Bioelectron. Med.* 4: 4.
148. Cani, P.D., Everard, A., and Duparc, T. (2013). Gut microbiota, enteroendocrine functions and metabolism. *Curr. Opin. Pharmacol.* 13 (6): 935–940.
149. Turroni, S., Brigidi, P., Cavalli, A., and Candela, M. (2018). Microbiota-host transgenomic metabolism, bioactive molecules from the inside. *J. Med. Chem.* 61 (1): 47–61.
150. Rothhammer, V., Mascanfroni, I.D., Bunse, L. et al. (2016). Type I interferons and microbial metabolites of tryptophan modulate astrocyte activity and central nervous system inflammation via the aryl hydrocarbon receptor. *Nat. Med.* 22 (6): 586–597.
151. O'Mahony, S.M., Clarke, G., Borre, Y.E. et al. (2015). Serotonin, tryptophan metabolism and the brain-gut-microbiome axis. *Behav. Brain Res.* 277: 32–48.
152. Zelante, T., Iannitti, R.G., Cunha, C. et al. (2013). Tryptophan catabolites from microbiota engage aryl hydrocarbon receptor and balance mucosal reactivity via interleukin-22. *Immunity* 39 (2): 372–385.
153. Cummings, J.H., Pomare, E.W., Branch, W.J. et al. (1987). Short chain fatty acids in human large intestine, portal, hepatic and venous blood. *Gut* 28 (10): 1221–1227.
154. Brown, D.M., Butler, D., Orman, N.R., and Davies, J.W. (1996). Gross solids transport in small diameter sewers. *Water Sci. Technol.* 33 (9): 25–30.
155. Kau, A.L., Ahern, P.P., Griffin, N.W. et al. (2011). Human nutrition, the gut microbiome and the immune system. *Nature* 474 (7351): 327–336.
156. Zhao, L., Zhang, F., Ding, X. et al. (2018). Gut bacteria selectively promoted by dietary fibers alleviate type 2 diabetes. *Science* 359 (6380): 1151–1156.
157. Machiels, K., Joossens, M., Sabino, J. et al. (2014). A decrease of the butyrate-producing species Roseburia hominis and Faecalibacterium prausnitzii defines dysbiosis in patients with ulcerative colitis. *Gut* 63 (8): 1275–1283.
158. Vinolo, M.A., Rodrigues, H.G., Hatanaka, E. et al. (2011). Suppressive effect of short-chain fatty acids on production of proinflammatory mediators by neutrophils. *J. Nutr. Biochem.* 22 (9): 849–855.
159. Vinolo, M.A., Rodrigues, H.G., Nachbar, R.T., and Curi, R. (2011). Regulation of inflammation by short chain fatty acids. *Nutrients* 3 (10): 858–876.
160. Furusawa, Y., Obata, Y., Fukuda, S. et al. (2013). Commensal microbe-derived butyrate induces the differentiation of colonic regulatory T cells. *Nature* 504 (7480): 446–450.
161. Arpaia, N., Campbell, C., Fan, X. et al. (2013). Metabolites produced by commensal bacteria promote peripheral regulatory T-cell generation. *Nature* 504 (7480): 451–455.
162. Al Nabhani, Z., Dulauroy, S., Marques, R. et al. (2019). A weaning reaction to microbiota is required for resistance to immunopathologies in the adult. *Immunity* 50 (5): 1276–1288 e5.
163. Singh, N., Gurav, A., Sivaprakasam, S. et al. (2014). Activation of Gpr109a, receptor for niacin and the commensal metabolite butyrate, suppresses colonic inflammation and carcinogenesis. *Immunity* 40 (1): 128–139.
164. Maslowski, K.M., Vieira, A.T., Ng, A. et al. (2009). Regulation of inflammatory responses by gut microbiota and chemoattractant receptor GPR43. *Nature* 461 (7268): 1282–1286.
165. Fukuda, S., Toh, H., Hase, K. et al. (2011). Bifidobacteria can protect from enteropathogenic infection through production of acetate. *Nature* 469 (7331): 543–547.

166. Nowarski, R., Jackson, R., Gagliani, N. et al. (2015). Epithelial IL-18 equilibrium controls barrier function in colitis. *Cell* 163 (6): 1444–1456.
167. Swanson, K.V., Deng, M., and Ting, J.P. (2019). The NLRP3 inflammasome: molecular activation and regulation to therapeutics. *Nat. Rev. Immunol.* 19 (8): 477–489.
168. Tedelind, S., Westberg, F., Kjerrulf, M., and Vidal, A. (2007). Anti-inflammatory properties of the short-chain fatty acids acetate and propionate: a study with relevance to inflammatory bowel disease. *World J. Gastroenterol.* 13 (20): 2826–2832.
169. Yoo, J.Y., Groer, M., Dutra, S.V.O. et al. (2020). Gut microbiota and immune system interactions. *Microorganisms* 8 (10): 1587.
170. Lewis, A.J., Seymour, C.W., and Rosengart, M.R. (2016). Current murine models of sepsis. *Surg. Infect.* 17 (4): 385–393.
171. Seemann, S., Zohles, F., and Lupp, A. (2017). Comprehensive comparison of three different animal models for systemic inflammation. *J. Biomed. Sci.* 24 (1): 60.
172. Murando, F., Peloso, A., and Cobianchi, L. (2019). Experimental abdominal sepsis: sticking to an awkward but still useful translational model. *Mediat. Inflamm.* 2019: e8971036.
173. Brooks, D., Barr, L.C., Wiscombe, S. et al. (2020). Human lipopolysaccharide models provide mechanistic and therapeutic insights into systemic and pulmonary inflammation. *Eur. Respir. J.* 56 (1).
174. Warren, H.S., Fitting, C., Hoff, E. et al. (2010). Resilience to bacterial infection: difference between species could be due to proteins in serum. *J. Infect. Dis.* 201 (2): 223–232.
175. Catorce, M.N. and Gevorkian, G. (2016). LPS-induced murine neuroinflammation model: main features and suitability for pre-clinical assessment of nutraceuticals. *Curr. Neuropharmacol.* 14 (2): 155–164.
176. Batista, C.R.A., Gomes, G.F., Candelario-Jalil, E. et al. (2019). Lipopolysaccharide-induced neuroinflammation as a bridge to understand neurodegeneration. *Int. J. Mol. Sci.* 20 (9): 2293.
177. Zhao, J., Bi, W., Xiao, S. et al. (2019). Neuroinflammation induced by lipopolysaccharide causes cognitive impairment in mice. *Sci. Rep.* 9 (1): 5790.
178. Hong, J., Yoon, D., Nam, Y. et al. (2020). Lipopolysaccharide administration for a mouse model of cerebellar ataxia with neuroinflammation. *Sci. Rep.* 10 (1): 13337.
179. Liang, X., Lin, T., Sun, G. et al. (2009). Hemopexin down-regulates LPS-induced proinflammatory cytokines from macrophages. *J. Leukoc. Biol.* 86 (2): 229–235.
180. Schabbauer, G. (2012). Polymicrobial sepsis models: CLP versus CASP. *Drug Discov. Today Dis. Model.* 9 (1): e17–e21.
181. Drechsler, S. and Osuchowski, M. (2021). Cecal ligation and puncture. *Methods Mol. Biol.* 2321: 1–8.
182. Rittirsch, D., Huber-Lang, M.S., Flierl, M.A., and Ward, P.A. (2009). Immunodesign of experimental sepsis by cecal ligation and puncture. *Nat. Protoc.* 4 (1): 31–36.

25 Oil Injections and ASIA Syndrome

Olga Vera-Lastra[1,2], Alberto Ordinola-Navarro[1,2], Abihai Lucas Hernández[1,2], Gabriela Medina[1,2], María P. Cruz-Domínguez[1,2], Gabriel M. Ramírez[3], and Luis J. Jara[4]

[1]Internal Medicine Department, Unidad Médica de Alta Especiad, Hospital de Especialidades, "Dr. Antonio Fraga Mouret", Centro Médico Nacional, "La Raza". Instituto Mexicano del Seguro Social, México City, México
[2]Internal Medicine Department, División de Estudios de Posgrado, Facultad de Medicina, Universidad Nacional Autónoma de México, México City, México
[3]Rheumatology Department, Hospital General de México, "Dr. Eduardo Liceaga", México City, México
[4]Research Division, Instituto Nacional de Rehabilitación, Mexico City, México

Highlights

- ASIA-MO is a model of genetic interaction, environment (adjuvant), and the immune system.
- ASIA-MO is the consequence of the illegal use of this substance in many countries of the world.
- ASIA-MO results from the injection of oily substances whose manifestations depend on the chemical structure, route, and administration site.
- ASIA-MO shares pathogenic mechanisms with activation of the innate and adaptive immune response as other entities of ASIA.
- ASIA-MO has pleomorphic manifestations: nonspecific and specific manifestations that meet criteria for autoimmune diseases.
- ASIA-MO treatment represents a challenge and requires a multidisciplinary approach.

Introduction

Autoimmune/inflammatory syndrome induced by adjuvants (ASIA) was described in 2011 by Shoenfeld and coworkers and encompassed a cluster of autoimmune diseases that develop among genetically prone individuals due to adjuvant agent exposure [1]. ASIA induced by mineral oil and other oily substances (ASIA-MO) occurs when oily-type modeling substances are infiltrated into the body for cosmetic purposes. This phenomenon has been reported in many countries, particularly in Eastern Europe, Asia, and Latin America. Despite its prevalence, such practices persist as

Autoimmune Disorders: Adjuvants and Other Risk Factors in Pathogenesis, First Edition.
Edited by Abdulla Watad, Nicola Luigi Bragazzi, and Yehuda Shoenfeld.

illegal in many parts of the world. Different modeling substances have been used for this objective: MO, liquid paraffin, and other oily substances [2–5]. MO are products obtained from the distillation of petroleum; these are primarily composed of hydrocarbons; they are mainly divided into two groups: mineral oil saturated hydrocarbons (MOSH) and mineral oil aromatic hydrocarbons (MOAH) [6]. MOSH consists of straight-chain, branched, and ring structures with carbon chain lengths greater than C16 [6–8]. MO may act as an adjuvant, a substance capable of prolonging or increasing the immune response, even producing a wide range of autoantibodies [9]. Experimental models with pristane allow us to explain the pathogenesis of ASIA-MO in humans [10].

The clinical manifestations of ASIA-MO are heterogeneous and vary from mild to severe, depending on the site of application of the MO injection [2]. Its treatment constitutes a significant challenge [2, 10]. This chapter analyzes the epidemiological, etiological, pathogenic, clinical manifestations, diagnostic, and treatment approaches of ASIA-MO.

Epidemiology

For a long time, foreign substances have been used for different reasons, ranging from medical to cosmetic purposes, which have shown an increase in recent years due to a trend to enhance appearance. The injection of modeling substances has been used since the nineteenth century to improve body contouring. In the 1960s, the use of paraffin as a modeling substance was very popular in Japan. In those years, complications were called "human adjuvant disease" by Miyoshi et al. [11]; these included the antecedent of injected paraffin or silicone that resolved after the implant material removal. However, more than a decade ago, Shoenfeld englobed four entities (Gulf War syndrome, siliconosis, macrophagic myofasciitis syndrome, and postvaccination phenomena). But of interest, those previously described syndromes such as Miyoshi's disease and Spanish toxic oil syndrome share clinical characteristics related to an adjuvant stimulus and could be englobed in ASIA [12, 13].

In the later years, an increase in surgical and nonsurgical cosmetic procedures has been reported; according to world records, the United States of America realized 4,310,180 procedures (leading country), while other countries, such as Colombia, Mexico, France, Brazil, and South Korea, present an increasing number of practice procedures per plastic surgeons [14]. Despite that, there is a high amount of noncountable procedures realized by nonprofessional workers, mostly in low-income countries [15–17].

Another contributing factor has been the "celebrity influence," with social media increasing in the past decade and information widely available via internet searchers. There has been an increase in lip fillers and butt enhancement or even transgender surgery [18].

Regarding nonsurgical procedures, the primary injectable substance has been botulin toxin, calcium hydroxyapatite, hyaluronic acid, and poly-L-lactic acid, while there has been an increase in facial rejuvenation treatments and nonsurgical fat reductions in recent years.

Most of these practices have been mainly in persons aged 35–60 years, representing 15% of surgical procedures in countries such as the United States. WHO accomplished more than one billion dollars of the total spending in 2019. Moreover, The Aesthetic Society highlights that man accounts for nearly 10% of all injectables procedures (9.6%) [19].

Of interest, in the past five years, the United States of America has presented an increase in buttock procedures up to 95%. With all that information and trends, injectables procedures have been increasing in the rest of the world, including various uses, since applying to increase the penis to facial procedures [20, 21].

While the Food and Drug Administration (FDA) has approved some substances such as hyaluronic acid, there are still many not authorized substances, such as biopolymers, silicone, methacrylate, and paraffin, among others. Many of these illegal practices are prevalent, particularly in Latin America, where numerous practitioners offer these procedures. This accessibility often motivates individuals to pursue their desired outcomes at a lower cost[15–17].

In this context, the lower prices, many available practitioners realizing the procedures, and the availability of ambulatory applications make this an increasing health problem due to the adverse effects. Sometimes, due to pain or fault, the patients delay seeking medical attention [22].

The use of these foreign substances opened the question that if it was possible that the substance would trigger an autoimmune response from the body? at the beginning, the American College of Rheumatology (ACR) did not find an association between breast implants and autoimmune rheumatic disease [17].

However, in the past decade that has changed, the ASIA includes the exposition to foreign substances that act as adjuvants, and it has been described that these can trigger an autoimmune response that could lead to different reactions, which goes from local pain or erythema to the formation of granulomas or even autoimmune disease, such as lupus or Sjögren's syndrome [23, 24].

Etiology

Mineral oils are products obtained from the distillation of petroleum. They are primarily composed of hydrocarbons, mainly divided into two groups: mineral-oil saturated hydrocarbon MOSH and mineral-oil aromatic hydrocarbons MOAH [25]. These hydrocarbons are divided depending on the atoms of carbon, between 10 and 50 for MOSH, these including paraffin and naphthene, while MOAH includes polycyclic aromatic hydrocarbons (PAH) [3].

There are specific standards for quality control of this substance. Therefore, the refining process of the oil has several steps, which include distillation, extraction, crystallization, purification, and solvent extraction. Moreover, a successive purification step removes impurities to reduce PAH levels to meet quality criteria [26].

The mineral oils are widely used in different sources; they are used in food, cosmetics, vaccines, or industrial applications such as oily tulles, patch tests, and laxatives [27].

In order to do these, mineral oils have been classified regarding the viscosity, high and medium Class I (allowed as food mineral oils), and medium and low viscosity Class II and III mineral oils, with lack of safety and controversy regarding daily intake [3].

Oily-type modelers are injected from 10 mL to 1 gallon per session, given their easy and economic access. The list is large and includes mineral oil, vegetable oil, olive oil, other cooking oil, Johnson oil, paraffin, liquid petroleum jelly, bovine fat, other animal fat, guaiacol, vitamins, liquid silicone, industrial silicone, industrial oil, and other biopolymers. Specifically, substances identified within mineral oils are as follows: (i) liquid paraffin of 15–50 carbons, a highly refined petroleum mineral oil consisting of a complex combination of hydrocarbons with sulfuric acid; (ii) Isoparaffin, a mixture of branched-chain aliphatic hydrocarbons with 18–70 carbons in the alkyl chain; (iii) Paraffin, a solid mixture of large crystals of hydrocarbons obtained from petroleum; (iv) Synthetic wax as paraffin wax, a C20 complex combination of hydrocarbons obtained from petroleum by solvent crystallization, and as synthetic hydrocarbon wax, obtained by the controlled polymerization of ethylene; (v) Microcrystalline wax, derived from petroleum and characterized by the fineness crystals. All of these are high-molecular-weight saturated aliphatic hydrocarbons. "Hydrogenated microcrystalline wax" is a microcrystalline wax that has been hydrogenated; (vi) Cera microcrystalline, a complex combination of long, branched-chain hydrocarbons obtained from residual oils by solvent crystallization. It consists predominantly of saturated straight and branched-chain hydrocarbons; (vii) Petrolatum, a complex combination of hydrocarbons obtained from dewaxing paraffinic residual oil as saturated crystalline and liquid hydrocarbons; (viii) Ozokerite, a complex combination of hydrocarbons produced by removing acidic materials; (ix) Ceresin, a combination of hydrocarbons purified with sulfuric acid and filtration through bone black; (x) Pristane (2,6,10,14-tetramethylpentadecane) mineral oil, incomplete Freund's adjuvant (IFA); and (xi) Squalene (2,6,10,15,19,23-hexamethyl-2,6,10,14,18,22-tetracosahexaene) [8, 27].

MOAH has been related to carcinogenic proprieties. MOSH seems relatively safe, but the illegal use has been related to different adverse effects, such as granulomas on the liver in rats (FISHER 344) and other adverse effects [3, 26].

The effects of the mineral oils would vary from the way of administration, quantity, and molecular structure, but besides the dose, the risk is still latent in some subjects. Besides that, these compounds can be combined with certain substances, which makes it difficult to determine the exact composition due to the absence of a validated measurement method. This, coupled with the illegal use of substances, makes this situation a more significant problem for detecting substances involved in the reactions. Most importantly, the use of these substances has resulted in death of people, primarily because of bacterial infections [17, 28], but in people where there is no fatal outcome, the quality of life has significantly declined. Besides this which seems to be a woman's problem, in the past decade, the "Aesthetic surgery report" mentioned an increase in the male population [29], and there have been severe cohorts that describe up to 30% of patients being male from 17 to 39 years old, with the involving substance being mineral oil [17, 28, 30].

Considering all of these, ASIA mineral oil (Asia-MO) is currently an increasing health problem not only for the female gender or in the low-middle-income countries.

Pathogenesis

ASIA-MO is a model where several factors interact: a genetically predisposed individual, an external factor (adjuvants), and their interaction with the immune system lead to a chronic inflammatory state (Figure 25.1). The concept "adjuvant" is essential to explain the problems because the patients develop the reaction after infiltration with contouring substances. An "adjuvant" is a substance capable of accelerating, lengthening, or increasing the immune response. Additionally, it can potentially induce or promote inadequate allergic or autoimmune responses that can cause adverse impacts on the health of individuals [9, 31]. The antigenic properties of adjuvant will be influenced by factors such as route of inoculation, frequency of administration, amount of

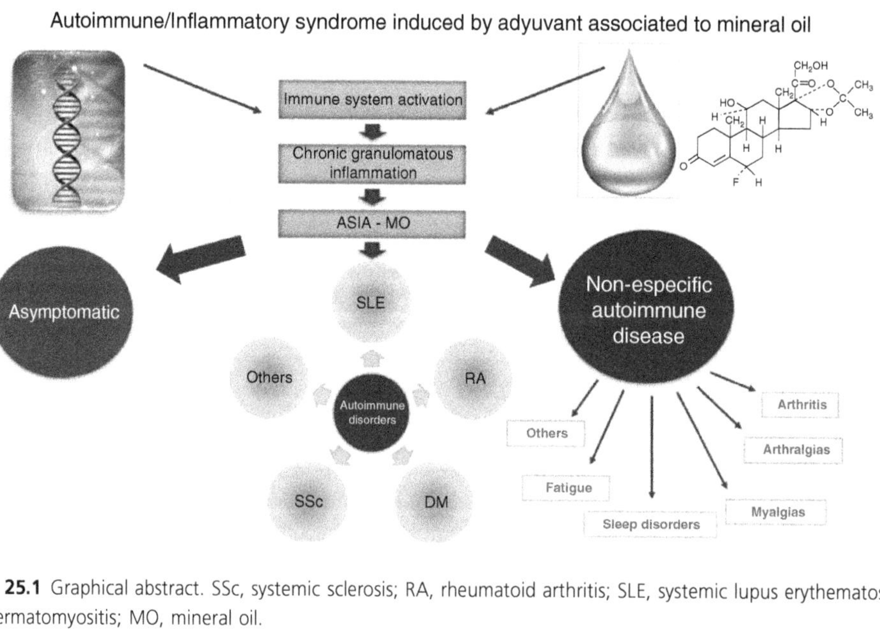

Figure 25.1 Graphical abstract. SSc, systemic sclerosis; RA, rheumatoid arthritis; SLE, systemic lupus erythematosus; DM, dermatomyositis; MO, mineral oil.

substance infiltrated, the characteristics of the substance, the site of infiltration, and the chemical structure of the MO, according to the animal models [32].

Even though MOs are widely utilized for different purposes as they are considered innocuous, there is evidence that exposure to these substances can be associated with the development of different diseases, including autoimmune phenomena. In the case of subcutaneous infiltration, the development of chronic inflammation has been identified [33].

Based on studies of experimental models in animals, especially with pristane, a typical oil used for experimental studies, a chronic inflammatory process of the granulomatous type has been demonstrated with activation of the innate and adaptive immune response. When tetramethylpentadecane or pristane is introduced into the peritoneal cavity, it induces systemic lupus erythematosus (SLE), arthritis, immune complex-mediated glomerulonephritis, and pulmonary capillaritis as well as autoantibodies. This murine model of lupus nephritis and autoantibody production depends strictly on signaling through the interferon (IFN)-I receptor [10].

The mechanisms associated with oils triggering the adaptive immune response are varied and complex; they generally involve the following steps: infiltration or deposition and location of the antigen; development of injury signals that act as coactivators of the immune response; activation of antigen-presenting cells; and activation of the innate immune response through toll-like receptors (TLR) and other receptors. Regarding humoral immunity, several mechanisms may account for how adjuvant substances interact with the immune system. The progressive release of certain antigens enhances the production of antibodies that block and keep antigen-presenting cells exposed to the antigen for long periods. The promotion of antigen translocation to the lymph nodes allows T cells to recognize these antigens. Soluble antigens are converted into tiny particles phagocyted by antigen-presenting cells, such as dendritic cells and macrophages. Specific injury signals stimulate the inflammatory reaction at the site of injection.

Moreover, MO infiltration induces the formation of granulomatous inflammation. This occurs due to secondary thickening in the dermis resulting from the accumulation of collagen fibers and a spontaneous induction of IL-1 by macrophages activated through the aggregation of inflammatory cells [34]. Additionally, there is interaction with toll-like receptors (TLRs), including the activation of NALP3 (inflammasomes). This mechanism bears similarity to those described in other ASIA models [35].

After applying contouring substances, two types of patients may be seen: those who develop an inflammatory response and those who do not show inflammation or will not develop this reaction. Because of this scenario, we undertook the task of studying the Th1, Th2, and Th17 inflammatory phenotypes of individuals who received infiltration of contouring substances. We found that patients with no inflammation showed a combined response pattern: Th1 (IL-1β, IFNγ)/Th2 (IL-5, IL-6, IL-13), with greater concentrations of IL-10 compared to those with inflammation. This suggests that the inflammatory process is controlled by an increase in IL-10, which most probably accounts for the absence of clinical manifestation in this group of individuals.

In patients with inflammation, we found an increased TNF-α First, there is a Th1 type of response, where antigen presenting cells are activated; T CD4 helper cells produce a clonal expan sion, and T CD8 cytotoxic cells develop; cytokines are produced that intensify cellular response, which ultimately translates into the final inflammatory effect [36].

Among the multiple alterations identified, sclerosing granulomas and the development of several autoantibodies, such as antichromatin and, most importantly, anti-DNA, have been recorded. This situation suggests that they are produced in response to hydrocarbons [37]. In fact, these substances have proven to be highly immunogenic [38].

In animal models, the development of T-cell induction-dependent arthritis has been observed, with induction of autoimmunity by different types of oils. Similarly, oily substances have resulted in producing a diversity of autoantibodies in human subjects [17].

Adjuvant effect mechanisms have been mainly described using aluminum; however, certain etiopathogenetic mechanisms could be extrapolated to contouring substances with this model. The infiltrated substances generate deposits that are antigenic traps at the site of injection, which in turn cause prolonged exposure, thus perpetuating the stimulus to the immune system and increasing the persistent presence of antigens at the injection site, and maintaining recruitment and activation of antigen-presenting cells. Later, other adjuvants, specifically pattern-recognition receptor ligands, induce innate immunity by antigen-presenting cell targets and by immunity induced by TLR, NOD-like receptors, RIG-1 receptors, and C-type lectin receptors. Signaling pathways lead to the activation of transcription factors, such as NF-kB and IRF3. The consequence of this process is the induction of cytokines and chemokines that play an essential role in the immune response's priming, expansion, and polarization mechanisms. When NLRs, such as NLRP3 and NLRC4, are activated, inflammasomes activate, resulting in IL-1b and IL-18 pro-inflammatory cytokines. Adjuvants can orchestrate antigen presentation to the major histocompatibility complex. These adjuvants are essential for intensifying and controlling the adaptive response, where T and B lymphocytes participate. Most of the antigens activate B cells through T helper lymphocytes. It is well known that the Th1 response causes a cell response that protects against intracellular pathogens; Th1 cells secrete IFN that in turn activates macrophages and induces B cells opsonization of antibodies. Th2 cells induce a humoral response, which is essential for the defense against extracellular pathogens. They secret cytokines, including IL-4, which promote the secretion of neutralizing antibodies by B cells. Th17 cells promote inflammation by activating neutrophiles and fibroblasts via IL-17/IL/23 [35].

The adjuvant mechanism of this disease caused by infiltration of modeling substances (mineral oil) is complex and perpetuated by the antigen's constant presence; however, the presence of a Th2 (IL-10) stimulation could somehow explain the absence of transient clinical manifestations or the delay in their presence.

Clinical manifestation

Clinical manifestations of ASIA-MO are pleomorphic and vary between mild and severe, including death. These manifestations depend on the site of application of the MO injections, and they can be divided into local or regional with further systemic extension. Systemic manifestations are nonspecific and specific for autoimmune diseases (AID) [2, 17, 39]. Table 25.1 shows the clinical spectrum of ASIA-MO.

The mean time between the injection and the onset of symptoms is 4.5± 4.3 years. The areas of the body where the modeling substances are mainly applied are buttocks (38–72%), breasts (12–16%), lower extremities (18–22%), and face (6–10%), depending on the concept of beauty of each individual. Hence, one of the main alterations observed is ulcers in the buttocks, legs, and breasts, producing chronic pain and infections; local manifestations include changes in skin color (hyperpigmentation), hardening, painful ulcers, and infections (Figure 25.2a,b,c). These are frequent causes of hospitalization and disability [17].

Likewise, these patients present the clinical manifestations of ASIA "per se," chronic fatigue, fever, dry eyes and dry mouth, cognitive impairment, musculoskeletal system disorders (arthralgias/arthritis, myalgias, and calcinosis), and sleep disturbances [2, 40–42]. Psychiatric disorders such as anxiety and depression, which have been found in up to 70% and 50%, respectively [43], may also share symptoms of secondary fibromyalgia. On the other hand, there are manifestations of defined disease of the connective tissue such as SLE, systemic sclerosis [44, 45], and other systemic disorders such as chronic kidney failure, interstitial lung diseases, and hypercalcemia, among others [46–48]. These clinical manifestations of ASIA-MO are similar to those observed in the analysis of the 300 international ASIA syndrome patients registry [48]. It can also observe acute manifestations given by the aspiration of mineral oil [49–52].

Regarding the injection of MO into the penis to increase its size, the clinical manifestations have a wide range of manifestations: from discrete edema or mass (80.7%) to extensive necrosis (28.9%), occasionally with scrotum involvement (5.0%) [5]. Besides, there is deformity of the male genital, which is described as penile paraffinomas lymphogranuloma of the penis [53].

Table 25.1 Clinical manifestations of ASIA associated with mineral oil.

Local manifestations	Systemic manifestations	
	Nonspecific/ASIA	**Specific manifestation for AID[a]**
Edema	Fever	Systemic lupus erythematosus
Erythema	Weight loss	Rheumatoid arthritis
Increased temperature	Fatigue	Systemic sclerosis
Induration ranging from panniculitis-like to severe wood-hard fibrosis	Chronic pain	Dermatomyositis
Scars • Atrophic • Hypertrophic	Arthralgias/Arthritis	Overlap syndrome
Discoloration • Hypopigmentation • Hyperpigmentation	Myalgia	Sjögren's syndrome
Necrosis	Cognitive impairment	Vasculitis
Ulceration	Adenopathy	Fibromyalgia
Exposure of the injected material	Hair loss	Autoimmune hemolytic anemia
Contractures	Oral ulcer	Autoimmune hepatitis
Calcification	Livedo reticularis	Ulcerative colitis
Abscesses	Nodules	Raynaud's phenomenon
Local infectious	Sicca syndrome	Still's disease
Fistulae	Sensitive neuropathy	Undifferentiated connective tissue syndrome
	Raynaud phenomenon	Systemic embolism (pulmonary)
Amputations		Other: depression, anxiety, fibromyalgia, thyroiditis

[a] AID, Autoimmune disease [2].

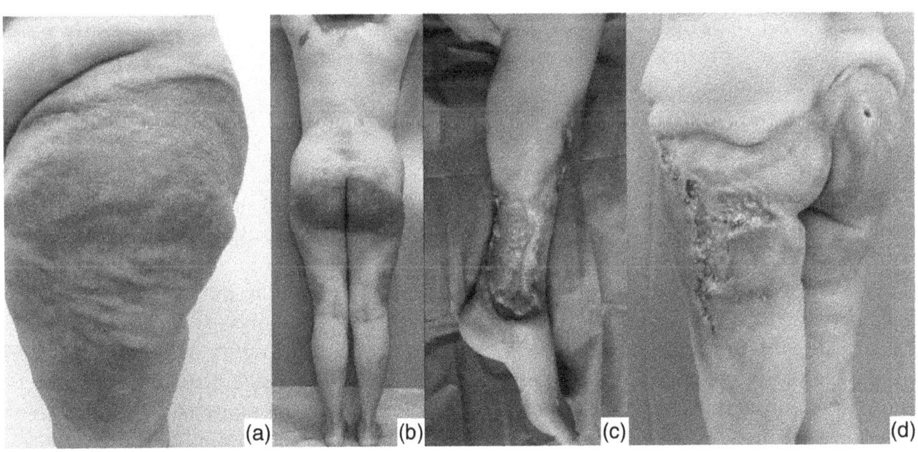

Figure 25.2 (a) Injection of mineral oil in buttocks and migration to thighs, with nodulations, hyperpigmentation, and hard skin. (b) Injection of mineral oil in the buttocks with the migration of the material to the legs and thighs and hyperpigmentation. (c) Injection of mineral oil in the thigh with deformation, ulcers, and fistulas. (d) Injection of mineral oil in the legs and presence of an ulcer.

Clinically, the lesion of granulomas is insidious, nonspecific, with progressive induration, fluctuating edema, and/or local inflammation of the affected area, which as time passes may be accompanied by necrosis, ulceration, and deformity [54]. On the other hand, the manifestations of applying mineral oil to increase the size of the penis have been a problem that is increasing, and they are urological and include mild manifestations until loss of the organ's function [55–61].

Diagnostic approach

To approach ASIA-MO is essential to obtain a complete history and physical examination. At present, in patients with autoimmune Rheumatic disease (ARD), it is essential to inquire about the history of injected substances for cosmetic purposes, use of silicone breast implants or vaccines, or other substance. An exhaustive medical history is essential for diagnosis, as the patient may omit part of the prior history due to fear or shame.

The diagnosis of ASIA-MO is based on the criteria published by Shoenfeld and Agmon-Levin in 2011. The presence of two major criteria, or one major and two minors, are sufficient for diagnosing ASIA [12]. Subsequently, Alijotas-Reig [13] proposed new diagnostic criteria for ASIA based only on objective clinical and laboratory data. For the diagnosis of ASIA-MO, it is important to carry out laboratory, imaging, and histological studies.

Laboratory studies

Autoantibodies are important for the diagnosis of ASIA-MO. Several autoantibodies have been reported: ANA, anti-ds-DNA, anti-Ro, anti-La, anticardiolipin, rheumatoid factor, anticentromere, and antineutrophil cytoplasmic autoantibodies (ANCA), among others. These autoantibodies have also been demonstrated in both animal and human models [34, 60]. In this regard, high levels of autoantibodies and SLE have been reported as a consequence of the intraperitoneal pristane injection in BALB/c mice (anti-Sm, anti-RNP, antiribosomal P, anti-Su, anti-ds-NA, and antichromatin) [10]. In general, it is suggested to perform the following laboratory tests: cell blood count, platelets, acute phase reactants, blood chemistry, urinalysis, or specific tests to identify diseases such as thyroiditis, hepatitis, pneumonitis, and other differential diagnoses. ASIA-MO patients frequently show anemia, thrombocytosis or thrombocytopenia, hypergammaglobulinemia, and an increase in C-reactive protein (CRP) and erythrocyte sedimentation rate (ESR). Physicians should remember that some of these patients might present prolonged fever, weight loss, and lymphadenopathies; they should be approached as having a fever of unknown origin [17].

Imaging studies

These studies are important to identify the spread of MO and other infiltrated substances throughout the body. Magnetic resonance imaging (MRI) of soft tissue is a valuable tool in detecting MO injected in different parts of the body. The location, amount, extension, and depth of damage caused by MO to the tissues and the presence of inflammatory activity can be observed. When MRI is not an option, ultrasound may be used to assess inflammation, measure the affected area, and estimate the amount of modeling agent injected. The main findings are increased density and echogenicity of the subcutaneous tissue [15]. Computerized tomography (CT) is another option, especially high-resolution CT, to investigate pulmonary affection, such as pneumonitis and other pulmonary manifestation, as well as lymphadenopathies. Mammography is another method for investigating breast involvement. Early paraffin injections appear as multiple, circumscribed, and noncalcified masses in the retroglandular and subpectoral regions. In contrast, late-stage paraffin injections (paraffinomas) show numerous multiple dense nodules with arc and ring calcifications [7]. When an ARD is present (RA, SLE, SSc, and DM), a specific protocol should be made for each entity.

Regarding imaging studies for complications on injection of MO in the penis, US and CT and MRI are recommended.

Ultrasound, which is a widely available and inexpensive technique, can be very useful for differential diagnosis. This imaging technique can also determine the involvement of structures such as the corpora cavernosa and regional lymph nodes and detect the formation of abscesses or fistulas. Furthermore, it can help identify the type of filler material, as specific echographic patterns have been described for some of these. The image in snowstorm pattern is observed, where a hyperechogenic region has a posterior acoustic shadow. This pattern is typical in nonabsorbable filler materials such as silicone oil, pure silicone, and OR liquid paraffin [59–62].

MRI seems to provide adequate imaging of the histological events occurring after paraffin oil injection in the subcutaneous tissues. Penile paraffinoma remains a clinical diagnosis, but MRI features may help plan an adequate surgical strategy and, in selected cases, establish the differential diagnosis with other penile diseases, including cancer [63, 64].

Histopathological studies

In ASIA-MO, a biopsy of the involved tissue (skin, subcutaneous tissue) is recommended in order to rule out infection, cancer, and other systemic affection. The histological features are chronic granulomatous inflammation (foreign body reaction), with foamy histiocytes or multinucleated giant cells with phagocytized foreign material, and the presence of "ghost spaces" or empty vacuoles previously occupied by MO. However, we can also find vasculitis, calcification, or specific manifestation of ARD such as dermatomyositis and SSc, among others [65, 66]. Regarding paraffinomas, the histological features are similar to granulomas due to silicone fluids, MO, and other substances [2, 66].

The spectrum of morphological changes in ASIA is extensive. The tissues show signs of immune inflammation, such as lymphohistiocytic infiltration, granulomatous inflammation, and scleroderma-like changes.

Treatment

Treatment should focus on systemic or local clinical manifestations, depending on the affected area: breast, buttocks, lower extremities, face, and genitalia (penis). In general, treatment is divided into medical and surgical. It may represent a dare, and the results can be displeasing [2].

Medical treatment

Treatment of patients with ASIA should be approached using a multidisciplinary strategy led by the rheumatologist or internist, including psychiatrist and psychologist, dermatologist, angiologist, plastic and general surgeon, infectious disease physician, neurologist, and rehabilitation specialist, among others [2, 15, 17]. Treatment varies according to the severity of the case, from proper wound care in mild cases to surgical treatment and systemic therapy. Medical treatment must be focused on pain control since this is one of the leading clinical manifestations. The use of analgesics, nonsteroidal anti-inflammatories (NSAIDs), and steroids is the cornerstone in treating this syndrome. In addition, since there is often depression or anxiety, assessment by a psychologist or psychiatrist is part of the multidisciplinary approach. If patients meet the criteria for fibromyalgia, they should be treated accordingly. Since these patients may experience concomitant infectious processes, treatment includes antibiotics, surgical debridement in some cases, and appropriate management for chronic skin ulcers, along with immunosuppressive therapy[2, 15, 17]. The latter aspect may be necessary in cases of ASIA associated with mineral oil; in patients developing the autoimmune disease with complications such as vasculitis, nephropathy, or thrombocytopenia; or in those who develop a definite autoimmune such as SLE, RA, or SSc; they should be treated according to the guidelines for these diseases [17]. Other medical therapies may include vitamin D

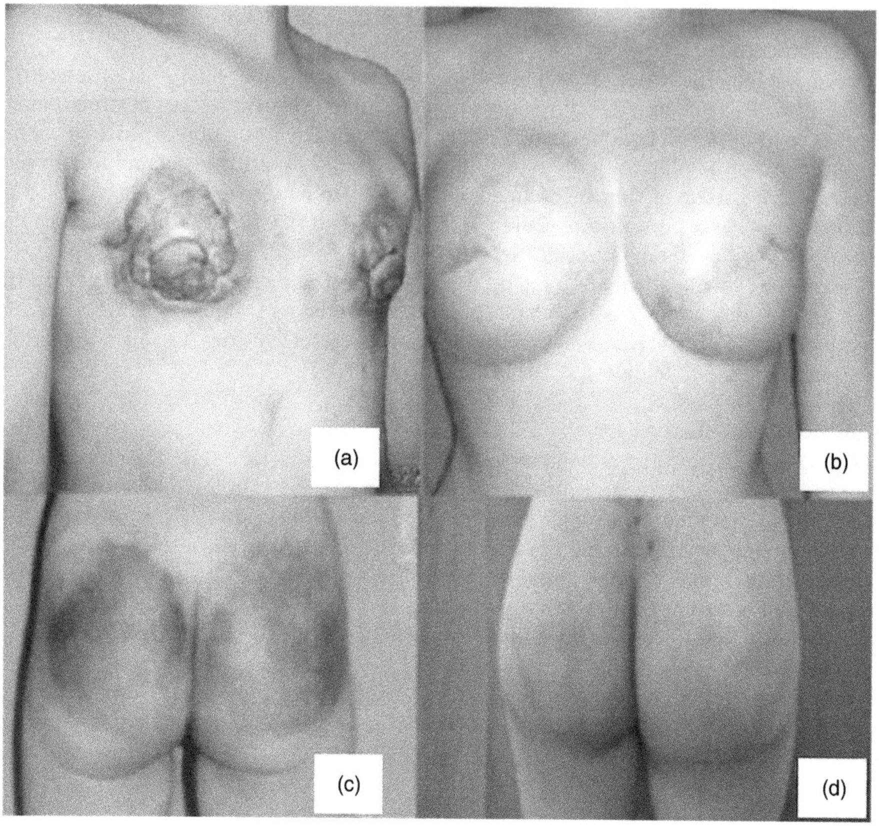

Figure 25.3 (a) Mild ASIA-MO observed after injection in both breasts. (b) Same patient as depicted in figure A, after undergoing multidisciplinary treatment with plastic surgery. (c) Mild ASIA-MO identified after injection in the buttocks. (d) Same patient as shown in figure C following multidisciplinary treatment with plastic surgery.

supplementation, as this deficiency is associated with autoantibodies in different diseases. Therefore, these patients could benefit from this treatment to avoid further development of autoantibodies coupled with its antifibrotic effects [66, 67].

Surgical treatment

The objectives of surgical treatment are the removal of the injected material, in this case, oil, both in the skin and in adjacent tissues to improve clinical manifestations; fewer relapses of the disease; better control of the immunologic response; and an acceptable functional and esthetic result [29, 68] (Figure 25.3).

Surgical treatment includes conservative local treatment, depending on the type of wound, inflammation or infection control, and moisture balance with adequate dressings. In certain circumstances, the use of negative pressure wound therapy (vacuum-assisted closure) may accelerate wound healing by promoting angiogenesis [69]. Other options include ultrasonic-assisted liposuction (UAL), open en bloc excision and primary closure, open *en bloc* excision, and microsurgical reconstruction angiogenesis [29]. Major skin disease will require significant skin removal with subsequent skin coverage. The removal of the injected material from the buttocks requires the application of expanders, flaps, grafts, and liposuction, among others. Reconstruction of defects arising after *en bloc excision* due to the infiltration of modeling substances is an option, especially in patients with severely impaired quality of life [29, 68].

The study by López-Mendoza et al. [29] identified a slight tendency of significant scores in the Euro-Qol-5ED tool (EQ-5D) in patients who underwent major excisions compared to those who underwent ultrasonic-assisted liposuction (UAL). In ASIA syndrome, excision of the infiltrated material is usually complex, representing a challenge with severe esthetic sequels, the goal of a total or near-total resection of the substance to have a more extended symptom-free period [68].

Conclusions

The injection of oily substances with cosmetic purposes is illegal; however, it continues to be a common practice in many countries (Eastern Europe, Asia, and Latin America), thus representing a serious health problem.

Mineral oil is an adjuvant that produces a chronic granulomatous inflammation, leading to local and systemic manifestations.

Treatment of ASIA-MO constitutes a great challenge for the physician and an ominous outlook for the patients.

In ASIA-MO, many aspects need to be investigated, such as genetic predisposition and interaction with different types of oils and other substances.

It is essential to spread the knowledge of ASIA-MO and other substances with cosmetic purposes to avoid this practice.

References

1. Borba, V., Malkova, A., Basantsova, N. et al. (2020). Classical examples of the concept of the ASIA syndrome. *Biomol. Ther.* 10 (10): 1436. https://doi.org/10.3390/biom10101436.
2. Vera-Lastra, O., Medina, G., Cruz-Domínguez, M.P. et al. (2018). Autoimmune/inflammatory syndrome induced by mineral oil: a health problem. *Clin. Rheumatol.* 37 (6): 1441–1448. https://doi.org/10.1007/s10067-018-4078-2.
3. De Siati, M., Selvaggio, O., Di Fino, G. et al. (2013). An unusual delayed complication of paraffin self-injection for penile girth augmentation. *BMC Urol.* 1 (13): 66. https://doi.org/10.1186/1471-2490-13-66.
4. Shariffuddin, F.N.A.A., Fam, X.I., Fatimah, M.N. et al. (2021). Massive penile lipogranuloma following olive oil injections. *Med. J. Malaysia* 76: 774–776.
5. Faveret, P.L.S. and Santiago, F. (2018). Surgical management of penile lesions secondary to foreign body reaction: a case report and systematic review. *Aesthet. Surg. J.* 38 (7): 770–780. https://doi.org/10.1093/asj/sjx203.
6. Chuberre, B., Araviiskaia, E., Bieber, T., and Barbaud, A. (2019). Mineral oils and waxes in cosmetics: an overview mainly based on the current European regulations and the safety profile of these compounds. *J. Eur. Acad. Dermatol. Venereol.* 33 (Suppl 7): 5–14. https://doi.org/10.1111/jdv.15946.
7. Peters, W. and Fornasier, V. (2009). Complications from injectable materials used for breast augmentation. *Can. J. Plast. Surg.* 17 (3): 89–96. https://doi.org/10.1177/229255030901700305.
8. Petry, T., Bury, D., Fautz, R. et al. (2017). Review of data on the dermal penetration of mineral oils and waxes used in cosmetic applications. *Toxicol. Lett.* 280: 70–78. https://doi.org/10.1016/j.toxlet.2017.07.899.
9. Israeli, E., Agmon-Levin, N., Blank, M. et al. (2009). Adjuvants and autoimmunity. *Lupus* 18 (13): 1217–1225. https://doi.org/10.1177/0961203309345724.
10. Reeves, W.H., Lee, P.Y., Weinstein, J.S. et al. (2009). Induction of autoimmunity by pristane and other naturally occurring hydrocarbons. *Trends Immunol.* 30 (9): 455–464. https://doi.org/10.1016/j.it.2009.06.003.
11. Miyoshi, K., Miyaoka, T., Kobayashi, Y. et al. (1964). Hypergammaglobulinemia by prolonged adjuvanticity in man: disorders developed after augmentation mammoplasty. *Ijishimpo* 22: 9–14.
12. Shoenfeld, Y. and Agmon-Levin, N. (2011). 'ASIA' – autoimmune/inflammatory syndrome induced by adjuvants. *J. Autoimmun. 36* (1): 4–8. https://doi.org/10.1016/j.jaut.2010.07.003.
13. Alijotas-Reig, J. (2015). Human adjuvant-related syndrome or autoimmune/inflammatory syndrome induced by adjuvants. Where have we come from? Where are we going? A proposal for new diagnostic criteria. *Lupus 24* (10): 1012–1018. https://doi.org/10.1177/0961203315579092.

14. Heidekrueger, P.I., Juran, S., Ehrl, D. et al. (2017). Global aesthetic surgery statistics: a closer look. *J. Plast. Surg. Hand Surg.* 51: 270–274. https://doi.org/10.1080/2000656X.2016.1248842.
15. Martínez-Villarreal, A.A., Asz-Sigall, D., Gutiérrez-Mendoza, D. et al. (2017). A case series and a review of the literature on foreign modelling agent reaction: an emerging problem. *Int. Wound J.* 14 (3): 546–554. https://doi.org/10.1111/iwj.12643.
16. De Almeida, A.T., Banegas, R., Boggio, R. et al. (2017). Diagnosis and treatment of hyaluronic acid adverse events: latin American expert panel consensus recommendations. *Surg. Cosmet. Dermatology.* 9 (3): 204–213. https://doi.org/10.5935/scd1984- 8773.20179302.
17. Vera-Lastra, O., Medina, G., Cruz-Dominguez Mdel, P. et al. (2012). Human adjuvant disease induced by foreign substances: a new model of ASIA (Shoenfeld's syndrome). *Lupus* 21 (2): 128–135. https://doi.org/10.1177/0961203311429317.
18. Tijerina, J.D., Morrison, S.D., Nolan, I.T. et al. (2019). Celebrity influence affecting public interest in plastic surgery procedures: Google trends analysis. *Aesthet. Plast. Surg. 43* (6): 1669–1680. https://doi.org/10.1007/s00266-019-01466-7.
19. Aesthetic Society The aesthetic society's cosmetic surgery national data bank: statistics 2019. *Aesthet. Surg. J.* 40: 1–26. https://doi.org/10.1093/ASJ/ SJAA144.
20. Seok, J., Hong, J.Y., Park, K.Y. et al. (2016). Delayed immunologic complications due to injectable fillers by unlicensed practitioners: our experiences and a review of the literature. *Dermatol. Ther.* 29 (1): 41–44. https://doi.org/10.1111/dth.12298.
21. Bjurlin, M.A., Carlsen, J., Grevious, M. et al. (2010). Mineral oil-induced sclerosing lipogranuloma of the penis. *J. Clin. Aesthet. Dermatol.* 3 (9): 41–44.
22. Gómez, B.T., Ramírez, G.M., Blancas, R.P. et al. (2010). Enfermedad por la infiltración de sustancias modelantes con fines estéticos. *Cir. Plast.* 20: 124–132.
23. Watad, A., Bragazzi, N.L., McGonagle, D. et al. (2019). Autoimmune/inflammatory syndrome induced by adjuvants (ASIA) demonstrates distinct autoimmune and autoinflammatory disease associations according to the adjuvant subtype: insights from an analysis of 500 cases. *Clin. Immunol.* 203: 1–8. https://doi.org/10.1016/j.clim.2019.03.007.
24. Bragazzi, N.L., Watad, A., Sharif, K. et al. (2017). Advances in our understanding of immunization and vaccines for patients with systemic lupus erythematosus. *Expert. Rev. Clin. Immunol.* 13 (10): 939–949. https://doi.org/10.1080/1744666X.2017.1361321.
25. Pirow, R., Blume, A., Hellwig, N. et al. (2019). Mineral oil in food, cosmetic products, and in products regulated by other legislations. *Crit. Rev. Toxicol.* 49 (9): 742–789. https://doi.org/10.1080/10408444.2019.1694862.
26. EFSA (2013). Scientific opinion on the safety assessment of medium viscosity white mineral oils with a kinematic viscosity between 8.5–11 mm^2/s at 100 °C for the proposed uses as a food additive. *EFSA J.* 11: 3073.
27. Yau, A.C.Y., Lönnblom, E., Zhong, J. et al. (2017). Influence of hydrocarbon oil structure on adjuvanticity and autoimmunity. *Sci. Rep.* 7 (1): 14998. https://doi.org/10.1038/s41598-017-15096-z.
28. Valdez, R.J.L., Merino, J.E., and Llanos, E.V. (2013). Enfermedad por modelantes. Comunicación de 10 casos. *Dermatol. Rev. Mex.* 57 (3): 159–164.
29. Lopez-Mendoza, J., Vargas-Flores, E., Mouneu-Ornelas, N. et al. (2021). Disease presentation and surgical treatment of patients with foreign-body granulomas and ASIA syndrome: case series. *Arch. Plast. Surg.* 48 (4): 366–372. https://doi.org/10.5999/aps.2020.02152.
30. Gordillo-Hernández, J., Alegre-Tamez, E., Torres-Baltazar, I. et al. (2013). Abordaje multidisciplinario de la enfermedad humana por infiltración de sustancias modelantes. *Cirugía Plástica Ibero-Latinoamericana 39* (3): 269–277. https://doi.org/10.4321/S0376-78922013000300009.
31. Kimber, I. and Dearman, R.J. (2010). An assessment of the ability of phthalates to influence immune and allergic responses. *Toxicology* 271 (3): 73–82. https://doi.org/10.1016/j.tox.2010.03.020.
32. Tuncel, J., Haag, S., Hoffmann, M.H. et al. (2016). Animal models of rheumatoid arthritis (i): pristane-induced arthritis in the rat. *PLoS One* 11: e0155936. https://doi.org/10.1371/journal.pone.0155936.
33. Vera-Lastra, O., Medina, G., Cruz-Dominguez del, M.P. et al. (2013). Autoimmune/inflammatory syndrome induced by adjuvants (Shoenfeld's syndrome): clinical and immunological spectrum. *Expert. Rev. Clin. Immunol.* 9 (4): 361–373. https://doi.org/10.1586/eci.13.2.

34. Cabral, A.R., Alcocer-Varela, J., Orozco-Topete, R. et al. (1994). Clinical, histopathological, immunological and fibroblast studies in 30 patients with subcutaneous injections of modelants including silicone and mineral oils. *Rev. Investig. Clin.* 46: 257–266.
35. Perricone, C., Colafrancesco, S., Mazor, R.D. et al. (2013). Autoimmune/inflammatory syndrome induced by adjuvants (ASIA) 2013: unveiling the pathogenic, clinical and diagnostic aspects. *J. Autoimmun.* 47: 1–16. https://doi.org/10.1016/j.jaut.2013.10.004.
36. Medrano-Ramírez, G., García-León, M.L., Priego-Blancas, R. et al. (2016). Papel de la respuesta Th1/Th 17 en los pacientes con enfermedad humana por aplicación de substancias modelantes. *Reumatol. Clin.* 12 (Supl E1): 37–110.
37. Kuroda, Y., Akaogi, J., Nacionales, D.C. et al. (2004). Distinctive patterns of autoimmune response induced by different types of mineral oil. *Toxicol. Sci.* 78 (2): 222–228. https://doi.org/10.1093/toxsci/kfh063.
38. Speil, C. and Rzepka, R. (2011). Vaccines and vaccine adjuvants as biological response modifiers. *Infect. Dis. Clin. N. Am.* 25 (4): 755–772. https://doi.org/10.1016/j.idc.2011.07.004.
39. Jara, L.J., García-Collinot, G., Medina, G. et al. (2017). Severe manifestations of autoimmune syndrome induced by adjuvants (Shoenfeld's syndrome). *Immunol. Res.* 65 (1): 8–16. https://doi.org/10.1007/s12026-016-8811-0.
40. Heppt, N., Hartmann, D.M., Reinholz, D.M. et al. (2015). Fillers and associated side effects. *HNO* 63 (7): 472–480. https://doi.org/10.1007/s00106-015-0030-9.
41. Tervaert JWC. Autoinflammatory/autoimmunity syndrome induced by adjuvants (ASIA; Shoenfeld's syndrome): a new flame. *Autoimmun. Rev.* 2018 17(12):1259–1264. https://doi.org/10.1016/j.autrev.2018.07.003.
42. Chan, J.L., Babadjouni, R., Sacks, W. et al. (2020). Symptomatic cervical tumoral calcinosis due to cosmetic body contouring mineral oil injections. *Cureus* 12 (11): e11743. https://doi.org/10.7759/cureus.11743.
43. Vera-Lastra, O., Hernadez, P.B., Sanchez-Rodriguez, A. et al. (2017). AB0991 prevalence of fibromyalgia and depression in patients with autoimmune/inflammatory syndrome induced by adjuvants compared to patients with systemic sclerosis. *Ann. Rheum. Dis.* 76 (Suppl 2): 1401.
44. Kumagai, Y., Shiokawa, Y., Medsger, T.A. Jr. et al. (1984). Clinical spectrum of connective tissue disease after cosmetic surgery. Observations on eighteen patients and a review of the Japanese literature. *Arthritis Rheum.* 27 (1): 1–12. https://doi.org/10.1002/art.1780270101.
45. Kumagai, Y., Abe, C., and Shiokawa, Y. (1979). Scleroderma after cosmetic surgery: four cases of human adjuvant disease. *Arthritis Rheum.* 22 (5): 532–537. https://doi.org/10.1002/art.1780220514.
46. Padilla, G.F., Mendoza, B.M., and Montenegro, A.P. (2014). Adjuvant induced autoimmune/inflammatory syndrome presenting as joint and lung manifestations. *Reumatol. Clin.* 10 (6): 406–408. https://doi.org/10.1016/j.reuma.2014.01.005.
47. Moraitis, A.G., Hewison, M., Collins, M. et al. (2013). Hypercalcemia associated with mineral oil-induced sclerosing paraffinomas. *Endocr. Pract.* 19 (2): e50–e56. https://doi.org/10.4158/EP12092.CR.
48. Bento, C., Velh, P., and Carvalho, N. (2015). Lots of steroids and vitamins, tons of complications. Hypercalcemia and nephrocalcinosis as important complications of performance-enhancing drugs. *Nefrologia* 35 (6): 598–600. https://doi.org/10.1016/j.nefro.2015.09.005.
49. Watad, A., Quaresma, M., Bragazzi, N.L. et al. (2018). The autoimmune/inflammatory syndrome induced by adjuvants (ASIA)/Shoenfeld's syndrome: descriptive analysis of 300 patients from the international ASIA syndrome registry. *Clin. Rheumatol.* 37 (2): 483–493. https://doi.org/10.1007/s10067-017-3748-9.
50. Wang, Y.X., Fang, Y., Guo, Y.F. et al. (2017). Analysis of 12 cases of exogenous lipoid pneumonia confirmed by pathology. *Zhonghua Jie He He Hu Xi Za Zhi* 40 (6): 445–449. https://doi.org/10.3760/cma.j.issn.1001-0939.2017.06.010.
51. Alvarez-Cordovés, M.M., Mirpuri-Mirpuri, P.G., Rocha-Cabrera, P. et al. (2013). Lipoid pneumonia: presentation of a case. *Semergen.* 39 (2): 110–112. https://doi.org/10.1016/j.semerg.2011.11.008.
52. Rajagopala, S. and Selvam, N. (2019). An unusual cause of respiratory distress. *Postgrad. Med. Postgrad. Med.* 65 (1): 38–40. https://doi.org/10.4103/jpgm.JPGM_496_17.
53. Morales-Raya, C., Calleja-Algarra, A., Tous-Romero, F., and Rivera-Díaz, R. (2017). Penile paraffinoma: should we perform ultrasound? *Actas Dermosifiliogr.* 108 (5): 478–480. https://doi.org/10.1016/j.ad.2016.11.007.
54. Bobik, O. Jr. and Bobik, O. Sr. (2011). Penile paraffinoma and ulcers of penis. *Bratisl. Lek. Listy* 112 (11): 653–654.

55. Pehlivanov G, Kavaklieva S, Kazandjieva J, et al. Foreign-body granuloma of the penis in sexually active individuals (penile paraffinoma). .*J. Eur. Acad. Dermatol. Venereol.* 2008 22(7):845–51. https://doi.org/10.1111/j.1468-3083.2008.02677.x.
56. Lee SW, Bang CY, Kim JH Penoscrotal reconstruction using groin and bilateral superomedial thigh flaps: a case of penile vaselinoma causing Fournier's gangrene.*Yonsei Med. J.* 2007; 48(4):723–6. https://doi.org/10.3349/ymj.2007.48.4.723.
57. Glicenstein J The first "fillers," vaseline and paraffin. From miracle to disaster. *Ann. Chir. Plast. Esthet.* 2007;52(2):157–61. https://doi.org/10.1016/j.anplas.2006.05.003.
58. Akkus E, Iscimen A, Tasli L, Hattat H Paraffinoma and ulcer of the external genitalia after self-injection of vaseline. *J. Sex. Med.* 2006 3(1):170–2. https://doi.org/10.1111/j.1743-6109.2005.00096.x.
59. Hohaus K, Bley B, Köstler E, Schönlebe J, Wollina U Mineral oil granuloma of the penis. *J. Eur. Acad. Dermatol. Venereol.* 2003 17(5):585–7. https://doi.org/10.1046/j.1468-3083.2003.00896.x.
60. Barker, T.T., Lee, P.Y., Kelly-Scumpia, K.M. et al. (2011). Pathogenic role of B cells in the development of diffuse alveolar hemorrhage induced by pristane. *Lab. Investig.* 91 (10): 1540–1550. https://doi.org/10.1038/labinvest.2011.108.
61. Menis, D., Castellanos-González, M., Llamas-Martín, R. et al. (2014). The utility of skin ultrasound for the diagnosis of complications of tissue filler materials. *Actas Dermosifiliogr.* 105 (8): 797–798. https://doi.org/10.1016/j.ad.2013.11.012.
62. Fernández, C.V., Álvarez, I.B., Centeno, A.F.T. et al. (2015). Ecografía cutánea y rellenos dermatológicos [Cutaneous ultrasound and dermal fillers]. *Actas Dermosifiliogr.* 106 (Suppl 1): 87–95. https://doi.org/10.1016/S0001-7310(16)30011-4.
63. Wortsman, X., Wortsman, J., Orlandi, C. et al. (2012). Ultrasound detection and identification of cosmetic fillers in the skin. *J. Eur. Acad. Dermatol. Venereol.* 26 (3): 292–301. https://doi.org/10.1111/j.1468--3083.2011.04047.x.
64. Cormio, L., Di Fino, G., Scavone, C. et al. (2014). Magnetic resonance imaging of penile paraffinoma: case report. *BMC Med. Imaging* 14: 39. https://doi.org/10.1186/1471-2342-14-39.
65. Zimmermann, U.S. and Clerici, T.J. (2004). The histological aspects of fillers complications. *Semin. Cutan. Med. Surg.* 23 (4): 241–250. https://doi.org/10.1016/j.sder.2004.09.004.
66. Radenska-Lopovok, S.G. and Volkova, P. (2018). Autoimmune/inflammatory syndrome induced by adjuvants [Article in Russian]. *Arkh. Patol.* 80 (5): 56–62. https://doi.org/10.17116/patol20188005156.
67. Colaris, M.J.L., van der Hulst, R.R., and Tervaert, J.W.C. (2017). Vitamin D deficiency as a risk factor for the development of autoantibodies in patients with ASIA and silicone breast implants: a cohort study and review of the literature. *Clin. Rheumatol.* 36 (5): 981–993. https://doi.org/10.1007/s10067-017-3589-6.
68. Mendoza, J.L., Tarriba, J.T., and Reyes, A.I. (2020). Microsurgical management of severe human adjuvant disease due to mineral oil injection. *Int. Microsurg. J.* 4: 1.
69. Ma, Z., Li, Z., Shou, K. et al. (2017). Negative pressure wound therapy: regulating blood flow perfusion and microvessel maturation through microvascular pericytes. *Int. J. Mol. Med.* 40 (5): 1415–1425. https://doi.org/10.3892/ijmm.2017.3131.

26 Metals in Dental Implants as a Trigger of Autoimmunity

Arad Dotan[1,2] and Yehuda Shoenfeld[1,3]
[1]Zabludowicz Center for Autoimmune Diseases, Sheba Medical Center, Tel-Hashomer, Israel
[2]Sackler Faculty of Medicine, Tel Aviv University, Tel Aviv, Israel
[3]Reichman University, Herzliya, Israel

The immune system is a highly complex network of biological processes that have the ability to respond toward foreign stimuli, including bacteria, viruses, parasites, fungi, as well as toxins, and other unfamiliar exogenous materials [1, 2]. The organization of cells and molecules of the immune system defends the organism from these foreign microbes and compounds [1]. These stimuli cause stimulation of the immune system, enabling a targeted response to protect the organism from infections and diseases [1]. This influence has a carousal role in survival, as adapting to changing environments and targeting foreign pathogens and substances that might harm the organism are essential requirements of the immune system [1, 2].

Various necessary factors are involved in stimulating the immune system's innate and acquired responses; these factors are commonly classified into three primary groups: genetic, epigenetic; environmental; and hormonal [3–5]. Nevertheless, the stimulation of the immune system may act as a double-edged sword; the described factors could deviate from their physiological association and contribute to the development of abnormal hyperstimulation that could result in the new onset of autoimmune diseases in genetically predisposed individuals [3–5]. Additionally, a lymphoma may develop in the long term due to the high pathological activity of the immune system, displaying as a chronic release of inflammatory mediators and the irregular proliferation of immune cells [6, 7].

In the past few decades, the rate of autoimmune diseases has been shown to be at an alarming rise worldwide [8]. Although genetic predisposition is undoubtedly a factor in developing an autoimmune disease, it alone cannot explain these changes on a worldwide scale [8]. Hence, there has been a focus on the environmental factors that are rapidly changing through new technology, industries, chemicals, drugs, and diets, rapidly being introduced in the fast-paced changing world [2].

It is well known that environmental factors have a substantial impact and even appear necessary for the loss of immune homeostasis and the development of autoimmunity [9]. Cigarette smoke, dietary factors, toxic chemicals, and infectious agents, such as viruses, bacteria, fungi, and parasites, are only a few examples of the numerous well-known environmental factors that have been shown to influence disease etiopathogenesis in animal modules and epidemiological studies [2, 4, 5, 8, 9].

Autoimmune Disorders: Adjuvants and Other Risk Factors in Pathogenesis, First Edition.
Edited by Abdulla Watad, Nicola Luigi Bragazzi, and Yehuda Shoenfeld.

Heavy metals are part of essential biochemical and physiological functions in numerous organisms, likewise in humans. Many of those roles include taking an instrumental part in oxidation–reduction reactions in crucial enzymes. However, a high dose of metal materials, primarily heavy metals, may have destructive effects by increasing the reactive oxygen species, contributing to epigenetic modifications, shifting the cytokine secretion to a pro-inflammatory profile, and contributing to abnormal activation of innate and adaptive immune cells.

In addition, some metal materials had also been shown to be related to autoimmunity [10–13]. Various metals are used for numerous purposes in different industries, such as medical, technological, and construction. These heavy metals are vastly used in many day-to-day life instruments, with which a significant part of modern society is in close contact. Some of these are certain jewelry, paint products, cosmetics products, batteries, and ceramics; thus, they may have an immense pathogenic potential in autoimmunity.

Some metals, such as aluminum, mercury, gold, copper, and nickel, can stimulate the immune system more drastically than others [13–21]. The effects of metals on autoimmune manifestations were investigated in humans [13, 16] as well as in animal modules [11, 21–24]. Accordingly, many interventions avoid these metals and use alternative materials to reduce the immune system's response toward foreign substances and to reduce the side effects of the treatment or procedure. However, the impact of the metals on the immune system can potentially evoke many manifestations, such as acute inflammation, typical skin lesions, chronic inflammation, and transplant rejection, as well as systemic and unspecific, for example, chronic fatigue, sleep problems, memory impairment, depression, and sensitivity to pain [13, 16]. Importantly, some studies had suggested improvement of symptoms following the removal of the metal implants [13, 16, 25].

Metals are used with excellent success and in numerous indications throughout various fields. In vaccinations, aluminum-based materials, such as aluminum hydroxide, aluminum phosphate, or potassium aluminum sulfate, are regularly used as adjuvants to invoke a robust immune stimulation [26]. This stimulation assists in improving the immune response to vaccine ingredients and the outcomes of the vaccination [26]. Crucially, there is no doubt that the immense benefits of vaccinations worldwide to prevent diseases minimize possible adverse effects of aluminum-based materials [27]. Nevertheless, some studies indicate that aluminum-based materials should be exchanged with nonaluminum adjuvants in order to reduce the chance of creating hyperstimulation of the immune system and contributing to an autoimmune manifestation [13, 16].

In the past, some metal implants, including gold Ti–aluminum–vanadium alloys, have been neglected; due to relatively poor bone-to-implant contact, their use was almost wholly abandoned [28]. Over the years, new types of dental crowns were developed to reduce side effects and improve the esthetic while maintaining for a more extended period [28]. In light of advances in the field, today, the most common dental crowns are porcelain crowns fused to seminoble and nonnoble metals, such as aluminum, chrome, and cobalt. However, even today, these metal components are significantly associated with immune manifestations, leading some patients to implant rejection and side effects [10, 12, 29–31]. Nowadays, nonmetallic dental crowns are being used more rapidly; these advanced crowns have biological advantages over fused porcelain crowns to metal and constitute a more esthetic treatment [32, 33].

A study by Vera Stejskal examined three individuals, one with chronic fatigue syndrome (CFS) and two with fibromyalgia, all suspected of a metal-mediated exposure as a trigger for their disease. After analyzing their disorders, the metal implants were removed, and a long-term health improvement had been recorded in follow-ups. The autoimmune/inflammatory syndrome induced by adjuvants (ASIA) is characterized by fibromyalgia and/or CFS, autoimmune diseases, and the production of autoantibodies. This syndrome may develop due to long-term exposure to materials that lead to adjuvant-mediated hyperstimulation of the immune system [3, 34, 35]. ASIA may assist in dipping understanding of the unspecific symptoms, CFS-like symptoms [12], similar to some patients with seminoble and nonnoble metal implants. We believe that nonmetallic dental crowns have an advantage in preventing such symptoms compared to dental implants fused with metal materials.

References

1. Delves, P.J. and Roitt, I.M. (2000). Advances in immunology: the immune system. *N. Engl. J. Med.* 343: 37–49.
2. Vojdani, A. (2014). A potential link between environmental triggers and autoimmunity. *Autoimmune Dis.* 2014: 437231.
3. Watad, A., Bragazzi, N.L., Amital, H., and Shoenfeld, Y. (2019). Hyperstimulation of Adaptive Immunity as the Common Pathway for Silicone Breast Implants, Autoimmunity, and Lymphoma of the Breast. *Isr. Med. Assoc. J.* 21 (8): 517–519.
4. Shoenfeld, Y., Blank, M., Abu-Shakra, M. et al. (2008). The mosaic of autoimmunity: prediction, autoantibodies, and therapy in autoimmune diseases–2008. *Isr. Med. Assoc. J.* 10: 13–19.
5. Shoenfeld, Y., Zandman-Goddard, G., Stojanovich, L. et al. (2008). The mosaic of autoimmunity: hormonal and environmental factors involved in autoimmune diseases–2008. *Isr. Med. Assoc. J.* 10: 8–12.
6. Goldin, L.R. and Landgren, O. (2009). Autoimmunity and lymphomagenesis. *Int. J. Cancer* 124: 1497–1502. https://doi.org/10.1002/IJC.24141.
7. Gibbs, G.W. and Labrèche, F. (2014). Cancer risks in aluminum reduction plant workers: a review. *J. Occup. Environ. Med.* 56 (5 Suppl): S40–S59.
8. Lerner, A., Jeremias, P., and Matthias, T. (2015). The world incidence and prevalence of autoimmune diseases is increasing. *Int. J. Cel. Dis.* 3: 151–155. https://doi.org/10.12691/IJCD-3-4-8.
9. Costenbader, K.H., Gay, S., Alarcón-Riquelme, M.E. et al. (2012). Genes, epigenetic regulation and environmental factors: which is the most relevant in developing autoimmune diseases? *Autoimmun. Rev.* 11: 604–609.
10. Bigazzi, P.E. (1994). Autoimmunity and heavy metals. *Lupus* 3: 449–453.
11. Bagchi, D. and Bagchi, M. (ed.) (2020). *Metal Toxicology Handbook*. CRC Press.
12. Bjørklund, G., Dadar, M., Chirumbolo, S. et al. (2020). Metals, autoimmunity, and neuroendocrinology: is there a connection? *Environ. Res.* 187: 109541.
13. Stejskal, V. (2014). Metals as a common trigger of inflammation resulting in non-specific symptoms: diagnosis and treatment. *Isr. Med. Assoc. J.* 16 (12): 753–758.
14. Pelletier, L., Pasquier, R., Rossert, J. et al. (1988). Autoreactive T cells in mercury-induced autoimmunity. Ability to induce the autoimmune disease. *J. Immunol.* 140 (3): 750–754.
15. Batista-Duharte, A., Lindblad, E.B., and Oviedo-Orta, E. (2011). Progress in understanding adjuvant immunotoxicity mechanisms. *Toxicol. Lett.* 203: 97–105.
16. Prochazkova, J., Sterzl, I., Kucerova, H. et al. (2004). The beneficial effect of amalgam replacement on health in patients with autoimmunity. *Neuroendocrinol. Lett.* 25 (3): 211–218.
17. Tomljenovic, L. and Shaw, C.A. (2012). Mechanisms of aluminum adjuvant toxicity and autoimmunity in pediatric populations. *Lupus* 21: 223–230. https://doi.org/10.1177/0961203311430221.
18. Lerner, A. (2012). Aluminum as an adjuvant in Crohn's disease induction. *Lupus* 21: 231–238.
19. Eggleston, D.W. (1984). Effect of dental amalgam and nickel alloys on T-lymphocytes: preliminary report. *J. Prosthet. Dent.* 51: 617–623.
20. Andrioli, M., Trimboli, P., Maio, D. et al. (2015). Systemic nickel allergic syndrome as an immune-mediated disease with an increased risk for thyroid autoimmunity. *Endocrine* 50 (3): 807–810.
21. Tournade, H., Guery, J.C., Pasquier, R. et al. (1991). Experimental gold-induced autoimmunity. *Nephrol. Dial. Transplant.* 6: 621–630.
22. Weening, J.J., Fleuren, G.J., and Hoedemaeker, P.J. (1978). Demonstration of antinuclear antibodies in mercuric chloride-induced glomerulopathy in the rat. *Lab. Invest.* 39 (4): 405–411.
23. Druet, E., Sapin, C., Günther, E. et al. (1977). Mercuric chloride-induced anti-glomerular basement membrane antibodies in the rat: genetic control. *Eur. J. Immunol.* 7: 348–351.
24. Balazs, T. (1987). Immunogenetically controlled autoimmune reactions induced by mercury, gold and d-penicillamine in laboratory animals: a review from the vantage point of premarketing safety studies. *Toxicol. Ind. Health* 3: 331–336.
25. Kristoffersen, A.E., Alræk, T., Stub, T. et al. (2016). Health complaints attributed to dental amalgam: a retrospective survey exploring perceived health changes related to amalgam removal. *Open Dent. J.* 10: 739.
26. Charerntantanakul, W. (2020). Adjuvants for swine vaccines: mechanisms of actions and adjuvant effects. *Vaccine* 38: 6659–6681. https://doi.org/10.1016/J.VACCINE.2020.08.054.

27. Karafillakis, E. and Larson, H.J. (2017). The benefit of the doubt or doubts over benefits? A systematic literature review of perceived risks of vaccines in European populations. *Vaccine* 35: 4840–4850. https://doi.org/10.1016/J.VACCINE.2017.07.061.
28. Gaviria, L., Salcido, J.P., Guda, T., and Ong, J.L. (2014). Current trends in dental implants. *J. Korean Assoc. Oral Maxillofac. Surg.* 40 (2): 50–60. https://doi.org/10.5125/jkaoms.2014.40.2.50.
29. Petrarca, C., Perrone, A., Verna, N. et al. (2006). Cobalt nano-particles modulate cytokine in vitro release by human mononuclear cells mimicking autoimmune disease. *Int. J. Immunopathol. Pharmacol.* 19: 11–14.
30. Biglia, A., Morandi, V., Monti, S. et al. (2020). Cobalt hip prosthesis intoxication mimicking an autoimmune disease. *Joint Bone Spine* 87: 652–654.
31. Shrivastava, R., Upreti, R.K., Seth, P.K., and Chaturvedi, U.C. (2002). Effects of chromium on the immune system. *FEMS Immunol. Med. Microbiol.* 34: 1–7.
32. Sailer, I., Makarov, N.A., Thoma, D.S. et al. (2015). All-ceramic or metal-ceramic tooth-supported fixed dental prostheses (FDPs)? A systematic review of the survival and complication rates. Part I: single crowns (SCs). *Dent. Mater.* 31: 603–623.
33. Pjetursson, B.E., Valente, N.A., Strasding, M. et al. (2018). A systematic review of the survival and complication rates of zirconia-ceramic and metal-ceramic single crowns. *Clin. Oral Implants Res.* 29 (Suppl 16): 199–214.
34. Watad, A., Bragazzi, N.L., McGonagle, D. et al. (2019). Autoimmune/inflammatory syndrome induced by adjuvants (ASIA) demonstrates distinct autoimmune and autoinflammatory disease associations according to the adjuvant subtype: Insights from an analysis of 500 cases. *Clin. Immunol.* 203: 1–8.
35. Shoenfeld, Y. and Agmon-Levin, N. (2011). "ASIA" – autoimmune/inflammatory syndrome induced by adjuvants. *J. Autoimmun.* 36: 4–8.

27 Conclusions: State of the Art and Prospects

Abdulla Watad[1,2,3,4,5], Nicola Luigi Bragazzi[6,7], and Yehuda Shoenfeld[8,9]

[1]Rheumatology Unit and Zabludowicz Center for Autoimmune Diseases, Sheba Medical Center, Tel-Hashomer, Israel
[2]Section of Musculoskeletal Disease, Leeds Institute of Molecular Medicine, University of Leeds, Leeds, United Kingdom
[3]Sackler Faculty of Medicine, Tel Aviv University, Tel Aviv, Israel
[4]Department of Internal Medicine 'B', Sheba Medical Center, Tel-Hashomer, Israel
[5]Institute of Oncology, Sheba Medical Center, Tel-Hashomer, Israel
[6]Laboratory for Industrial and Applied Mathematics (LIAM), Department of Mathematics and Statistics, York University,Toronto, Canada
[7]Postgraduate School of Public Health, Department of Health Sciences (DISSAL), University of Genoa, Genoa, Italy
[8]Reichman University, Herzliya, Israel
[9]Zabludowicz Center for Autoimmune Diseases, Sheba Medical Center, Tel-Hashomer, Israel

This book – *Autoimmune Disorders: Adjuvants and Other Risk Factors in Pathogenesis* – embarks on a multifaceted journey, unraveling the intricate connections between adjuvants and autoimmune responses. It casts a critical eye on the emergence of the autoimmune/inflammatory syndrome induced by adjuvants (ASIA syndrome) while acknowledging the remarkable benefits that vaccines confer upon public health. With each chapter, the book delves into different facets of this complex interplay, underlining the paramount importance of informed medical decision-making.

While the book probes into the potential for adjuvants to trigger autoimmune responses, it does so within the broader context of vaccines' monumental impact on global health. It is paramount to acknowledge that vaccines have been the cornerstone of disease prevention, saving countless lives and eradicating some of the most virulent infectious diseases. The overwhelming majority of vaccine recipients experience only the protective effects, with any side effects being exceedingly rare.

"The Hyperstimulation Syndrome" introduces the core concept that sets the stage for understanding ASIA syndrome. It elucidates how immune responses can be hyperstimulated by various stimuli, initiating discussions about the delicate balance between immune activation and regulatory mechanisms.

In "Genetics, Immunization, and Autoimmunity," the genetic landscape that influences immune responses is unveiled. While genetic factors can influence susceptibility to autoimmune reactions, they are only part of the intricate puzzle that encompasses this complex syndrome.

Autoimmune Disorders: Adjuvants and Other Risk Factors in Pathogenesis, First Edition.
Edited by Abdulla Watad, Nicola Luigi Bragazzi, and Yehuda Shoenfeld.

As the narrative unfolds in "Adjuvants (History, Role, and Side Effects)," the historical context of adjuvants in vaccine development is explored. The chapter acknowledges the role adjuvants play in enhancing immune responses, while simultaneously investigating potential side effects, placing them in the broader perspective of vaccine benefits.

"The Frequently Food Additives as a Trigger of Autoimmunity" extends the discussion beyond vaccines, examining the potential impact of commonly used food additives on autoimmune responses. This exploration underscores the broader range of factors that can potentially influence the immune system's behavior.

Shifting the focus to medical interventions, "Silicone Implant Incompatibility Syndrome" delves into the intricate connection between silicone implants and autoimmune responses. This chapter emphasizes the challenges of foreign materials interacting with the body and their implications for immune system reactivity.

"Mesh and Autoimmunity" scrutinizes mesh implants' role in potentially inducing autoimmune reactions, contributing to a broader conversation about the unintended consequences of surgical interventions.

The realm of vaccines returns in "Vaccines, Vaccinosis, and Autoimmunity," where the concept of vaccinosis is dissected. While vaccines have revolutionized disease prevention, this chapter navigates the delicate balance between immune enhancement and potential autoimmune triggers.

"Sustained Immune Activation in ASIA Syndrome – A Bridge to Lymphomagenesis" bridges chronic immune responses in ASIA syndrome to the potential development of lymphomas. This chapter delves into the intricate connections between prolonged immune activation and serious health outcomes.

"Chronic Fatigue Syndrome" spotlights the intersection of chronic fatigue syndrome and the ASIA syndrome, pushing the boundaries of understanding the links between immune dysregulation and debilitating health conditions.

"Autoantibodies Against the Autonomic System: β2AR Ab" unravels autoantibodies targeting the autonomic system, revealing the complex immune pathways involved and the potential convergence of autoimmunity and autonomic functions.

"Postural Orthostatic Tachycardia Syndrome (POTS) as a Part of ASIA Syndrome" showcases POTS within the context of ASIA syndrome, unveiling the systemic implications of autoimmune responses on autonomic functions.

"Role of Small-Fiber Neuropathy in the Pathogenesis of ASIA Syndrome" dives into the neural realm, dissecting the impact of small-fiber neuropathy on the development of ASIA syndrome. This chapter intertwines neural pathways and immune responses in the intricate web of autoimmune disorders.

From the world of art, "Tattoo as a Trigger of ASIA Syndrome" unearths potential connections between tattoos and autoimmune responses. The immune reactions to tattoo ink open a dialogue about personal expression and potential health risks.

Environmental factors are examined in "Sick Building Syndrome as a Part of ASIA Syndrome," spotlighting sick building syndrome within the context of ASIA syndrome. This chapter expands the discussion to encompass the broader impact of environmental influences on autoimmune responses.

"Gulf War Syndrome (GWS) and ASIA Syndrome" navigates the potential connection between Gulf War syndrome and ASIA syndrome, bridging overlapping symptoms and immune responses in the pursuit of understanding systemic autoimmune manifestations.

The complexities of vaccinations in individuals with preexisting autoimmune disorders are dissected in "Vaccinations in Patients with Autoimmune Diseases," offering guidance through the intricate landscape of balancing immune reactions and potential autoimmune triggers. "Immune Checkpoints and Autoimmunity" ventures into the territory of immune checkpoints, shedding light on their potential connection to autoimmunity. This chapter delves into the nuanced regulation of immune responses and their potential for tipping the balance.

"Metals and Autoimmunity" investigates metals as potential triggers of autoimmunity, unraveling the intricate connections between metal exposure and immune system dysregulation, within the broader context of environmental influences.

Expanding the scope, "Bisphenol and Autoimmunity" includes bisphenol and its potential contribution to autoimmune responses. This chapter underscores the impact of environmental compounds on immune balance, delving into contemporary environmental challenges. "Sarcoid as a Proof of Concept of the Hyperstimulation Syndrome" presents sarcoidosis as a case study, illustrating the hyperstimulation syndrome concept. By scrutinizing immune responses in sarcoidosis, this chapter reinforces the idea of immune system hyperactivation. Similarly, "Sjögren's Syndrome as a Proof of Concept of the Hyperstimulation Syndrome" uses Sjögren's syndrome to exemplify the hyperstimulation syndrome. Through the lens of immune responses targeting moisture-producing glands, this chapter underscores the systemic implications of immune dysregulation.

"Gluteal Biopolymer Injections as a Case of ASIA Syndrome" shifts focus to cosmetic interventions, investigating gluteal biopolymer injections' potential contribution to ASIA syndrome. By dissecting the relationship between elective procedures and autoimmune responses, this chapter engages in a broader discourse about the consequences of aesthetic enhancements.

"The Chemical and Social Landscape of the Modern World and Increased Risk of ASIA" broadens the perspective to the contemporary chemical and social landscape. This chapter unravels how modern lifestyles and environmental exposures might elevate the risk of ASIA syndrome, urging a holistic understanding of potential triggers.

"Oil Injections and ASIA Syndrome" delves into the realm of oil injections and their potential connection to ASIA syndrome. By uncovering the immune responses ignited by foreign substances, this chapter unravels the intricate web of potential autoimmune triggers.

"Dental Implants as a Trigger of Autoimmunity" revisits medical interventions, turning the focus to dental implants and their potential role in inducing autoimmune responses. This chapter navigates the complex terrain of restorative dentistry and its ties to immune system dysregulation.

In the grand tapestry of "The Link Between Adjuvants and Autoimmunity (ASIA Syndrome)," every chapter contributes a thread of knowledge, intricately weaving adjuvants, autoimmune responses, and their multifaceted interactions. Throughout this exploration, the book underscores the profound impact of vaccines on public health, emphasizing that their benefits far outweigh potential side effects. By inviting medical professionals, researchers, and readers to journey through this multidisciplinary landscape, the book fosters a deeper understanding of the complex relationship among immunology, public health, and individual well-being.

Index

Please Note: Entries in *italics* refer to figures, entries in **bold** refer to tables.

8-OHdG *see* 8-hydroxydeoxyguanosine

AAb *see* autoantibodies
acellar pertussis combination vaccines, 21–22
acetylcholinesterase (AChE) inhibitors, Gulf War Syndrome, 169
AChE *see* acetylcholinesterase
ACPAs *see* anticitrullinated protein antibodies
acute lymphomas, postvaccination, 97
adaptive immunity, bisphenol A, 232–234
ADHD *see* attention deficit/hyperactivity disorder
adjuvant-induced autoimmunity, 8, 9–11, 87–88, 270–271
  see also Autoimmune/inflammatory Syndrome Induced by Adjuvants
adjuvants
  classification, 16–18
  definition, 15
  etymology, 16
  history of, 18–19
  lipophilicity, 98–100, **99**
  mechanisms, 19–20
  safety and side effects, 20–24
  see also nutritional adjuvants; *specific adjuvants...*; vaccine adjuvants
α1AdR *see* α1-adrenergic receptors
α2AdR *see* α2-adrenergic receptors
β1AdR *see* β1-adrenergic receptors
β2AdR *see* β2-adrenergic receptors
α1AdR *see* α1-adrenergic receptors
α2AdR *see* α2-adrenergic receptors
β1AdR *see* β1-adrenergic receptors
β2AdR *see* β2-adrenergic receptors
α1-adrenergic receptors (α1AdR), 118, 130
α2-adrenergic receptors (α2AdR), 130
β1-adrenergic receptors (β1AdR), 118
β2-adrenergic receptors (β2AdR), 118
ADs *see* autoimmune diseases
adult-onset Still's disease (AOSD), 202
adverse events
  acetylcholinesterase inhibitors, 169
  aluminum-adjuvanted vaccines, 20–22
  biopolymer injections, 284–297, **285–286**
  emulsion-adjuvanted vaccines, 22–23
  gluten, 32, 32–33
  immune checkpoint inhibitors, 192–195
  mesh implants, 69–72
  novel adjuvants, 23–24
  pesticides, 169
  vaccine adjuvants, 20–24, 86–88
AID *see* autoimmune diseases
AIRD *see* autoimmune rheumatic diseases
Akureyri disease (Iceland disease), 109
ALCL *see* anaplastic large cell lymphoma
allergic reactions, 71, 156, 306
aluminum, 7, 8, 100, 203–205, 207, 209–210, 214
aluminum-adjuvanted vaccines, **16**, 17, 20–22, 98–101, **99**, 270–271
ALVAL *see* aseptic lymphocytic (lymphocyte-dominated) vasculitis-associated lesions
ANA *see* antinuclear antibodies
analogy, 81
anaplastic large cell lymphoma (ALCL), 4, 97, 100–101
ANCAs *see* antineutrophil cytoplasmic antibodies
animal models, 93–96, 120–122, 169–170, 256, 312–313
ANS *see* autonomic nervous system
anthrax vaccines, 170–171
anti-angiotensin II type 1 receptor (anti-AT1R) autoantibodies, 119–120
anti-AT1R *see* anti-angiotensin II type 1 receptor
anti-bisphenol A antibodies, 235
anticitrullinated protein antibodies (ACPAs), 206
anti-endothelin receptor type A (anti-ETAR) autoantibodies, 120
anti-ETAR *see* anti-endothelin receptor type A
antigen-presenting cells (APCs), bisphenol A, 230–231
anti-GPCR antibodies, 117–127, **121**, 130–131
anti-idiotype immune responses, 9–10
anti M3 receptor autoantibodies, 120
antimony, 203, 211
antineutrophil cytoplasmic antibodies (ANCAs), 100
antinuclear antibodies (ANA), 131, 172, 193
antiphospholipid syndrome (APS), 131, 237
AOSD *see* adult-onset Still's disease
APCs *see* antigen-presenting cells
apoptosis-associated speck-like protein containing a C-terminal caspase-recruitment domain (ASC), 75

Autoimmune Disorders: Adjuvants and Other Risk Factors in Pathogenesis, First Edition.
Edited by Abdulla Watad, Nicola Luigi Bragazzi, and Yehuda Shoenfeld.

Index

APRIL ligand, 202
APS *see* antiphospholipid syndrome
arthralgia, immune checkpoint inhibitors, 192
arthritis *see* inflammatory arthritis; rheumatoid arthritis
AS03-adjuvanted vaccines, **16**, 17, 99
ASC *see* apoptosis-associated speck-like protein containing a C-terminal caspase-recruitment domain
aseptic lymphocytic (lymphocyte-dominated) vasculitis-associated lesions (ALVAL), 76
ASIA *see* Autoimmune/inflammatory Syndrome Induced by Adjuvants
ASIA-MO *see* Autoimmune/inflammatory Syndrome Induced by Adjuvants, mineral oils
atezolizumab (Tecentriq), 192
atopic diseases, mesh-mediated disease, 71
attention deficit/hyperactivity disorder (ADHD), 36–37
atypical poliomyelitis, 109
auramine O, 36
autoantibodies (AAb), 117–127, **121**, 130–131, 139, 172, 193, 253–254
autoimmune diseases (ADs/AID)
  animal models, 93–96
  development, 73–76, *74*
  foreign bodies, 3–4, 73–76
  genetics, 7–9
  immune checkpoint inhibitors, 194–195
  and intestinal permeability, 306–307
  lymphoproliferative disorders, 4, 93–96
  metals, 3–4, 201–223, 337–340
  postvaccination, 8–11, 87–88, 170–171
  POTS associations, 131–132
  relative lymphomagenic risks, 93, **94**
  see also specific diseases...
autoimmune dysautonomia, 63–66, 117–127, **123**, 139–140, **139**
autoimmune exocrinopathy, 120
Autoimmune/inflammatory Syndrome Induced by Adjuvants (ASIA), 7–14, **8**, 72–76, **76**, **92**, 93–96, 112–113, 213–214, 305–321
autoimmune rheumatic diseases (AIRD), 181–190
autoimmune sialadenitis, 202–203
autonomic nervous system (ANS), 117–127
avelumab (Bavencio), 192
azathioprine, 256
AZB *see* azoximer bromide
azo food dyes, 36
azoximer bromide (AZB/polyoxidonium), 23–24

bacterial-derived adjuvants, **16**, 17
Bavencio *see* avelumab
β1-adrenergic receptors (β1AdR), 118
β2-adrenergic receptors (β2AdR), 118
biomarkers, Gulf War Syndrome, 171–172
biomaterials *see specific materials...*
biopolymer injections, 283–303
biopsy, small-fiber neuropathy, 140
bisphenol A (BPA), 225–246
  adaptive immunity, 232–234
  as an adjuvant, 227
  antibodies, 235
  autoimmunity, 228–240
  direct mechanisms, 228–234
  endocrine disruption, 225–227, 235–236
  epigenetic alterations, 236
  healthcare exposures, 227
  humoral immunity, 234
  indirect mechanisms, 234–236
  innate immunity, 228–232
  pathophysiology, 225–241
  protein disulfide isomerase, 234–235
BPA *see* bisphenol A
Bradford–Hill criteria, 78–80
brain defects, Gulf War Syndrome, 171
BRI *see* building-related illness
building-related illness (BRI), 156
  see also sick building syndrome
butterfly wings technique, 295

cadmium, 204–208, 210, 211, 212
CaHA *see* calcium hydroxyapatite
calcinosis cutis, 204
calcium hydroxyapatite (CaHA), **285**
Canadian consensus criteria, chronic fatigue syndrome, 111
cancer, immune checkpoint inhibitors, 191–199
caramel color class IV, 36
carbamates, Gulf War Syndrome, 169
CARD *see* caspase-recruitment domains
cardiac autoimmunity, 239
caspase-recruitment domains (CARD), 75
causation
  analogy, 80
  Bradford–Hill criteria, 78–80
  coherence, 80
  consistency, 80
  experimental evidence, 80
  Gulf War Syndrome, 168–171
  Koch's postulates, 78
  mesh-mediated disease, 78–81
  sarcoidosis, 248–249, **250**
  sick building syndrome, 156–159
  temporality, 80
  see also etiology; pathophysiology
CD *see* celiac disease
cecal ligation and puncture model (CLP), 312–313
celiac disease (CD), 32–34, 131
cellular immunity, bisphenol A, 228–234
cemiplimab (Libtayo), 192
central nervous system (CNS) alterations, Gulf War Syndrome, 171
central sensitivity syndrome, 112
cerebral blood flow, Gulf War Syndrome, 171
CFA *see* complete Freund's adjuvant
CFS *see* chronic fatigue syndrome
challenge-dechallenge-rechallenge evidence, mesh, 79–80
chemical warfare agents, 169–170
childhood stress, 309
cholinergic neurotransmission, 120
chromium, systemic lupus erythematosus, 206
chronic Epstein–Barr virus syndrome, 110
chronic fatigue syndrome (CFS), 70, 107–115, 122, 173, 338
chronic inflammation
  animal models, 312–313
  Gulf War Syndrome, 170, 171–172

lymphoproliferative disorders, 4, 91–106
mesh, 2–4, 73–76
metals, 3–4
neurogenic switching, 162
POTS, 131
programmed cell death protein-1 95–96
self-reactive clones, 101
silicone breast implants, 2, 3–4, 53–54
Chronic Multisystem Illness (CMI), 167
see also Gulf War Syndrome
classification
chronic fatigue syndrome, 108–112
small-fiber neuropathy, 140
vaccine adjuvants, 16–18
claudins, 307–308
cleaning agents, 308
clioquinol, 209
clone immunodominancy, 96
CLP *see* cecal ligation and puncture model
CMI *see* Chronic Multisystem Illness
CMV *see* cytomegalovirus
CNS *see* central nervous system
coherence, 80
colchicine, 295–297
colitis, 35, 36
collagen injections, **285**
combination vaccines, 21–22, 88, 186
complete Freund's adjuvant (CFA), 99
components, tattoos, 148–149
consistency, 80
conventional buildings, sick building syndrome, 159
copper, 204–210, 212
cortical thymocyte marker of *Xenopus* (CTX), 307
corticosteroids, 196, 256
Coxsackie B3 virus, 239
CpG hypomethylation, 236
CpG oligodeoxynucleotides (ODNs), **16**, 17
Crohn's disease, 37
cross-linked nanoparticles, 35
cross-reactivity, 10
CTLA-4 *see* cytotoxic T lymphocyte antigen-4
CTX *see* cortical thymocyte marker of *Xenopus*
cuprizone, 208–209
cyclophosphamide, 122
cyclosarin, 169
CYP P450 inhibition, 236
cytokine-based adjuvants, 18
cytomegalovirus (CMV), 107, 269
cytotoxic T lymphocyte antigen-4 (CTLA-4), 95–96, 191–192

damage-associated molecular patterns (DAMPs), 232
DAMPs *see* damage-associated molecular patterns
delivery systems, classification, 18
dental implants, 337–340
depression, 120, 169
dermatopolymyositis, influenza vaccination, 183–184
detergents, 308
dextran sulfate sodium (DSS)-induced colitis, 35
diagnosis
ASIA, **76**, **92**
chronic fatigue syndrome, 107–108, 111
Gulf War Syndrome, 168–173
mesh-mediated disease, 72
mineral oil reactions, 330–331
postural orthostatic tachycardia syndrome, 131–132
sarcoidosis, 248–253
small-fiber neuropathy, 140–142, **141**
differential diagnosis, postural orthostatic tachycardia syndrome, 131–132
diffuse large B-cell lymphoma (DLBCLs), 94, 273
diisopropyl fluorophosphate, 169–170
diptheria combination vaccines, 21–22, 88, 186
direct mechanisms, bisphenol A, 228–234
DLBCLs *see* diffuse large B-cell lymphoma
DSS *see* dextran sulfate sodium
durvalumab (Imfinzi), 192
dysautonomia, 63–66, 117–127, 139–140, **139**
animal models, 120–122
clinical associations, 118–120, **121**
genetic susceptibility, 120, **123**
historical perspectives, 117–118
treatment, 122–123

EAE *see* experimental autoimmune encephalomyelitis
early-life stress, 309–310
EBV *see* Epstein–Barr virus
effort syndrome, 108–109
emulsifiers, 31, 37–38, 100, 308
emulsion-adjuvanted vaccines, **16**, 17, 22–23, 37–38
endocrine autoimmunity, bisphenol A, 237–239
endocrine disruption, bisphenol A, 225–227, 235–236
environmental factors, 305–321
epithelial tight junctions, 307–309
Gulf War Syndrome, 168
gut–brain axis, 310–312
intestinal permeability, 306–307
microplastics, 308–309
sarcoidosis, 248–249, **250**
Sjögren's syndrome, 266–267
stress, 309–310
epidemiology
ASIA clinical manifestations, **161**
chronic fatigue syndrome, 107
Gulf War Syndrome, 167 168, **171**
lymphomas and autoimmune diseases, 93, **94**
mineral oils, 324–325
sick building syndrome, **157**
epigenetic alterations, 211, 236
epithelial tight junctions, 307–309, 311
epitope breadth, 96
Epstein–Barr virus (EBV), 4, 107, 110, 119, 268
ERs *see* estrogen receptors
estrogen receptors (ERs), 225–228, 235–236
etiology
foreign body reactions, 73–76
Gulf War Syndrome, 168–171
mesh-mediated disease, 72–76, 78–81
mineral oils, 325–326
sarcoidosis, 247–248, **250**
sick building syndrome, 156–159
silicone implant incompatibility syndrome, 52, 53
small-fiber neuropathy, **136**, 137–139
see also pathophysiology

experimental autoimmune encephalomyelitis (EAE), 209
explantation
  biopolymers, 290–297, **291–294**
  silicone breast implants, 56–57

fatigue, 70, 168
  see also chronic fatigue syndrome
FBR *see* foreign body reactions
Febricula, 108
ferroptosis, 35
FGFR-3 *see* fibroblast growth factor receptor-3
fibroblast growth factor receptor-3 (FGFR-3) autoantibodies, 139
fibromyalgia (FM), 118–119, 120–123, 173, 184, 338
fillers, 283–303, **285–286**, **291–294**, 323–336
Fluad*R vaccine, 22–23
FM *see* fibromyalgia
food additives, 29–50, *39*, **40**
food colorants, 31–32, 36–37
food emulsifiers, 31, 37–38
foreign body reactions (FBR), 73–76, 97–100, 143–144, 147–153, 284–297
  see also mesh implants; silicone breast implants
Fukuda definition, chronic fatigue syndrome, 111

GAD *see* glutamic acid decarboxylase
gastrointestinal disease, 71, 120, 239–240
GBS *see* Guillain–Barré syndrome
GCS *see* glucocorticosteroids
genetic susceptibility, 7–9
  autoimmune dysautonomia, 120, **123**
  celiac disease, 33, 34
  chronic fatigue syndrome, 112
  emulsifier sensitivity, 38
  Gulf War Syndrome, 171, 173
  nanoparticle sensitivity, 35
  sarcoidosis, 254
  silicone implant incompatibility syndrome, 8, 54–55
  Sjögren's syndrome, 265
genomic instability, 95
gliadins, 32–33
glucocorticoids, 309–310
glucocorticosteroids (GCS), 256
glutamic acid decarboxylase (GAD) vaccines, 205
gluteal biopolymer injections, 283–303, **291–294**
gluten, 30, 32–33
gold alloys, 338
G-protein-coupled receptors (GPCRs), 117–123, **121**, 130–131, 311
Graves' disease, 117–118
green buildings, sick building syndrome, 159
Guillain–Barré syndrome (GBS), 8, 98
Gulf War Syndrome (GWSy), 8, 167–180, **174**
gut–brain axis, 310–312
gut microbiomes, 172, 210, 235, 310–312
gut permeability, 32, 33, 34, 38, 306–307
GWSy *see* Gulf War Syndrome

H1N1 vaccinations, 8–9, 10
Haemophilus influenzae (*H. influenzae*) vaccines, 22–23
Hashimoto's disease, 186
HBV *see* hepatitis B
HCV *see* hepatitis C virus
heart rate variability (HRV) testing, **141**, 142
heavy metals, 7, 8, 100, 201–223, 337–340
  see also specific elements...
helper T-cells, bisphenol A, 232–234
hematologic malignancies, 97–101
  see also foreign body reactions
hepatitis B (HBV) vaccines, 22, 88, 184–185
hepatitis C virus (HCV), 268–269
HHV-6 *see* human herpes virus
H. influenzae see Haemophilus influenzae
histopathology, mineral oil reactions, 331
HLA *see* human leukocyte antigen
hormonal disruption, 225–227, 235–239, 272–273
household cleaning agents, 308
HPV *see* human papilloma virus
HRV *see* heart rate variability
HTLV-1 *see* human T-cell leukemia virus
human herpes virus (HHV-6), 107, 119
human papilloma virus (HPV) vaccines, 88, 131, 185–186
human T-cell leukemia virus (HTLV-1), 268, 269
humoral disturbances, Gulf War Syndrome, 172
humoral immunity, 234
hyaluronic acid, **285**, 323–336
hydroxychloroquine, 256
8-hydroxydeoxyguanosine (8-OHdG), 156

IA *see* inflammatory arthritis
IBD *see* inflammatory bowel disease
Iceland disease *see* Akureyri disease
ICIs *see* immune checkpoint inhibitors
ID *see* intradermal
idiopathic environmental intolerance (IEI), 156
idiopathic thrombocytopenic purpura (ITP), 8, 88
IEI *see* idiopathic environmental intolerance
IEQ *see* indoor environmental quality
IFA *see* incomplete Freund's adjuvant
ILCs *see* innate lymphoid cells
IM *see* intramuscular
imaging studies, mineral oil reactions, 330–331
Imfinzi *see* durvalumab
immune checkpoint inhibitors (ICIs), 191–199, 271–272
immune hyperstimulation, 1–6, 73–76, 202–203, 265, 266–267, 273–274
immune-modulatory antibodies, 191–199
  see also immune checkpoint inhibitors
immune potentiators, **16**, 17
immune related adverse events (irAEs), 191–199
immunodominant clones, 96
immunostimulatory complexes (ISCOMS), 99
immunosuppresive therapy, sarcoidosis, 254–256
inactivated polio vaccine (IPV), 21–22
incomplete Freund's adjuvant (IFA), 99
indirect mechanisms, bisphenol A, 234–236
indoor environmental quality (IEQ), 155–166
  see also sick building syndrome
inflammasomes, 75, 97, 203, 267
inflammatory arthritis (IA), 193
inflammatory bowel disease (IBD), 32, 35, 37, 71, 209–210
influenza vaccines, 22–23, 88, 182–184
innate immunity, 228–232

innate lymphoid cells (ILCs), 231
instrumental methods, 140–142, **141**
Intanza*R vaccine, 22–23
interleukin-based adjuvants, 18
intestinal permeability, 306–307
intradermal (ID) vaccines, 22–23
intramuscular (IM) vaccines, 22–23
intravenous immunoglobulin (IVIG), 122–123, 196
in vitro effects, biopolymers, 284
ipilimumab (Yervoy), 192
IPV *see* inactivated polio vaccine
irAEs *see* immune related adverse events
ISA 51 *see* Montanide ISA*TM51
ischemic cerebral disease, 70
ISCOMS *see* immunostimulatory complexes
ITP *see* idiopathic thrombocytopenic purpura
IVIG *see* intravenous immunoglobulin

kaleidoscope phenomenon, 94
Keytruda *see* pembrolizumab
Koch's postulates, 78

laboratory testing, 72, 140, 330
laser evoked potentials, **141**
LD-SFN *see* length-dependent small-fiber neuropathy
lead, 203, 210, 211
leflunomide, 256
legislation, 159–160
  see also regulation
length-dependent small-fiber neuropathy (LD-SFN), 140
Libtayo *see* cemiplimab
lindane *see* organochlorine
lipid particles, **16**, 17
lipid sorting, 98
lipophilicity, adjuvants, 98–100, **99**
lipopolysaccharide (LPS), 99, 312
liposomes, **16**, 17
liquid silicone, **285**
livedo reticularis, mesh-mediated disease, 70
liver function, bisphenol A, 236
LPS *see* lipopolysaccharide
lymph nodes, 70
lymphomagenesis, 91–106, 273–274
lymphoproliferative disorders, 4, 72, 91–106, **94**, 273–274

mAChR *see* muscarinic acetylcholine receptors
macrophagic myofasciitis syndrome (MMF), 7, 8, 100, 214
MALT *see* mucosa-associated lymphoid tissue lymphomas
manganese, thyroid disease, 212
MAPK *see* mitogen activated protein kinase
MCS *see* multiple chemical sensitivity
ME *see* myalgic encephalomyelitis
measles–mumps–rubella (MMR) vaccinations, 88
memory responses, foreign body reactivity, 75–76
Mentanil Yellow, 36
mercury, 203, 212, 337–338
mesh implants, 2–4, 67–84, 75
metals, 7, 8, 100, 148–149, 201–223, 337–340
  see also specific elements...
methotrexate, 256
methylation, 101
MF59-adjuvanted vaccines, 17, 22–23, 99
MGB *see* microbiota-gut-brain
microbial-derived adjuvants, **16**, 17
microbial transglutaminase (mTG), 31, 33–34
microbiome, 172, 210, 235, 310–312
microbiota-gut-brain (MGB) axis, 310–312
microparticles, **16**, 17
microplastics, 308–309
migration, silicone gel particles, 2
mineral oil aromatic hydrocarbons (MOAH), 325–326
mineral oils, 323–336
mineral oil saturated hydrocarbons (MOSH), 325–326
mineral salts, **16**, 17, 21–22
mitogen activated protein kinase (MAPK), 202–203
MMF *see* macrophagic myofasciitis syndrome
MMR *see* measles–mumps–rubella
MOAH *see* mineral oil aromatic hydrocarbons
models
  sarcoidosis, 256
  see also animal models
molecular mimicry, 10, 225–227, 235–236
monophosphoryl lipid A (MPL-A), **16**, 17, 99
Montanide ISA*TM51 (ISA 51) vaccine, 23
MOSH *see* mineral oil saturated hydrocarbons
MPL-A *see* monophosphoryl lipid A
MS *see* multiple sclerosis
mTG *see* microbial transglutaminase
mucosa-associated lymphoid tissue lymphomas (MALT), 93–94
mucosal adjuvants, **16**, 17
multiple chemical sensitivity (MCS), 156, 173
multiple sclerosis (MS), 131, 207–209
muscarinic acetylcholine receptors (mAChR), 118, 130
myalgia, 192–193
myalgic encephalomyelitis (ME), 110, 119–120, 122
  see also chronic fatigue syndrome
MyD88 pathyway, 202–203
myocarditis, 239
myositis, 194

nAchR *see* nicotinic acetycholine receptors
nanoemulsions, 37–38
nanoparticles (NPs), **16**, 17, 31, 34–36
narcolepsy, 8–9, 10
NCA *see* neurocirculatory asthenia
neoplasms, and sustained immune activation, 273–274
nerve agents, and Gulf War Syndrome, 169–170
NETs *see* neutrophil extracellular traps
neurocirculatory asthenia (NCA), 108–109
neurogenic switching, 162
neuroinflammation, 171
neurological syndromes, 70, 168, 169–171, 194, 240
neutrophil extracellular traps (NETs), 231
NHL *see* non-Hodgkin lymphomas
nickel, 204–207
nicotinic acetycholine receptors (nAchR), 130
night sweats, mesh-mediated disease, 70
nivolumab (Opdivo), 192
NLD-SFN *see* non-length-dependent small-fiber neuropathy
NLRP3 *see* NOD-like receptor protein 3

NOD-like receptor protein 3 (NLRP3) inflammasomes, 75, 97, 203, 267
non-Hodgkin lymphomas (NHL), 93–94
non-length-dependent small-fiber neuropathy (NLD-SFN), 140
novel adjuvants, 23–24
NPs *see* nanoparticles
nutritional adjuvants, 29–50
  and ASIA, 29–30, *39*, **40**
  emulsifiers, 31, 37–38
  food colorants, 31–32, 36–37
  gluten, 30, 32–33
  increasing usage, 30
  microbial transglutaminase, 31, 33–34
  nanoparticles, 31, 34–36

occludin, 307–308
ODNs *see* CpG oligodeoxynucleotides
oil adjuvants, 37–38, 99–100, **99**
  see also mineral oils
OP *see* organophosphates
Opdivo *see* nivolumab
Orange II, 36
organochlorine (lindane), 169
organophosphates (OP), 169, 173
organ-specific events, immune checkpoint inhibitors, 195
oxidative stress, 76, 95, 232

pain, 70, 168
palladium, systemic sclerosis, 211
p-anilinoaniline, 36
paraffin, **285**
paraoxonase, 173
pararosaniline, 36
parvovirus B19, 107
pathophysiology
  ASIA, 9–11
  autoimmune dysautonomia, 117–122
  bisphenol A, 225–241
  emulsifiers, 37–38
  food colorants, 36–37
  foreign body reactions, 73–76, *75*
  gluten, 32
  Gulf War Syndrome, 8, 171–172
  mesh-mediated disease, 73–76, *75*
  microbial transglutaminase, 33
  mineral oils, 326–328
  nanoparticles, 34–35
  postvaccination syndromes, 9–11
  silicone breast implants, 53–54, 63–64
  small-fiber neuropathy, **136**, 137–139
pattern recognition receptors (PRRs), 20, 75–76, 202–203
PB *see* pyrostigmine bromide
PCI *see* peritoneal contamination and infection
PD-1 *see* programmed cell death protein-1
PDI *see* protein disulfide isomerase
PDMS *see* polydimethylsiloxane
Pediarix*R vaccine, 21–22
pembrolizumab (Keytruda), 192
Pentacel*R vaccine, 22
Pentaxim*R vaccine, 22
peripheral immune abnormalities, Gulf War Syndrome, 172
peritoneal contamination and infection (PCI) model, 312
pesticides, Gulf War Syndrome, 168–169
phagocytosis, bisphenol A, 229–230
pharmacokinetics, adjuvant lipophilicity, 98–100, **99**
plastics, 308–309
plausibility, mesh-mediated disease, 78
PLGA *see* polyethylenimine-coated poly lactic-co-glycolic acid
PLLA *see* poly-L-lactic acid
PMMA *see* polymethyl methacrylate
PMR *see* polymyalgia rheumatica
pneumococcal vaccinations, 184
poliovirus vaccines, 21
polyacrylamide hydrogels, **285**
polydimethylsiloxane (PDMS), 101
polyethylenimine-coated poly lactic-co-glycolic acid (PLGA) nanoparticles, 35
poly-L-lactic acid (PLLA), **286**
polymethyl methacrylate (PMMA), **286**
polymyalgia rheumatica (PMR)-like syndromes, immune checkpoint inhibitors, 193
polyneuropathic small-fiber neuropathy, 140
polyoxidonium *see* azoximer bromide
polypropylene (PP) mesh, 2–4, 67–84, *75*
postinfection conditions, 118–119, 267–270
posttranslational modification of proteins (PTMP), 33
postural orthostatic tachycardia syndrome (POTS), 108, 112, 118–120, 122, 129–135, 150
postvaccination acute lymphomas, 97
postvaccination autoimmunity, 7–11, 87–88, 100, 118–119, 170–171, 214
POTS *see* postural orthostatic tachycardia syndrome
PP *see* polypropylene
pregnancy, 205
premature ovarian failure, 238
prenatal stress (PRS), 309–310, 313
prevalence
  ASIA clinical manifestations, **161**
  Gulf War Syndrome, 167–168, **174**
  immune checkpoint inhibitor reactions, 192–195
  sick building syndrome, **157**, **161**
pristane, 99, 213
pristane *see* tetramethylpentadecane
programmed cell death protein-1 (PD-1), 95–96, 192
protein disulfide isomerase (PDI), 234–235
protein fragmentation, 211
PRRs *see* pattern recognition receptors
PRS *see* prenatal stress
PTMP *see* posttranslational modification of proteins
pyrethroids, Gulf War Syndrome, 169
pyrexia, mesh-mediated disease, 70
pyrostigmine bromide (PB), and Gulf War Syndrome, 170

QS-21 adjuvant, 99
QSART *see* quantitative ship motor axon reflex testing
QST *see* quantitative sensory testing
quadrivalent human papilloma virus vaccines, 88, 131, 185–186
quantitative sensory testing (QST), **141**, 142

quantitative ship motor axon reflex testing (QSART), **141**, 142
questionnaires, small-fiber neuropathy, 140

RA *see* rheumatoid arthritis
radiological assessments, 72
reactive oxygen species (ROS), 76, 95, 232
Red 40, 36
regulations, 88–89, 159–160
regulatory T cells (Treg), 95
removal
  mineral oils, 332–333
  silicone breast implants, 56–57
rheumatoid arthritis (RA), 8, 120, 183, 184, 185, 206–207
rhodamine B, 36
rituximab, 94, 122
ROS *see* reactive oxygen species
Royal Free disease, 109

Saccharomyces cerevisiae, 269
safety
  aluminum-adjuvanted vaccines, 20–22
  emulsion-adjuvanted vaccines, 22–23
  novel adjuvants, 23–24
  pesticides, 169
  vaccine adjuvants, 20–24, 86–89
  see also adverse events
sarcoidosis, 142–143, 149, 195, 247–264, 250, **250–251**
sarin, 169
SARS-CoV-2 9, 10–11, 119, 120, 270
SBIs *see* silicone breast implants
SBS *see* sick building syndrome
SCFAs *see* short-chain fatty acids
self-adjuvating lipopeptide vaccines, 37
self-reactive clones, and lymphomagenesis, 101
semivolatile organic compounds (SVOCs), 157, 159
sensory symptoms, small-fiber neuropathy, 139–140, **139**
serological assessments, 72, 140, 171–172
SFN *see* small-fiber neuropathy
Shoenfeld's syndrome *see* Autoimmune/inflammatory Syndrome Induced by Adjuvants
short-chain fatty acids (SCFAs), 311
Sicca syndrome, 193–194, 265–266, 269
  see also Sjögren's syndrome
sick building syndrome (SBS), 155–166, **157**, **161**
side effects *see* adverse events
SIGBIC *see* silicone-induced granuloma of the breast implant capsule
SIIS *see* silicone implant incompatibility syndrome
silica nanoparticles, 34–35
silicone, 53, 100, **285**
silicone breast implants (SBIs), 2, 3–4, 8, 51–66, 63–66, 100–101, 118, 120, **121**, 143–144, 271
silicone implant incompatibility syndrome (SIIS), 51, 54–62, 101, 143–144, 150
silicone-induced granuloma of the breast implant capsule (SIGBIC), 4
silicosis, 271
silver, 204–205
SIR *see* standard incidence ratios
Sjögren's syndrome (SjS/SS), 70, 93, 101, 120, 122, 131, 143, 149, 193–194, 202–203, 213, 237, 265–281, 271, 272
  as ASIA, 266
  immune hyperstimulation, 266–267
  postinfection, 267–270
  vaccinations, 270–271
SjS *see* Sjögren's syndrome
SLE *see* systemic lupus erythematosus
sleep disorders, 120, 168
small-fiber neuropathy (SFN), 132, **136**, 137–146, **141**, 150, 250, **251**
smoking, 206
specificity of association, 80
sphingomyelins, 98
squalene, 99, 170–171
squalene nanoemulsions, 37
stress, 309–310, 313
subjective night sweats, 70
superoxide dismutase, 201
surfactants, 31, 37–38, 308
surgical resections, 295, 332–333
sustained immune activation, and lymphomagenesis, 91–106
SVOCs *see* semivolatile organic compounds
systemic lupus erythematosus (SLE), 8, 88, 120, 131, 182–186, 195, 202–205, 237
systemic sclerosis, 120, 122, 211
systemic symptoms, mesh implants, 70–71
systems vaccinology, 20

T1DM *see* type 1 diabetes mellitus
TAMPs *see* tight junction-associated MARVEL proteins
Tapanui outbreak, 110
tartrazine, 36
tattoos, 147–153
T-cells, 95–96, 232–234
Tecentriq *see* atezolizumab
temporality, 80
testosterone, 272
tetanus combination vaccines, 21–22, 186
tetramethylpentadecane (pristane), 99, 213
Theiler's virus induced demyelination (TVID), 240
thrombotic thrombocytopenia, 10–11
thyroid disease, 211–212, 238
tight junction-associated MARVEL proteins (TAMPs), 307
titanium dioxide, 35
Toll-like receptor 4 (TLR4), 4, 75–76
Toll-like receptor (TLR) agonists, **16**, 17
TPSO *see* transporter protein
transient reporter potential channel VI (TRPV1), 74
transporter protein (TPSO), 171
treatment
  autoimmune dysautonomia, 122–123
  biopolymer injection events, 290–297, **291–294**
  immune checkpoint inhibitor side effects, 195–196
  mineral oil reactions, 331–333
  postural orthostatic tachycardia syndrome, 132
  sarcoidosis, 255–256
  small-fiber neuropathy, 142
  tattoo-induced ASIA, 150

Treg *see* regulatory T cells
trisulfated heparin disaccharide (TS-HDS) autoantibodies, 139
TRPV1 *see* transient reporter potential channel VI
TS-HDS *see* trisulfated heparin disaccharide
TVID *see* Theiler's virus induced demyelination
type 1 diabetes mellitus (T1DM), 205–206, 238–239

urinary 8-hydroxydeoxyguanosine, 156

vaccinations, 85–89, 97, 170–171, 181–190, 270–271
see also specific vaccines...
vaccine adjuvants, 15–27, 37–38, 86–89, 97–100, **99**
vaccine-induced immune thrombotic thrombocytopenia (VITT), 10–11
vaccinosis, 86–88
see also vaccinations
vagal tone, 310–311
vascular complications, 70, 194–195
vasculitis, 194
virus-like particles (VLPs), **16**, 17
VITT *see* vaccine-induced immune thrombotic thrombocytopenia
VLPs *see* virus-like particles
VOCs *see* volatile organic compounds
volatile organic compounds (VOCs), 157, 159

World Trade Center attack, 10

xanthene food dyes, 36

Yellow 6, 36
Yervoy *see* ipilimumab

zinc, 211–212, 211–213

www.ingramcontent.com/pod-product-compliance
Lightning Source LLC
LaVergne TN
LVHW062206200926
848484LV00006B/1330